Robbins and Cotran
Atlas of Pathology

THIRD EDITION

Robbins and Cotran
Atlas of Pathology

Edward C. Klatt, MD

Professor of Pathology
Biomedical Education Program Director
Department of Biomedical Sciences
Mercer University School of Medicine
Savannah, Georgia

ELSEVIER
SAUNDERS

1600 John F. Kennedy Blvd.
Ste 1800
Philadelphia, PA 19103-2899

ROBBINS AND COTRAN ATLAS OF PATHOLOGY,
THIRD EDITION

ISBN: 978-1-4557-4876-1
International Edition ISBN 978-0-323-2-8080-8

Library of Congress Cataloging-in-Publication Data

Klatt, Edward C., 1951- , author.
  Robbins and Cotran atlas of pathology / Edward C. Klatt. – Third edition.
    p. ; cm.
  Atlas of pathology
  Includes index.
  ISBN 978-1-4557-4876-1 (pbk. : alk. paper) – ISBN 978-0-323-28080-8 (E-ISBN)
  I. Title. II. Title: Atlas of pathology.
  [DNLM: 1. Pathology–Atlases. QZ 17]
  RB33
  616.07022'2–dc23
                                                                    2014031172

Executive Content Strategist: William Schmitt
Content Development Specialist: Laura Schmidt
Publishing Services Manager: Catherine Jackson
Senior Project Manager: Mary Pohlman
Design Direction: Ashley Miner

Printed in China

Last digit is the print number: 9 8 7 6 5 4 3 2 1

Working together
to grow libraries in
developing countries

www.elsevier.com • www.bookaid.org

This third edition of the atlas accompanying the Robbins series of texts has been updated with the addition of over 400 new images that increase the depth and breadth for coverage of subject areas in pathology, enhancing its usefulness to the entire series. This atlas remains organized into chapters that closely follow the section on Diseases of Organ Systems in the ninth edition of the "big" *Robbins and Cotran Pathologic Basis of Disease*. The atlas is designed to complement the *Pathologic Basis of Disease, Basic Pathology,* and *Robbins' Pocket Companion* texts by providing even more examples of disease processes. The atlas reflects the knowledge base of the Robbins series primarily in a visual format, and because most students are "visual learners" they will readily take advantage of this study aid. The gross, microscopic, and radiologic images used for the figures as presented in this atlas are designed to reinforce one another, as well as those present in other works in the Robbins

series. In addition, there are examples of normal organs and tissues for review and orientation.

Each figure is accompanied by a brief description that provides the key points illustrated by the figure. For initial and more complete study, the learner is directed to the Robbins texts. The labels and descriptions provided for the figures will guide the learner in a discovery process while perusing these figures. Though concise, the figure descriptions cumulatively yield a considerable volume of reading, but that reading is highly compartmentalized to aid review and reflection. Correlations with findings from clinical history, physical examination, and clinical laboratory testing are included in many of the descriptions. The atlas author pursues an integrative approach to medical education, combining elements of basic science, clinical, and behavioral subjects into learning materials that promote a flowering of knowledge to benefit those in need of health care.

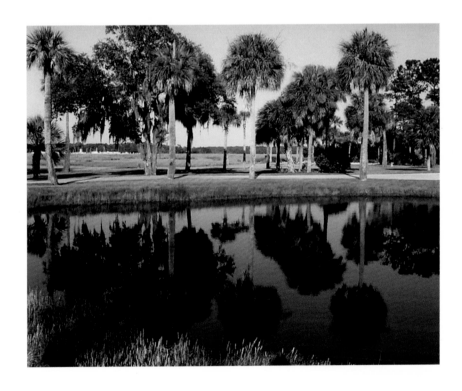

Acknowledgments

The author is indebted to the stalwart figures who have fundamentally contributed to the development of the entire Robbins series, starting with the founding author Dr. Stanley Robbins, continuing with Dr. Ramzi Cotran, and ongoing with Dr. Vinay Kumar. These lead authors have set the standard of excellence that characterizes this series. In addition, there have been and continue to be numerous contributing authors who have made the Robbins series into the valuable tool it remains for medical education. Just as no single monarch butterfly completes a migration, so too medical educators build on the work of colleagues over many generations.

Persons associated with the publisher, Elsevier, require special thanks including the Content Development Specialist, Laura Schmidt, and Senior Project Manager, Mary Pohlman. Of course, none of this work would be possible without the support and vision provided by Mr. William Schmitt, Executive Content Strategist for Medical Textbooks.

Edward C. Klatt, MD

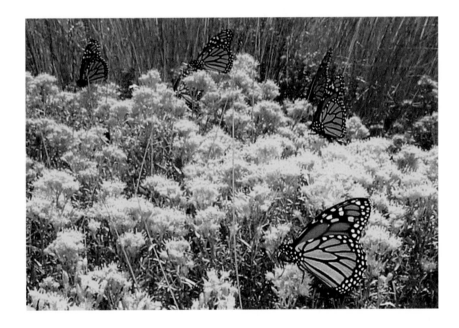

To all who strive for improving the health of everyone.

Contributors

Arthur J. Belanger, MHS, PA(ASCP)
Autopsy Service Manager
Yale University School of Medicine
New Haven, Connecticut

John Blackmon, MD
Associate Professor of Pathology
Florida State University College of Medicine
Tallahassee, Florida

Professor David Y. Cohen
Director of Pathology
Herzliyah Medical Center
Herzliyah-on-Sea, Israel

Richard M. Conran, MD, PhD, JD
Professor of Pathology
Uniformed Services University of the Health Sciences
Bethesda, Maryland

Todd Cameron Grey, MD
Chief Medical Examiner, State of Utah
Associate Professor of Pathology
University of Utah
Salt Lake City, Utah

Ilan Hammel, DSc
Professor and Chairman
Department of Pathology
Sackler Faculty of Medicine
Tel Aviv University
Tel Aviv, Israel

M. Elizabeth H. Hammond, MD
Professor of Pathology and
    Adjunct Professor of Internal Medicine
University of Utah School of Medicine
Salt Lake City, Utah

Sate Hamza, MD
Assistant Professor
University of Manitoba
Winnipeg, Manitoba, Canada

Walter H. Henricks, MD
Staff Pathologist and
    Director of Laboratory Information Services
The Cleveland Clinic Foundation
Cleveland, Ohio

Lauren C. Hughey, MD
Associate Professor of Dermatology
University of Alabama at Birmingham
Birmingham, Alabama

Carl R. Kjeldsberg, MD
Professor of Pathology and Medicine
University of Utah School of Medicine
Chief Executive Officer and Chairman
ARUP Laboratories
Salt Lake City, Utah

Nick Mamalis, MD
Professor of Ophthalmology and Visual Sciences
John A. Moran Eye Center
University of Utah
Salt Lake City, Utah

Professor John Nicholls
Clinical Professor
Department of Pathology
The University of Hong Kong
Pok Fu Lam, Hong Kong, SAR

Sherrie L. Perkins, MD, PhD
Professor of Pathology
University of Utah School of Medicine
Director of Hematopathology Laboratory
ARUP Laboratories
Salt Lake City, Utah

Mary Ann Sens, MD, PhD
Professor and Chair of Pathology
University of North Dakota School of Medicine
    and Health Sciences
Grand Forks, North Dakota

Shane Silver, MD, FRCPC
Dermatologist
203 Edmonton Street
Winnipeg, Manitoba

Hiroyuki Takahashi, MD, PhD
Associate Professor
Department of Pathology
The Jikei University School of Medicine
Tokyo, Japan

Amy Theos, MD
Associate Professor of Dermatology
University of Alabama Medical Center
Birmingham, Alabama

Omid Zargari, MD
Consultant Dermatologist
Pars Clinic
Rasht, Iran

Contents

Blood Vessels

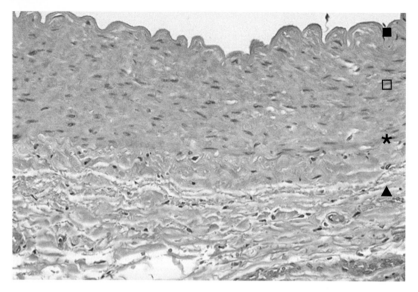

Figure 1-1 Normal artery, microscopic

This is a muscular artery in longitudinal section showing a thin intima (■) on top of the internal elastic lamina. Below this is the thick media (□), with layers of circular smooth muscle and interspersed elastic fibers to withstand the arterial pressure load and dampen the pressure wave from left ventricular contraction. The media is bounded by the external elastic lamina (★). Outside the media is the adventitia (▲), which merges with surrounding supporting connective tissue.

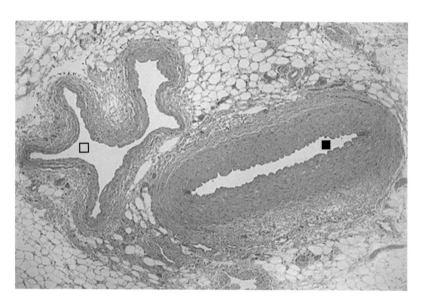

Figure 1-2 Normal artery and vein, microscopic

Seen here in cross-section is a normal artery (■) with a thick, smooth muscle wall alongside a normal vein (□) with a thin, smooth muscle wall, running in connective tissue in a fascial plane between muscle bundles of the lower leg. The larger arteries and veins are often grouped, along with a nerve, into a neurovascular bundle to supply a body region. More distal areas of regional blood flow and the blood pressure are regulated by alternating vasoconstriction and dilation of small muscular arteries and arterioles.

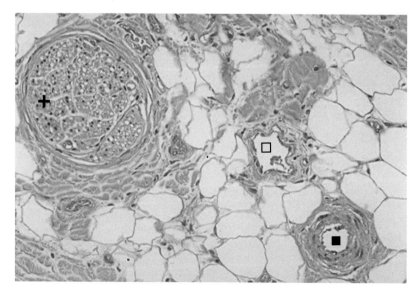

Figure 1-3 Normal arteriole and venule, microscopic

A normal arteriole (■) is alongside a normal venule (□) and a small peripheral nerve (✚), all in cross-section, grouped into a loose neurovascular bundle. The major point of blood pressure regulation is at the arteriolar level. Exchange of solutes and gases with diffusion into tissues occurs at the capillary level. The diminished vascular pressure of the venules, along with the intravascular oncotic pressure exerted by plasma proteins, brings interstitial fluids back into the venules. Not seen here are the normally inconspicuous lymphatic channels that scavenge what little residual fluid is exuded from capillaries and not recovered into the venous system, preventing edema.

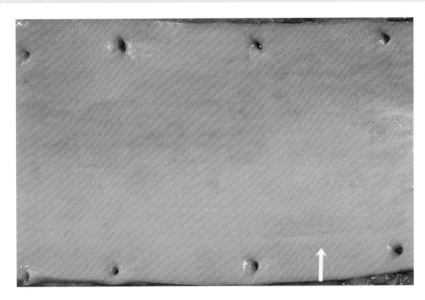

Figure 1-4 Atherosclerosis, gross
Shown is an adult aorta that is as normal as possible. The intimal surface is quite smooth, with only occasional small, pale yellow, fatty lipid streaks visible (↑).Such fatty streaks may initially appear in the aortas of children. (The faint reddish staining in this autopsy specimen comes from hemoglobin that leaked from red blood cells after death.) With a healthy lifestyle and without additional risk factors, these intimal fatty lesions are unlikely to progress. The lipid streaks can serve as precursors for atheroma formation. Major risk factors advancing atheroma formation include increased serum LDL cholesterol, decreased HDL cholesterol, hypertriglyceridemia, diabetes mellitus, hypertension, and smoking.

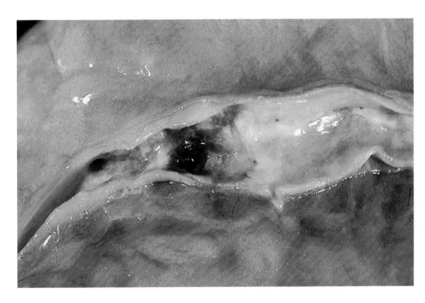

Figure 1-5 Atherosclerosis, gross
This coronary artery opened longitudinally shows yellowish atheromatous plaques over much of its intimal surface. There is focal hemorrhage into a plaque, a complication of atherosclerosis that can acutely narrow the lumen. Endothelial dysfunction that impairs vasoreactivity or induces a thrombogenic surface or abnormally adhesive surface to inflammatory cells may initiate thrombus formation, atherosclerosis, and the vascular lesions of hypertension. Advanced atheromas can be complicated by erosion, ulceration, rupture, hemorrhage, aneurysmal dilation, calcification, and thrombosis. Arterial narrowing may lead to tissue ischemia, and marked or prolonged loss of blood supply may lead to infarction. This may lead to acute coronary syndromes involving the heart.

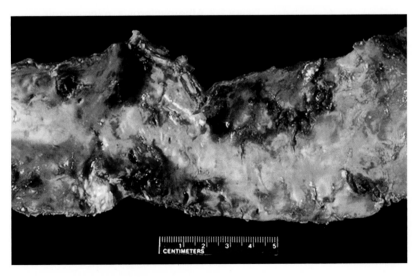

Figure 1-6 Atherosclerosis, gross
Severe aortic atherosclerosis involving nearly the entire intimal surface is shown, with ulceration of the atheromatous plaques along with formation of overlying mural thrombus. This degree of atherosclerosis may develop when atherogenesis proceeds over many years or with significant risk factors driving more accelerated atherosclerosis, such as hyperlipidemia, diabetes mellitus, smoking, hypertension, and obesity. Mitigating these risk factors through adoption of a healthy lifestyle with increased exercise and reduced caloric intake can halt the progression of atherosclerosis, and atheromas can even regress over time, with reduced likelihood of complications.

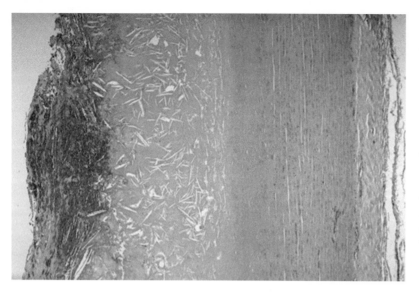

Figure 1-7 Atherosclerosis, microscopic
This cross-section of aorta shows a large overlying advanced atheroma containing numerous cholesterol clefts, resulting from breakdown of lipid imbibed into foam cells. The luminal surface at the far left shows ulceration of its fibrous cap with hemorrhage. Despite this ulceration, which predisposes to mural thrombus formation, atheromatous emboli are rare (or at least, clinically significant complications from them are infrequent). The thick medial layer is intact, and the adventitia appears normal at the right. As atheromas become larger, they can be complicated by ulceration, which promotes overlying thrombosis. Organization of the thrombus further increases the size of the plaque.

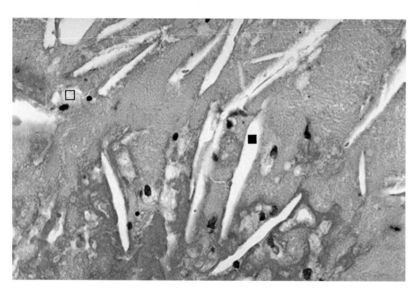

Figure 1-8 Atherosclerosis, microscopic
This high-magnification view of the necrotic center of an aortic atheroma shows foam cells (□) and cholesterol clefts (■). In the process of atheroma formation, endothelial injury leads to increased permeability, leukocyte adhesion, and release of cytokines that attract blood monocytes, which become macrophages that accumulate lipids, becoming foam cells. Macrophages readily ingest oxidized LDL cholesterol through their scavenger receptors. Macrophages also generate cytokines driving cellular recruitment. An increased serum LDL level increases the amount of oxidized LDL, promoting this process. In contrast, HDL cholesterol tends to promote mobilization of lipid in an atheroma and transport to the liver.

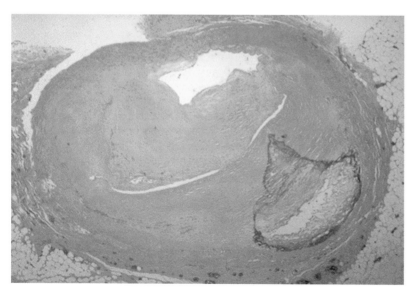

Figure 1-9 Atherosclerosis, microscopic
This severe degree of coronary arterial narrowing results from smooth muscle cell migration and proliferation within the intima to form an enlarging fibrofatty atheroma. Shown here is a "complex" atheroma, so designated because of the large area of bluish calcification at the lower right with this H&E stain. Complex atheromas can have calcification, thrombosis, or hemorrhage. Calcification would make coronary angioplasty to dilate the lumen more difficult. Reducing the radius of an artery by half increases the resistance to flow 16-fold. When the degree of narrowing is 70% or more, angina is often present. Such patients are at great risk for acute coronary syndromes, including myocardial infarction and sudden death from dysrhythmias.

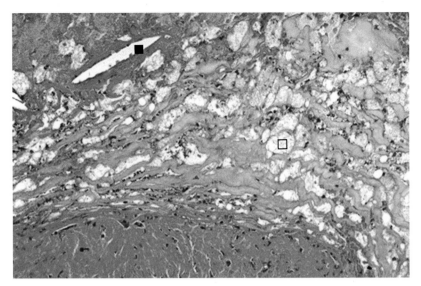

Figure 1-10 Atherosclerosis, microscopic
This coronary artery cross-section shows residual smooth muscle in the media with overlying atheroma composed of extensive lipid deposition in lipophages (□) and a cholesterol cleft (■) from breakdown of those cells. Such plaques are prone to rupture, hemorrhage, and thrombosis. Platelets become activated and adhere to sites of endothelial injury, then release cytokines such as platelet-derived growth factor that promote smooth muscle proliferation, and the adherent platelet mass increases the size of the plaque while narrowing the residual arterial lumen. Use of antiplatelet agents such as aspirin helps reduce platelet "stickiness" and slows platelet participation in atheroma formation. Daily exercise is even better.

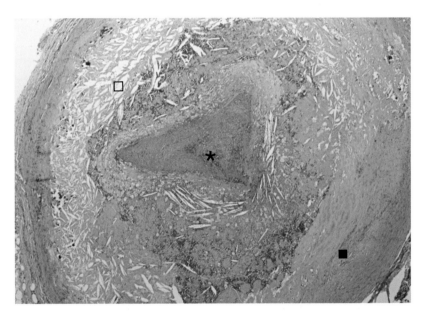

Figure 1-11 Atherosclerosis, microscopic
This coronary artery cross-section shows severe occlusive atherosclerosis. The atheromatous plaque is circumferential and markedly narrows the remaining lumen. Note the prominent cholesterol clefts within this atheroma. This advanced atheromatous process involves the arterial media (■) and the overlying intima (□) with numerous cholesterol clefts. The remaining lumen has become occluded by a recent thrombus (★) that fills it. Thrombosis is often the basis for acute coronary syndromes, including unstable angina, sudden death, and acute myocardial infarction.

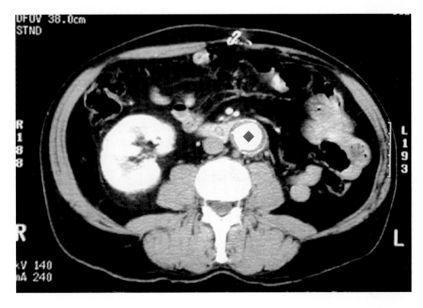

Figure 1-12 Atherosclerosis, CT image
Contrast enhancement leads to an aortic lumen (♦) highlighted by bright attenuation of the blood, with darker gray mural thrombus seen around the periphery of the lumen. This abdominal aorta has severe atherosclerosis, and it is slightly dilated. Mural thrombus can form atop advanced atheromas, and thrombus can organize and narrow the lumen further, or portions may break off and embolize distally to occlude smaller arterial branches in the systemic circulation. This aortic wall also has focal thin, bright areas of atheromatous calcification. (The left kidney is absent from prior nephrectomy. The right kidney is brightly attenuated as intravenous contrast material flows through it.)

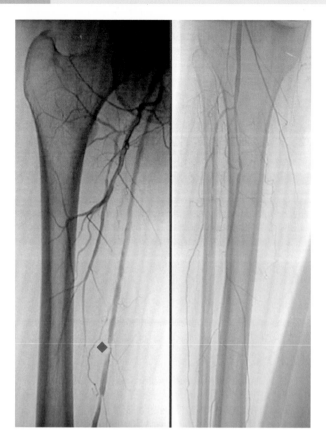

◄ **Figure 1-13 Atherosclerosis, angiogram**
This patient's type 1 diabetes mellitus, poorly controlled for many years, led to claudication (pain with exercise) in the right lower extremity. This angiogram reveals multiple areas of atherosclerotic narrowing (◆) involving femoral arterial branches. The upper leg with femur is in the *left panel,* and the lower leg with tibia and fibula is in the *right panel.* The arterial lumens appear dark with the digital subtraction imaging technique shown here.

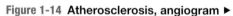

Figure 1-14 Atherosclerosis, angiogram ►
There are multiple areas of atherosclerotic narrowing involving branches of the right femoral artery in this patient with poorly controlled diabetes mellitus who developed severe peripheral vascular disease with claudication. On physical examination, peripheral pulses are decreased or even absent with this degree of arterial occlusion. The risk for tissue ischemia and possible gangrenous necrosis is increased.

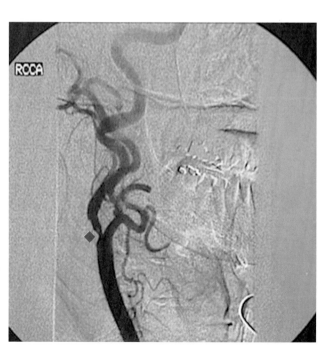

◄ **Figure 1-15 Atherosclerosis, angiogram**
The degree of atherosclerotic narrowing (◆) in this right internal ca-rotid artery can produce mental status changes, including transient ischemic attacks, which could presage a stroke from ischemia to one or more areas of the brain. On physical examination, a bruit may be auscultated over such an area of large arterial narrowing, caused by faster turbulent flow of blood distal to the region of nar-rowing (Bernoulli principle).

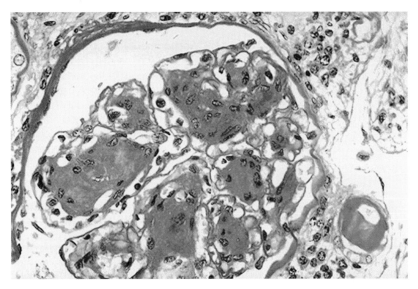

Figure 1-16 Hyaline arteriolosclerosis, microscopic
Another form of arteriosclerosis (hardening of the arteries) in addition to atherosclerosis is hyaline arteriolosclerosis, typically seen in kidneys and brain. It is shown here involving the markedly thickened arteriole at the lower right of this glomerulus with PAS stain. This change often accompanies benign nephrosclerosis, leading to progressive loss of nephrons and eventual renal atrophy. Hyaline arteriolosclerosis is also seen in elderly individuals, who are often normotensive. More advanced arteriosclerotic lesions may occur in persons with diabetes mellitus or hypertension.

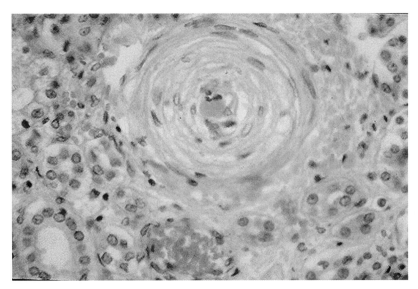

Figure 1-17 Hyperplastic arteriolosclerosis, microscopic
The hyperplastic form of arteriolosclerosis is prominent in this arteriole. It has an "onion skin" appearance from concentric, laminated intimal and smooth muscle proliferation with marked narrowing of the arteriolar lumen. Affected arterioles also may undergo fibrinoid necrosis (necrotizing arteriolitis), and there may be local hemorrhage. Surrounding tissues may show focal ischemia or infarction. This lesion is associated with malignant hypertension, with diastolic blood pressure greater than 120 mm Hg. Such malignant hypertension may occur de novo or may complicate long-standing "essential" hypertension.

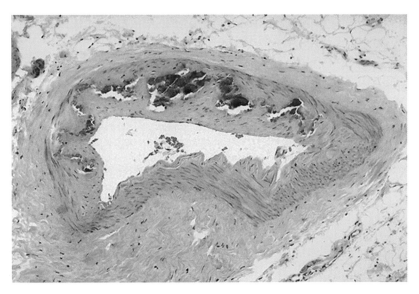

Figure 1-18 Medial calcific sclerosis, microscopic
Mönckeberg medial calcific sclerosis is the most insignificant form of arteriosclerosis (atherosclerosis and arteriolosclerosis are significant because of arterial luminal narrowing). It is more common in the elderly. Note the purplish blue calcifications involving only the media; the lumen appears unaffected by this process. No significant clinical consequences occur in most patients, and it is usually an incidental finding. Recall this process when you see calcified muscular arteries on a radiograph of the pelvic region, although other regions such as the neck or breast may also be involved.

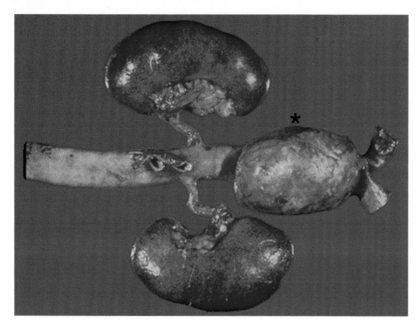

Figure 1-19 Aortic aneurysm, gross
Atherosclerosis involving the intima and media may focally weaken the wall of the aorta so that it bulges out to form an aneurysm. A classic atherosclerotic aortic aneurysm typically occurs in the abdominal portion distal to the renal arteries, as shown here (★). Aortic aneurysms tend to enlarge over time, and those with a diameter greater than 5 to 7 cm are more likely to rupture. Aneurysms may also form in the larger arterial branches of the aorta, most often the iliac arteries. On physical examination, there may be a palpable pulsatile abdominal mass with an atherosclerotic aortic aneurysm. Increased expression of matrix metalloproteinases that degrade extracellular matrix components such as collagen is observed in aortic aneurysms.

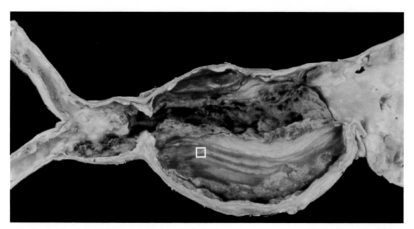

Figure 1-20 Aortic aneurysm, gross
This aorta has been sectioned longitudinally to reveal a large abdominal atherosclerotic aortic aneurysm distal to the renal arteries (at the right) and proximal to the iliac bifurcation (at the left). This bulging aneurysm, 6 cm in diameter, is filled with abundant layered mural thrombus (□). Note the rough atheromatous surface of the aortic lumen.

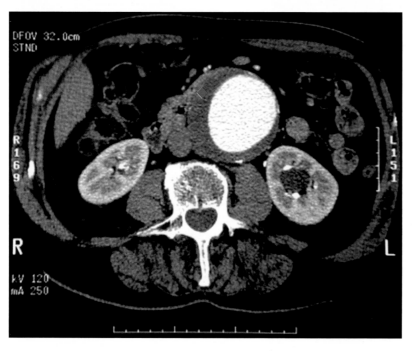

Figure 1-21 Aortic aneurysm, CT image
Contrast enhancement reveals an abdominal atherosclerotic aortic aneurysm that extends distal to the level of the renal arteries past the takeoff of the inferior mesenteric artery. Note the bright contrast material in the blood filling the open aortic lumen, whereas the surrounding mural thrombus (◆) has decreased (darker) attenuation. The total aortic diameter here is about 7 to 8 cm, in great danger of rupture. A pulsatile abdominal mass was palpable in this patient. Although atherosclerotic aneurysms are more common in the abdominal aorta, they can also be found in the thoracic aorta.

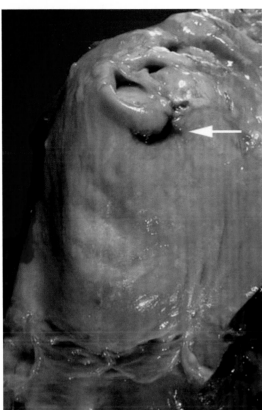

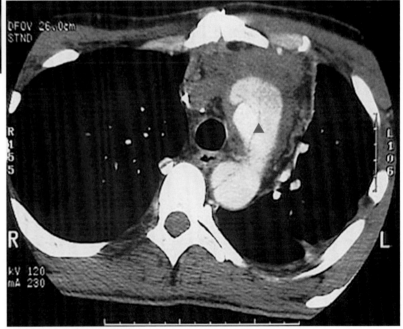

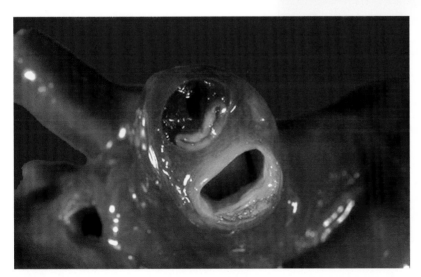

◄ Figure 1-22 Aortic dissection, gross
There is an intimal tear (◄) located 7 cm above the aortic valve and proximal to the great vessels in this aorta with marked atherosclerosis. Risk factors for this aortic dissection include atherosclerosis, hypertension, and cystic medial degeneration. When the tear occurs, the systemic arterial blood under pressure can begin to dissect into the aortic media. From there, the blood may re-enter the aorta at a distal site through another tear, or it may dissect through the wall of the aorta and rupture into adjacent tissues or body cavities. Proximal ruptures may reach the pericardial cavity, with hemopericardium. There may be rupture into a pleural cavity, with hemothorax. With distal dissection, rupture into the abdominal cavity produces hemoperitoneum.

Figure 1-23 Aortic dissection, CT image ►
The contrast enhancement shows a dissection involving the aortic arch. The thin, dark linear segments (▲) mark extension of blood into the aortic media. There is extension of this dissection to involve the left common carotid artery. Aortic dissections may be diagnosed with CT, transesophageal echocardiography, MRI, or angiography. Angiography is preferred before surgical repair.

◄ Figure 1-24 Aortic dissection, gross
The right common carotid artery is compressed by blood dissecting upward from a tear with aortic dissection. Blood may also dissect to involve the coronary arteries. Patients with aortic dissection may have symptoms of sudden, severe chest pain (for distal dissection) or may demonstrate findings that suggest a stroke (with carotid compression from proximal dissection) or myocardial ischemia (with coronary arterial compression from proximal dissection). Pain may be absent in proximal dissections.

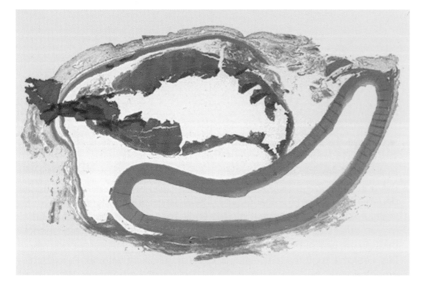

Figure 1-25 Aortic dissection, microscopic
This cross-section of aorta shows a red blood clot splitting the media and compressing the aortic lumen. This occurred as a result of aortic dissection in which there was a tear in the intima of the aortic arch, followed by dissection of blood at high pressure out into and through the muscular wall to the adventitia. This blood dissecting out can lead to sudden death from hemothorax, hemopericardium, or hemoperitoneum. Severe knifelike chest pain may be present.

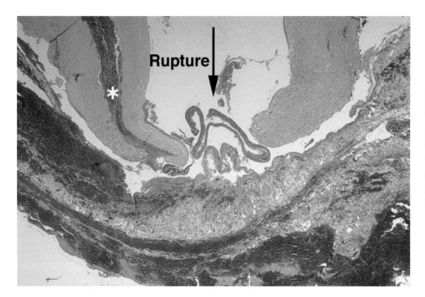

Figure 1-26 Aortic dissection, microscopic
The tear (↓) in this aorta extends through the media, but blood also dissects along the media (★). Medical management can be undertaken; but with leakage or rupture, surgical repair of the dissection can be performed with closure of the tear and placement of a synthetic graft or endovascular stent.

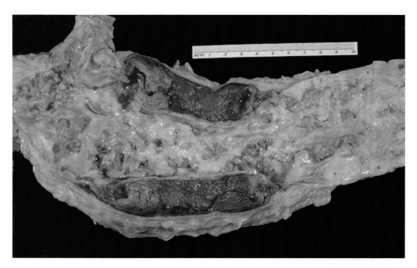

Figure 1-27 Aortic dissection, gross
This aorta opened longitudinally shows an area in the thoracic portion of limited dissection that is organizing within the media. The red-brown thrombus can be seen on both sides of the section as it extends around the aorta. The intimal tear would have been at the left. This creates a "double lumen" to the aorta. This aorta shows severe atherosclerosis, which was the major risk factor for dissection in this patient.

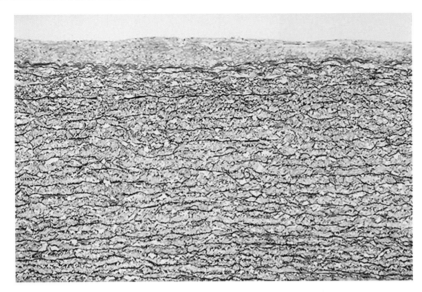

Figure 1-28 Normal aorta, microscopic
This longitudinal section through the normal aorta with an elastic tissue stain shows the intima at the top. The thick aortic media shows parallel dark elastic fibers, here highlighted by the elastic stain. The smooth muscle fibers are between the elastic fibers, and both of these fibers give the aorta great strength and resiliency, allowing the pulse pressure of left ventricular systole to be transmitted distally.

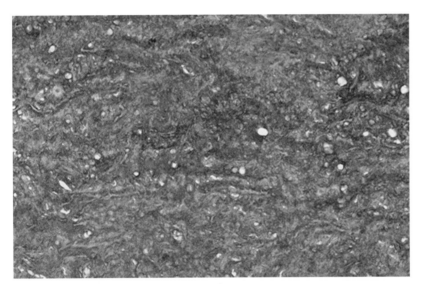

Figure 1-29 Aorta, cystic medial degeneration, microscopic
This mucin stain of the aortic media shows pink elastic fibers that, instead of running in parallel arrays, are disrupted by pools of blue mucinous ground substance. This is typical for Marfan syndrome affecting connective tissues containing elastin. This causes the connective tissue weakness that explains the propensity for aortic dissection, particularly when the aortic root dilates beyond 3 cm in diameter. Dilation of the aortic root can lead to aortic insufficiency. Patients with Marfan syndrome can undergo proximal aortic graft and aortic valve prosthesis placement to prevent aortic dissection.

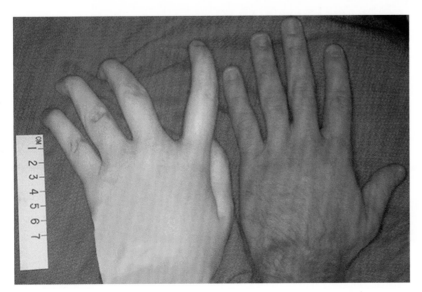

Figure 1-30 Arachnodactyly, gross
The hand on the left exhibits arachnodactyly in a young woman with Marfan syndrome, and the hand on the right belongs to a normal man. Both individuals were of the same height, 188 cm. Marfan syndrome is an autosomal dominant condition in which there is a mutation in the fibrillin-1 (FBN1) gene. The mutant gene's protein product disrupts normal microfibril assembly, producing a "dominant negative" effect. As a consequence, there are abnormalities of connective tissues, particularly tissues with an elastic component, such as the aorta, chordae tendineae, and ligaments of the crystalline lens of the eye.

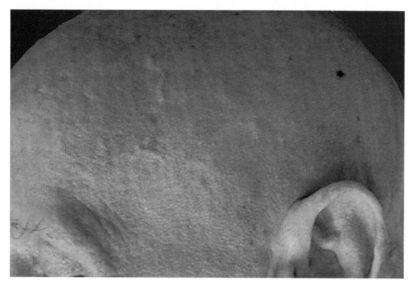

Figure 1-31 Giant cell (temporal) arteritis, gross

Giant cell arteritis is the most common of the vasculitides and usually involves branches of the external carotid artery, most often the temporal artery, although the vertebral arteries, coronary arteries, and aorta may be involved occasionally. Giant cell arteritis may lead to a visible firm, palpable, painful temporal artery that courses over the surface of the scalp. The inflammation is often focal. The involved arterial segment may be excised for diagnosis or therapy. Other branches of the external carotid artery provide collateral flow. A feared complication is occlusion of the ophthalmic arterial branch leading to blindness.

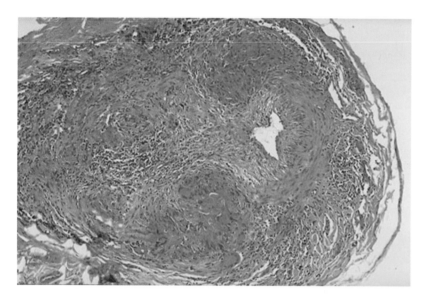

Figure 1-32 Temporal arteritis, microscopic

Temporal arteritis is one manifestation of giant cell arteritis, which can affect mainly branches of the external carotid artery, but sometimes also the great vessels at the aortic arch and coronaries. It is uncommon in individuals younger than 50 years. The erythrocyte sedimentation rate (ESR) is often markedly elevated (≥100 mm/hr). Half of patients have polymyalgia rheumatica. The cause is related to a cell-mediated immune response. The result is granulomatous inflammation of the media with a narrowed arterial lumen, as shown here. There may be active inflammation with mononuclear infiltrates and giant cells, or fibrosis in more chronic lesions.

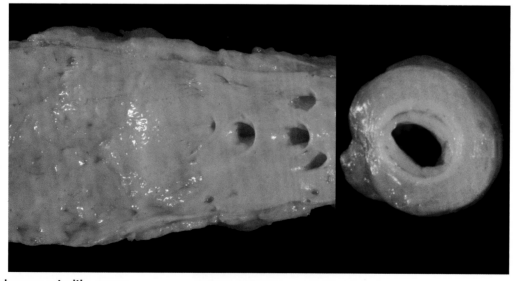

Figure 1-33 Takayasu arteritis, gross

An uncommon granulomatous arteritis, Takayasu arteritis typically involves the aortic arch but may involve the distal aorta, shown in the *left panel,* and renal and coronary arteries. There is marked luminal narrowing, mainly from intimal thickening, seen in cross-section of the carotid artery in the *right panel*. Luminal narrowing produces flow restriction with decreased pulses, often in the upper extremities and neck.

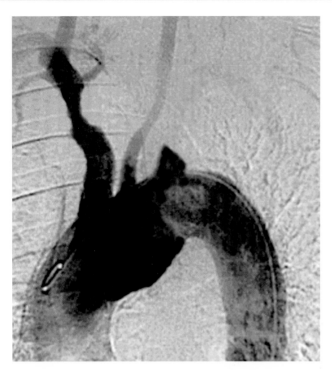

Figure 1-34 Takayasu arteritis, angiogram
The arch of the aorta, filled with dark-appearing intraluminal contrast medium, shows aneurysmal dilation. The left subclavian artery is completely occluded, appearing cut off near its origin, and would be detectable from markedly reduced blood pressure in the left arm. The right innominate artery has irregular narrowing. Patients often have visual problems and neurologic changes. Less frequent involvement of the distal aorta can lead to lower extremity claudication. Pulmonary arterial involvement may lead to pulmonary hypertension and cor pulmonale. The disease course is variable. Most affected patients are younger than 50 years, typically women younger than 40 years. Prevalence is highest in East Asia, especially Japan. Microscopic findings are similar to the findings of giant cell arteritis, with more chronic changes, including fibrosis, giant cells, and lymphocytic infiltrates in the arterial walls.

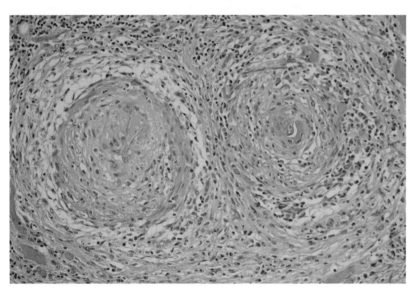

Figure 1-35 Polyarteritis nodosa (classic), microscopic
At low magnification, these muscular arteries show severe vasculitis with few acute and many chronic inflammatory cell infiltrates, along with necrosis of the vascular walls and occlusion of the lumens. The classic form of polyarteritis nodosa (PAN) involves mainly small to medium-sized arteries anywhere in the body, but more often in the renal and mesenteric arteries. The serum antineutrophil cytoplasmic autoantibody (ANCA) test result is usually negative (but more likely to be positive with microscopic polyangiitis). Clinical manifestations include malaise, fever, weight loss, hypertension, abdominal pain, melena, myalgias, arthralgias, and peripheral neuritis.

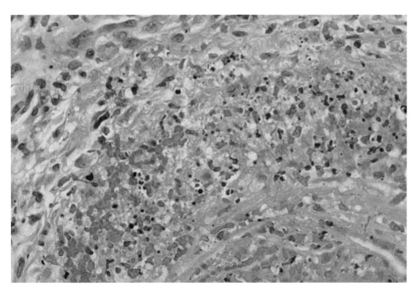

Figure 1-36 Polyarteritis nodosa (classic), microscopic
This is a higher magnification of the arterial wall with acute PAN in its classic form. In time, the lesion may heal with fibrosis and vascular luminal narrowing. The disease most often strikes young adults and may have an acute, subacute, or chronic course of exacerbations and remissions. Involvement of mesenteric arteries can lead to abdominal pain from bowel ischemia or infarction. Renal involvement can lead to renal failure. A third of patients with PAN are infected with hepatitis B virus. Therapy with corticosteroids and cyclophosphamide produces remissions or cures in 90% of cases, which would otherwise prove fatal.

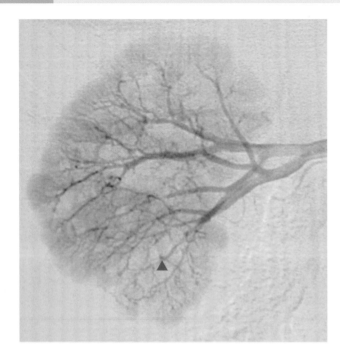

◄ **Figure 1-37 Polyarteritis nodosa (classic), angiogram**
This angiogram of the right kidney shows arterial wall irregularity along with distal microaneurysm formation in vessels that exhibit abrupt termination (▲). Classic PAN has a segmental distribution of transmural vascular inflammation that can acutely weaken arterial walls, leading to microaneurysm formation. As this vasculitis heals, there is vascular fibrosis with luminal narrowing and, possibly, obliteration, leading to areas of ischemic necrosis in affected organs. Various stages of inflammation are present at the same time, even in the same vessel.

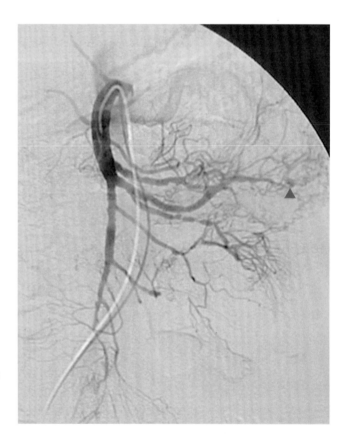

Figure 1-38 Polyarteritis nodosa (classic), angiogram ►
This angiogram of the superior mesenteric artery shows arterial wall irregularity along with distal microaneurysm formation (▲) with abrupt termination in small distal arteries. Reduction in arterial flow can lead to ischemia and infarction of tissues. Acute and chronic changes may coexist within the same arterial distribution. The ANCA result is usually negative with classic PAN.

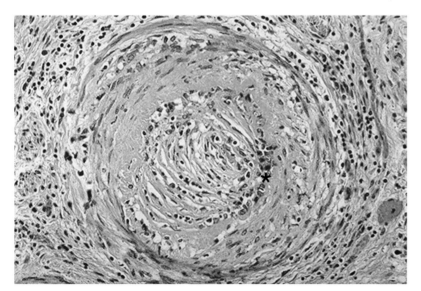

◄ **Figure 1-39 Vasculitis, chronic, microscopic**
This muscular artery exhibits vasculitis with chronic inflammatory cell infiltrates. The endothelial cells (★) have proliferated, and the lumen is absent. Often, vasculitis is a feature of an autoimmune disease, such as systemic lupus erythematosus, as was present in this patient. A more chronic form of classic PAN could appear very similar to this. In general, vasculitides are uncommon, and the various forms are often confusing and difficult to diagnose and classify.

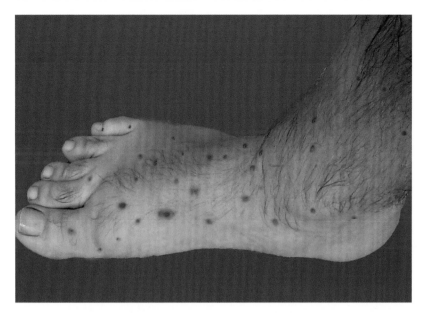

◄ Figure 1-40 Granulomatosis with polyangiitis, gross

Arterioles, capillaries, and venules are uniformly involved in granulomatosis with polyangiitis, in contrast to larger vessels in classic PAN. Granulomatosis manifests with palpable purpura, seen here on the foot. There is pulmonary capillaritis and necrotizing glomerulonephritis. Leukocytoclasis is often present. The ANCA result is positive in 70% of patients, but immune deposition is difficult to show (pauci-immune injury). Clinical findings include hemoptysis, arthralgia, abdominal pain, hematuria, proteinuria, and myalgia. Type III hypersensitivity re-action to drugs, infections, and neoplasms may be a precipitating event. A similar pattern of hypersen-sitivity angiitis is seen in Henoch-Schönlein purpura, vasculitis with autoimmune diseases, and essential mixed cryoglobulinemia.

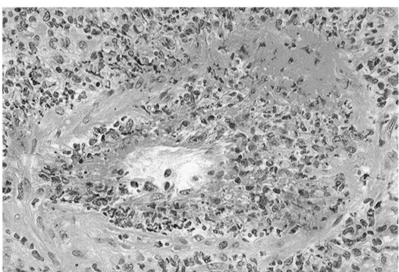

◄ Figure 1-41 Granulomatosis with polyangiitis, microscopic

This vasculitis is seen to involve a renal artery branch. Necrotizing granulomatous vasculitis is destroying the arterial media. Antineutrophil cy-toplasmic autoantibody (ANCA) can be present. In this patient, the perinuclear ANCA serology (p-ANCA or anti-myeloperoxidase [MPO], or cytoplasmic ANCA [c-ANCA] or anti-proteinase 3 [PR3]) is positive. This ANCA-associated vasculi-tis most often involves the kidneys and the lungs.

Figure 1-42 Thromboangiitis obliterans, angiogram ►

In this extremity the small muscular arterial branches have a corkscrew (◆) appearance, along with areas of narrowing, typical for changes from Buerger disease. This rare form of vasculitis has segmental, thrombosing, acute, and chronic inflammation of medium-sized and small arteries, principally the tibial and radial arteries. The inflammation can extend to adjacent veins and nerves. This condition is most often seen in young adults who are heavy cigarette smok-ers. There may be severe pain. Late complications include chronic ulcerations of the toes, feet, or fingers and frank gangrene.

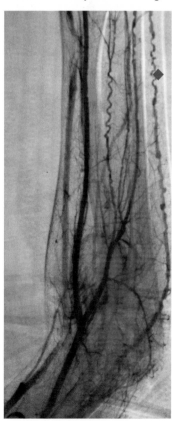

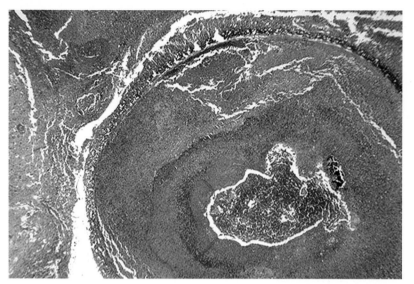

Figure 1-43 Infectious arteritis, microscopic
Parenchymal tissue infection can spread to vessels, as with pneumonia. Septicemia and septic emboli, as from endocarditis, may also lead to this complication. The infection is typically bacterial or fungal, such as *Staphylococcus aureus* or *Aspergillus* species. The infection can weaken or destroy the vascular wall and lead to aneurysm formation or hemorrhage. An aneurysm formed in such a manner is known as a *mycotic aneurysm*. The bacterial infection involving the muscular artery shown here is leading to necrosis, marked by an irregular luminal outline, along with inflammation and hemorrhage of the media and adventitia.

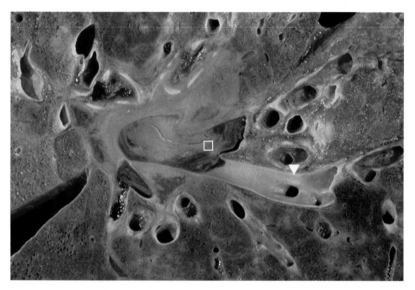

Figure 1-44 Invasive aspergillosis, gross
Aspergillus is a fungal organism that has a tendency to form thrombi (□) and invade vessels, even large pulmonary arterial branches as shown. The thrombus is formed of fungal hyphae with platelets and fibrin, shown here filling the lumen of a pulmonary arterial branch. Dissemination through the vascular system to other organs and pulmonary infarction can occur. Extensive pulmonary arterial occlusion with thrombi or emboli, or reduction in size of the pulmonary vascular bed from restrictive or obstructive lung diseases, can lead to pulmonary hypertension, which, if chronic, can promote pulmonary arterial atheroma (▼) formation.

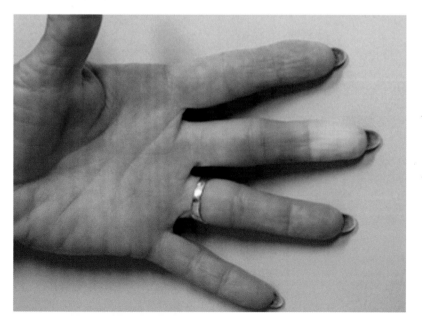

Figure 1-45 Raynaud phenomenon, gross
The "red, white, and blue" changes shown represent Raynaud phenomenon, which can be a primary exaggerated vasomotor activity without an underlying disease, typically in younger women. In older persons, an underlying disease, such as an autoimmune disease, hyperviscosity, or scleroderma should be sought. Progression to ischemia and ulceration is rare.

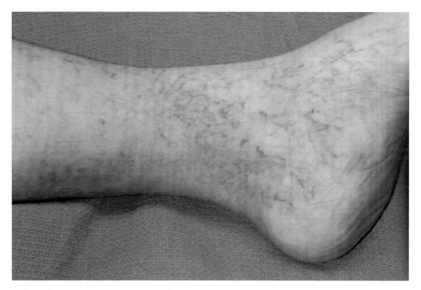

Figure 1-46 Varicose veins, gross
The prominent superficial veins shown here on the lower leg are varicosities, a common problem, particularly with aging and in individuals whose occupation involves prolonged standing, which increases hydrostatic pressure and exacerbates the problem. The venous valves may become incompetent over the years. Muscular atrophy with less muscle tone to provide a massage effect on the large superficial veins is a risk factor. Also, the skin becomes less elastic with aging. Although there may be vascular stasis and thrombosis with local edema and pain, these superficial veins typically do not give rise to thromboemboli.

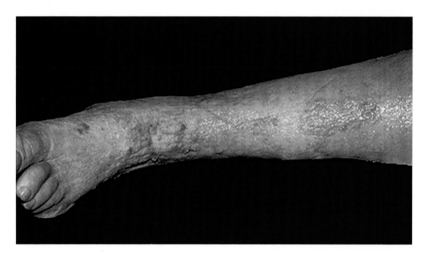

Figure 1-47 Stasis dermatitis, gross
The rough, thickened appearance to the skin surface is accompanied by brownish discoloration. Ulceration also is possible. Years of poor circulation with vascular stasis from poor cardiac function lead to chronic edema and venous pooling of blood with extravasation of red blood cells that leads to collection of dermal hemosiderin to give the skin this brown appearance. Pruritus and edema may be present.

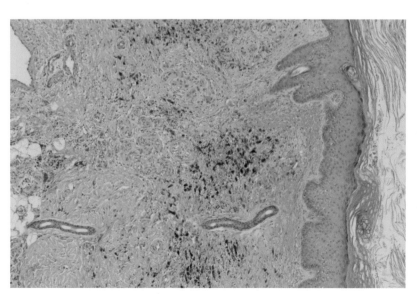

Figure 1-48 Stasis dermatitis, microscopic
Beneath the hyperkeratotic and acanthotic epidermis at the right can be seen bright red recent hemorrhage admixed with dark-brown hemosiderin granules and proliferating, thickened vascular channels. Middle-aged to elderly persons are mainly affected, or those with impaired vascular flow after surgery or trauma. The medial ankle is most often involved. Venous Doppler studies may reveal underlying venous thrombosis. There is an increased risk for contact dermatitis and cellulitis.

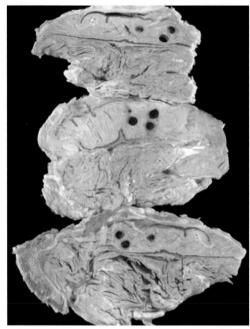

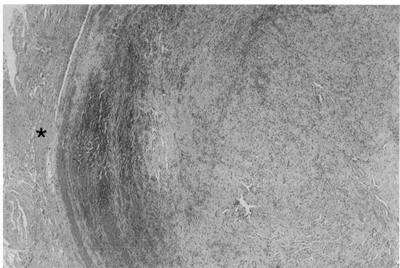

Figures 1-49 and 1-50 Phlebothrombosis, gross and microscopic ↑

Large dark-blue thrombi are seen in deep leg veins at the left. At the right is a large venous thrombus seen at low power. Note the thin muscular wall (★) typical of a vein. The thrombus displays varying degrees of organization, reflecting its propagation over time. Note the layering of the red blood cells and fibrin (lines of Zahn) at the periphery on the left, whereas there is organization of the thrombus on the right with granulation tissue and capillary proliferation, which result in the attachment of the thrombus to the vessel wall.

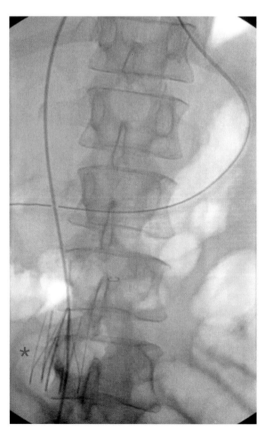

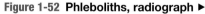

◄ Figure 1-51 Inferior vena cava filter, radiograph

This angiogram view in the lower abdominal region reveals the placement of an inferior vena cava (IVC) filter (✱) to prevent massive and potentially fatal pulmonary thromboembolism in a patient who had a prior episode of thromboembolism and who underwent a Doppler ultrasound of the lower extremities that revealed thromboses in the larger leg veins, the usual source for such large, potentially fatal emboli. The metal struts of the filter extend to the venous intima and block passage of potentially life-threatening large thromboemboli to the pulmonary arteries.

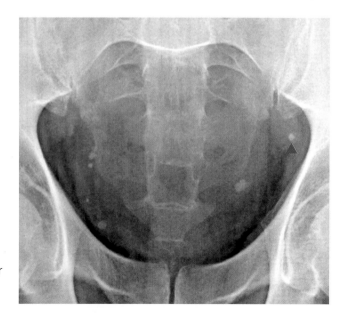

Figure 1-52 Phleboliths, radiograph ►

This abdominal plain film reveals multiple small, discrete bright densities (▲) in the pelvis. These are phleboliths, or small calcifications of veins, which are a common finding in middle-aged to older adults. Phleboliths have no significance but must be distinguished from other objects, such as urinary tract calculi.

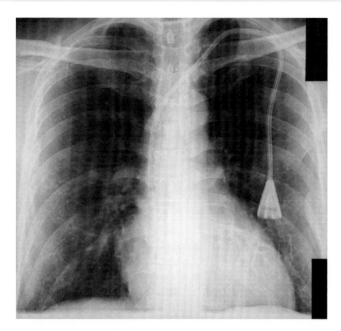

Figure 1-53 Central vascular catheter, radiograph
This chest radiograph shows the proper position for a central line placed through the right subclavian vein that passes into the superior vena cava down to the right atrium. A central line can be used to monitor fluid status and cardiac function in the patient.

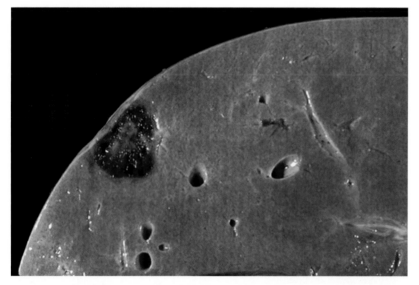

Figure 1-54 Hemangioma, gross
This benign circumscribed lesion is just beneath the capsule of the liver. About 1 person in 50 has such a neoplasm in the liver, which is typically an incidental finding, because most are 1 cm or less in diameter. They can sometimes be multiple. Hemangiomas are common pediatric neoplasms and may manifest at birth. One third of all hemangiomas occur in the liver. It is unlikely that malignant transformation would occur in such a hemangioma.

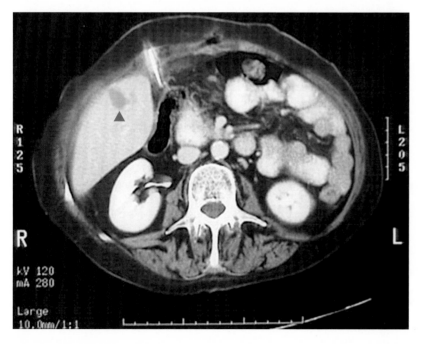

Figure 1-55 Hemangioma, CT image
This abdominal CT scan with oral and intravenous contrast shows a small lesion (▲) in the lower right lobe of the liver. The lesion has rounded margins and decreased central attenuation compared with the adjacent hepatic parenchyma. This is consistent with a small hemangioma that is an incidental finding unlikely to be clinically significant.

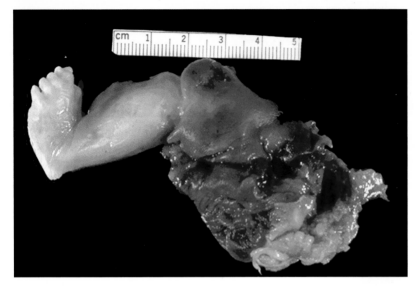

Figure 1-56 Congenital hemangioma, gross
The left lower extremity is shown here at 19 weeks' gestation. There is a reddish mass lesion involving the fetus's pelvic region and extending down the extremity. This is a congenital hemangioma. Although the neoplasm was histologically benign, its large size with increased vascular flow through the blood vessels resulted in congestive heart failure and fetal demise.

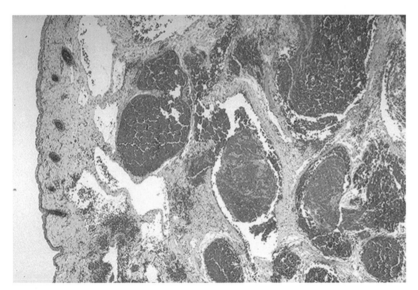

Figure 1-57 Hemangioma, microscopic
Beneath the skin surface at the left are many large vascular channels filled with numerous red blood cells. This cavernous hemangioma has large, dilated vascular spaces that extend to the underlying adipose tissue. A reddish "mole" on the skin that is small and round and raised may also represent a hemangioma. The vascular channels, which may vary in size and shape, are lined by flat endothelial cells. On physical examination these lesions appear to change slowly over time, if at all, and seem to have been present as long as the patient can remember. A capillary hemangioma has smaller vascular channels; it is most common on the skin and may grow rapidly in infancy before regressing.

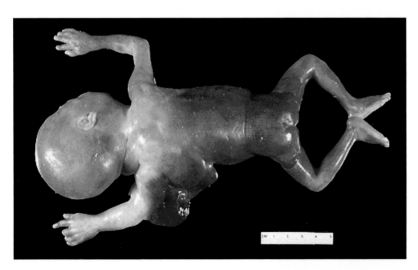

Figure 1-58 Congenital lymphangioma, gross
There is a large mass involving the left upper arm and left side of the chest of this fetus at 18 weeks' gestation. This congenital neoplasm is composed of irregular vascular channels resembling lymphatics—a lymphangioma. Smaller lymphangiomas are incidental findings, but larger ones may produce a mass effect, and they may be difficult to remove because, although histologically benign, they do not have distinct borders and may infiltrate into surrounding soft tissues.

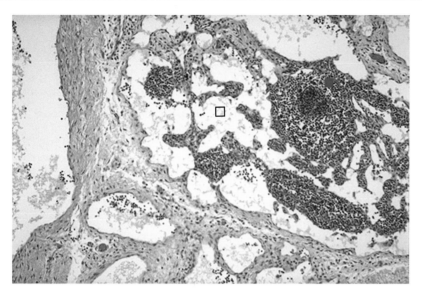

Figure 1-59 Lymphangioma, microscopic
Large, irregular lymphatic spaces (□) are lined by a thin endothelium. Note the absence of red blood cells within these vascular channels. The adjacent stroma has lymphoid nodules (■). Lymphangiomas appearing in children tend to involve the head, neck, and chest regions. A cystic hygroma composed of cavernous lymphatic channels is a pediatric head, neck, or upper chest lesion; a variant of cystic hygroma is present with monosomy X (Turner syndrome).

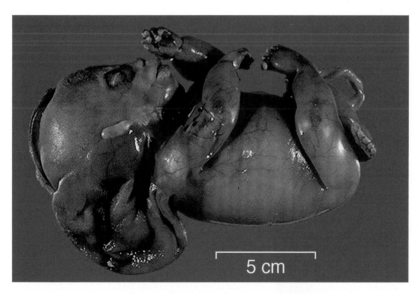

Figure 1-60 Cystic hygroma, gross
One very characteristic feature of a fetus with monosomy X (Turner syndrome, with 45,X gonadal dysgenesis karyotype) is the cystic hygroma of the posterior neck region. This lesion is not a true neoplasm but represents developmental failure of lymphatics to form and drain properly. This structure eventually forms the "web neck" feature of women with Turner syndrome. Note the gray coloration seen here from prolonged intrauterine fetal demise in this 18-week fetus. Microscopically, the cystic hygroma consists of irregularly dilated lymphatic spaces in the soft tissues of the posterior neck.

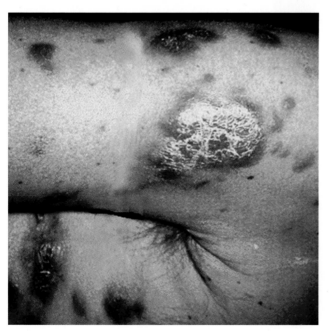

Figure 1-61 Kaposi sarcoma, gross
Endemic forms of Kaposi sarcoma (KS) were seen before the AIDS epidemic, but they were uncommon. The epidemic form of KS seen with AIDS usually appears in men who have sex with men and is rare in other groups at risk for HIV infection. The risk factor for KS is infection with human herpesvirus 8 (HHV-8), known as the *Kaposi sarcoma–associated herpesvirus* (KSHV), which can be sexually transmitted. The seroprevalence of HHV-8 is 5% to 10% of the general population, but 20% to 70% in men who have sex with men. The lesions can start as small reddish to red-purple plaques or patches on one or more areas of the skin. Over time the lesions may become nodular, larger, and more numerous. In patients who test positive for HIV, KS is diagnostic of AIDS. The use of antiretroviral therapy markedly decreases the incidence of KS.

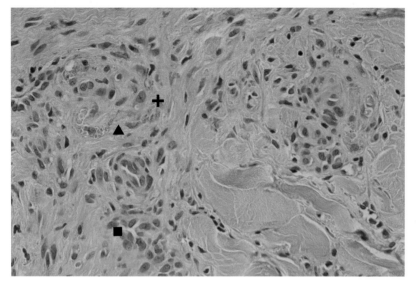

Figure 1-62 Kaposi sarcoma, microscopic
The atypical endothelial cells (■) of KS that line the irregular vascular spaces are shown here. The lesions characteristically have deposits of hemosiderin granules (✚) and faint, pale pink hyaline globules (▲).

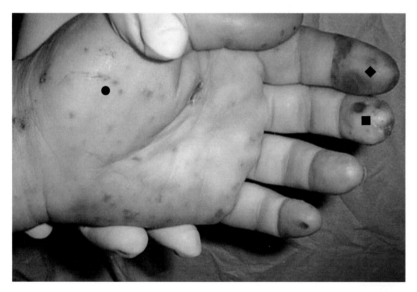

Figure 1-63 Petechiae, gross
The multiple small nodular red hemorrhages (■) seen here on the hand (Janeway lesions) resulted from peripheral embolization of fragments of a left-sided valvular vegetation in a patient with infective endocarditis. The irregular reddish purple mottled areas (◆) of skin represent livedo reticularis from ischemia after embolization to medium-sized arteries. The smaller pinpoint hemorrhages (●) can be termed *petechiae* and represent bleeding from small vessels. Petechial hemorrhages are classically found when a coagulopathy is caused by a low platelet count. They can also appear after sudden hypoxia.

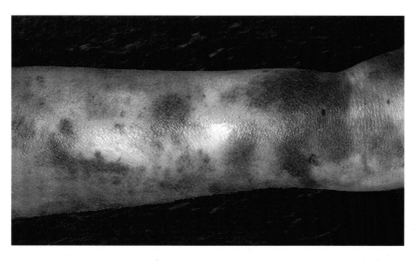

Figure 1-64 Purpura, gross
The blotchy areas of hemorrhage in the skin are called *ecchymoses* (singular, *ecchymosis*). Ecchymoses are larger than petechiae. In between in size are hemorrhages called *purpura*. The terms *ecchymosis* and *purpura* are often used interchangeably. Extravasation of red blood cells outside of vessels leads to ecchymoses and purpura. They can appear with coagulation disorders and most often when there are few platelets or nonfunctional platelets. In the setting of normal tissues subjected to sufficient blunt trauma to rupture small blood vessels and produce soft-tissue bleeding, the process would be called a *contusion*.

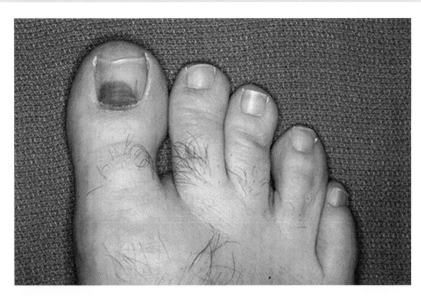

Figure 1-65 Hematoma, gross
A localized collection of blood outside the vascular system within tissues is known as a *hematoma.* Shown is a small hematoma under the toenail after trauma. The hematoma, no longer connected to the circulation, has a bluish appearance from the deoxygenated blood within it. The blood is gradually broken down and recycled. The iron in the hemoglobin in hemorrhages contained within the body is not lost. The pressure effect from a hematoma can be trivial, as in this patient; can produce pain; or can cause serious disease if in an enclosed space, such as the cranial cavity. Blood collecting outside the vasculature can press on vessels to reduce blood flow, or cause vasospasm.

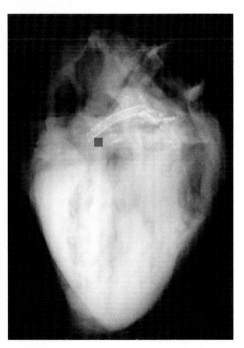

Figure 1-66 Coronary stent, radiograph
This postmortem radiograph reveals the presence of a right coronary artery stent (■) that is made of wire mesh. Percutaneous transluminal coronary angioplasty is a common procedure done to try to restore blood flow when a focal stenosis is present in one or more major coronary arteries. Placement of a stent helps to keep the artery open longer after the angioplasty procedure. Lifestyle changes help in preventing future stenoses. Drug-eluting stents help prevent recurrence of atheroembolic events. The drugs include paclitaxel and sirolimus. Sirolimus is a natural macrocyclic lactone that inhibits the activation of the mammalian target of rapamycin (mTOR) to arrest the cell cycle and prevent proliferation of cells, such as smooth muscle cells and inflammatory cells that participate in atheroma formation. The drug paclitaxel inhibits the disassembly of microtubules to suppress cellular proliferation.

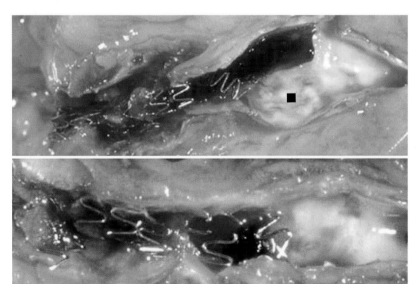

Figure 1-67 Coronary stent, gross
These panels show examples of coronary arterial stents placed to keep the artery lumen patent longer after angioplasty. Note the placement of the wire stent within the lumen of these atherosclerotic coronary arteries opened at autopsy. Percutaneous transluminal coronary angioplasty works best with focal coronary arterial stenosis. Note the atheroma formation on the luminal surfaces (■).

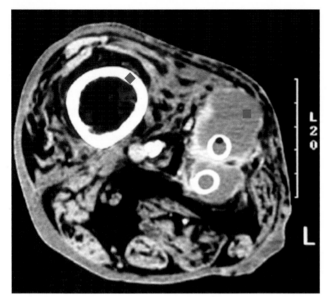

Figure 1-68 Peripheral vascular disease, grafts, CT image
In this patient with severe peripheral vascular disease from complications of diabetes mellitus, there are two circular, bright-appearing femoropopliteal polytetrafluoroethylene (PTFE) grafts within the diseased arteries, which are aneurysmally dilated surrounding the grafts and showing thrombosis and fluid collection (■). Note the bright femoral bone (◆). Endovascular placement of grafts and stents can be done to restore blood flow. Peripheral vascular disease may be marked by findings such as pallor, coolness, paresthesias, and paralysis if severe. Pulses may be reduced or absent. Pain may initially be present with exercise, but pain at rest is an ominous sign. Decreased tissue perfusion predisposes to nonhealing ulcerations with even minor trauma. Continued tissue ischemia may lead to gangrenous necrosis.

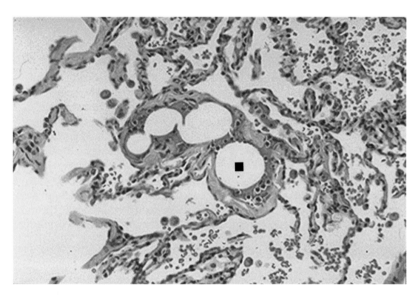

Figure 1-69 Fat embolism, microscopic
The rounded clear spaces (■) seen in the small pulmonary arterial branch in this section of lung represent fat globules and are characteristic of fat embolism. Fat embolism syndrome is most often a consequence of trauma with long bone fractures. It can also be seen with extensive soft-tissue trauma, burn injuries, and severe fatty liver, and very rarely after orthopedic procedures. The onset may be delayed on average 1 to 3 days after trauma and is marked by severe dyspnea. The mechanism may be mechanical release of fat droplets, or biochemical alterations with coalescence of blood lipids. The result is widespread obstruction of the pulmonary vascular bed.

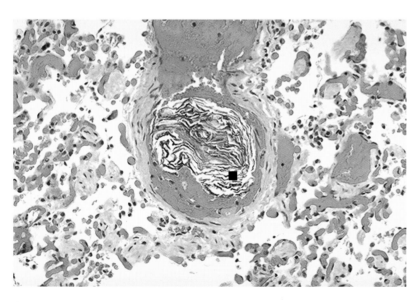

Figure 1-70 Amniotic fluid embolism, microscopic
Seen here are epithelial squames (■) in a peripheral pulmonary artery as a consequence of amniotic fluid embolism. This is a rare complication seen at term during or shortly after labor in pregnancy and can result in sudden death. The amniotic fluid may gain access to uterine veins after a tear in the placental membranes and embolize to the lungs through the venous return into the pulmonary capillary bed, producing acute dyspnea with cyanosis and shock. Fetal squames, lanugo hair, vernix, and mucin all can embolize to occlude small pulmonary arteries extensively as part of this process.

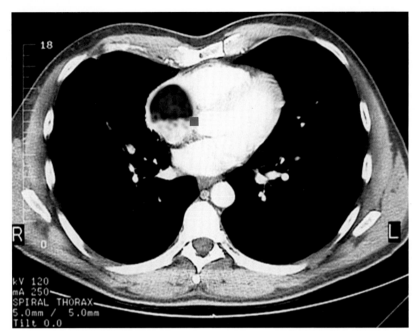

Figure 1-71 Air embolism, CT image
There is decreased attenuation with a layering effect (■) of air and blood in the right atrium consistent with venous air embolism. This uncommon process typically starts with laceration that involves a vein. Negative venous pressure draws air into the wound and into the vein. The air soon reaches the vena cava, then the right atrium, where it produces an occlusion. The pump loses its "prime." At least 100 mL of air is usually required. Surgical procedures and vascular lines may also predispose to air embolism. Air embolism involving arteries may occur in individuals such as divers who have diffusion of nitrogen into tissues under increased pressure; small bubbles form when the pressure decreases on decompression with surfacing. Such bubbles can occlude small arteries, producing tissue ischemia.

The Heart

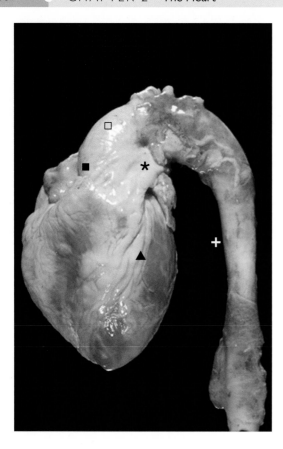

◄ **Figure 2-1 Normal heart and aorta, gross**
From this anterior view, the aortic root (■), aortic arch (□), and thoracic aorta (✚) can be seen. The pulmonic trunk (✶) is present. The anterior descending coronary artery (▲) is on the anterior surface of the heart. Note the smooth epicardial surface with yellowish epicardial adipose tissue.

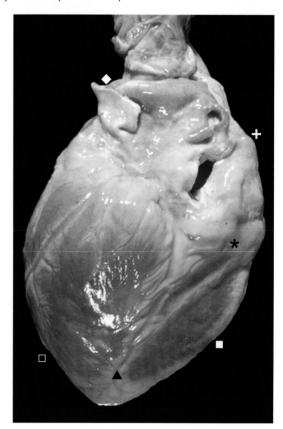

Figure 2-2 Normal heart, gross ►
The posterior surface of the heart has the right coronary artery (✶), which becomes the posterior descending artery (▲). Note the right ventricle (■) and the left ventricle (LV) (□), and the right atrium (✚) and the left atrium (◆).

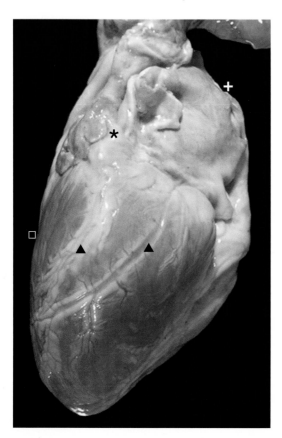

◄ **Figure 2-3 Normal heart, gross**
This is the appearance of the left lateral aspect of the heart with the left atrial appendage (✚) and LV (□). The circumflex artery (✶) gives off marginal branches (▲). The normal adult heart weighs about 250 to 300 g in women and 300 to 350 g in men. The LV, averaging 1.3 to 1.5 cm in thickness, produces the cardiac output that serves the systemic circulation. The right ventricle, 0.3 to 0.5 cm in thickness, works under a lower pressure to supply the pulmonary circulation. The ejection fraction (EF) is the amount of blood ejected from the LV with each heart beat and is normally more than 55%. An EF can be calculated with an echocardiogram, a left ventriculogram done during a cardiac catheterization, or a nuclear study called a MUGA scan. The method of calculating the EF involves tracing the dimensions of the LV at the end of its contraction period (systole) and at the end of its relaxation period (diastole).

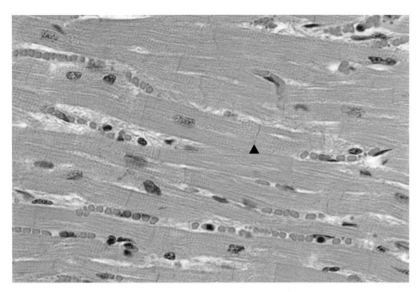

Figure 2-4 Normal myocardium, microscopic
Normal cardiac muscle in longitudinal section shows a syncytium of myocardial fibers (cardiac myocytes) with centrally located nuclei. Cardiac myocytes are a form of striated muscle with units called *sarcomeres* that contain the contractile proteins myosin and actin. Faint dark-pink intercalated discs (▲) traverse myocytes, forming mechanical and electrical couplings through gap junctions. Red blood cells appear in single file in the numerous capillaries between the myocardial fibers. There are numerous mitochondria and abundant myoglobin.

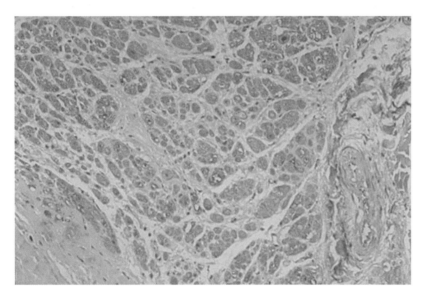

Figure 2-5 Normal conduction system, microscopic
The cardiac conduction system, difficult to observe histologically in humans, consists of specialized myocytes that conduct electrical impulses more readily than surrounding myocardial fibers. The neural differentiation of myocytes in the cross-section of atrioventricular node shown here is highlighted by this S100 immunohistochemical stain. The initial pacemaker of the heart is the sinoatrial node in the right atrium, and the specialized conducting myocytes spread excitation pulses, leading to a wave of depolarization through the atria, which is then conducted through the atrioventricular node and down the bundle of His into the ventricles.

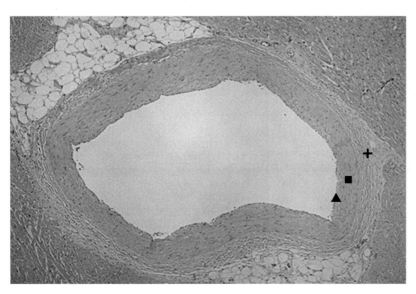

Figure 2-6 Normal coronary artery, microscopic
Three major coronary branches (left anterior descending, left circumflex, and right coronary) supply blood to the heart. The intima (▲) is normally thin and indistinct. The media (■) with smooth muscle forms the bulk of the artery. The adventitia (✛) is outside the media and merges with surrounding epicardial adipose and connective tissue. Distally, major branches of the coronary artery bifurcate to smaller branches. Shown is a distal coronary artery branch with a prominent lumen that is adjacent to myocardium. Such arteries anchored in myocardium are less likely to have turbulent blood flow and to develop atherosclerosis. Atherosclerosis tends to develop in the proximal portions of major coronary arteries.

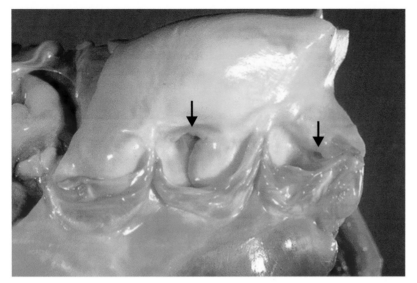

Figure 2-7 Normal aortic valve, gross
The aortic valve, similar to the other semilunar valve—the pulmonic valve—has three thin, delicate cusps. The coronary artery orifices (↓) can be seen just above the aortic valve cusps. The endocardium is smooth; beneath it can be seen the red-brown myocardium. The aorta above this valve displays a smooth intimal surface with no atherosclerosis.

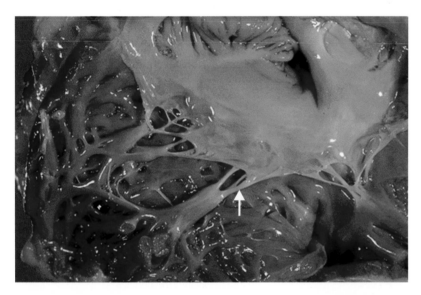

Figure 2-8 Normal tricuspid valve, gross
The leaflets of the atrioventricular valves (mitral and tricuspid) are thin and delicate. Similar to the mitral valve, the leaflets shown here have thin chordae tendineae (↑) that tether the leaflet margins to the papillary muscles of the ventricular wall below the valve. The right atrium can be seen above the valve.

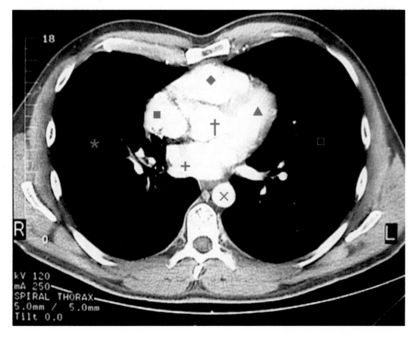

Figure 2-9 Normal heart, CT image
This normal chest CT scan in "bone window" shows the right lung (✱), left lung (□), right atrium (■), right ventricle (◆), left atrium (✚), LV (▲), aortic root (†), and descending aorta (✖) in the upper chest. The lungs, filled with air, have greatly decreased attenuation (less brightness), consistent with "air density" for radiographs. The chest wall is normal.

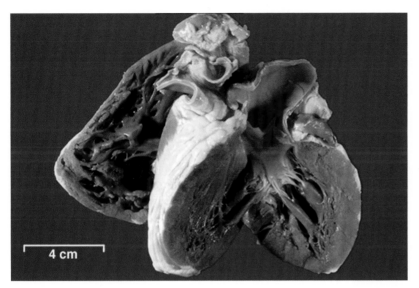

Figure 2-10 Brown atrophy, gross
Virtually all cardiac diseases lead to an enlarged heart. Here is a rare example of brown atrophy in which the heart is small, with chocolate-brown myocardium. In this condition, there is excessive lipochrome (lipofuscin) deposition within the myocardial fibers. Aging and malnutrition may favor this process, a form of cellular autophagocytosis. Antioxidants may protect against such injury. In the normal aging process the amount of lipofuscin increases within myocardial fiber cytoplasm, but not to the degree shown here.

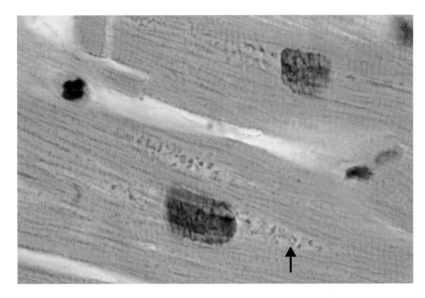

Figure 2-11 Lipofuscin, microscopic
The stippled, finely granular, intracytoplasmic, golden-brown pigment (↑) that lies primarily in a perinuclear location within these myocytes is lipofuscin (lipochrome) pigment. This "wear-and-tear" pigment represents the remnants of long-term autophagocytosis and cell remodeling accompanying free radical formation and lipid peroxidation. With the small amounts shown here, which increase with aging, there is no significant pathologic effect.

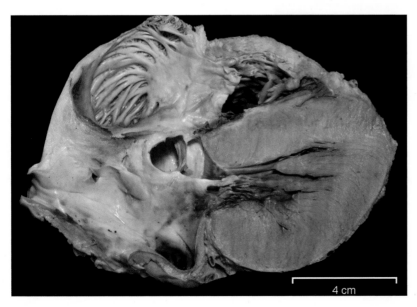

Figure 2-12 Cardiac hypertrophy, gross
Note prominent concentric left ventricular hypertrophy. The number of myocardial fibers does not increase, but their size can increase in response to an increased workload, leading to marked thickening of the LV. Increased pressure load from systemic hypertension is the most common cause of left ventricular hypertrophy. An increased volume load from aortic regurgitation can also lead to hypertrophy. Some degree of cardiac chamber dilation also accompanies ventricular failure. A relatively decreased capillary density, increased fibrous tissue, and synthesis of abnormal proteins predispose to heart failure.

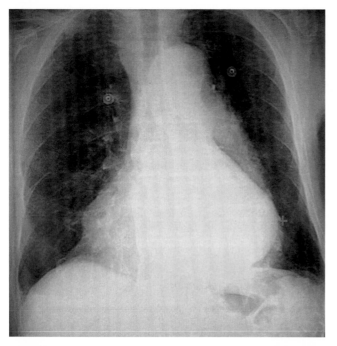

Figure 2-13 Cardiomegaly, radiograph
This PA chest radiograph shows marked cardiomegaly, with the left heart border (✛) appearing far into the left chest. Ordinarily the cardiac shadow occupies about half the distance across the chest from one rib margin to the other. The most common cause of an enlarged heart is ischemic heart disease. Systemic hypertension is also a frequent cause. Intrinsic disease of the myocardium may produce a cardiomyopathy. Pulmonary hypertension can lead to cor pulmonale with initial right-sided enlargement. Eventually, failure of the left or right ventricle leads to failure of the opposite ventricle, and there is more likely to be global cardiac enlargement with long-standing disease.

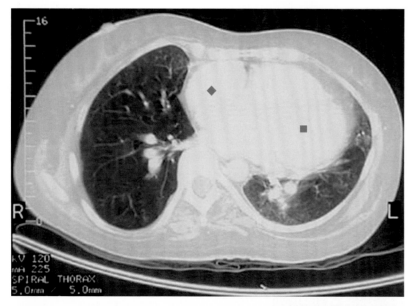

Figure 2-14 Cardiomegaly, CT image
Note the large size of the heart, with the left side of the heart filling much of the left chest cavity, in this patient with cardiomegaly. Right (◆) and left (■) ventricles are dilated. In this lung window, the interstitial markings within the lungs appear more prominent from vascular congestion.

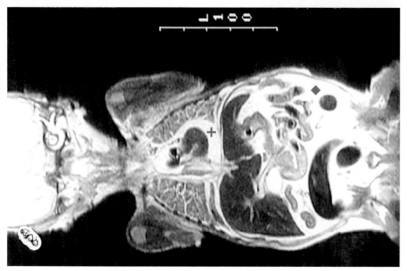

Figure 2-15 Heart failure and effusions, MRI
This T2-weighted MRI image of a neonate in coronal view shows a bright pericardial effusion (✛) around the heart. There is also ascites with bright fluid (◆) around the intra-abdominal organs in the peritoneal cavity. Such effusions can occur with hydrops, and heart failure from causes such as anemia, infection, and congenital cardiac anomalies.

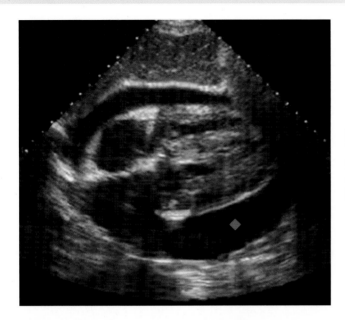

Figure 2-16 Heart failure and effusion, ultrasound
This ultrasound image of a neonate shows a large area of diminished echogenicity (◆) around the heart. This effusion is a fluid collection that is most often a serous transudate with congestive heart failure, leading to perinatal hydrops.

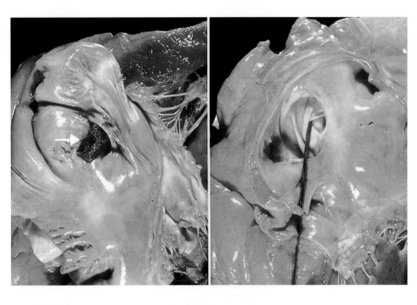

Figure 2-17 Patent foramen ovale, gross
The *right panel* shows a probe patent foramen ovale in an adult interatrial septum. A metal probe lifts the septum secundum and reveals the abnormal opening. Normally, left atrial pressure keeps the foramen closed, but if right atrial pressure increases with pulmonary hypertension (acutely with pulmonary embolus), the foramen may open and even allow a *thromboembolus* (→), shown in the *left panel,* to go from right to left. This is a rare *paradoxical* embolus, so called because a thromboembolus arising within the venous circulation can travel to the systemic circulation.

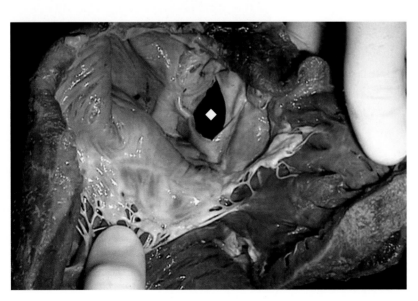

Figure 2-18 Atrial septal defect, gross
This large (◆) atrial septal defect (ASD) led to a left-to-right shunt and pulmonary hypertension with increased pulmonary arterial pressures that eventually caused reversal and right-to-left shunt, resulting in marked right ventricular hypertrophy, a complication known as *Eisenmenger complex.* The examiner's finger (lower left) holds a markedly thickened right ventricular free wall below the tricuspid valve, and the finger (right) holds the interventricular septum below the mitral valve. About 90% of ASDs such as this one are secundum defects. Primum defects account for 5% of ASDs and are often associated with an anterior mitral leaflet cleft. The remainder are sinus venosus defects near the entrance of the superior vena cava.

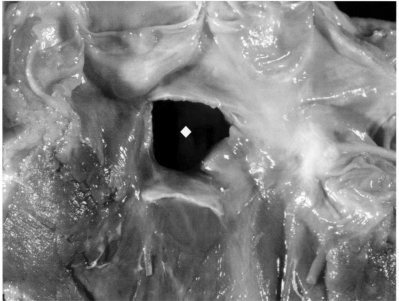

◀ **Figure 2-19 Ventricular septal defect, gross**
There is a large ventricular septal defect (VSD) (◆) just below the aortic valve. A third of VSDs are isolated defects without accompanying anomalies, but many diagnosed perinatally or in infancy are part of multiple anomalies. This VSD involves the membranous septum, as are 90% of VSDs, whereas 10% occur in the muscular interventricular septum. About half of small VSDs may eventually close. A large VSD with a significant left-to-right shunt leads to cardiac failure, and if not corrected surgically the shunt leads to pulmonary hypertension with cor pulmonale and eventual reversal to a right-to-left shunt (Eisenmenger complex). VSDs increase the risk for endocarditis.

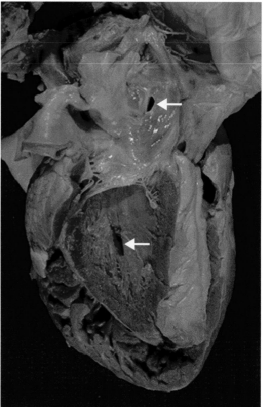

Figure 2-20 Atrial septal defect and ventricular septal defect, gross ▶
The heart is opened on the left side with the left ventricular free wall reflected superiorly to reveal two defects (◀) including both an ASD and a muscular VSD. Such small defects do not produce significant left-to-right shunting, but they do increase the risk for infective endocarditis, and a holosystolic murmur may often be audible on auscultation of the chest.

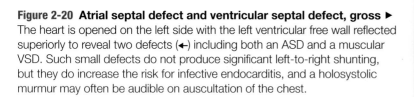

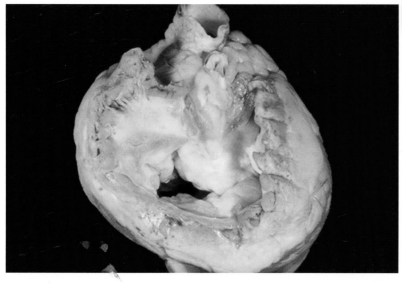

◀ Figure 2-21 Endocardial cushion defect, gross
A severe defect is shown in which there is only a single large atrioventricular valve, as visible superiorly, that separates a single ventricle from a single atrium. This patient was able to survive with this two-chambered heart because a small amount of residual interventricular septum provided some direction to flow of oxygenated and unoxygenated blood, and because of pulmonic stenosis, which protected the lungs from the shunting. (This is an explanted heart from a cardiac transplantation procedure, so most of the atria are not present.)

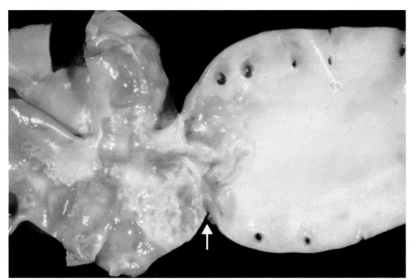

Figure 2-22 Aortic coarctation, gross
This aorta from an adult is opened longitudinally to reveal a region of narrowing (↑). There was increased turbulence that led to increased atherosclerosis. Males are affected twice as often as females. Coarctation is a common feature of monosomy X (Turner syndrome), however. Coarctation is categorized in relation to the ductus arteriosus. The preductal form with proximal aortic tubular hypoplasia is also known as the *infantile* form because of symptoms appearing in early childhood. The postductal form becomes symptomatic later in life, with findings related to diminished blood flow to lower extremities, but hypertension in the upper body.

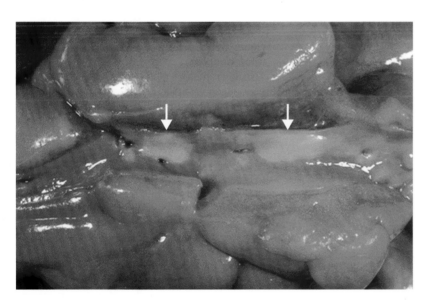

Figure 2-23 Coronary atherosclerosis, gross
A minimal amount of coronary atherosclerosis, with a few scattered yellow lipid plaques (↓), is shown on the intima of the opened coronary artery traversing the epicardial surface of a heart. The degree of atherosclerosis here is not great enough to cause significant luminal narrowing but could be the harbinger of worse atherosclerosis to come, if plaques continue to enlarge. Atherosclerosis is initiated with endothelial damage and inflammation with leukocyte elaboration of cytokines, such as tumor necrosis factor (TNF), interleukin-1 (IL-1), and interferon-γ (IFN-γ). This process is promoted by uptake of increased circulating oxidized LDL cholesterol into macrophages.

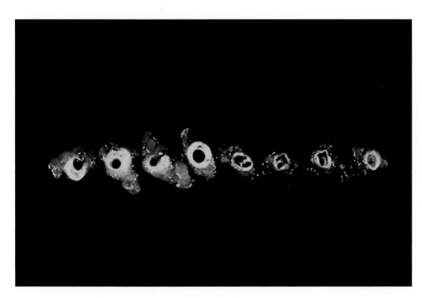

Figure 2-24 Coronary atherosclerosis, gross
These cross-sections of the left anterior descending coronary artery show atherosclerosis with more pronounced luminal narrowing at the left, the more proximal portion of this artery. Atherosclerosis is generally worse at the origin of a coronary artery and in the first few centimeters, where turbulent blood flow is greater. This turbulent flow over many years promotes endothelial injury that favors inflammation with insudation of lipids to promote formation of atheromas. With lifestyle modifications, this process is reversible.

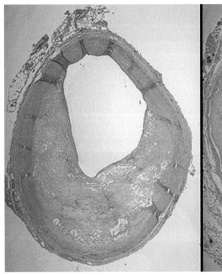
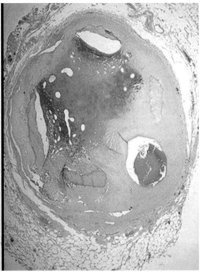

Figure 2-25 Coronary atherosclerosis, microscopic

The coronary artery in the *left panel* is narrowed by 60% to 70%, on the verge of producing angina, which could then be precipitated by transient vasoconstriction. Acute coronary syndromes from marked ischemia are more likely to occur when luminal narrowing reaches 70%. The coronary artery in the *right panel* has even more severe occlusion, with evidence for previous thrombosis and organization of the thrombus leading to recanalization, such that there are only three small lumens remaining.

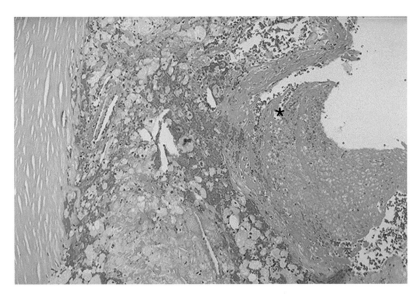

Figure 2-26 Coronary atherosclerosis, microscopic

This atheromatous plaque shows endothelial denudation with plaque disruption and overlying thrombus (★) formation from platelet aggregation. Note the composition of the plaque base with foam cells, cholesterol clefts, and areas of hemorrhage. Such a plaque complicated by rapid overlying thrombus formation can lead to an acute coronary syndrome resulting in an ischemic cardiac event. The first sign of ischemic heart disease may be angina pectoris, a symptom complex characterized by recurrent acute episodes of substernal or precordial chest pain. Occlusive coronary atherosclerosis increases the risk for subsequent myocardial infarction (MI).

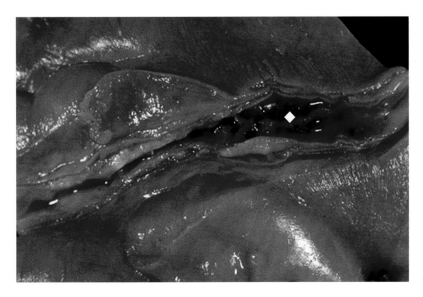

Figure 2-27 Coronary thrombosis, gross

One of the severe complications of coronary atherosclerosis, shown here with thickened arterial walls with yellow-tan plaques that narrow the arterial lumen, is thrombosis. The dark red thrombus (◆) occludes this anterior descending coronary artery, opened longitudinally. The thrombotic occlusion leads to ischemia or infarction of the myocardium supplied by the artery. One possible outcome of coronary thrombosis is sudden death. Other complications include ongoing arrhythmias and congestive heart failure.

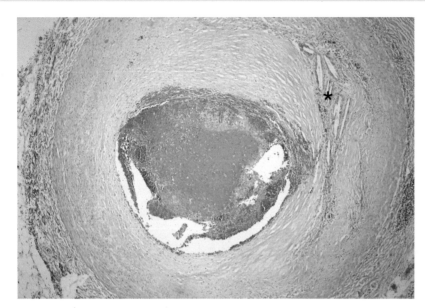

Figure 2-28 Coronary thrombosis, microscopic
The recent thrombus shown here nearly occludes the remaining small lumen of this coronary artery already narrowed from severe atherosclerosis. Note the fibrointimal proliferation (✱) with cholesterol clefts. Endothelial damage with platelet activation promotes thrombosis. A small dose of aspirin taken each day helps reduce platelet function, making the platelets less sticky and less prone to participate in thrombotic events.

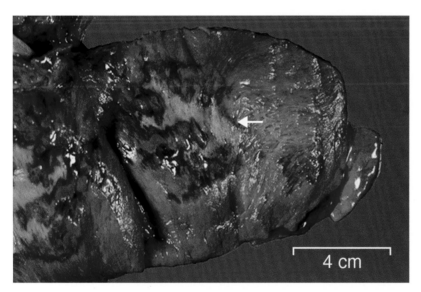

4 cm

Figure 2-29 Myocardial infarction, gross
The interventricular septum is sectioned to reveal an extensive acute MI. The dead muscle is tan-yellow, with a surrounding hyperemic border (←). This appearance is characteristic of an infarction that is 3 to 7 days old. Serum creatinine kinase (CK), specifically the CK-MB isozyme more specific to heart, and troponin I are released from damaged myofibers and start to increase 3 to 4 hours after the initial ischemic event. CK-MB peaks about 1 day later, then declines to negligible levels by 3 days. The troponin I level remains increased for 10 to 14 days. Serum myoglobin can be increased starting 3 hours after MI, but it is not specific for myocardium.

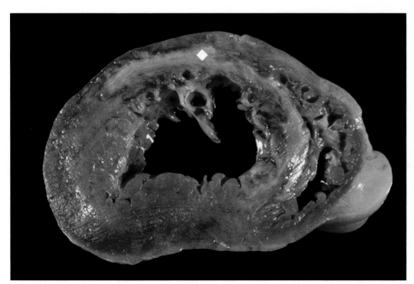

Figure 2-30 Myocardial infarction, gross
This axial section reveals a large MI involving the anterior left ventricular wall and interventricular septum in the distribution of the left anterior descending coronary artery. Note the yellowish area (◆) of necrosis with the hyperemic border that is nearly transmural. Radionuclide imaging would show decreased uptake into this region. Echocardiography would show diminished ventricular wall motion with such a large infarction, and the EF would be decreased. Electrocardiographic changes could include ST segment elevation followed by T wave inversion and by development of Q waves.

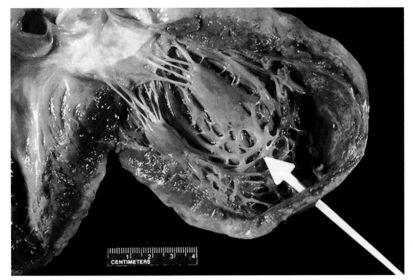

Figure 2-31 Myocardial infarction, gross
In cross-section, the point of rupture of the left ventricular free wall myocardium is shown at the (↑). In this case, an MI 3 weeks prior accounts for the ventricular wall thinning shown here; a subsequent MI occurred and ruptured through an already thinned ventricular wall 3 days later. The mitral valve with chordae tendineae and the papillary muscles appear normal here. Rupture is most likely to occur 3 to 7 days after a transmural infarction, when the necrotic muscle is soft and before any significant amount of organization with ingrowth of capillaries and fibroblasts has occurred.

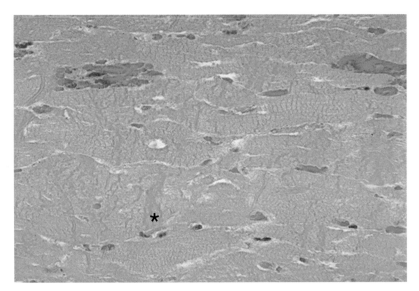

Figure 2-32 Myocardial infarction, microscopic
The earliest histologic change seen with acute MI during the first 24 hours is contraction band necrosis. These myocardial fibers are beginning to lose cross-striations, and the nuclei are not clearly visible in most of the myocytes shown here. Note the many irregular, darker pink, wavy contraction bands (★) extending across the fibers. Serologic markers for infarction include nonspecific myoglobin and the more specific markers of cardiac muscle injury, including CK-MB and troponin I. Use of thrombolytic agents, percutaneous transluminal coronary angioplasty, and coronary arterial bypass grafting are methods to help restore blood flow and prevent further damage.

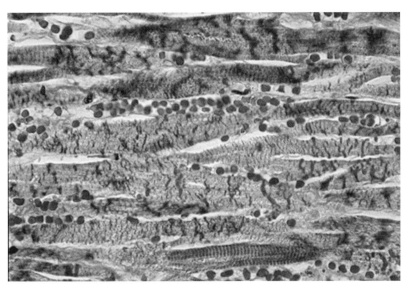

Figure 2-33 Myocardial infarction, microscopic
This trichrome stain shows the appearance of an early acute MI, less than 1 day old, with prominent reddish contraction band necrosis. Coagulative necrosis with karyolysis has led to loss of the nuclei. If the area of infarction remains small, the MI may be "silent" without signs or symptoms and detectable only with electrocardiography or serum cardiac muscle enzyme elevation. The myocardial irritability after an MI leads to electrical conduction disturbances with arrhythmias such as sinus bradycardia, heart block, asystole, and ventricular fibrillation.

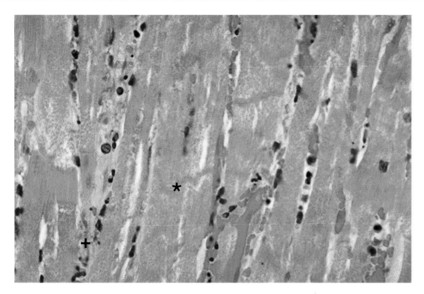

Figure 2-34 Myocardial infarction, microscopic
This early acute MI is 1 to 2 days old. There is loss of cross-striations, and some contraction bands (★) are seen. The cardiac fiber nuclei have undergone karyolysis and are no longer visible. Some neutrophils (✚) are beginning to infiltrate into this necrotic myocardium. The loss of the nuclei represents an irreversible form of cellular injury. Reperfusion of such damaged muscle may lead to increased production of toxic free radicals that can potentiate further myocardial damage. Thrombolytic therapy to treat acute coronary thrombosis is most beneficial within 30 minutes of the initial arterial occlusion.

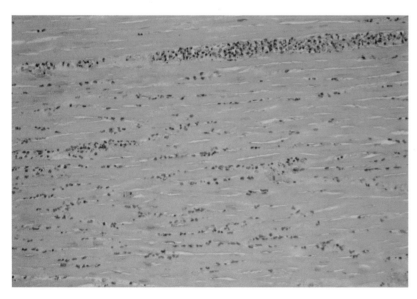

Figure 2-35 Myocardial infarction, microscopic
This early acute MI is 2 to 3 days old. There is increasing infiltration by neutrophils into the myocardium. With ongoing coagulative necrosis, the outlines of myofibers remain, but their nuclei have undergone dissolution. At this point CK-MB is decreasing while troponins remain elevated. The extent of infarction determines residual ventricular function. A large infarct may severely reduce EF and lead to acute congestive heart failure with pulmonary congestion and edema.

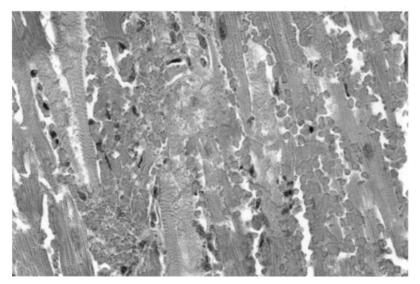

Figure 2-36 Myocardial infarction, microscopic
The extensive hemorrhage in this acute MI may represent the hyperemic border, but if extensive may be the result of a reperfusion injury. The vulnerable ischemic but not yet infarcted myocardium is at greatest risk for this injury, because endothelial swelling reduces blood flow to these areas. Reperfusion injury may be mediated by oxidative stress, calcium overload, and/or acute inflammation.

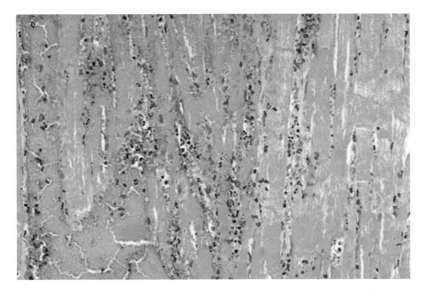

Figure 2-37 Myocardial infarction, microscopic

There is extensive acute inflammation with neutrophils infiltrating into these myofibers undergoing coagulative necrosis. This MI is 3 to 4 days old. There is an extensive acute inflammatory cell infiltrate, and the myocardial fibers are so necrotic that the outlines of them are only barely visible. Clinically, such an acute MI is marked by changes in the electrocardiogram and by an increase in troponins. In addition to chest pain, patients with MI may have a rapid, weak pulse; hypotension; diaphoresis; and dyspnea from acute left-sided congestive heart failure.

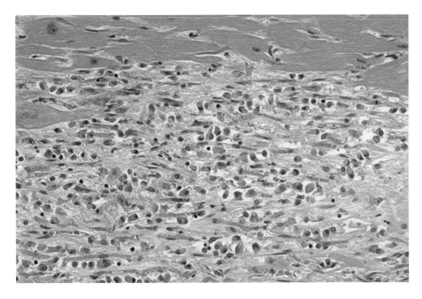

Figure 2-38 Myocardial infarction, microscopic

Toward the end of the first week after the initial ischemic event that triggered infarction, healing of the MI becomes more prominent, with numerous capillaries, fibroblasts, and macrophages filled with hemosiderin. The granulation tissue shown here becomes most prominent 2 to 3 weeks after onset of infarction. This area of granulation tissue is nonfunctional and noncontractile, reducing the EF, but it is unlikely to rupture.

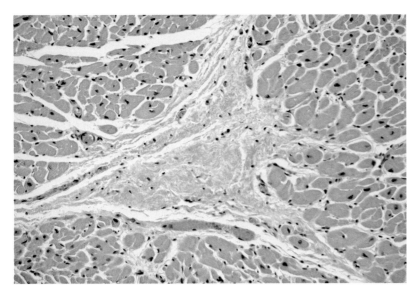

Figure 2-39 Myocardial infarction, microscopic

Two to 3 weeks after the onset of MI, healing at the site of myocardial necrosis is well under way, and there is more extensive collagen deposition. This remote MI has a dense collagenous scar after 2 months, shown here as an irregular pale area surrounded by surviving myocardial fibers. The size of the MI determines the residual EF and clinical findings. As expected, larger MIs are more likely to become complicated by heart failure and arrhythmias.

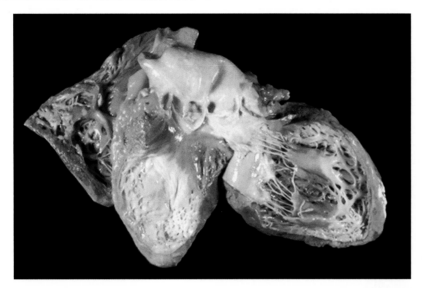

Figure 2-40 Myocardial infarction, gross
The left ventricular free wall is on the right and the interventricular septum is at the center, with the right ventricle at the left. A remote MI has extensively involved the anterior left ventricular free wall and septum, shown here as the white appearance of the endocardial surface in the areas of extensive scarring. Involvement of the right ventricle is uncommon. This scarred area is noncontractile, and the EF and cardiac output are reduced. The papillary muscles here appear to be mostly spared.

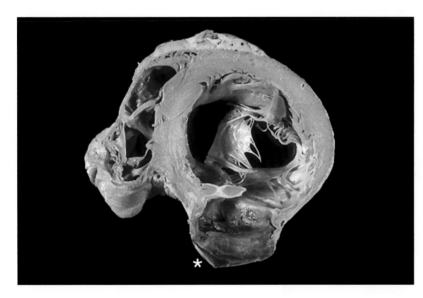

Figure 2-41 Myocardial infarction, gross
This axial cross-section reveals a ventricular aneurysm (★) with a very thin wall that visibly bulges out. The stasis in this aneurysm has predisposed to the mural thrombus filling it. A previous extensive transmural MI involving the free wall of the LV reduced the thickness of the myocardial wall. This infarction was so extensive that, after healing, the ventricular wall was replaced by a thin band of collagen, forming an aneurysm. The aneurysm represents noncontractile tissue that reduces stroke volume and strains the remaining myocardium.

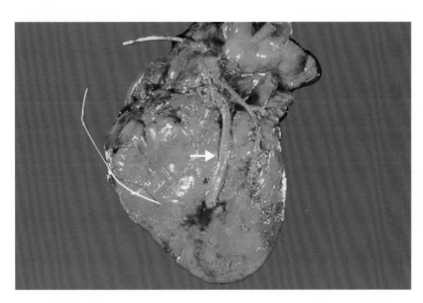

Figure 2-42 Coronary artery bypass grafting, gross
This patient underwent myocardial revascularization for ischemic heart disease. Coronary artery bypass grafting (CABG) with autogenous vein (saphenous vein) grafts is shown here. The largest graft (→) runs down the center of the heart to anastomose with the left anterior descending artery distally. Another graft extends in a Y fashion just to the right of this to marginal branches of the circumflex artery. A white temporary pacing wire to treat arrhythmias extends from the mid left surface, and a Swan-Ganz catheter that extended to a peripheral pulmonary artery to measure wedge pressure, equivalent to left atrial pressure, emerges from the right atrium.

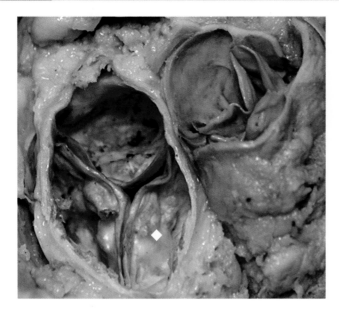

Figure 2-43 Calcific aortic stenosis, gross
An aortic valve need not be bicuspid to calcify. A normal tricuspid aortic valve may undergo slowly progressive dystrophic calcification over many years, so-called "senile calcific aortic stenosis." Nodules of calcification (◆) are shown on these cusps, as viewed in the aortic outflow tract at the lower left (compare with pulmonic valve at upper right). Calcium deposition leads to progressive stenosis with reduced cusp excursion, and pulse pressure is diminished. This increased ventricular pressure load leads to left ventricular hypertrophy. As the cross-sectional area of the remaining valve outlet approaches 1 cm^2, sudden left ventricular failure may occur.

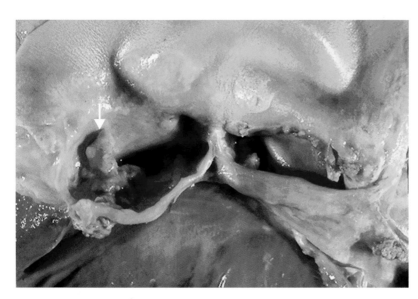

Figure 2-44 Bicuspid aortic valve, gross
The valve here has been opened with the aortic outflow above and the left ventricular myocardium below. Bicuspid aortic valve is a common congenital cardiac defect, seen in 1% of the population. Most bicuspid valves are prone to undergo calcification, but patients can remain asymptomatic until middle age, when the stenosis reaches a critical point at which congestive heart failure rapidly ensues. The dense irregular nodules of calcification (↓) shown are present on both valve surfaces. The increasing pressure gradient leads to left ventricular hypertrophy and eventually to left-sided congestive heart failure marked by pulmonary congestion and edema.

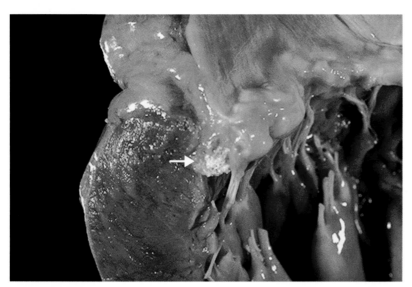

Figure 2-45 Mitral annular calcification, gross
A relatively uncommon but benign condition that may appear on radiographic studies is mitral valve ring calcification, shown here as the circular white deposit (→) in cross-section. It is most common in older adults, particularly women older than 60 years. This process produces a doughnut-shaped ring of calcification around the mitral valve annulus. In severe cases there may be valvular regurgitation with a murmur heard on auscultation of the chest. The red-brown myocardium of the left ventricular wall shown here is completely normal.

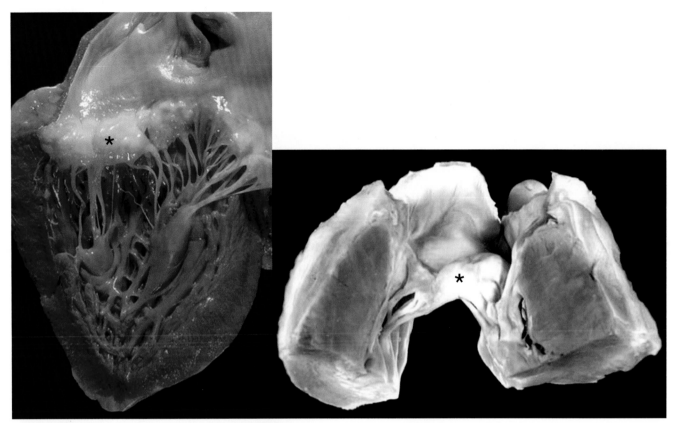

Figures 2-46 and 2-47 Myxomatous degeneration with floppy mitral valve, gross
The leaflets of the mitral valve are ballooned upward (★). This is characteristic of floppy mitral valve with mitral valve prolapse. The chordae tendineae anchoring the leaflets to the ventricle become elongated and thin. There is microscopic myxomatous degeneration of the valve, which weakens the connective tissue. Most patients are asymptomatic. There may be an audible heart murmur in the form of a midsystolic click. In more severe cases, mitral regurgitation can occur, with a late systolic or holosystolic murmur. Mitral valve prolapse may occur, and rupture of the chordae is possible, leading to the appearance of acute valvular insufficiency. As a sporadic condition it affects 3% of the population. It can also occur with Marfan syndrome.

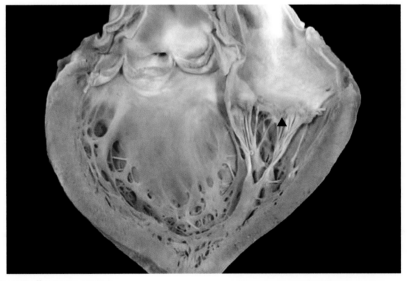

Figure 2-48 Rheumatic heart disease, gross
Acute rheumatic fever (ARF) can produce pancarditis, but shown here are the characteristic small verrucous vegetations (▲) of rheumatic endocarditis located over areas of fibrinoid degeneration on the valve cusp margins. These vegetations, composed of platelets and fibrin and located at the valve closure line, are usually no more than 2 mm in size but may produce an audible murmur. These lesions are not likely to embolize and do not produce significant valvular deformity at this early stage of rheumatic valvulitis.

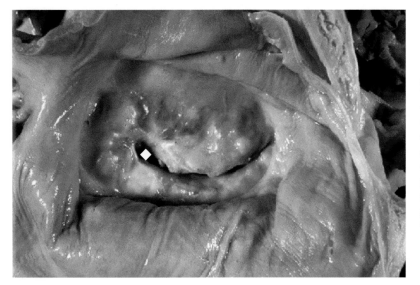

◀ **Figure 2-49 Rheumatic heart disease, gross**

This mitral valve is shown from above the inflow from a dilated left atrium and shows the typical fish-mouth shape following chronic rheumatic valvulitis with scarring and narrow valve opening (◆). There can be both stenosis and insufficiency, with the former predominating. The mitral valve is most often affected with rheumatic heart disease (RHD); followed by mitral and aortic valves together; then aortic alone; then mitral, aortic, and tricuspid valves together.

Figure 2-50 Rheumatic heart disease, gross ▶

In time, chronic rheumatic valvulitis may develop by organization of acute and recurrent endocardial inflammation along with fibrosis, as shown here affecting the mitral valve, as viewed from the opened LV, with the aortic valve at the top. Note the shortened and thickened chordae tendineae (←). This complication can take decades to become slowly symptomatic. Valvular stenosis can lead to prominent left atrial enlargement, which predisposes to mural thrombus formation and systemic embolization.

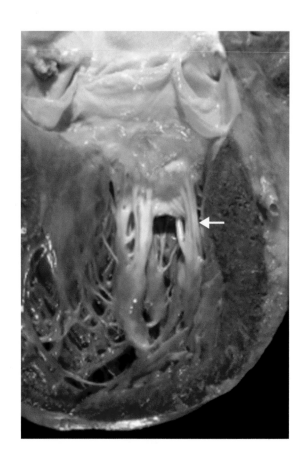

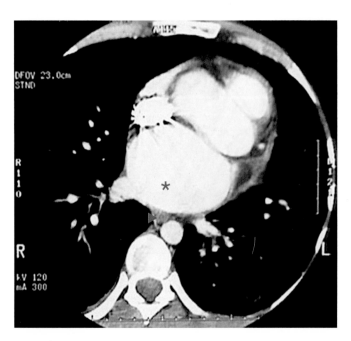

◀ **Figure 2-51 Rheumatic heart disease, CT image**

Chronic rheumatic valvulitis can produce either valvular insufficiency or stenosis, and an element of both may be present simultaneously, but stenosis usually predominates. Because the mitral valve is most often involved, a common finding is marked left atrial enlargement. In this chest CT with contrast the enlarged left atrium (✱) displaces the adjacent esophagus (▶) and leads to dysphagia.

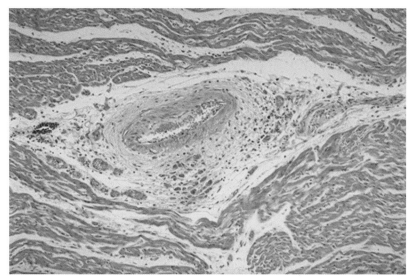

Figure 2-52 Rheumatic heart disease, microscopic

The Aschoff nodule of ARF typically occurs in the myocardial interstitium. It is a nodular perivascular collection of mainly mononuclear inflammatory cells. This manifestation of RHD occurs 10 days to 6 weeks after group A streptococcal pharyngitis. This carditis results from molecular mimicry and immunologic cross-reaction with the streptococcal capsular M protein. The endocardium, myocardium, and epicardium can be affected, producing a pancarditis. Serologic markers of rheumatic fever may include antistreptolysin O, antihyaluronidase, and anti–DNase B.

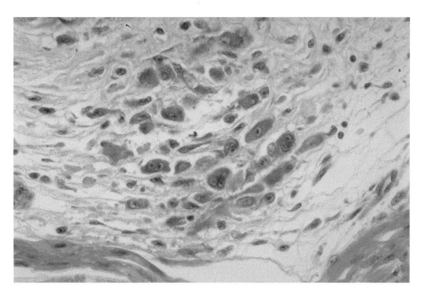

Figure 2-53 Rheumatic heart disease, microscopic

The most characteristic cellular component of this Aschoff nodule is the Aschoff giant cell. These appear here as large cells with two or more nuclei that have prominent nucleoli. Scattered mononuclear inflammatory cells accompany them and can be occasional neutrophils. Such inflammation can occur not only in myocardium, but also in endocardium (including valves) and epicardium. Involvement of all three cardiac layers is termed *pancarditis*. Myocardial involvement leads to death in about 1% of patients with ARF. RHD is now so uncommon that the number of streptococcal infections needed to treat to prevent one case of RHD is over 10,000.

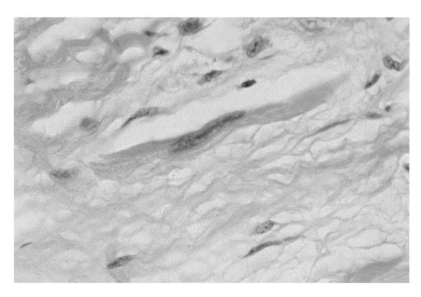

Figure 2-54 Rheumatic heart disease, microscopic

This long, thin cell with an elongated nucleus, which occurs with acute rheumatic carditis, is the Anichkov myocyte. Signs and symptoms of ARF are most likely to appear in children. Extracardiac manifestations may include "major" Jones criteria: subcutaneous nodules, erythema marginatum, fever, and polyarthritis. "Minor" criteria include arthralgia, fever, previous RF, leukocytosis, elevated sedimentation rate, and C-reactive protein.

There is a propensity for reactivation of RF with subsequent episodes of group A streptococcal pharyngitis. Chronic RHD is usually the result of multiple recurrent episodes of ARF.

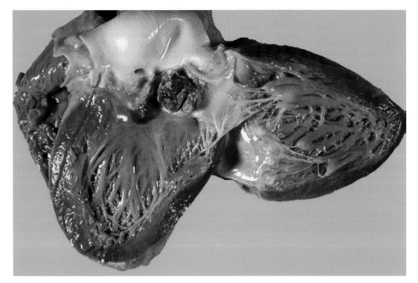

Figure 2-55 Infective endocarditis, gross
The aortic valve shows a large, irregular, reddish tan vegetation. Virulent organisms, such as *Staphylococcus aureus,* produce an acute bacterial endocarditis within days, similar to the lesion shown here, whereas some organisms, such as the viridans group of *Streptococcus,* produce a more slowly developing subacute bacterial endocarditis. Endocarditis is marked by fever with heart murmur. Predisposing risks for endocarditis include bacteremia and previously damaged or deformed valves, but endocarditis can involve anatomically normal valves.

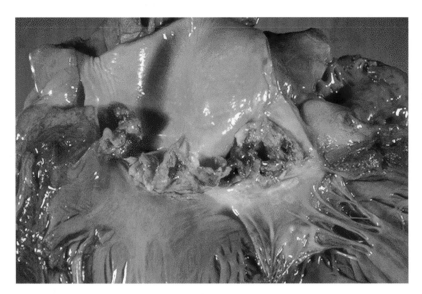

Figure 2-56 Infective endocarditis, gross
The more virulent bacteria causing the acute bacterial form of infective endocarditis can lead to serious valvular destruction, as shown here involving the aortic valve. Irregular reddish tan vegetations overlie valve cusps that are being destroyed by the action of the proliferating bacteria. Portions of the vegetation can break off and become septic emboli that travel to other organs, leading to foci of infarction or infection.

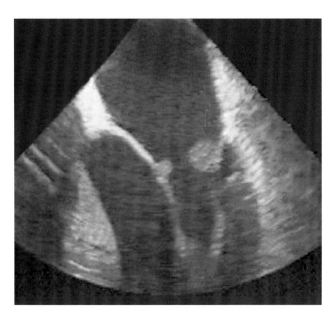

Figure 2-57 Valvular vegetations, ultrasound
The large valvular vegetation (↓) represents a conglomeration of bacteria with fibrin and platelets. Vegetations may interfere with valve motion to cause an audible murmur or interfere with blood flow. The friable vegetations of infective endocarditis are prone to break apart and embolize to cause vascular occlusion at distant sites. Thus, left-sided vegetations may underlie cerebrovascular strokes, whereas right-sided lesions predispose to pulmonary infarcts and abscesses.

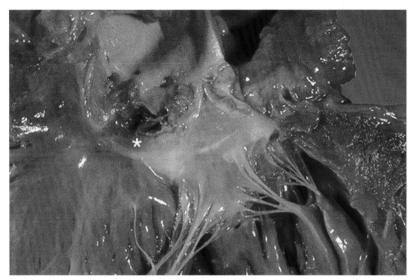

Figure 2-58 Infective endocarditis, gross
In this subacute endocarditis with less virulent Streptococcus pyogenes, the inflammation is not as florid, but it is persistent and shows how the infection tends to spread from the valve surface. Vegetations can be seen here involving the endocardial surfaces, and the infection is extending into the underlying myocardium (★). Blood culture is required to diagnose the causative organism, which is most often a bacterium, but in 10% of cases, no organism may be identified.

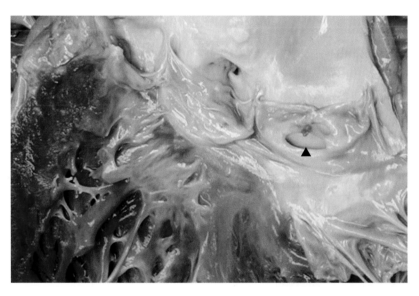

Figure 2-59 Infective endocarditis, gross
Healing of infective endocarditis may leave residual valve damage. Shown here is a larger fenestration (▲) of an aortic valve cusp as a consequence of healed infective endocarditis, with partial destruction of another cusp. The result of this valvular damage is aortic insufficiency and a jet lesion with adjacent focal endocardial fibrosis of the left ventricular myocardium from regurgitant flow. A murmur may be audible. Larger fenestrations may cause valvular insufficiency.

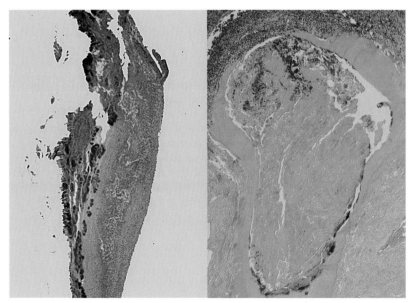

Figure 2-60 Infective endocarditis, microscopic
The valve leaflet in the *left panel* has friable vegetations composed of fibrin and platelets (pink) mixed with inflammatory cells and bacterial colonies (blue). The friability explains how portions of the vegetation can break off and embolize. In the *right panel* a septic embolus fills the lumen of a small artery showing inflammation and necrosis. Left-sided endocarditis can be complicated by embolization to the systemic circulation, whereas right-sided embolization affects the lungs. Cardiac valves are relatively avascular, so high-dose, prolonged antibiotic therapy is needed to eradicate the infection.

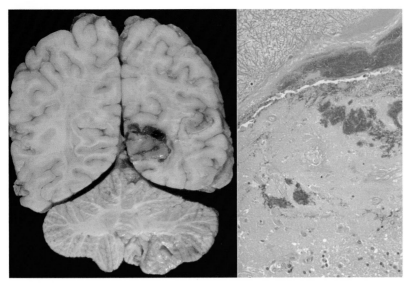

Figure 2-61 Mycotic aneurysm, gross and microscopic

Septic embolization from infective endocarditis spreads the infection to other parts of the body. Left-sided valvular lesions shower emboli to the systemic circulation, and embolic lesions can subsequently lodge in organs such as the brain, spleen, and kidneys. Shown here is an embolic infarct involving a cerebral hemisphere in the *left panel,* which microscopically shows features of a mycotic aneurysm in the *right panel,* with destruction of an arterial wall by the blue bacterial colonies.

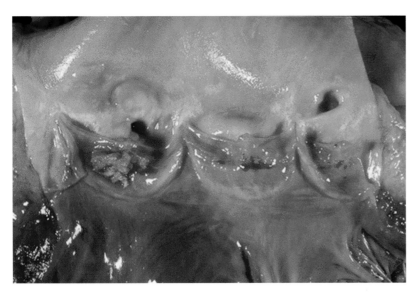

Figure 2-62 Nonbacterial thrombotic endocarditis, gross

The small pink vegetation on the leftmost aortic cusp margin represents the typical finding with nonbacterial thrombotic endocarditis (NBTE), or so-called *marantic endocarditis.* This is one form of noninfective endocarditis. NBTE tends to occur in individuals with a hypercoagulable state (e.g., Trousseau syndrome, a paraneoplastic syndrome associated with malignancies) and in very ill patients. These vegetations are rarely larger than 0.5 cm. They are very prone to embolize, however. Patients with NBTE often have concomitant venous thromboembolic disease. Note the normal right and left coronary artery orifices above the valve cusps.

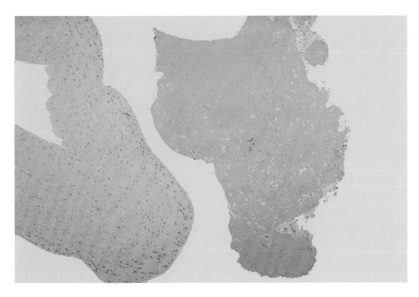

Figure 2-63 Nonbacterial thrombotic endocarditis, microscopic

The valve is on the left, and a bland vegetation is to the right. It appears pink because it is composed of fibrin and platelets, but it is sterile without blue-staining organisms. It displays about as much morphologic variation as a brown paper bag. Such bland vegetations are typical of the noninfective forms of endocarditis (NBTE, Libman-Sacks, rheumatic). The vegetations of NBTE, although small, are friable and prone to embolize.

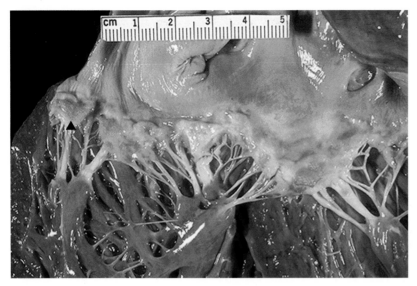

Figure 2-64 Libman-Sacks endocarditis, gross

Flat, pale tan, spreading vegetations (▲) are visible over the mitral valve surface. They even spread onto the adjacent chordae tendineae. This patient has systemic lupus erythematosus. These vegetations can occur on any valve or even on endocardial surfaces. These vegetations appear in about 4% of patients with systemic lupus erythematosus and rarely cause problems because they are not large and rarely embolize. Note also the thickened, shortened, and fused chordae tendineae that represent remote RHD.

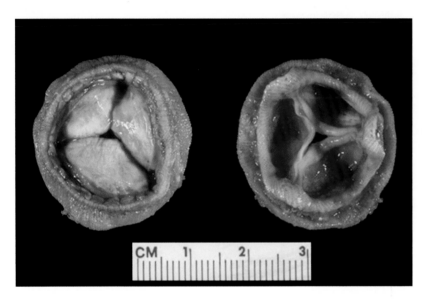

Figure 2-65 Porcine bioprosthesis, gross

A porcine bioprosthesis is shown with the undersurface at the left and the outflow side at the right. There are three cusps sewn into a synthetic ring. The main advantage of this bioprosthesis is the lack of need for continued anticoagulation. The drawback of this type of prosthetic heart valve is the limited life span of the prosthetic cusps, on average 5 to 10 years (but sometimes shorter), because of wear and subsequent dystrophic calcification that reduces cusp motion and leads to stenosis.

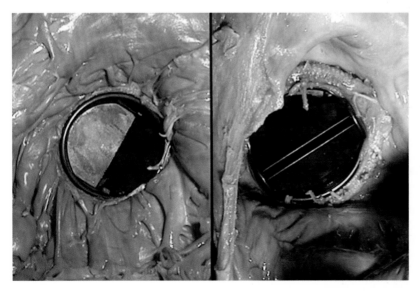

Figure 2-66 Mechanical valve prosthesis, gross

This mechanical valve prosthesis is the tilting disc variety, and the one shown here replaces the native mitral valve. Such mechanical prostheses last indefinitely from a structural standpoint, but the patient requires continuing anticoagulation because the exposed nonbiologic surfaces are prone to thrombosis. The inferior aspect is shown in the *left panel* with the left ventricular chamber below. The outflow tract from this prosthesis is shown in the *right panel,* with the two leaflets tilted outward toward the left atrium. Another prosthetic complication is infective endocarditis, which is most prone to involve the ring.

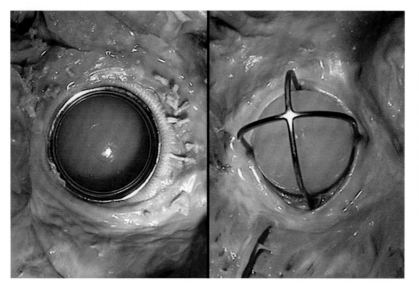

Figure 2-67 Mechanical prosthesis, gross
The mitral mechanical valve prosthesis shown is of the older ball-and-cage variety, which had the complication of hemolysis. Although these mechanical prostheses last indefinitely from a structural standpoint, the patient requires continuing anticoagulation to prevent thrombosis. The superior aspect (here the left atrium) is shown in the *left panel,* and the inflow into the LV is shown in the *right panel.*

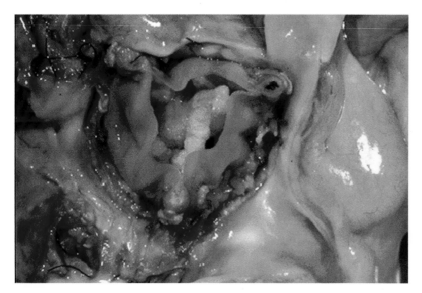

Figure 2-68 Porcine bioprosthesis, gross
This bioprosthesis, a porcine artificial heart valve, is sutured in place with blue-green sutures around the valve ring. The valve cusps are still pliable, but the valve has become infected with large vegetation filling the valve orifice. This is an uncommon complication of valve prostheses.

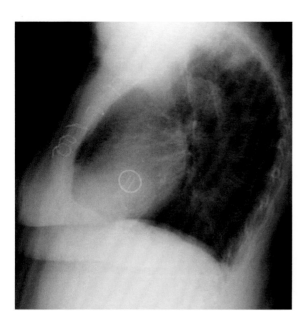

Figure 2-69 Mechanical prosthesis, radiograph
This chest radiograph in lateral view reveals the presence of a bileaflet, tilting disc, mechanical aortic valve prosthesis. The two leaflets are open and on edge.

Figure 2-70 Pacemaker, gross ▶
The right ventricle and atrium are opened to reveal a pacemaker wire (◀) that extends to the apex to embed on the septum in the right ventricle. Pacemakers aid in maintaining a rhythm in hearts prone to arrhythmias.

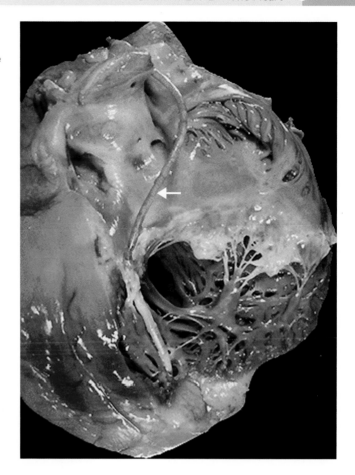

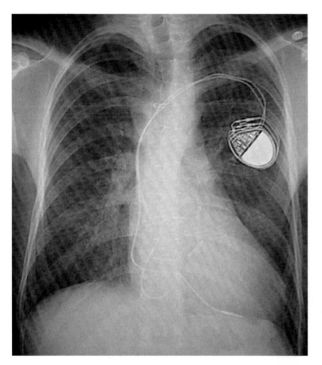

◀ Figure 2-71 Pacemaker, radiograph
A cardiac pacemaker battery implanted under the skin on the left chest wall is visible in this chest radiograph. The leads from the battery extend down to the right atrium and the apex of the right ventricle.

Figure 2-72 Dilated cardiomyopathy, gross ▶
This very large heart has a globoid shape because all the chambers are dilated. It felt very flabby at autopsy, and the myocardium in life was poorly contractile. This is a *cardiomyopathy,* a term used to denote conditions in which the myocardium functions poorly, and the heart is typically large and dilated, but there is often no characteristic histologic finding. Many cases are idiopathic. In 30% to 50% of cases dilated cardiomyopathy is familial. Some cases may occur after myocarditis, whereas others may appear in the peripartum period with pregnancy. Some cases occur as a consequence of chronic alcohol abuse.

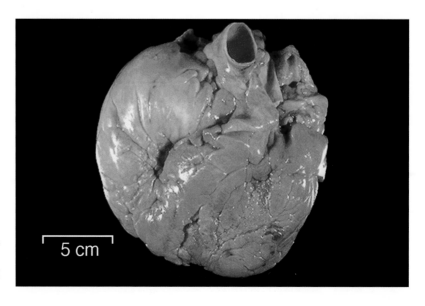
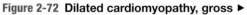
5 cm

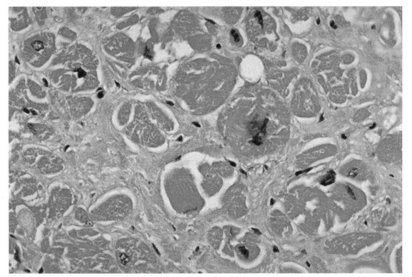

Figure 2-73 Cardiomyopathy, microscopic
The myocardium in many cases of cardiomy-opathy shows hypertrophy of myocardial fibers, which have prominent dark enlarged nuclei as shown here, along with interstitial fibrosis. Systolic dysfunction ensues. This same appearance could follow ischemic injury, in which case the term *ischemic cardiomyopathy* could be applied. In most cases of idiopathic dilated cardiomy-opathy, the coronary arteries show little or no atherosclerosis.

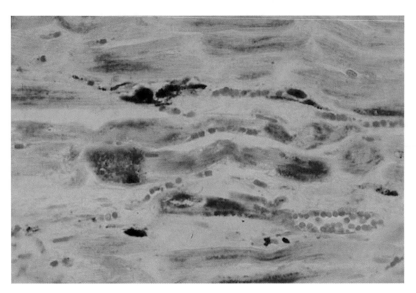

Figure 2-74 Dilated cardiomyopathy, microscopic
Some forms of cardiomyopathy lead to de-creased ventricular compliance with impaired ventricular filling during diastole. It may be idiopathic or the result of an identifiable cause, such as hemochromatosis, with excessive iron deposition, shown here with Prussian blue iron stain. The iron deposition leads to myocardial dysfunction with cardiac heart enlargement and failure. Iron overload can accompany hereditary hemochromatosis or transfusion-dependent anemias.

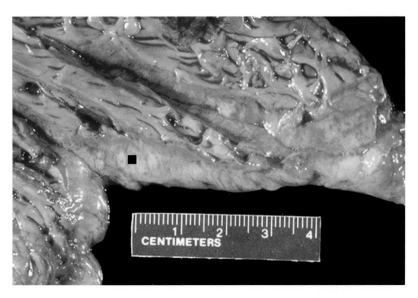

Figure 2-75 Arrhythmogenic right ventricular cardiomyopathy, gross
There is extensive fatty replacement (■) of the right ventricular myocardium (and sometimes the left as well), so that grossly the ventricular wall of the dilated heart is yellowish, as shown here. These fatty areas correspond to diffuse high–signal intensity areas on MRI. This condi-tion has an incidence of 1 in 10,000, and may be familial, with an autosomal dominant pattern of transmission with mutations in genes encoding for desmosomal proteins such as plakoglobin affecting gap junctions. The median age of onset is 33 years. There is progressive right ventricular failure.

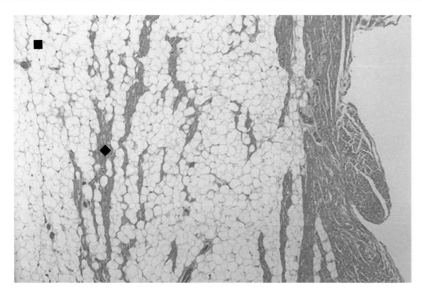

Figure 2-76 Arrhythmogenic right ventricular cardiomyopathy, microscopic

There is segmental loss of myocardium in the muscular wall, with replacement by adipose (■) and fibrous (◆) tissue. Within the fat are strands of residual cardiac myocytes. The subendocardial layer at the right is preserved. This condition is associated with dysrhythmias that can lead to syncope or even sudden death from heart failure. The pathogenesis of this condition involves abnormal desmosome proteins with uncontrolled apoptosis of myocardium, muscular degeneration with fibrofatty replacement, and inflammation.

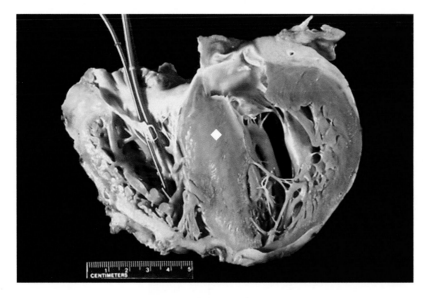

Figure 2-77 Hypertrophic cardiomyopathy, gross

Shown here is an explanted heart (the atria with venous connections, along with great vessels, remained behind to connect to the new heart provided by someone with empathy to make transplantation possible). Note the marked left ventricular hypertrophy and asymmetric bulging of a very large interventricular septum (◆) into the left ventricular chamber. One in 500 persons is affected, and about half of cases are familial, although various gene mutations may be responsible for this disease. Children and adults can be affected, and sudden death can occur, typically from an arrhythmia. Pacemaker wires enter the right ventricle here.

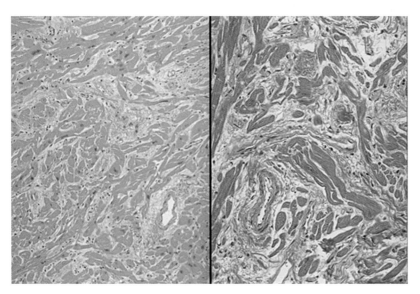

Figure 2-78 Hypertrophic cardiomyopathy, microscopic

This myocardium shows myofiber disarray with a hypertrophic cardiomyopathy, typically within the interventricular septum. In the *left panel* with H&E stain and in the *right panel* with trichrome stain are sections of myocardium showing these irregular myofibers with surrounding collagen. Such abnormal areas predispose to arrhythmias. Many cases are caused by mutations in genes encoding for sarcomeric proteins, such as β-myosin heavy chain, troponin T, myosin-binding protein C, and α-tropomyosin. Clinical findings are related to reduced ventricular compliance with impaired left ventricular diastolic filling. Functional left ventricular outflow obstruction may also occur.

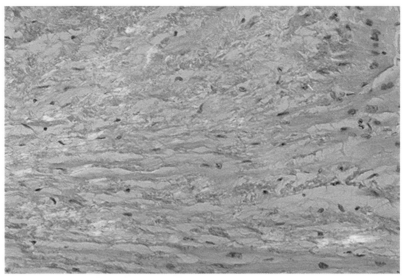

Figure 2-79 Amyloidosis with cardiomyopathy, microscopic

Amorphous deposits of amyloid have a characteristic "apple green" birefringence with Congo red stain under polarized light micros-copy, as shown here. Amyloid is orange-red with Congo red stain on routine light microscopy. Cardiac amyloidosis is a nightmare for anesthesiologists when intractable arrhythmias may occur during surgery. Underlying causes include AL amyloid with multiple my-eloma, AA amyloid with chronic inflammatory conditions, and senile cardiac amyloid derived from serum transthyretin protein. Other causes of diastolic dysfunction include endomyocardial fibrosis with dense collagen deposition in endocardium and subendocardium, and endocardial fibroelastosis with fibroelastic thickening of the LV in children younger than 2 years.

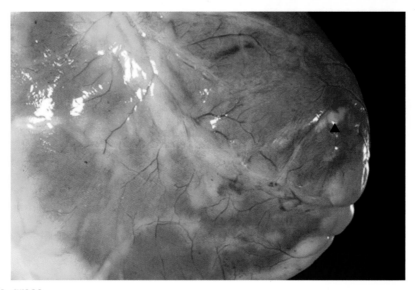

Figure 2-80 Myocarditis, gross

The epicardial surface of the heart shows small yellowish microabscesses (▲) that may appear in patients with sepsis and who have hematogenous spread of infection. They may also represent emboli from an infective endocarditis in which small portions of cardiac vegetation have embolized into the coronary arteries. Myocarditis caused by other microorganisms can give a similar pattern of focal inflammation with necrosis. Patients with myocarditis can have fever, chest pain, dyspnea from left-sided heart failure, and peripheral edema from right-sided heart failure. Arrhythmias may lead to sudden death.

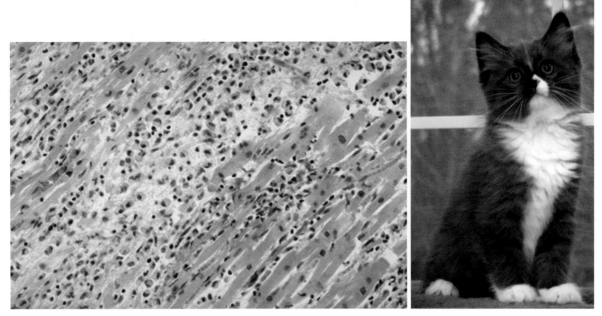

Figures 2-81 and 2-82 Myocarditis, microscopic and host

This florid myocarditis has myofiber inflammation with necrosis. There are mainly mononuclear cells mixed with some scattered neutrophils. The pattern is that of a patchy myocarditis consistent with *Toxoplasma gondii* infection (intense cuteness in the right panel belies definitive host status; beware of cat litter with *T. gondii* cysts), which is most likely to occur in immunocompromised patients, although no free tachyzoites or pseudocysts with bradyzoites are shown here. Immunosuppression also increases the risk for cytomegalovirus and other opportunistic infections.

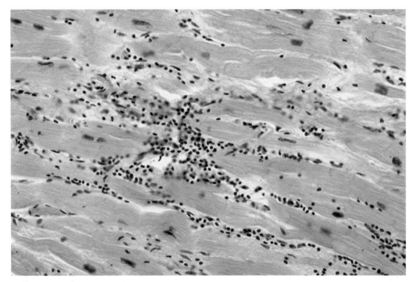

Figure 2-83 Myocarditis, microscopic

The interstitial lymphocytic infiltrates shown are characteristic for viral myocarditis, the most common type of myocarditis. There is usually little accompanying myofiber necrosis. Many of these cases are probably subclinical, but findings may include fever and chest pain. In severe cases, cardiac failure leads to dyspnea and fatigue. The first manifestation may be arrhythmia, which can cause sudden death in young individuals. A late sequela may be dilated cardiomyopathy. The most common viral agents are coxsackieviruses A and B. Individuals infected with HIV can have similar findings. About 5% of patients with Lyme disease develop myocarditis.

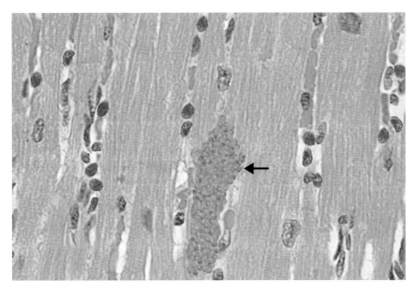

◄ **Figure 2-84 Chagasic myocarditis, microscopic**

A pseudocyst (◄) in this myocardium contains many intracellular amastigotes of *Trypanosoma cruzi,* along with interstitial lymphocytic infiltrates; an acute myocarditis rarely occurs. Most deaths in acute Chagas disease are from heart failure. The acute symptoms resolve spontaneously in virtually all patients, who then enter the asymptomatic or indeterminate phase. Chronic Chagas disease becomes apparent years or even decades later, when there is heart failure from dilation of several cardiac chambers with fibrosis, thinning of the ventricular wall, aneurysm formation (especially at the left ventricular apex), and mural thrombosis.

Figure 2-85 Myocarditis, microscopic ►

A granuloma with a giant cell (↑) is shown here, along with myocyte necrosis. No infectious organisms can be found, so the term applied here is *giant cell myocarditis.* This is a rare, idiopathic form of myocarditis that occurs mostly in young to middle-aged adults. It has a poor prognosis.

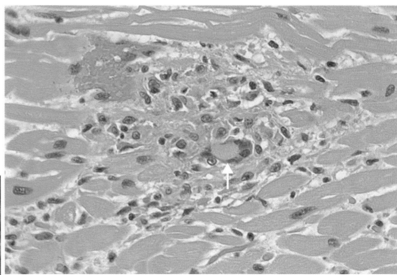

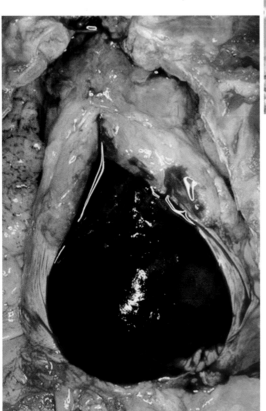

◄ **Figure 2-86 Hemopericardium, gross**

Dark blood is noted in the pericardial sac opened at autopsy. Severe blunt force trauma to the chest (often from rapid deceleration with impact) causes a rupture of the myocardium or coronary arteries with bleeding into the pericardial cavity. The extensive collection of blood in this closed space leads to cardiac tamponade from impaired ventricular filling. An aortic dissection proximally may also result in hemopericardium, as the blood dissects into the pericardial space.

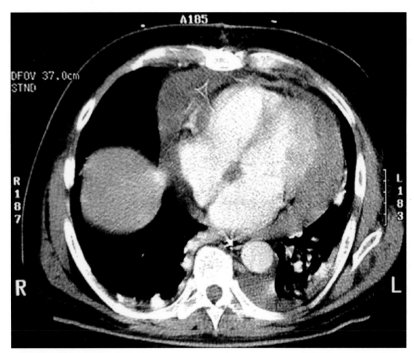

Figure 2-87 Pericardial effusion, CT image

This chest CT scan shows a large effusion (✛) within the pericardial sac around the heart. The dome of the liver appears at the right. Effusions in body cavities can occur from right-sided heart failure. An acute serous pericarditis, with minimal inflammatory exudate but significant transudation of fluid, could produce a similar finding.

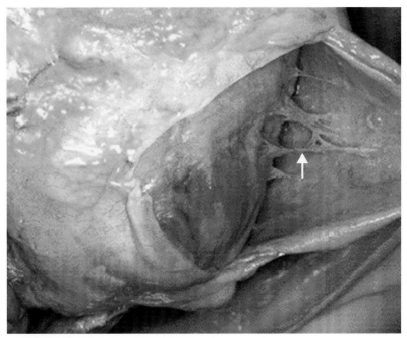

Figure 2-88 Fibrinous pericarditis, gross

A window of adherent pericardium is reflected to reveal thin strands (↑) of fibrinous exudate extending from the epicardial surface to the pericardium, typical for fibrinous pericarditis. A clinical finding is a friction rub (heard by the student on the night of the patient's admission to the hospital, but inaudible with increasing serous fluid collection when the attending physician examines the patient on morning rounds, and the term *serofibrinous pericarditis* is more appropriate). Diffuse fibrinous pericarditis is more typical of systemic conditions, such as uremia or systemic lupus erythematosus, whereas focal pericarditis may overlie a transmural MI (Dressler syndrome).

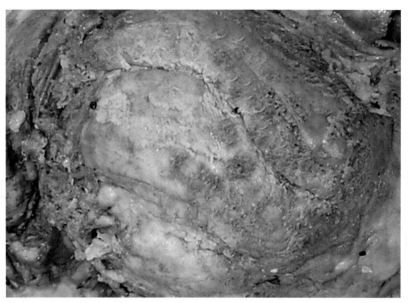

Figure 2-89 Fibrinous pericarditis, gross

The epicardial surface of this heart shows a rough exudate typical for fibrinous pericarditis. These surfaces have a shaggy exudate formed by the organizing strands of fibrin, described as bread-and-butter pericarditis, although the appearance is more reminiscent of buttered bread dropped onto a carpet. The fibrin can result in an audible friction rub on auscultation, as the strands of fibrin on epicardium and pericardium rub against each other. In general, some degree of serous effusion also accompanies fibrinous exudation. The volume of fluid is usually not large enough to produce cardiac tamponade, however. Most cases resolve without significant collagenization, so there is no significant interference with ventricular wall motion.

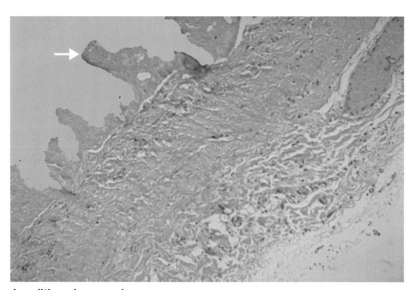

Figure 2-90 Fibrinous pericarditis, microscopic

The pericardial surface shows strands of pink fibrin (→) extending outward to the left. There is minimal underlying inflammation. Eventually the fibrin can be organized and cleared, although sometimes adhesions may remain. Fibrinous pericarditis results from inflammation or vascular injury that leads to exudation of fibrin, typically with some accompanying fluid. Causes include an underlying MI, uremia, rheumatic carditis, autoimmune diseases (although these are most often mostly serous), radiation to the chest, and trauma.

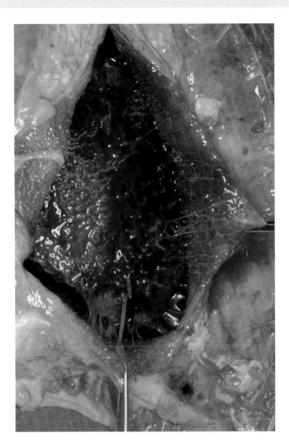

◄ Figure 2-91 Hemorrhagic pericarditis, gross
The pericardium is opened and reflected to reveal a pericarditis that has not only fibrin strands, but also dark-red hemorrhage. Termed *hemorrhagic pericarditis,* it is really just fibrinous pericarditis with hemorrhage. This is the result of more severe inflammation or vascular injury, but it is not so acute as to be merely termed a hemopericardium. Without inflammation, blood in the pericardial sac would be called *hemopericardium.* Causes include epicardial metastases, tuberculosis, bleeding diatheses, and cardiac surgery.

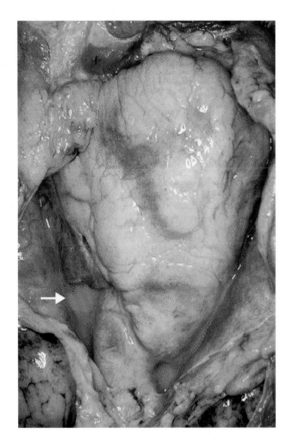

Figure 2-92 Purulent pericarditis, gross ►
The pericardial sac has been opened and reflected. Yellowish exudate (→) that has pooled in the lower pericardial sac is shown here. A bacterial organism is usually implicated in this process, and the infection has typically spread from the adjacent lungs. A purulent pericarditis can have variable components of fibrinous exudate and serous effusion. If the inflammation is severe, it could even become hemorrhagic.

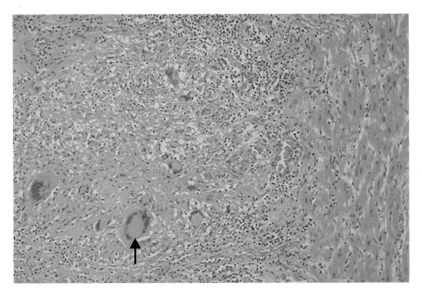

◄ Figure 2-93 Tuberculous pericarditis, microscopic
Pericarditis from *Mycobacterium tuberculosis* infection can produce extensive granulomatous inflammation with resultant calcification that can encircle the heart and severely restrict cardiac motion (so-called *constrictive pericarditis*). Granulomatous inflammation over the surface of the heart with Langhans giant cells (↑) is shown, with myocardial cells at the right. This is a chronic process developing over weeks to months.

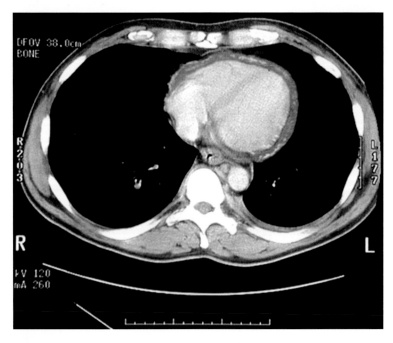

Figure 2-94 Constrictive pericarditis, CT image

In this chest CT scan a thickened pericardium encases the heart. Areas of brighter calcification (✚) can be seen within the thickening and calcification of the pericardium that constrict cardiac movement. This leads to a so-called constrictive pericarditis with a clinical finding of pulsus paradoxus with an exaggerated decrease (<10 mm Hg) in the amplitude of the arterial pulsation during inspiration and an increased pulse amplitude during expiration. Constrictive pericarditis is uncommon because most forms of pericarditis heal without significant scarring. A tuberculous pericarditis or severe purulent pericarditis may lead to this complication.

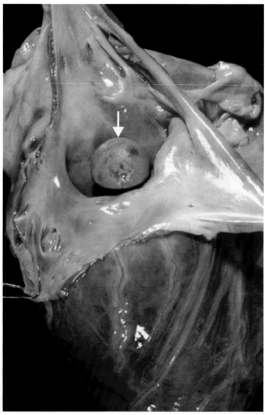

Figure 2-95 Cardiac myxoma, gross

The left atrium is opened to reveal the most common primary cardiac neoplasm—a myxoma (↓). These benign masses are attached to an atrial wall in more than 90% of cases, but they also can arise on a valve surface or ventricular wall. Myxomas can produce a ball-valve effect by intermittently occluding an atrioventricular valve orifice to produce clinical findings resembling a transient ischemic attack. Elaboration of IL-6 by the tumor may produce fever and malaise. Embolization of fragments of the tumor may also occur. Myxomas are easily diagnosed with echocardiography. Surgical removal is easily accomplished.

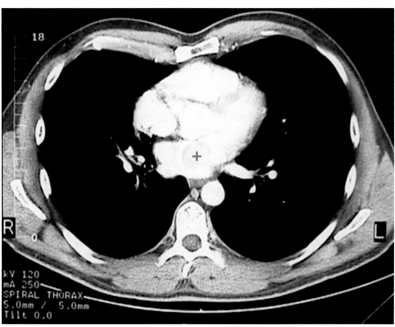

Figure 2-96 Cardiac myxoma, CT image

This chest CT scan reveals a faint circumscribed left atrial myxoma (✚) in a patient with a history of syncope. Although they are uncommon, myxomas are the most common primary cardiac tumor, and most are found in the atria, where larger ones may cause focal outflow obstruction. Portions of the myxoma may break off and embolize, often to the brain to produce clinical findings of a stroke. Myxomas are thought to arise from primitive multipotent mesenchymal cells.

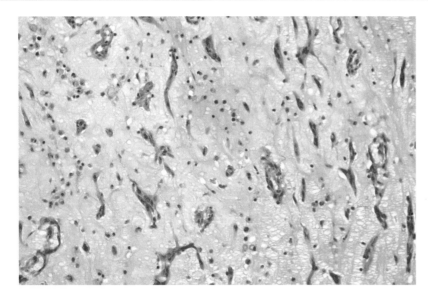

Figure 2-97 Cardiac myxoma, microscopic
This high-power microscopic appearance of a cardiac myxoma shows minimal cellularity. Only scattered clusters of short, thin spindle cells with scant pink cytoplasm are present within a loose myxoid stroma. Although most myxomas occur sporadically, about 10% of cases are associated with the familial autosomal dominant Carney syndrome, with a mutated *PRKAR1A*, or with McCune-Albright syndrome and *GNAS1* activating mutations. Syndromes are suggested by the presence of multiple cardiac or extracardiac myxomas.

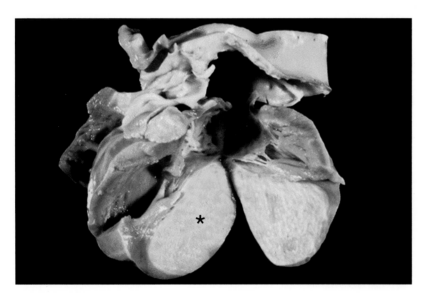

Figure 2-98 Cardiac rhabdomyoma, gross
This 2-year-old child died suddenly. At autopsy, this large, firm, white, circumscribed tumor mass (★) protruded into the LV, which obstructed blood flow. Although rare, cardiac rhabdomyomas are the most common primary cardiac tumor in infants and children; they typically arise in the left ventricular wall or intraventricular septum. Half result from sporadic mutations; half occur from *TSC1* or *TSC2* mutations with tuberous sclerosis. On echocardiography, they are hyperechoic masses. Some may regress, suggesting that they are hamartomas and not true neoplasms.

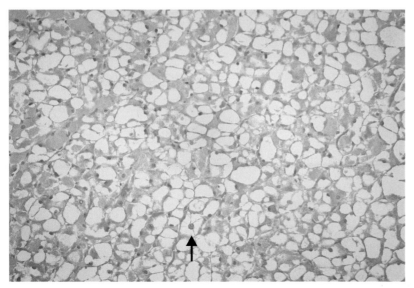

Figure 2-99 Cardiac rhabdomyoma, microscopic
The tumor cells have prominent vacuolation and distinct cell borders; a variable number of pink myofibers are present that contain abundant glycogen, with PAS stain. Spider cells (↑) are shown that have a centrally located nucleus with radial extensions to the cell wall; they are positive for ubiquitin on immunostaining, suggesting an apoptotic pathway accounting for regression of the tumor in some cases. The malignant counterpart, a rhabdomyosarcoma, is a very rare neoplasm in adults.

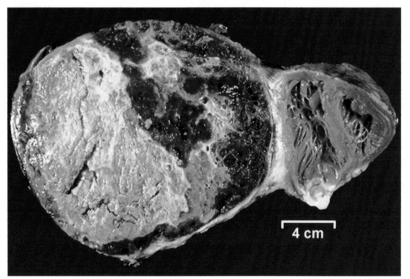

4 cm

Figure 2-100 Cardiac angiosarcoma, gross
This variegated, hemorrhagic mass arises in the epicardium in the groove between the right atrium and right ventricle. Although rare, it is one of the most common primary malignancies in the heart. The neoplastic cells are oblong to spindle shaped, form ill-defined vascular spaces, and are positive for vimentin and CD34 but negative for cytokeratin. The differential diagnosis includes Kaposi sarcoma, which usually manifests with multiple nodules that rarely exceed 2 cm in size. Mesotheliomas tend to encase the heart and are CD34 negative. In this case, complete resection, along with orthotopic cardiac transplantation, was performed. There is a great tendency for cardiac sarcomas to recur locally.

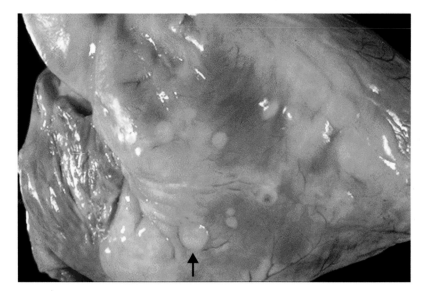

Figure 2-101 Cardiac metastases, gross
Metastases to the heart are more common than primary cardiac tumors but are still rare overall (only about 5% to 10% of all malignancies have cardiac metastases, usually when widespread metastases are present). Pale, white-tan nodules (↑) of metastatic tumor are shown here over the surface of the epicardium. Metastases may lead to pericardial inflammation with effusions, including hemorrhagic pericarditis. Another pattern of cardiac involvement can be seen with bronchogenic carcinomas with contiguous spread to the heart.

CHAPTER

3

Hematopathology

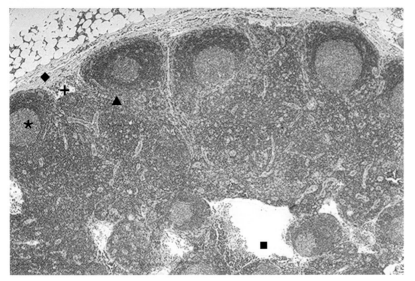

Figure 3-1 Normal lymph node, microscopic
This benign reactive lymph node has a well-defined connective tissue capsule (◆), and beneath that a subcapsular sinus (✚) where afferent lymphatics drain lymph fluid from tissues peripheral to the node. The lymph may contain macrophages and dendritic cells, both forms of antigen-presenting cells, carrying antigens to the node. Beneath the subcapsular sinus is the paracortical zone (▲) with lymphoid follicles having pale germinal centers with a predominance of B lymphocytes. In the germinal centers (★), immune responses to antigens are generated, assisted by a darker mantle zone of mainly T lymphocytes. Central to the follicles are sinusoids extending to the hilum of the node. The efferent lymphatics drain out the hilum (■).

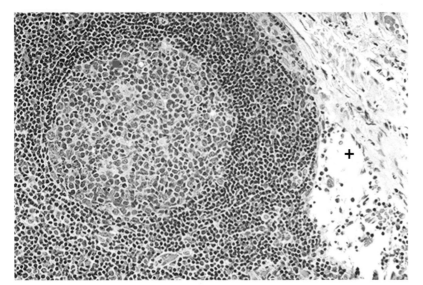

Figure 3-2 Normal lymph node, microscopic
At high magnification, a lymph node follicle with a germinal center (■) contains larger lymphocytes undergoing cytokine activation. At the lower right is the subcapsular sinus (✚). Leukocytes are often identified and classified by CD (clusters of differentiation) markers for specific cellular proteins. The center of the lymphoid follicle—the germinal center—is where CD4 helper lymphocytes and antigen-presenting cells (macrophages and follicular dendritic cells) interact with B lymphocytes, leading to an antibody-mediated immune response.

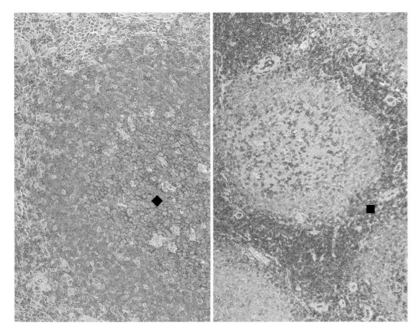

Figure 3-3 Normal lymph node, microscopic
The nature of the cell population and function of a lymph node are shown in the *left panel* with an immunohistochemical stain for CD20, a B-cell marker. Note the larger number of B cells staining with the red-brown reaction product within the germinal center (◆) of a lymph node follicle, with additional B cells scattered in the interfollicular zone. The node in the *right panel* has been stained for CD3, a T-cell marker. Note the larger number of T cells around (■) the germinal center of a follicle, with additional T cells extending into the paracortex.

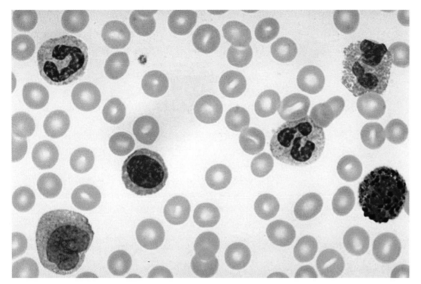

Figure 3-4 Normal white blood cells, microscopic

The normal types of leukocytes that are routinely observed on the peripheral blood smear are shown here, including a segmented neutrophil, band neutrophil, eosinophil, basophil, lymphocyte, and monocyte. The red blood cells (RBCs) appear normal, and there is a normal platelet present. A complete blood count includes a total white blood cell (WBC) count. The types of leukocytes may be enumerated by a machine that measures size and chemical characteristics. A manual WBC differential count is performed by examining the peripheral blood smear with Wright-Giemsa stain by light microscopy.

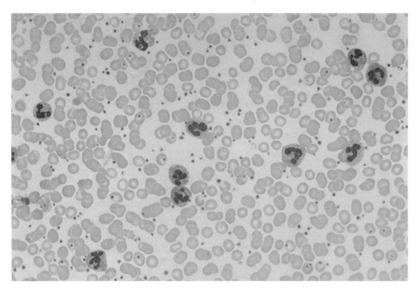

Figure 3-5 Leukocytosis, microscopic

Many granulocytes, both segmented neutrophils and band neutrophils, are present in this peripheral blood smear. An elevated WBC count with neutrophilia suggests inflammation or infection. A very high WBC count (>50,000/mm^3) that is not a leukemia is known as a leukemoid reaction—much more pronounced than just the left shift with bandemia and the occasional metamyelocyte with acute inflammation. An accompanying increase occurs in acute-phase reactants in the plasma, such as C-reactive protein (CRP). Inflammatory cytokines, such as tumor necrosis factor (TNF) and interleukin-1 (IL-1), stimulate proliferation and differentiation of marrow granulocytic cells.

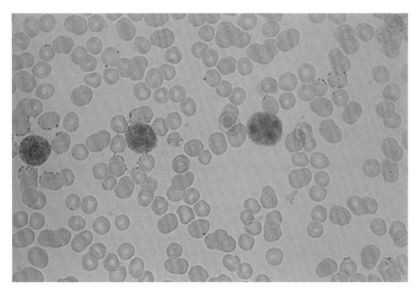

Figure 3-6 Leukocyte alkaline phosphatase test, microscopic

Distinguishing leukemoid reaction from chronic myelogenous leukemia (CML) may be done with the leukocyte alkaline phosphatase (LAP) stain. Seen here are neutrophils with red granular cytoplasmic staining for LAP. The abnormal myeloid cells in CML are not as differentiated as the normal myeloid cells. Counting granulocytic cells staining with LAP yields a score. A high LAP score is seen with a leukemoid reaction, whereas a low LAP score suggests CML. A leukemoid reaction is typically a transient but exaggerated bone marrow response to inflammatory cytokines, such as IL-1 and TNF, which stimulate bone marrow progenitor cells.

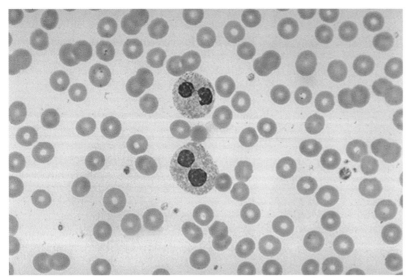

Figure 3-7 Pelger-Huët anomaly, microscopic
If most of the neutrophils appear bilobed on a peripheral blood smear, this is indicative of an uncommon inherited condition known as *Pelger-Huët anomaly.* This is the heterozygous form. The homozygous form, marked by neutrophils displaying just a single round nucleus without lobation, may be associated with abnormal neutrophil function. Be aware of this condition when the "band" count is reported as high but the WBC count is normal, or the patient shows no signs of infection or inflammation. True band neutrophils have a bridge of chromatin between the lobes. In the setting of myelodysplasia, these bilobed neutrophils represent pseudo–Pelger-Huët cells.

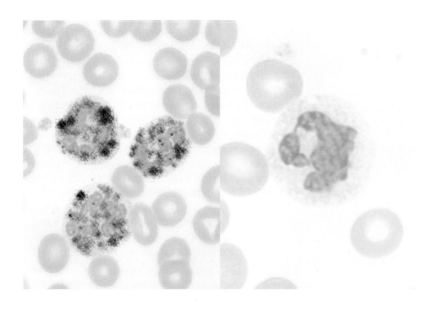

Figure 3-8 Chronic granulomatous disease, microscopic
The nitroblue tetrazolium (NBT) slide test aids in screening for defects in NADPH oxidase. Patient neutrophils are exposed to a stimulus, incubated with NBT, and made into a smear on a slide. The neutrophils with dark cytoplasmic granules of reaction product are counted. Normally, more than 95% of the granulocytes are positive as shown in the *left panel.* In chronic granulomatous disease (CGD), there is an absent or reduced function of the respiratory burst, the intracellular process in neutrophils dependent on NADPH oxidase, which produces oxygen free radicals used to kill phagocytized organisms. In the abnormal NBT test in CGD in the *right panel,* less than 5% of neutrophils stain.

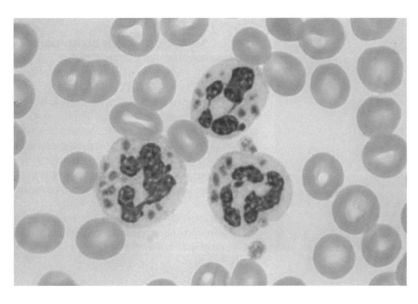

Figure 3-9 Chédiak-Higashi syndrome, microscopic
A history of recurrent bacterial infections and giant granules seen in peripheral blood leukocytes is characteristic of Chédiak-Higashi syndrome. This disorder results from a mutation in the *LYST* gene on chromosome 1q42 that encodes a protein involved in intracellular trafficking of proteins. Microtubules fail to form properly, and the neutrophils do not respond to chemotactic stimuli. Giant lysosomal granules fail to function. Soft-tissue abscesses with *Staphylococcus aureus* are common. Other cells affected by this disorder include platelets (bleeding), melanocytes (albinism), Schwann cells (neuropathy), natural killer cells, and cytotoxic T cells (aggressive lymphoproliferative disorder).

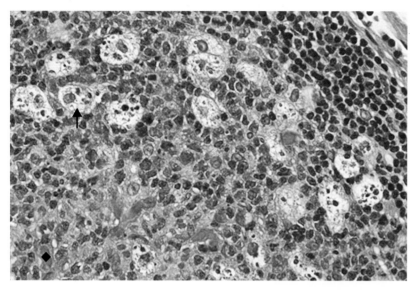

Figure 3-10 Lymphadenitis, microscopic
Lymphadenitis is a pronounced reactive change in a lymph node, with a large follicle and germinal center showing prominent macrophages (↑) with irregular cytoplasmic debris (tingible body macrophages). Blood vessels (◆) are also more prominent. Multiple shapes and sizes of leukocytes are present, indicative of a polymorphous population of cells, or polyclonal immune response, typical for a benign process reacting to multiple antigenic stimulants. In general, lymph nodes in a benign reactive process are more likely to enlarge quickly, are often tender on palpation during physical examination, and diminish in size after the infection.

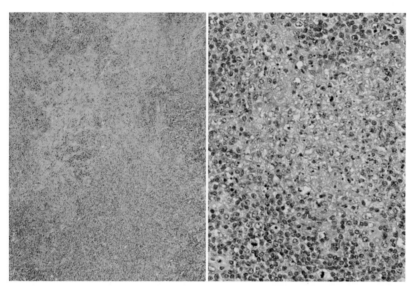

Figure 3-11 Lymphadenitis, necrotizing, microscopic
The reactive change in the lymph node shown here is primarily necrotizing, with a radiating stellate pattern seen in the *left panel.* Necrotic leukocytes in a central abscess are seen surrounded by still viable lymphocytes in the *right panel.* More advanced lesions may have granulomatous features. This necrotizing inflammatory process is caused by *Bartonella henselae,* a gram-negative rod. A cat scratch may introduce the organisms, which induce a papule at the inoculation site then regional lymphadenopathy within 1 to 2 weeks, followed by resolution in 2 to 4 months.

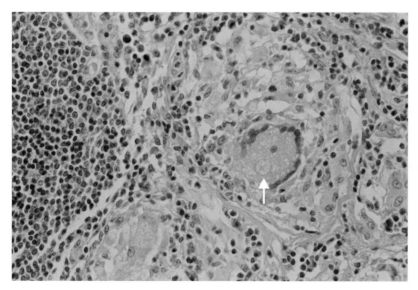

Figure 3-12 Granulomatous lymphadenitis, microscopic
Infectious agents such as *Mycobacteria* and dimorphic fungi *("Crypto, Histo, Blasto, Cocci")* may become disseminated and involve tissues of the mononuclear phagocyte system, such as lymph nodes. When there is no evidence for infection, then sarcoidosis should be considered, particularly when noncaseating granulomas are present, as shown here. Note the asteroid body (↑) in the Langhans giant cell, an uncommon but characteristic feature of sarcoid granulomas.

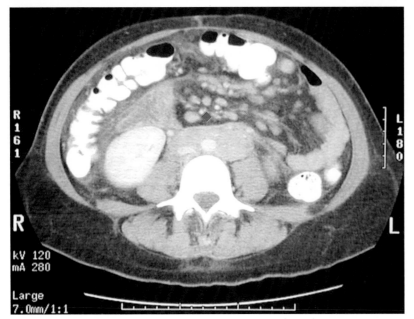

Figure 3-13 Lymphadenopathy, CT image

Note the prominent mesenteric lymph nodes (◆) in this patient with mesenteric lymphadenitis. Benign and malignant processes can lead to lymph node enlargement. Infections are a common cause for lymphadenopathy because lymph draining from the site of infection reaches regional lymph nodes. The lymph fluid carries antigens and antigen-presenting cells to the node. Antigens may also circulate out of the regional node and be carried around the body by the bloodstream, reaching other lymphoid tissues in which clones of memory lymphocytes may be present that can react to specific antigens. After the infection or inflammatory process has subsided, the stimulated nodes diminish in size.

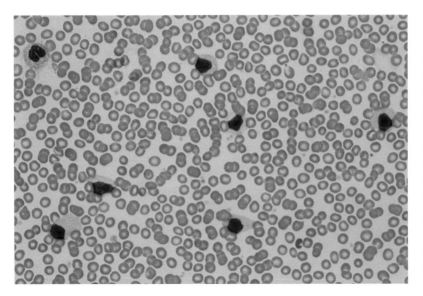

Figure 3-14 Infectious mononucleosis, microscopic

Epstein-Barr virus (EBV) infection transmitted by close human contact, often through saliva, most often in adolescents and young adults, causes infectious mononucleosis ("mono") with fever, sore throat, generalized lymphadenopathy, splenomegaly, and absolute lymphocytosis. EBV-infected B cells elicit a cell-mediated immune response with CD8+ cytotoxic T cells that appear in the peripheral blood as atypical lymphocytes, shown here with abundant pale blue cytoplasm, and they proliferate in lymphoid tissues. Initially IgM antibodies are formed, both "heterophile" antibodies detected by a screening monospot test and more specific antibodies against EBV capsid antigens.

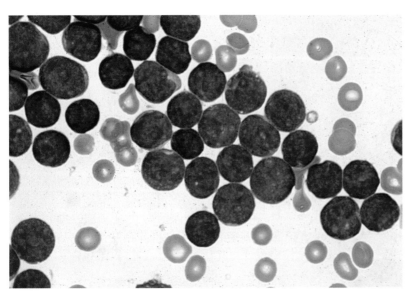

Figure 3-15 Acute lymphoblastic leukemia, microscopic

The white blood cells seen here are leukemic blasts—very immature leukocytes with large nuclei that contain multiple nucleoli. These abnormal lymphocytes are indicative of acute lymphoblastic leukemia (ALL). These cells have the B-cell markers CD10, CD19, and CD22, as well as transcription factor PAX5. About 85% of ALLs are precursor B-cell neoplasms. The cells of ALL originate in the marrow but often circulate to produce leukocytosis. Patients with ALL often have generalized lymphadenopathy along with splenomegaly and hepatomegaly. Bone pain is common. ALL is more common in children than adults. Many children with ALL respond well to treatment, and many are curable.

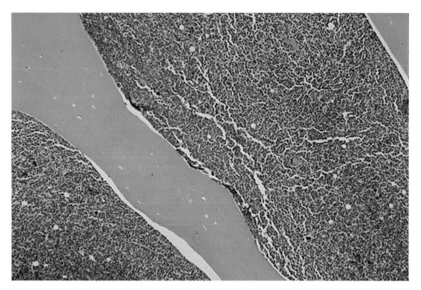

Figure 3-16 Leukemia, microscopic
Neoplastic proliferation of leukocytes results in a highly cellular marrow. The marrow between the pink bone trabeculae shown here is nearly 100% cellular, and it consists of the leukemic cells of ALL that have virtually replaced or suppressed normal hematopoiesis. There is a near absence of adipocytes. The bone spicules are unlikely to become affected by the leukemic process. Although the marrow is quite cellular, there can be peripheral blood cytopenias. This explains the usual leukemic complications of infection (diminished normal leukocytes), hemorrhage (fewer platelets), and anemia (decreased RBCs) that often appear in the clinical course of leukemia.

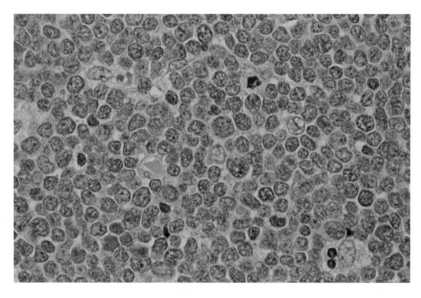

Figure 3-17 Lymphoblastic lymphoma, microscopic
Lymphoblastic features may be present in the non-Hodgkin lymphoma (NHL) that mimics the leukemia of the same name, and both may coexist as lymphoblastic leukemia or lymphoma. Multiple mutations underlie their development. Shown here are large primitive cells resembling pre-B, pre-T cells (lymphoblasts). About 85% of these malignancies are B-cell malignancies, and most manifest as leukemia. The remaining cases have a T-cell origin, and over half manifest as a thymic mediastinal mass in teenage boys. ALL is the most common childhood malignancy. These neoplastic cells are terminal deoxynucleotidyl transferase (TdT), CD1, CD2, CD5, and CD7 positive.

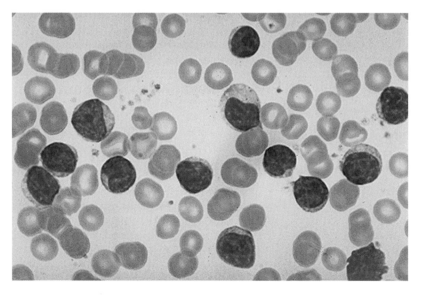

Figure 3-18 Chronic lymphocytic leukemia, microscopic
These mature-appearing lymphocytes in the peripheral blood are markedly increased in number. This form of leukocytosis is indicative of chronic lymphocytic leukemia (CLL), a disease most often seen in older adults, with a male-to-female ratio of 2:1. The cells often mark with CD19, CD20, CD23, and CD5 (a T-cell marker). Monoclonal immunoglobulin is displayed on cell surfaces, but there is unlikely to be a marked increase in circulating immunoglobulin. The peripheral leukocytosis is highly variable. CLL responds poorly to treatment, but it is indolent. In 15% to 30% of patients, there is transformation to a more aggressive lymphoid proliferation.

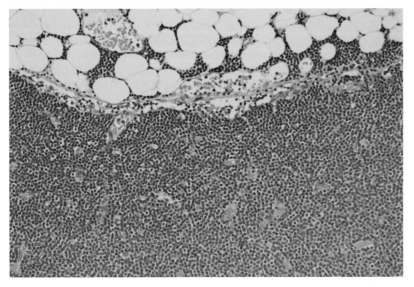

Figure 3-19 Small lymphocytic lymphoma, microscopic

At low power, the normal architecture of this lymph node is obliterated and is replaced by an infiltrate of small (mature-appearing) neoplastic lymphocytes. The infiltrate extends through the capsule of the node and into the surrounding adipose tissue. This pattern of malignant lymphoma is diffuse, and no lymphoid follicles are identified. Small lymphocytic lymphoma (SLL) is the tissue phase of CLL. The molecular and biochemical characteristics of these SLL cells are identical to those of CLL. About 5% to 10% of SLL cases transform to a diffuse large B-cell lymphoma (DLBCL; Richter syndrome).

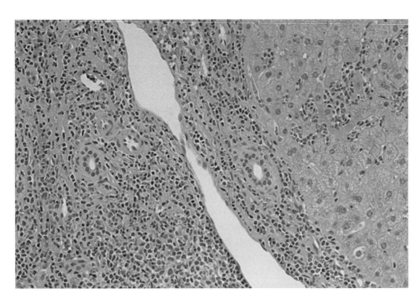

Figure 3-20 Small lymphocytic lymphoma, microscopic

These infiltrates within the liver are composed of small lymphocytes. The tissue involvement of CLL is called *small lymphocytic lymphoma.* Liver, spleen, and lymph nodes may become enlarged, although organ function is often not markedly diminished because the progression of disease is slow, and CLL-SLL has an indolent course. Chromosomal translocations are rare in CLL-SLL, although the immunoglobulin genes of some CLL-SLL patients are somatically hypermutated, and there may be a small immunoglobulin "spike" in the serum. An autoimmune hemolytic anemia appears in about one sixth of CLL-SLL patients.

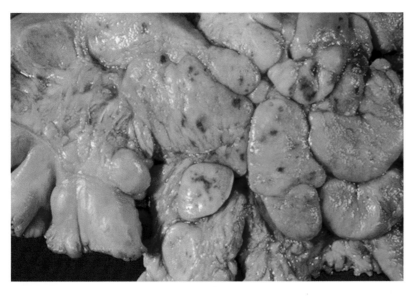

Figure 3-21 Non-Hodgkin follicular lymphoma, gross

This cross-section through the mesentery reveals multiple enlarged lymph nodes that abut one another and are nearly confluent. In contrast to carcinoma metastases, lymph nodes involved with lymphoma tend to have little necrosis and only focal hemorrhage. They grossly maintain a solid, fleshy tan appearance on sectioning. Low-grade NHL such as this tends to involve multiple lymph nodes at multiple sites, whereas high-grade NHL tends to be more localized. High-grade NHL may involve a single lymph node, a localized group of lymph nodes, or an extranodal site.

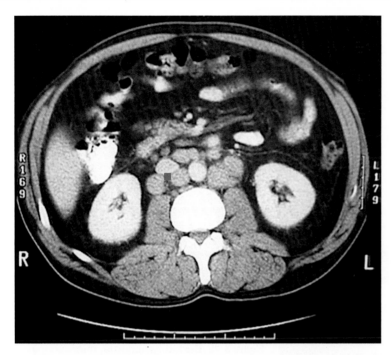

Figure 3-22 Follicular lymphoma, CT image
This abdominal CT scan with contrast enhancement shows prominent periaortic lymphadenopathy (■) involving multiple nodes in a patient with low-grade non-Hodgkin follicular lymphoma. This appearance could represent any lymphoid neoplasm, however. Lymphadenopathy is the hallmark of many lymphoid neoplasms. Leukemia describes neoplasms with extensive bone marrow involvement and often peripheral leukocytosis. Lymphoma describes proliferations arising as discrete tissue masses either in lymph nodes or at extranodal sites. Hodgkin lymphoma (HL) is clinically and histologically distinct from the NHLs, is treated in a unique fashion, and is important to distinguish. All HLs and two thirds of NHLs manifest with nontender nodal enlargement. Plasma cell neoplasms composed of terminally differentiated B cells most commonly arise in the bone marrow, rarely involve lymph nodes, and rarely have a leukemic phase.

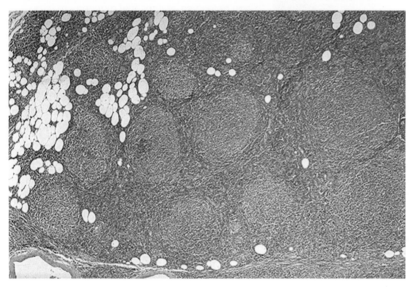

Figure 3-23 Follicular lymphoma, microscopic
The capsule of this lymph node has been invaded, and lymphoma cells extend into the surrounding adipose tissue. The follicles are numerous and irregularly shaped, giving the nodular appearance seen here. This is a follicular form of B-cell lymphoma. The markers CD19, CD20, and CD10 are often present. In 90% of patients, a karyotype shows the t(14;18) translocation, which brings the IgH gene locus into juxtaposition with the *BCL2* gene, leading to overexpression of the BCL2 protein, which inhibits apoptosis and promotes survival and accumulation of the abnormal lymphocytic cells. Mutations in *MLL2* encoding for histone methyltransferase, an epigenetic regulator of gene expression, are often present. One third to one half of cases may transform to DLBCL.

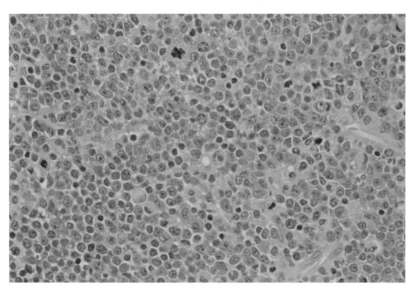

Figure 3-24 Diffuse large B-cell lymphoma, microscopic
Many NHLs in adults are large-cell lymphomas such as the one shown here at medium power. Most are sporadic and of B-cell origin. The cells seen here are large, with large nuclei having prominent nucleoli and moderate amounts of cytoplasm. Mitoses are frequent. The cells often mark with CD10, CD19, and CD20 but are negative for TdT. The *BCL2* gene may be activated. Dysregulation of *BCL6,* a DNA-binding zinc-finger transcriptional regulator required for the formation of normal germinal centers, is often present. DLBCL tends to be localized (low stage), but with more rapid nodal enlargement and a greater propensity to be extranodal than low-grade NHL.

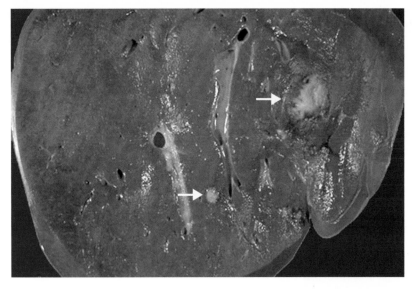

Figure 3-25 Diffuse large B-cell lymphoma, gross
Large-cell NHLs have a propensity to involve extranodal locations. The Waldeyer ring of oro-pharyngeal lymphoid tissues, including tonsils and adenoids, is often involved, as are extranodal sites, such as liver, spleen, gastrointestinal tract, skin, bone, and brain. Marrow involvement occurs late in the course, and leukemia is rare. Seen here on cut surface of liver are two rounded pale tan mass lesions (→). The color can range from white to tan to red, often intermixed. DLBCL can be associated with immunosuppressed states, such as AIDS from HIV infection, whereas another subset arises with Kaposi sarcoma herpesvirus (KSHV) infection and leads to body cavity involvement marked by malignant pleural or peritoneal effusions. These aggressive neoplasms may respond to multiagent chemotherapy.

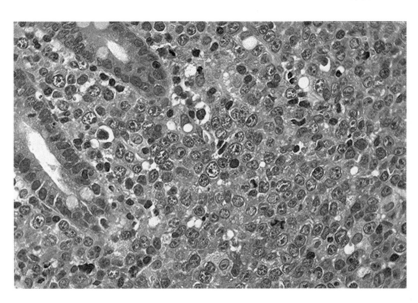

Figure 3-26 Burkitt lymphoma, microscopic
Seen here in small intestinal mucosa are large infiltrating cells of Burkitt lymphoma (BL), one of the most common lymphomas in Africa, which most often appears in children and young adults and involves extranodal sites, particularly the mandible or the abdomen. In the United States, abdominal involvement is the most common presentation. The cells mark for CD10, CD19, and CD20, BCL6, and surface IgM. Mitoses and apoptosis with cellular debris cleared by large macrophages producing a "starry sky" pattern are prominent features. All forms of BL are associated with t(8;14) of the *MYC* gene on chromosome 8 to the IgH locus. Latent EBV infection occurs in essentially all endemic tumors, about 25% of HIV-associated tumors, and 15% to 20% of sporadic cases.

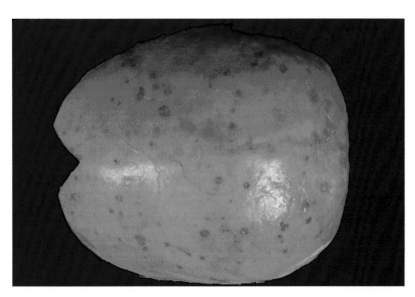

Figure 3-27 Multiple myeloma, gross
This skull shows the characteristic rounded "punched-out" lesions of multiple myeloma. The focal areas of plasma cell proliferation result in bone lysis to produce these multiple lytic lesions. Such lesions can produce bone pain. A solitary lesion is termed *plasmacytoma*. Myeloma results from a monoclonal proliferation of well-differentiated plasma cells often capable of producing light-chain and heavy-chain immunoglobulins. Proliferation and survival of these cells depend on elaboration of IL-6 by plasma cells and marrow stromal cells. Cytogenetic abnormalities may include t(6;14) or t(11;14), which juxtaposes the IgH locus with the cyclin D3 gene or cyclin D1 gene, respectively.

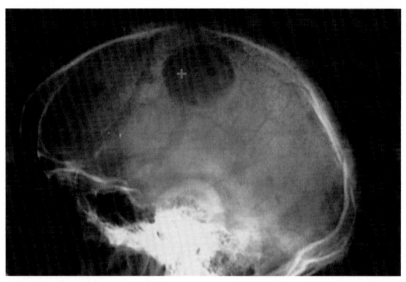

Figure 3-28 Multiple myeloma, radiograph

The "punched-out" circular lytic lesions (✚) in the skull seen here are the result of multiple myeloma in an older adult. These bone lesions consist of a neoplastic proliferation of plasma cells that can lead to hypercalcemia and an elevated serum alkaline phosphatase. A serum monoclonal globulin spike is typical. Increased production of immunoglobulin light chains can lead to excretion of the light chains in the urine, termed *Bence Jones proteinuria*. The diminished amount of normal circulating immunoglobulin increases the risk for infections, particularly with bacterial organisms, such as *Streptococcus pneumoniae, Haemophilus influenzae, Staphylococcus aureus,* and *Escherichia coli.*

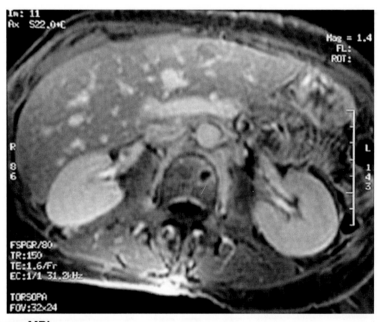

Figure 3-29 Multiple myeloma, MRI

The rounded lucency (▲) seen here in a vertebral body on a T2-weighted MRI scan is one focus of plasma cells in a patient with multiple myeloma. This patient had lesions in multiple bone sites and bone pain. The total serum immunoglobulin level is often increased, with an immunoglobulin spike (of M protein) seen on serum protein electrophoresis, and monoclonal bands of a single heavy-chain or light-chain class on immunoelectrophoresis of serum. Half of myelomas produce IgG, and a fourth produce IgA. In 60% to 70% of patients, increased light chains (either kappa or lambda), known as *Bence Jones proteins,* are produced and excreted in the urine, are toxic to renal tubules, and can lead to tubular injury with renal failure. The excessive light-chain production may lead to the AL form of amyloidosis, with deposition of amyloid in many organs.

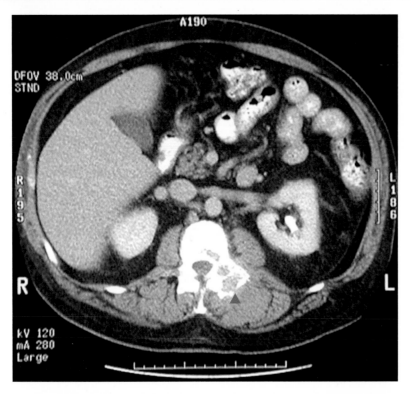

Figure 3-30 Plasmacytoma, CT image
The destructive, expansile lytic lesion (▲) involving the L2 vertebral pedicle on the left on this abdominal CT scan is a solitary plasmacytoma. Bones in the axial skeleton are most often involved with plasma cell neoplasms. The focal lesions typically begin in the medullary cavity, erode cancellous bone, and progressively destroy the bony cortex, leading to pathologic fractures, typically vertebral compressed fractures. The bone lesions appear radiographically as "punched-out" defects, usually 1 to 4 cm in diameter. About 3% to 5% of plasma cell neoplasms are solitary, but many progress to myeloma. Cytokines produced by the tumor cells include MIP1α, which upregulates the receptor activator of NF-κB ligand (RANKL), an osteoclast-activating factor.

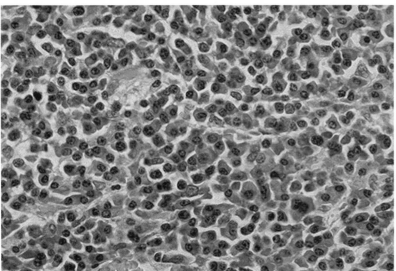

Figure 3-31 Multiple myeloma, microscopic
In this bone marrow biopsy section, as in most myeloma cases, there are sheets of plasma cells that are very similar to normal plasma cells, with eccentric nuclei and abundant pale purple cytoplasm. In fewer cases, the myeloma cells may also be poorly differentiated. Usually the plasma cells are differentiated enough to retain immuno-globulin production, but in less than 1% of cases, there is no increase in circulating immunoglobulin. Myelomas are typically detected by an immuno-globulin spike on protein electrophoresis or by the presence of Bence Jones proteins (light chains) in the urine. Immunoelectrophoresis characterizes the type of monoclonal immunoglobulin being produced.

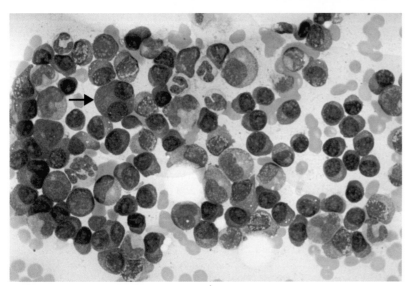

Figure 3-32 Multiple myeloma, microscopic
A smear of bone marrow aspirate has neoplastic plasma cells constituting more than 30% of the cellularity. There are numerous well-differentiated plasma cells with eccentric nuclei and a peri-nuclear halo of clearer cytoplasm (representing the Golgi apparatus). Larger abnormal plasma cells, including one double-nucleated form (→), are present. Clear cytoplasmic droplets contain immunoglobulin. This neoplasm is typically well differentiated, with easily recognizable plasma cells, most of which are hardly distinguish-able from normal plasma cells except by their increased numbers. Plasma cell leukemia is rare.

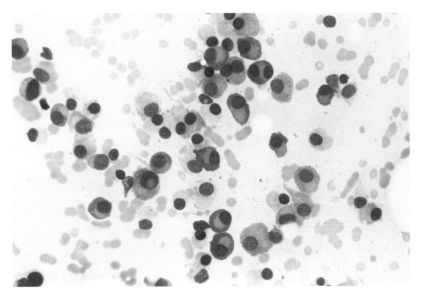

Figure 3-33 Waldenström macroglobulinemia, microscopic

This form of B-cell lymphoma, called *lymphoplasmacytic lymphoma,* shown here in a bone marrow smear, is seen in older adults and is widely distributed. It has plasmacytoid differentiation so that many cells resemble plasma cells and can secrete immunoglobulin, usually as an IgM paraproteinemia. Acquired mutations in *MYD88* encoding part of the NF-κB signaling pathway are nearly always present. Anemia is typically present. Lymphadenopathy, splenomegaly, and/or hepatomegaly may be present. Peripheral blood, skin, and gastrointestinal tract may be involved.

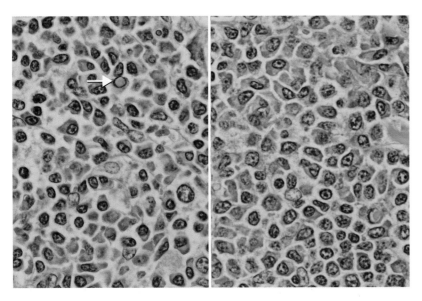

Figure 3-34 Lymphoplasmacytic lymphoma, microscopic

Note the small lymphocytes along with plasmacytoid cells and few large transformed cells. Plasmacytoid cells mark with CD138, but are CD5, CD10, and CD23 negative. There are characteristic PAS-positive intranuclear inclusions (➔) known as *Dutcher bodies.* Many of these neoplasms secrete substantial amounts of monoclonal IgM, with Waldenström macroglobulinemia, leading to a hyperviscosity syndrome with clinical findings that include reduced vision, headaches, dizziness, coagulopathy, and cryoglobulinemia with cold agglutinins and hemolytic anemia.

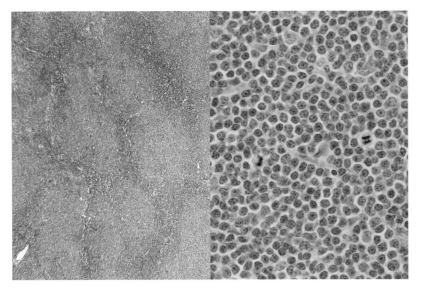

Figure 3-35 Mantle cell lymphoma, microscopic

At low power *(left panel),* there is a vaguely nodular pattern effacing the lymph node architecture, and at high power *(right panel),* the slightly large lymphocytes have folded (cleaved) nuclei. In addition to pan–B-cell markers CD19 and CD20, these cells mark with CD5 and CD22, but not CD23. The characteristic karyotypic abnormality is t(11;14) with fusion of the cyclin D1 gene on chromosome 11 to the immunoglobulin heavy-chain promoter-enhancer region on chromosome 14, leading to increased cyclin D1 expression with loss of cell cycle regulation. Most cases involve lymph nodes and spleen, but 20% are associated with leukemia. Some may involve the gastrointestinal tract with submucosal polypoid nodules.

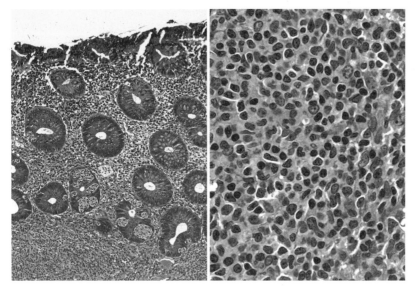

Figure 3-36 Marginal zone lymphoma, microscopic
The extranodal lymphoma seen here involving gastric mucosa is known as a *mucosa-associated lymphoid tissue* (MALT) lesion and is composed of small round to irregular lymphocytes *(right panel)* resembling those seen in the marginal zone of lymphoid follicles. Some of the cells may be plasmacytoid. The cells tend to invade epithelium as small nests *(left panel)*. MALT lesions often arise in areas of chronic inflammation, such as gastritis with *Helicobacter pylori* infection, sialadenitis with Sjögren syndrome, and Hashimoto thyroiditis. MALT lesions are indolent and may regress after elimination of a predisposing inflammatory stimulus or by local excision. The initial polyclonal expansion may acquire t(11;18) or t(14;18) and evolve to monoclonal lymphoma.

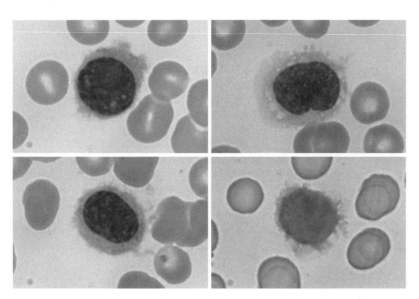

Figure 3-37 Hairy cell leukemia, microscopic
This collage of peripheral blood smears depicts abnormal lymphocytes with indistinct cytoplasmic borders and surface projections, giving the cells a "hairy" appearance. The red cytoplasmic staining seen at the lower right is tartrate-resistant acid phosphatase (TRAP) positivity. This uncommon B-cell proliferation occurs mostly in older men. Hairy cells usually express pan–B-cell markers CD19 and CD20, surface IgH, CD11c, CD25, and CD103. Activating mutations in *BRAF* are present in 90% of patients. Clinical manifestations include splenomegaly, often massive. Hepatomegaly is less common and not marked. Lymphadenopathy is rare. Hairy cell leukemia (HCL) often has an indolent course, and chemotherapy can produce long-lasting remission.

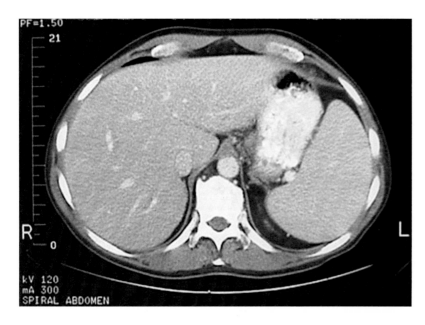

Figure 3-38 Hairy cell leukemia, CT image
This abdominal CT scan with contrast enhancement shows marked splenomegaly in a 55-year-old man with HCL. The liver is only slightly increased in size. The spleen has uniform attenuation, typical for diffuse lymphoid neoplasms, which are often diffusely infiltrative and rarely necrotic or hemorrhagic. The clinical findings of HCL most often result from splenic and bone marrow involvement, with pancytopenia in over half of patients from decreased marrow function and increased splenic sequestration of peripheral blood cells (secondary hypersplenism). In contrast to many other leukemias, a peripheral leukocytosis in HCL is uncommon.

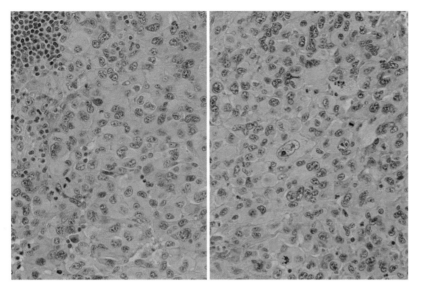

Figure 3-39 Anaplastic large cell lymphoma, microscopic
Shown are sheets of large cells, some with curved (horseshoe-shaped) nuclei, multiple nucleoli, and abundant cytoplasm that contains vacuoles. These lymphoid cells mark with CD30, Ki-1, epithelial membrane antigen (EMA), and anaplastic lymphoma kinase (ALK). Anaplastic large cell lymphoma (ALCL) accounts for 5% of NHLs in adults and 25% of large cell lymphomas in children. It often manifests with extranodal multiorgan involvement (skin, bone marrow, soft tissues, liver) along with fever.

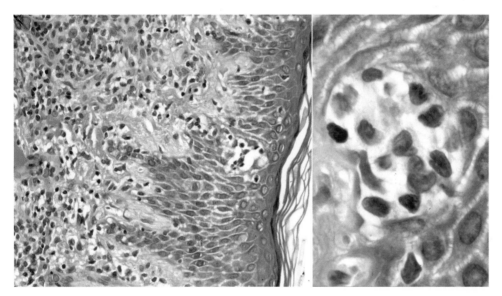

Figure 3-40 Mycosis fungoides, microscopic
Mycosis fungoides is the most common form of cutaneous lymphoma, a local or generalized T-cell neoplasm of CD4 helper cells. Note the small cells with convoluted nuclei infiltrating the dermis *(left panel)* and extending into epidermis as Pautrier microabscesses *(right panel)*. An inflammatory premycotic phase progresses through a plaque phase to a tumor phase on the skin. The course of the disease tends to be indolent.

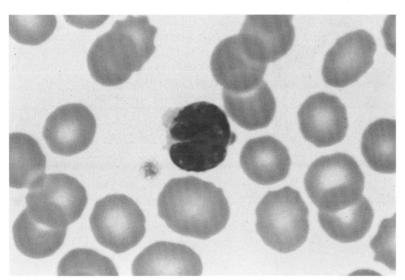

Figure 3-41 Sézary syndrome, microscopic
Disease progression of mycosis fungoides is characterized by extracutaneous spread, most commonly to lymph nodes and bone marrow. Sézary syndrome occurs when skin involvement is manifested by generalized exfoliative erythroderma and an associated leukemia of Sézary cells, also known as Sézary-Lutzner cells, with characteristic cerebriform nuclei. Note the appearance of the deep-clefted, cerebriform nucleus in this circulating lymphocyte. Late in the course of this disease, transformation to a large T-cell lymphoma often occurs.

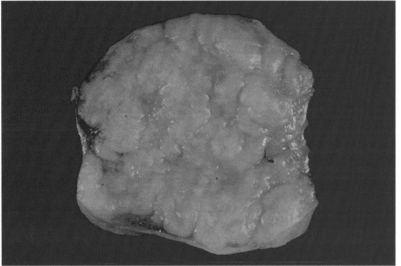

Figure 3-42 Hodgkin lymphoma, gross
An enlarged 5-cm lymph node (from a patient with lymphadenopathy) is shown. A lymph node should normally be soft and pink and less than 1 cm in size. This lymph node is involved with HL, but this gross appearance could pass for NHL as well, with a slightly lobulated, tan-to-pink cut surface and no or minimal necrosis and hemorrhage. On physical examination, nodes involved with a neoplasm are usually nontender. HL, similar to NHL, can involve a single node, a group of nodes, or multiple lymph node sites. HL may also be extranodal and involve sites such as bone marrow, spleen, and liver.

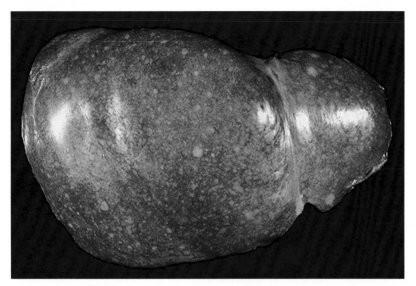

Figure 3-43 Hodgkin lymphoma, gross
Shown is a liver that is involved with HL. The staging of HL is very important in determining therapy. It is important to determine whether the patient has only a single lymph node region involved, multiple node regions, or extranodal involvement. HL typically occurs with contiguous spread. Grossly and radiographically, mass lesions are often present. This picture could probably suffice for a diagnosis of extranodal NHL hepatic disease as well.

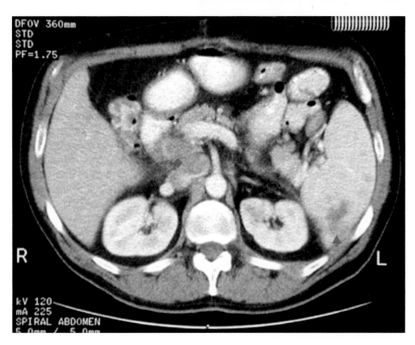

Figure 3-44 Hodgkin lymphoma, CT image
This abdominal CT scan reveals one larger (▲) and several smaller, more darkly attenuated splenic mass lesions representing extranodal involvement by HL. There is also prominent lymphadenopathy (◆). Staging of HL is important to determine therapy and prognosis and is often done by radiographic means, with CT used to document lymphadenopathy or extranodal lesions, ultrasonography to determine size and lesions of liver and spleen, and chest radiography. Many patients respond to chemotherapy, particularly younger patients, patients with a lower stage of disease, and those with absence of constitutional symptoms. After therapy, about 5% of patients develop myelodysplastic syndromes (MDSs), acute myelogenous leukemia (AML), or carcinomas, particularly of the lung.

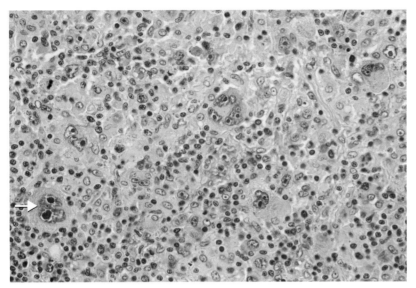

Figure 3-45 Hodgkin lymphoma, microscopic
The classic microscopic finding with HL is the Reed-Sternberg (RS) cell. The large multinucleated cells (→) shown in this effaced lymph node typically constitute only 1% to 5% of the cellular mass of the neoplasm, with the remainder composed of reactive cells and connective tissue. Clinical findings in about 40% of patients may include constitutional ("B") symptoms, such as fever, night sweats, and weight loss. Some patients have pruritus. Ingestion of alcohol may cause pain at involved sites.

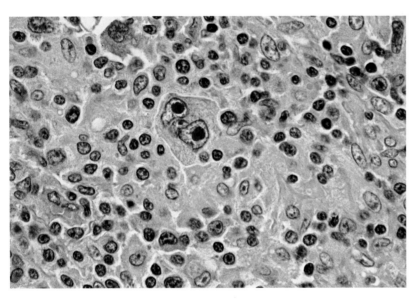

Figure 3-46 Hodgkin lymphoma, microscopic
The prototypical Reed-Sternberg cell is bilobed with mirror-image halves, and the large nuclei have an "owl eye" appearance from prominent nucleoli (as large as a small lymphocyte). These cells are often multinucleated with abundant cytoplasm. The Reed-Sternberg cells mark with PAX5, CD15, and CD30, but not CD20 or CD45. They secrete cytokines that promote proliferation of additional reactive cells, forming the bulk of the tumor mass. Reactive cells include lymphocytes, macrophages, eosinophils, and fibroblasts. Cell-mediated immunity is often reduced, as evidenced by anergy with skin testing and more frequent and severe infections.

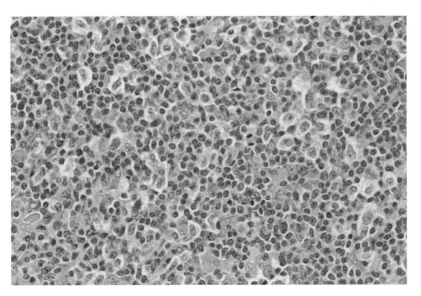

Figure 3-47 Hodgkin lymphoma, microscopic
There are scattered large cells with a surrounding prominent clear space, an artifact of formalin fixation. These are lacunar cells, the mononuclear variants of the Reed-Sternberg cell that are often seen in HL; they are most characteristic of the nodular sclerosis type of HL. Note the background of reactive cells that compose most of the cellular mass of HL, which accumulate as a consequence of cytokine release by Reed-Sternberg cells, including IL-5, IL-6, IL-13, TNF, and granulocyte-macrophage colony-stimulating factor (GM-CSF). EBV DNA is found in some patients. Laboratory findings include anemia, leukocytosis, and an elevated erythrocyte sedimentation rate.

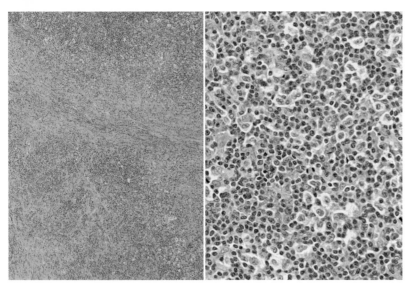

Figure 3-48 Hodgkin lymphoma, nodular sclerosis, microscopic
Note the prominent bands of pink collagenous tissue contributing to the fibrosis dividing the cellular infiltrate in the *left panel* low-power field in this lymph node. Nodular sclerosing HL is the most common form of HL, constituting about two thirds of cases, and is most common in young adults. The background infiltrate of cells has lymphocytes, plasma cells, eosinophils, and macrophages. Scattered Reed-Sternberg cells and also large lacunar cells with pale cytoplasm, seen in the *right panel,* are common in this type of HL. Histologic diagnosis is typically made from biopsy of involved tissue. Most nodular sclerosis cases are the lower stages I or II.

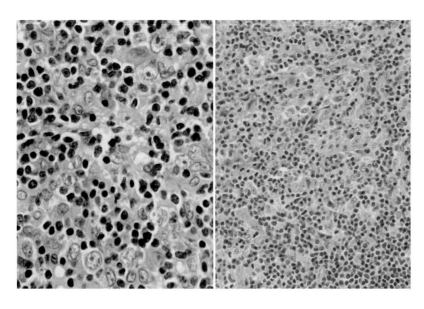

Figure 3-49 Hodgkin lymphoma, mixed cellularity, microscopic
Many different cell types are visible here, including small lymphocytes, eosinophils, and macrophages *(right panel).* There are often many lacunar cells *(left panel)* and Reed-Sternberg cells. This subtype of HL is more common in men and strongly associated with EBV infection. Compared with the lymphocyte predominance and nodular sclerosis subtypes, mixed cellularity subtype is more likely to be associated with older age, systemic symptoms such as night sweats, and weight loss. Although more than half of cases of HL of this histologic type are the higher stage III or IV, the prognosis is still good.

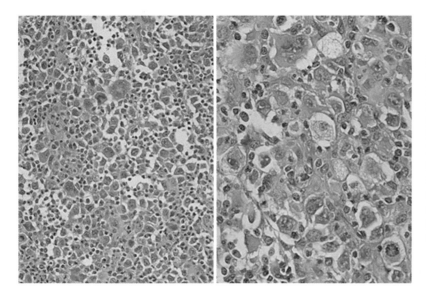

Figure 3-50 Hodgkin lymphoma, lymphocyte depletion, microscopic
Many Reed-Sternberg variants are present here. Few lymphocytes or other reactive cells are found. The lymphocyte depletion type of HL is the least common form. It may resemble large-cell NHL. Lymphocyte depletion HL most often occurs in older patients, particularly men, or in association with HIV infection. It is often associated with EBV infection. Advanced stage and systemic symptoms are frequent, and the overall outcome is less favorable than with other subtypes.

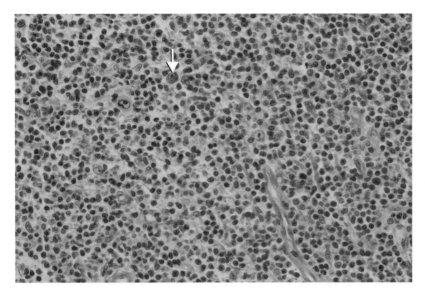

Figure 3-51 Hodgkin lymphoma, lymphocyte predominance, microscopic

The background of lymphocytes and paucity of Reed-Sternberg cells make this nonclassic type of HL difficult to distinguish from small cell lymphomas. Variant lymphocytic and histiocytic (L&H; "popcorn") cells with multilobulated or large nuclei (↓) mark for CD20 and BCL6 but not for CD15, CD30, or EBV. In contrast, the lymphocyte-rich form of HL has reactive lymphocytes constituting most of the cellular infiltrate. In most cases, lymph nodes are diffusely effaced, but vague nodularity resulting from the presence of residual B-cell follicles can sometimes be seen. The lymphocyte rich variant has frequent mononuclear variants and Reed-Sternberg cells. It is associated with EBV in about 40% of patients and has a very good to excellent prognosis.

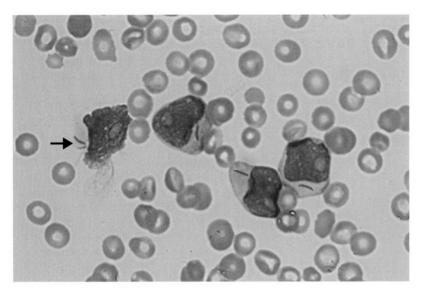

Figure 3-52 Acute myelogenous leukemia, microscopic

AML arises when acquired genetic alterations inhibit terminal myeloid differentiation, leading to replacement of normal marrow elements with undifferentiated blasts exhibiting one or more types of early myeloid differentiation. This peripheral blood smear shows large, immature myeloblasts with nuclei that have fine chromatin and multiple nucleoli. A distinctive feature of these blasts is the linear red Auer rod (→) composed of crystallized azurophilic granules. AML is most prevalent in young adults. Subclassifications of AML are based on cellular morphology. The M2 type seen here, the most common, has prominent Auer rods with a range of immature to mature myeloid cells present.

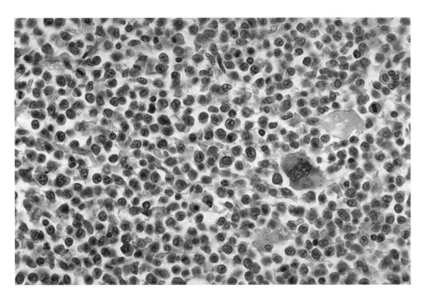

Figure 3-53 Acute myelogenous leukemia, microscopic

This bone marrow biopsy specimen has one lone large megakaryocyte, and remaining cells are mainly immature myeloid precursors. Thus this marrow is essentially 100% cellular, but with leukemic blasts almost exclusively filling the marrow—more than the 20% or more blasts needed for diagnosis—displacing and replacing normal hematopoiesis (a myelophthisic process) or suppressing stem cell division. Leukemic patients are prone to anemia, thrombocytopenia, and granulocytopenia, and all the complications that ensue, particularly complications of bleeding and infection. Molecular changes in AML often include CD33 overexpression; mutations in kinase FLT3 suggest a worse prognosis.

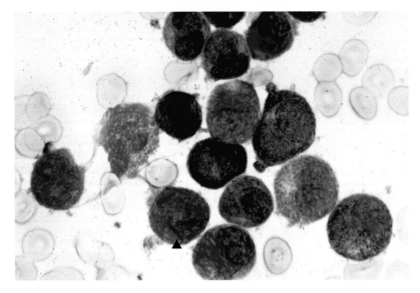

Figure 3-54 Acute promyelocytic leukemia, microscopic

This M3 variant of AML with cells resembling promyelocytes shows numerous coarse cytoplasmic azurophilic cytoplasmic granules and Auer rods (▲). The characteristic t(15;17) karyotypic abnormality with M3 results in fusion of the retinoic acid receptor α-gene on chromosome 17 with the *PML* gene on chromosome 15, leading to blockage of myeloid differentiation at the promyelocytic stage. For this reason, treatment with retinoic acid, a vitamin A analogue, helps overcome the block. Cell death with release of the granules into the peripheral blood can cause disseminated intravascular coagulation.

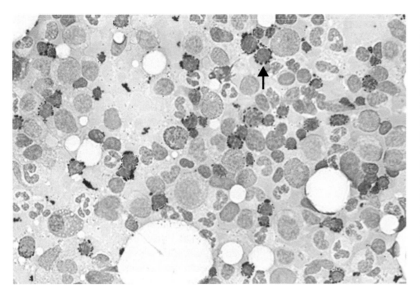

Figure 3-55 Myelodysplasia, microscopic

MDSs are clonal stem cell disorders leading to impaired cell proliferation and differentiation. MDS may be primary (idiopathic) in the elderly or secondary to chemotherapy or radiation therapy (tMDS). Precursor erythroid, myeloid, and megakaryocytic cells appear abnormal. Bone marrow findings include dyserythropoietic changes with nuclear abnormalities, ringed sideroblasts (↑) in erythroid precursors (shown here with iron stain), hypogranulation and hyposegmentation in myeloid precursors, increased myeloblasts, and reduced numbers of disorganized nuclei within megakaryocytes. There are peripheral blood cytopenias, and most patients initially have anemia. There is risk for transformation of MDS to AML.

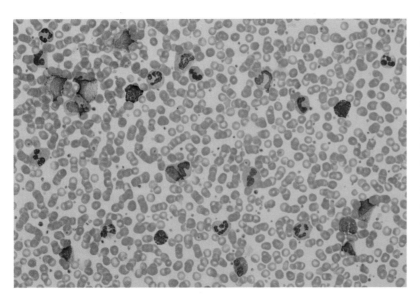

Figure 3-56 Chronic myelogenous leukemia, microscopic

This peripheral blood smear shows immature myeloid cells and band neutrophils. CML is a myeloproliferative disorder, and in contrast to AML, there are less than 10% circulating blasts. CML is most prevalent in middle-aged adults. A useful test to help distinguish CML from leukemoid reaction is the LAP score, which should be low with CML and high with a leukemoid reaction. CML may also involve the spleen, liver, and lymph nodes, often with accompanying extramedullary hematopoiesis. Because some cases arise from malignant transformation in a pluripotent cell line, there may also be erythroid and megakaryocytic involvement.

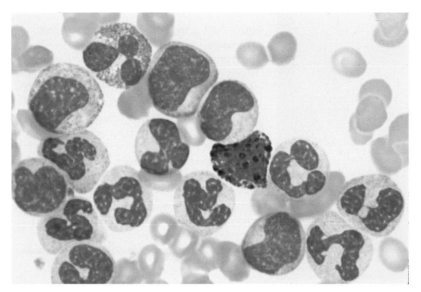

Figure 3-57 Chronic myelogenous leukemia, microscopic

Often in CML, the numbers of basophils and eosinophils, and bands and immature myeloid cells (metamyelocytes and myelocytes), are increased. Myeloid cells of CML also have the Philadelphia chromosome (Ph1) on karyotyping from a translocation of a portion of the q arm of chromosome 22 to the q arm of chromosome 9, designated t(9;22). This translocation brings the C-ABL proto-oncogene on chromosome 9 in approximation with the BCR (breakpoint cluster) gene on chromosome 22. The hybrid BCR-ABL fusion gene encodes a tyrosine kinase that has growth-promoting effects through nuclear stimulation.

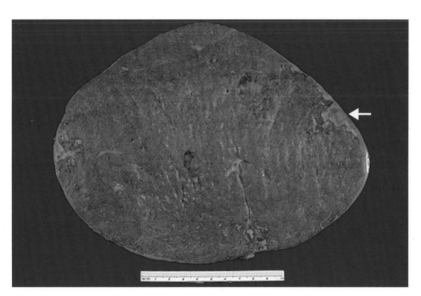

Figure 3-58 Myeloproliferative disorder, gross

This large spleen (the ruler is 15 cm long) has subcapsular yellow-tan infarcts (◄). Massive splenomegaly is usually indicative of myeloproliferative disorders, including CML, polycythemia vera, essential thrombocytosis, and primary myelofibrosis. These disorders may "blast out" to an acute leukemia. They often terminate in marrow fibrosis, with pancytopenia, extramedullary hematopoiesis, and splenomegaly. Although congestive splenomegaly is unlikely to exceed 1000 g, a spleen larger than 1000 g suggests underlying myeloproliferative, lymphoproliferative, or hematopoietic disorders. Chronic infections such as malaria or leishmaniasis also may produce marked splenomegaly. Secondary hypersplenism follows.

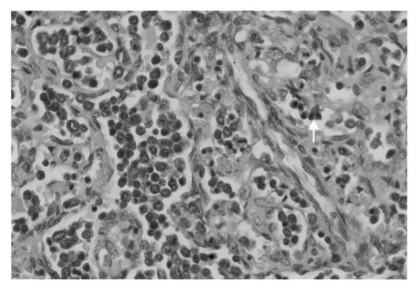

Figure 3-59 Myeloproliferative disorder, microscopic

This high magnification view of the spleen shows extramedullary hematopoiesis, a proliferation of RBCs and other hematopoietic precursors (↑), usually in the organs of the mononuclear phagocyte system, which often accompanies a myeloproliferative disorder involving bone marrow. Peripheral blood findings in myeloproliferative disorders include leukoerythroblastosis and giant platelets. As the disease progresses to myelofibrosis from secretion of cytokines such as transforming growth factor–β and platelet-derived growth factor, there is pancytopenia, and the patient is at risk for infection, bleeding, and high-output congestive heart failure. Some myeloproliferative disorders evolve to AML.

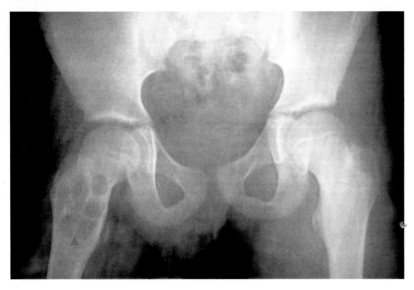

Figure 3-60 Langerhans cell histiocytosis, CT image
There are several forms of Langerhans cell histiocytosis (LCH), a proliferative disorder of immature dendritic cells with features of macrophages. The acute disseminated form, known as *Letterer-Siwe disease,* is seen in children younger than 2 years who have mainly cutaneous lesions and visceral involvement. A unifocal to multifocal form called *eosinophilic granuloma* mainly involves bones in children and young adults. A multilocular eosinophilic granuloma of bone (▲) is seen here in the right upper femur. These lesions can be unilocular and multilocular. If the pituitary stalk is involved, there is a Hand-Schüller-Christian triad of skull lesions with diabetes insipidus and exophthalmos.

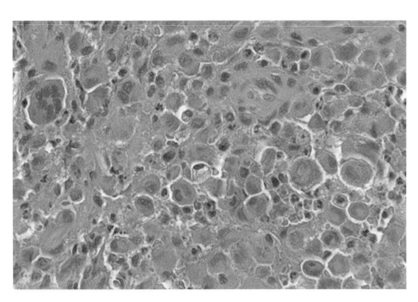

Figure 3-61 Langerhans cell histiocytosis, microscopic
Eosinophilic granuloma of bone is one form of LCH. The characteristic cell is an oval to round, macrophage-like cell, interspersed with inflammatory cells, including eosinophils. Eosinophilic granuloma is most common in children and young adults. This lesion forms within the marrow cavity and can expand to cause erosion of bone, which produces pain or pathologic fracture. Some lesions heal spontaneously by fibrosis, whereas others may require curettage. Sites of involvement with more disseminated forms of LCH include skin, lymph nodes, spleen, liver, lungs, and bone marrow.

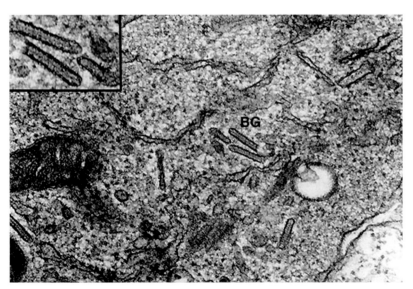

Figure 3-62 Langerhans cell histiocytosis, EM
Birbeck granules *(BG)* (*inset* shows several at higher magnification) are seen here in a Langerhans cell from a patient with histiocytosis X, one of the forms of peculiar neoplastic proliferations known as the Langerhans cell histiocytoses. The cells express HLA-DR, S-100, and CD1a. They have abundant, often vacuolated cytoplasm and vesicular nuclei containing linear grooves or folds. Pulmonary LCH is most often seen in adult smokers, can regress spontaneously on cessation of smoking, and usually involves a polyclonal population of Langerhans cells, suggesting it is a reactive hyperplasia rather than a true neoplasm.

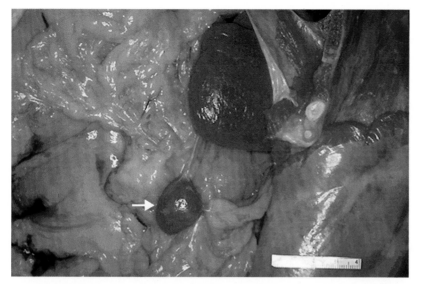

Figure 3-63 Normal spleen with accessory spleen, gross
The normal spleen in the left upper quadrant seen here is accompanied by a smaller accessory spleen (→). An accessory spleen is common and is usually just an incidental finding. An accessory spleen can undergo all the changes that the larger spleen can. There is also an uncommon condition known as *splenosis* that occurs when portions of a disrupted spleen (usually from blunt abdominal trauma) implant on peritoneal surfaces and grow and continue to function, even after the damaged spleen has been removed ("born again" spleen).

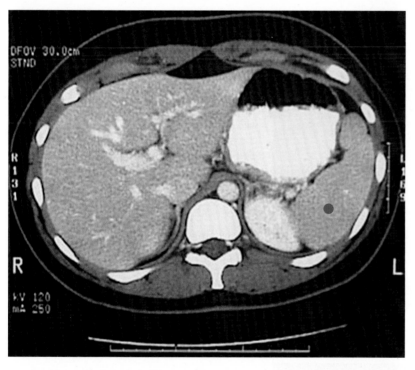

Figure 3-64 Normal spleen, CT image
An abdominal CT scan with intravenous contrast (and oral contrast in the stomach) shows the normal size and position of the spleen (●). The attenuation (brightness) of the normal spleen and liver are similar. The spleen acts as a filter, removing old RBCs and RBC inclusions, such as Heinz bodies and Howell-Jolly bodies, as the RBCs move through sinusoids. Splenic phagocytes also actively remove other particulate matter from the blood, such as bacteria, cell debris, and WBCs. The spleen also acts as a storage area for about one third of circulating platelets. Abnormal macromolecules produced with some inborn errors of metabolism, such as Gaucher disease and Niemann-Pick disease, may accumulate in splenic phagocytes and lead to splenomegaly.

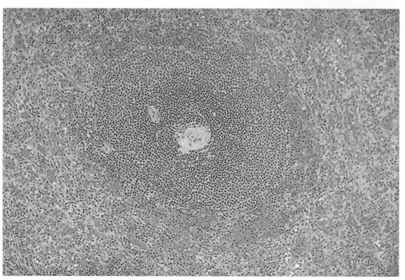

Figure 3-65 Normal spleen, microscopic
Note the small lymphocytes centered on the splenic arteriole at the center, forming the white pulp. Around this is the red pulp composed of many splenic sinusoids. The spleen, a key part of the immune system, has dendritic cells in periarterial lymphatic sheaths that trap antigens and present them to T lymphocytes, where T and B cells interact at the edges of white pulp follicles, generating antibody-secreting plasma cells found mainly within the sinuses of red pulp. The lack of splenic function from splenectomy or with autoinfarction (sickle cell disease) leads to susceptibility to disseminated infection with encapsulated bacteria, such as pneumococcus, meningococcus, and *Haemophilus influenzae*.

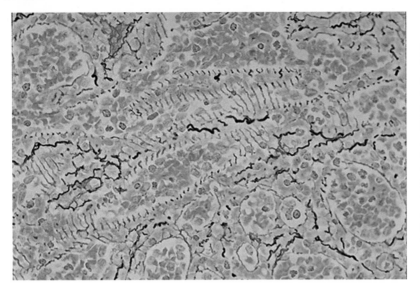

Figure 3-66 Normal spleen, microscopic
The normal structure of splenic red pulp in normal spleen is shown here with a reticulin stain. The "barrel ribs" of reticulin fibers outline longitudinal sinusoids in the red pulp through which the blood flows. RBCs must squeeze through slit pores in the sinusoids, and in so doing must deform. RBCs with abnormal shape or size, such as spherocytes or elliptocytes or sickled cells, cannot do so and may be removed from circulation. RBCs with immunoglobulin or complement bound to their surfaces are more likely to be removed in the spleen, a process termed *extravascular hemolysis.*

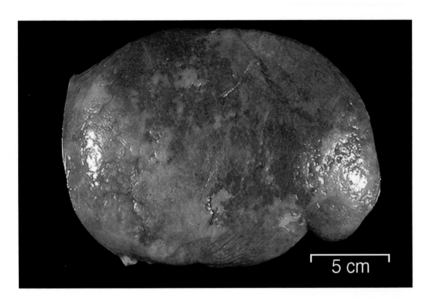

Figure 3-67 Congestive splenomegaly, gross
One of the most common causes of splenomegaly is portal hypertension with hepatic cirrhosis. It may also result from right-sided cardiac failure with cor pulmonale. Micronodular cirrhosis from chronic alcohol abuse or macronodular cirrhosis after hepatitis B or C infection may lead to portal hypertension. This spleen also shows irregular tan-white fibrous plaques over the purple capsular surface. This "sugar icing" is termed *hyaline perisplenitis.* The increased portal venous pressure causes dilation of sinusoids, with slowing of blood flow from the cords to the sinusoids that prolongs the exposure of the blood cells to the cordal macrophages, resulting in excessive trapping and destruction (hypersplenism).

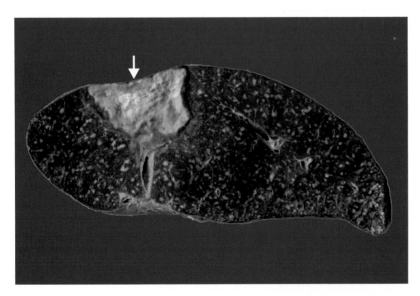

Figure 3-68 Splenic infarction, gross
This splenic infarct (↓) is a consequence of systemic arterial embolization in a patient with infective endocarditis involving either aortic or mitral valve. Clinical findings include left upper quadrant pain and splenic enlargement. Portions of the friable vegetations have embolized to the spleen through the splenic artery branch from the celiac axis and then to the peripheral splenic artery branches. Most splenic infarcts are ischemic and caused by emboli from either vegetations on valves or mural thrombi in the heart. They are based on the capsule, pale, and wedge shaped. The remaining splenic parenchyma of dark red pulp has pinpoint pale malpighian corpuscles of white pulp.

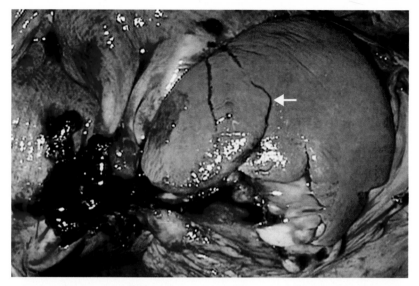

Figure 3-69 Splenic trauma, gross
Splenic rupture results most often from blunt force injury with abdominal trauma. Shown here are two large capsular lacerations (←) in a patient who was involved in a motor vehicle collision. Note the dark red hematoma formation at the left resulting from the splenic rupture. The hemorrhage can extend into the peritoneal cavity to produce hemoperitoneum. Enlargement of the spleen from predisposing conditions that render the spleen prone to rupture even with minor trauma include infectious mononucleosis, malaria, typhoid fever, and lymphoid neoplasms.

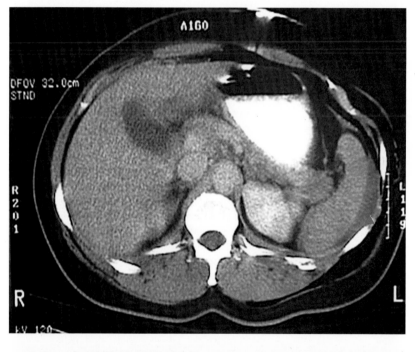

Figure 3-70 Splenic trauma, CT image
This abdominal CT scan with contrast enhancement shows a hematoma (▲) lateral to a ruptured spleen from blunt force abdominal trauma. The peritoneal lavage performed on this patient yielded bloody fluid, a clue to the diagnosis. The spleen may need to be surgically removed after such injury with splenic capsular rupture because the capsule is difficult to repair. Splenic preservation is desirable to preserve immune function, particularly in children.

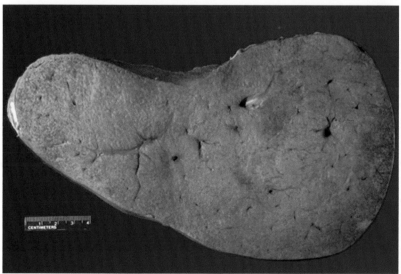

Figure 3-71 Gaucher disease, gross
This enlarged spleen is pale and has a firm feel. This young patient had an inborn error of metabolism with lack of the enzyme glucocerebrosidase, resulting in accumulation of storage product in cells of the mononuclear phagocyte system. There are three types of Gaucher disease. The most common, type 1 (99% of patients), is the non-neurologic form in which the affected individual has normal intelligence and lives into adulthood. Type 2 is the neuronopathic form, which is lethal in infancy. Type 3 has a course intermediate between the other types.

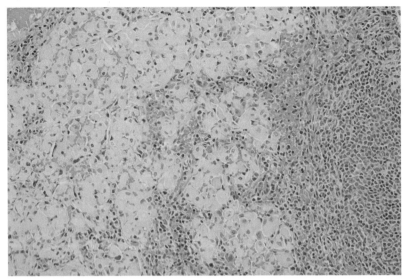

Figure 3-72 Gaucher disease, microscopic
Gaucher disease is a type of lysosomal storage disease with accumulation of the nonmetabolized storage product mainly in the large, pale macrophages shown in red pulp, with residual white pulp at the right. Numerous clusters of these macrophages enlarge the spleen, an appearance typical of a storage disease. This accumulation in marrow may produce a mass effect with bone pain, deformity, and fracture; pancytopenia can occur. Other tissues of the mononuclear phagocyte system, including lymphoid tissues and liver, may also be involved. Perivascular accumulation of macrophages in type 2 Gaucher disease leads to neuronal loss.

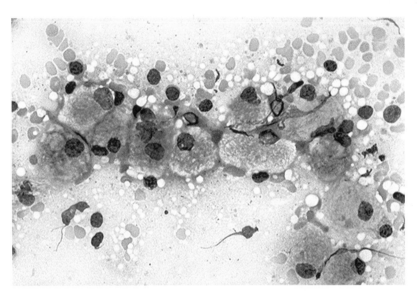

Figure 3-73 Gaucher disease, microscopic
The delicate cytoplasm of Gaucher cells in a bone marrow smear resembles crinkled tissue paper from the abundance of accumulated cytoplasmic lipid. As in many genetic diseases resulting from enzymatic abnormalities, enzyme activity, in this case glucocerebrosidase activity, in peripheral blood leukocytes or skin fibroblasts can be measured to confirm the diagnosis. As in many genetic diseases, multiple allelic mutations in Gaucher disease complicate detection because there is often no single genetic test to detect all cases. Different alleles may lead to different enzymatic activities, with variable severity of the disease.

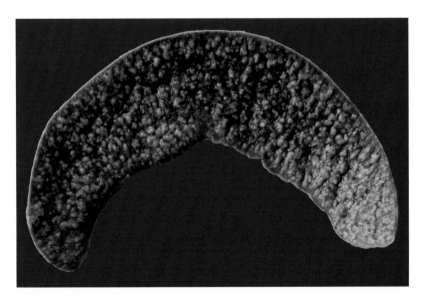

Figure 3-74 *Mycobacterium avium* complex infection, gross
Seen here in this cross-section of spleen are numerous small white nodules representing ill-formed granulomas. This patient had disseminated *Mycobacterium avium* complex (MAC) infection, and organs of the mononuclear phagocyte system are often involved. MAC infection is most likely to occur in immunocompromised persons, such as those with HIV infection.

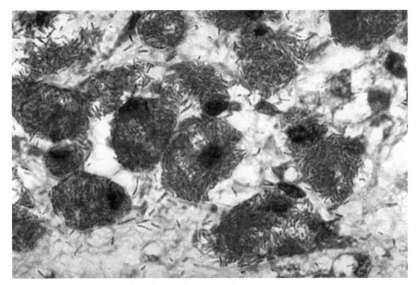

Figure 3-75 *Mycobacterium avium* complex infection, microscopic
There are numerous red bacilli filling and expanding the cytoplasm of numerous macrophages in this case of MAC infection. An immunodeficiency state leads to reduced cell-mediated immunity to battle the mycobacteria.

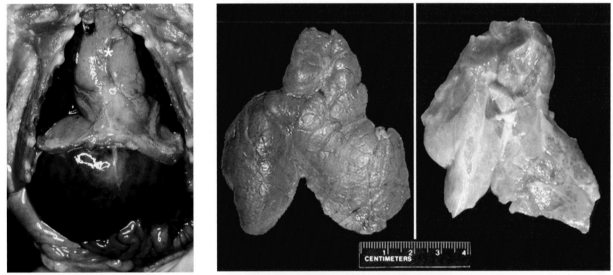

Figures 3-76 and 3-77 Normal thymus in situ, gross, and comparison of normal fetal and adult thymus, gross
The normal pink thymus (★) in the anterior mediastinum of the chest is prominent in late fetal life *(left panel),* in infancy *(middle panel),* and in childhood. There is eventual atrophy with fatty replacement, shown with the smaller adult thymus in the *right panel.* In development of the immune system, the thymus is an important place to which marrow stem cells migrate, undergo maturation with selection, and give rise to T lymphocytes.

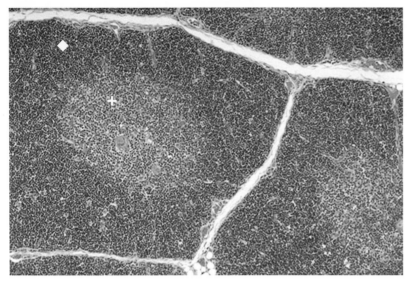

Figure 3-78 Normal thymus, microscopic
The normal third-trimester thymus of a fetus seen here at low magnification is well populated with T lymphocytes. There is a well-defined cortex (◆) and medulla (✚). Hassall corpuscles composed of epithelial cells are in the center of the medullary regions. In embryonic development of the immune system, progenitor cells of marrow origin migrate to the thymus and give rise to mature T cells that are exported to the periphery. The thymic production of T cells slowly declines during adulthood as the organ atrophies. In addition to the thymocytes and epithelial cells, macrophages, dendritic cells, few B lymphocytes, rare neutrophils and eosinophils, and scattered myoid (muscle-like) cells are found within the thymus.

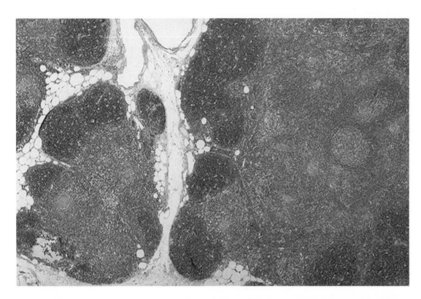

Figure 3-79 Thymic hyperplasia, microscopic
About two thirds to three fourths of patients diagnosed with myasthenia gravis (MG) have thymic hyperplasia, as shown here at low magnification. Ordinarily the thymus in an adult is composed mostly of adipose tissue, with a few clusters of lymphocytes and residual Hassall corpuscles. Here the lymphoid tissue is abundant, with lymphoid follicles present. The follicular hyperplasia seen in this case of thymic hyperplasia with MG is associated with autoantibody production. The acetylcholine receptor antibodies diminish the receptor function in the skeletal muscle motor end plates, leading to the onset of muscular weakness, particularly with repetitive muscular contraction.

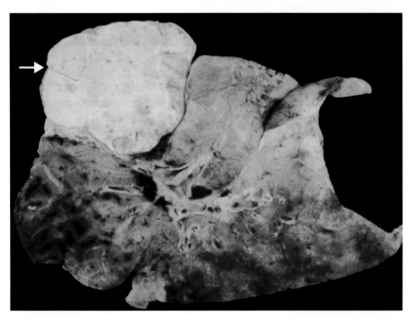

Figure 3-80 Thymoma, gross
Thymomas arising in the anterior mediastinum can compress adjacent structures as they enlarge. Seen here anterior to the lung is a discrete but lobulated tan-white mass (→) that proved to be a thymoma. Benign and malignant thymomas usually arise in adults older than 40 years. Most are found in the anterosuperior mediastinum, but sometimes they occur in the neck, thyroid, pulmonary hilus, or elsewhere. They account for only 20% to 30% of tumors in the anterosuperior mediastinum because this is also a common location for the nodular sclerosis type of HL and certain forms of NHL, such as T-cell lymphoblastic lymphoma.

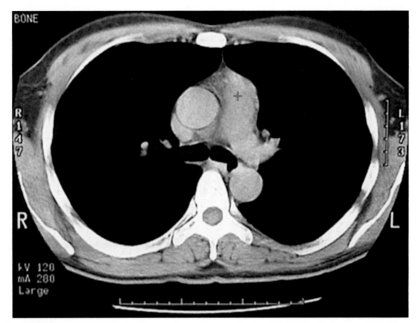

Figure 3-81 Thymoma, CT image

This chest CT scan in bone window shows a thymoma (✛) of the anterosuperior mediastinum. It is arising in the left aspect of the thymus anterior and to the left of the aortic arch. Thymomas can be slow growing and act in a benign fashion, but malignant thymomas can be locally invasive. Thymomas that are cytologically malignant are termed *thymic carcinoma.* About 40% of thymomas are found when symptoms occur from impingement on mediastinal structures, and another 30% to 45% are present with MG. The remainder are discovered incidentally during imaging studies or during cardiothoracic surgery.

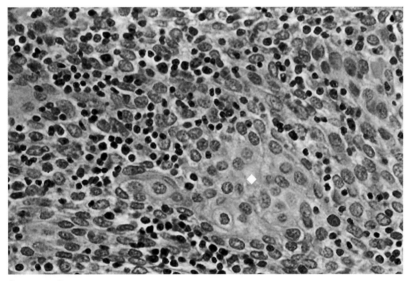

Figure 3-82 Thymoma, microscopic

A thymoma contains epithelial elements (◆), with a background of small round lymphocytes that are not neoplastic themselves. One third to one half of all thymomas occur in association with MG. The neoplastic epithelial elements of this thymoma display minimal pleomorphism, but this tumor was locally invasive and a malignant thymoma. About 10% of thymomas are associated with systemic paraneoplastic syndromes other than MG, including Graves disease, pure RBC aplasia, polymyositis, Cushing syndrome, and pernicious anemia.

Red Blood Cell Disorders

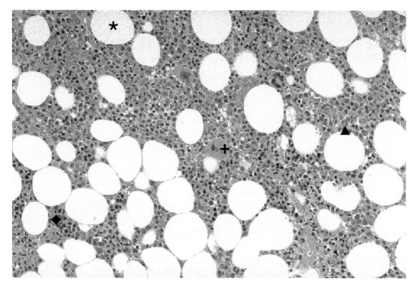

Figure 4-1 Normal bone marrow, microscopic
At medium-power magnification, normal marrow is seen to be a mixture of hematopoietic elements and adipose tissue. This marrow was taken from the posterior iliac crest of a middle-aged person; marrow is about 50% cellular at age 50 years, declining by 10% per decade thereafter. In very elderly individuals, most remaining hematopoiesis is concentrated in vertebrae, sternum, and ribs. The erythroid islands (◆) and granulocytic precursors (▲) form the bulk of the hematopoietic components, admixed with steatocytes (★). The large multinucleated cells are megakaryocytes (✚). Small numbers of lymphocytes, mainly memory B cells, and plasma cells secreting immunoglobulins are present.

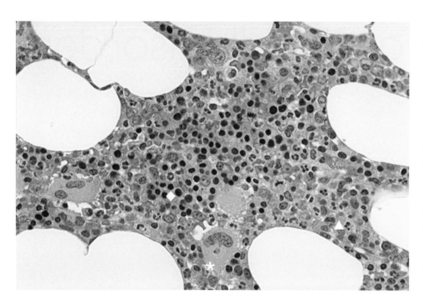

Figure 4-2 Normal bone marrow, microscopic
At higher magnification, megakaryocytes (★), erythroid islands (◆), and granulocytic precursors (▲) are present. The normal myeloid-to-erythroid ratio is about 2:1 to 3:1. A high proliferation rate from CD34+ stem cells differentiating into various colony-forming units under the influence of c-KIT ligand is needed because granulocytes last less than 1 day in circulation, platelets less than 1 week, and red blood cells (RBCs) about 120 days. Erythropoietin stimulates RBC production, thrombopoietin platelet formation, granulocyte-macrophage colony-stimulating factor, granulocyte and monocyte-macrophage proliferation, and granulocyte colony-stimulating factor neutrophil production.

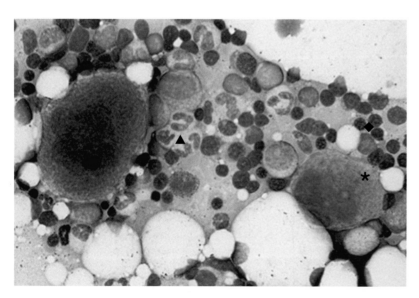

Figure 4-3 Normal bone marrow smear, microscopic
In this normal bone marrow smear at high magnification, megakaryocytes (★), erythroid precursors (◆), and granulocytic precursors (▲) are present. Erythroid precursors are nucleated, but the nucleus is normally lost before mature RBCs are released into the circulation. Newly released RBCs, called *reticulocytes,* have a slightly increased mean corpuscular volume (MCV) and increased RNA content that imparts a slightly basophilic appearance, and this RNA can be precipitated by supravital staining for identification and enumeration (the "retic" count). Platelets are formed by budding off megakaryocyte cytoplasm.

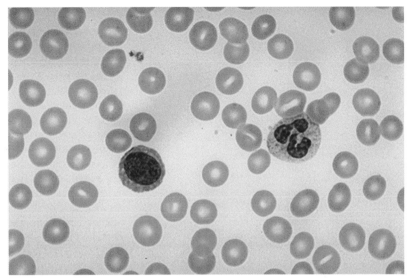

Figure 4-4 Normal peripheral blood smear, microscopic

These are happy, normal RBCs with a zone of central pallor about one third the size of the RBC diameter. These RBCs show minimal variation in size (anisocytosis) and shape (poikilocytosis). A small blue-staining platelet is present. A normal mature lymphocyte on the left can be compared with a segmented neutrophil (polymorphonuclear leukocyte) on the right. An RBC is about two thirds the size of a normal lymphocyte. The hemoglobin in RBCs supplies most of the oxygen-carrying capacity:

$$O_2 \text{ content} = 1.34 \times \text{hemoglobin} \times \text{saturation} + (0.0031 \times Po_2)$$

With hemoglobin 15 g/dL, Po_2 100 mm Hg, and O_2 saturation 96%, the O_2 content of the blood is 19.6 mL O^2/dL on leaving the pulmonary capillaries.

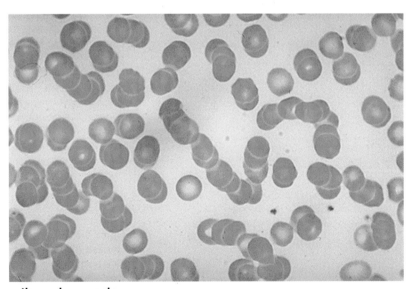

Figure 4-5 Rouleaux formation, microscopic

The RBCs here have stacked together in long chains (known as *rouleaux formation*). This phenomenon occurs with an increase in serum proteins, particularly fibrinogen, C-reactive protein, and globulins. Such long chains of RBCs achieve sedimentation more readily when left to stand in a column. This is the mechanism for measuring the erythrocyte sedimentation rate (ESR, or often called the "sed rate"), which increases nonspecifically when inflammation is present and with an increase in the acute-phase serum proteins. The sed rate is a nonspecific indicator of an inflammatory process.

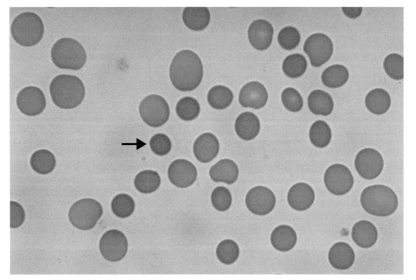

Figure 4-6 Hemolytic anemia, microscopic
This peripheral blood smear shows many smaller RBCs lacking central pallor—spherocytes (→). There are some larger, bluish-staining reticulocytes from increased marrow release to compensate for RBC loss. This patient had an autoimmune hemolytic anemia from antibody coating the RBC surface membranes. Subsequently, portions of RBC membranes are removed, mostly in the spleen, decreasing RBC size (microcytosis). Reduction in size or number of RBCs results in anemia. The bone marrow can respond to anemia with increased erythropoiesis, indicated by an elevated reticulocyte count. The increased RBC turnover with rapid recycling leads to uncerjugated (indirect) hyperbilirubinemia.

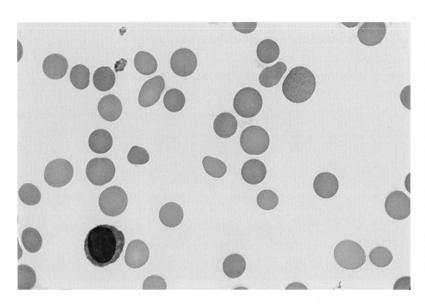

Figure 4-7 Hereditary spherocytosis, microscopic
The size of many of these RBCs is quite small, with lack of the central zone of pallor and loss of the biconcave shape. These RBCs are known as *spherocytes*. In hereditary spherocytosis, an autosomal dominant condition most frequent in northern Europeans, there is a lack of key RBC cytoskeletal membrane proteins such as spectrin or ankyrin. This lack produces membrane instability that forces the cell to take the smallest volume possible—a sphere. In the laboratory, this is shown by increased osmotic fragility. The spherocytes do not survive in circulation for as long as normal RBCs. Note the reticulocyte from increased bone marrow production of RBCs.

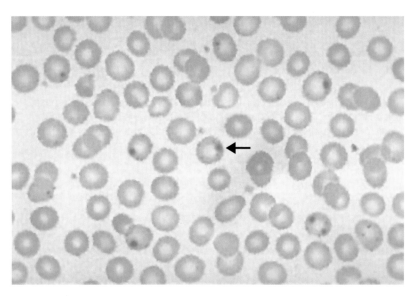

Figure 4-8 Glucose-6-phosphate dehydrogenase (G6PD) deficiency, microscopic
This peripheral blood smear with methylene blue stain shows RBC Heinz body inclusions (←) in G6PD deficiency. The defect is in the hexose monophosphate (HMP) shunt, which helps protect RBCs from oxidation. This X-linked disorder, found in 12% of male African Americans, is also seen in individuals from the Mediterranean region, including Italy, Greece, and Turkey. It is asymptomatic until stress occurs from infection or ingestion of an oxidizing drug. Older RBCs exposed to oxidizing agents such as primaquine, sulfa drugs, members of the nitrofurantoin family, aspirin, and phenacetin undergo hemolysis. Foods such as fava beans may have a similar effect. Laboratory findings include anemia, reticulocytosis, indirect hyperbilirubinemia, and decreased haptoglobin.

Cellulose Acetate pH 8.4

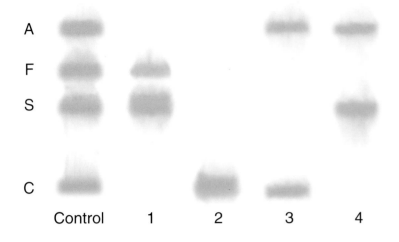

A

F

S

C

Control   1   2   3   4

Figure 4-9 Hemoglobin electrophoresis, cellulose acetate
The hemoglobin in RBCs can be analyzed by multiple methods to determine the types of hemoglobin present to diagnose hemoglobinopathies. Shown here in lane 1 is an infant with sickle cell anemia (hemoglobin S [Hgb S]) and significant Hgb F production; the heterozygous state of sickle cell trait is shown in lane 4. Lane 2 illustrates homozygous, and lane 3 heterozygous Hgb C disease.

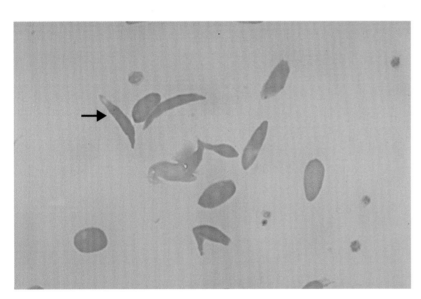

Figure 4-10 Sickle cell anemia, microscopic
Many sickled RBCs (→) in the peripheral blood are present in sickle cell crisis. The abnormal Hgb S is prone to polymerization with tactoid formation when oxygen tension is low, and the RBCs change shape to long, thin sickle forms that do not exchange oxygen well and are prone to stick together, plugging smaller vessels and leading to decreased blood flow with ischemia from decreased oxygen delivery to tissues, with clinical findings such as acute abdominal pain, chest pain, and back pain. Hemoglobin electrophoresis in sickle cell disease shows 90% to 95% Hgb S, 1% to 3% Hgb A2, and 5% to 10% Hgb F. In sickle cell trait, there is 40% to 45% Hgb S, 55% to 60% Hgb A1, and normal amounts (1% to 3%) of Hgb A2, and the RBCs have no or minimal sickling.

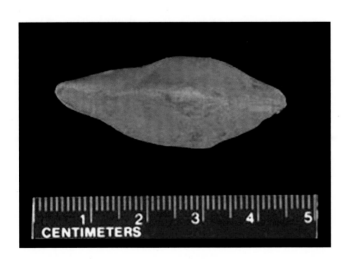

Figure 4-11 Sickle cell anemia, gross
The β-globin gene defect with Hgb S is a single point mutation with glu → val substitution. Although in early childhood the spleen may be enlarged with sickle cell anemia, continual stasis and trapping of abnormal RBCs in the spleen leads to extensive infarctions, which eventually reduce the size of the spleen tremendously by adolescence. This is called *autosplenectomy.* Seen here is the remnant of spleen in a teenage patient with sickle cell anemia. Lack of a spleen predisposes to infections, particularly with encapsulated bacterial organisms such as pneumococcus. In African Americans, the gene frequency for Hgb S is about 1 in 25, with a carrier rate of 1 in 12, and a 1 in 625 chance for sickle cell disease.

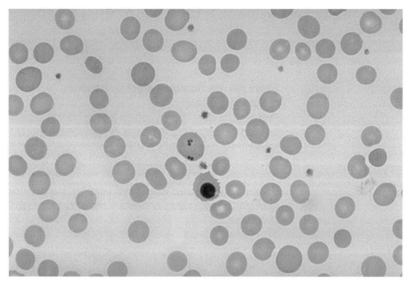

Figure 4-12 Howell-Jolly bodies, microscopic
The RBC in the center of this peripheral blood smear field contains two dark-blue Howell-Jolly bodies, or inclusions of nuclear chromatin remnants. There is also a nucleated RBC just beneath this RBC. Abnormal and aging RBCs approaching their 120-day life span are typically removed by the spleen. The appearance of increased poikilocytosis, anisocytosis, and RBC inclusions on a peripheral blood smear suggests that the spleen is absent. The presence of a nucleated RBC is typical for hemolysis with increased RBC turnover, so that the bone marrow is stressed to release not only reticulocytes, but also RBC precursors.

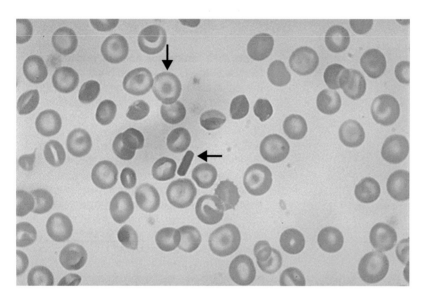

Figure 4-13 Hemoglobin SC disease, microscopic
This patient has both Hgb S and Hgb C present within RBCs. With SC disease, the RBCs may sickle, but not as commonly or as severely as with Hgb SS disease (sickle cell anemia), although there is a chronic hemolytic anemia. The Hgb C leads to the formation of target cells—RBCs that have a central reddish dot within the zone of pallor (↓), as shown in this peripheral blood smear. The rectangular RBC (←) is indicative of an Hgb C crystal, which is also characteristic of Hgb C disease, which arose in West Africa. The abnormal β-globin gene has an amino acid substitution at position 6 (β6Glu-Lys).

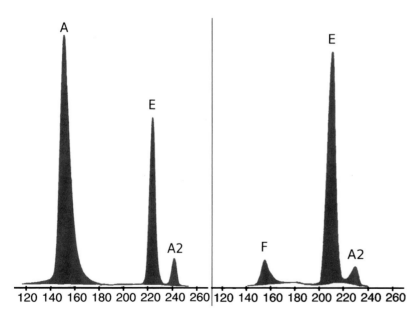

Figure 4-14 Hemoglobin E disease, capillary electrophoresis
One of the world's most common hemoglobinopathies is Hgb E. This disorder arose in Southeast Asia. The resulting anemia tends to be mild, even with homozygous disease shown in the right panel. There is sufficient Hgb A1 with heterozygous disease (left panel) that only mild microcytosis in peripheral blood RBCs is usually present. The abnormal β-globin gene has an amino acid substitution at position 26, with lysine substituted for glutamic acid.

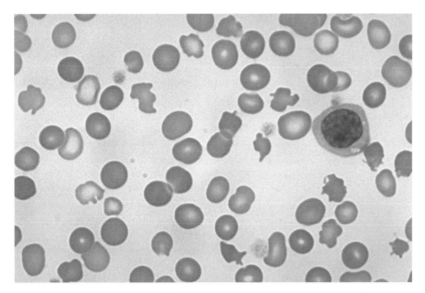

Figure 4-15 β-Thalassemia major, microscopic
This peripheral blood smear shows marked poikilocytosis (abnormally shaped RBCs) and some anisocytosis (variation in RBC size), although many are small (microcytosis). This patient has β-thalassemia, a hereditary disorder with deficient β-globin chain synthesis that leads to ineffective erythropoiesis and a chronic, microcytic anemia. Some of these RBCs resemble jigsaw puzzle pieces. Patients who are severely affected (β-thalassemia major) have increased iron absorption, leading to hemochromatosis. Iron overload is worsened if multiple transfusions of RBCs are given to treat chronic anemia. Each unit of packed RBCs contains 250 mg of iron.

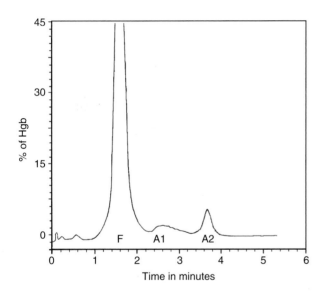

Figure 4-16 β-Thalassemia major, hemoglobin electrophoresis
This high-performance liquid chromatography (HPLC) analysis of RBCs shows very little normal hemoglobin A1, whereas most is F and A2, characteristic for β-thalassemia from deficient β-globin chain synthesis. There is insufficient production of Hgb F and A2 to completely compensate for reduced A1. There are many β-globin gene mutations underlying this disorder, and most involve splice sites, leading to mRNA transcripts that do not function normally. The residual function and β-globin production determine the severity of the anemia.

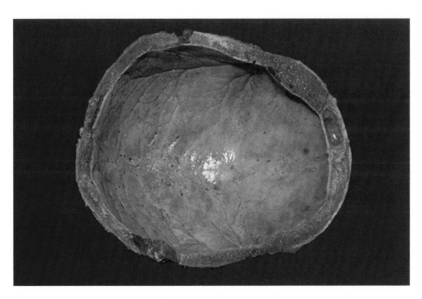

Figure 4-17 β-Thalassemia major, gross
Severe, chronic anemias (e.g., thalassemias and sickle cell anemia) can increase the bone marrow proliferative response to produce RBCs. This drive for erythropoiesis may increase the mass of marrow and lead to an increase in marrow in places, such as the skull seen here, where it is not normally found. Such an increase in marrow in skull may lead to "frontal bossing" or forehead prominence because of the skull shape change. Bone deformity with fracture may occur elsewhere.

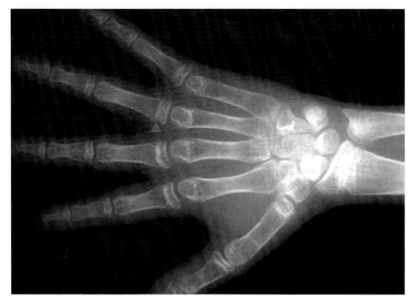

Figure 4-18 β-Thalassemia major, radiograph
This patient has β-thalassemia major, an inherited disorder of β-globin chain synthesis leading to ineffective erythropoiesis with marked expansion of marrow spaces to compensate. The result can be bony prominence with prominent epiphyseal regions (▲), as seen in this 20-year-old man. The hemochromatosis can lead to dilated cardio-myopathy, hepatic failure, hypogonadism, and "bronze" diabetes mellitus from iron deposition in islets of Langerhans.

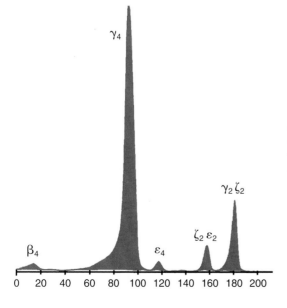

Figure 4-19 α-Thalassemia major, microscopic
α-Thalassemia major can lead to a severely hydropic stillborn fetus. Predominantly hemoglo-bin Bart's production from lack of α-globin chain synthesis results in marked anisocytosis and poikilocytosis of RBCs, with expansion of eryth-ropoiesis and the presence of many immature RBCs in the peripheral blood, as evidenced by polychromasia (◆), nucleated RBCs (▲), and even erythroblasts (□). α-Thalassemia major occurs when all four α-globin chain genes have a muta-tion. α-Thalassemia minor, which leads to a mild microcytic anemia, results from the presence of mutations involving only two α-globin chains.

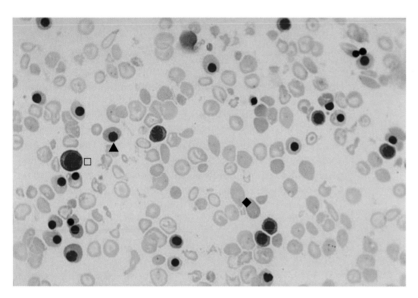

Figure 4-20 α-Thalassemia major, capillary electrophoresis
In this sample of fetal RBCs, the largest component is a tetramer of gamma chains, or hemoglobin Bart's, characteristic for lack of α-globin chain production. Embryonic hemoglobins ε and ζ are present here, but they do not persist after birth and cannot compensate. The tetramer of β chains forms Hgb H, which may be seen in small amounts in neonates with α-Thalassemia minor. Larger amounts (10% to 25%) of Hgb H persist in persons with three abnormal α-globin chains (Hgb H disease).

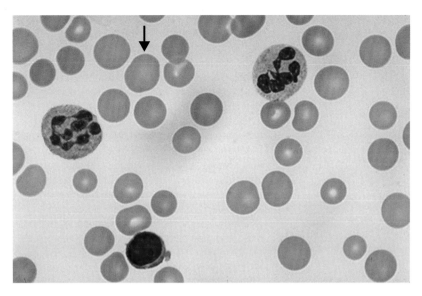

Figure 4-21 Megaloblastic anemia, microscopic

Hypersegmented neutrophils are present here along with macro-ovalocytes (↓) in a patient with pernicious anemia. The neutrophil at the left has eight lobes instead of the usual three or four. Such anemias can be caused by folate or vitamin B$_{12}$ deficiency. The increased size of the RBCs (macrocytosis) is hard to appreciate in a blood smear. Compare the RBCs with the lymphocyte at the lower left center. There is a markedly increased MCV. The MCV can be mildly increased in individuals recovering from blood loss or hemolytic anemia because the newly released RBCs, the reticulocytes, are increased in size over normal RBCs, which decrease in size slightly with aging.

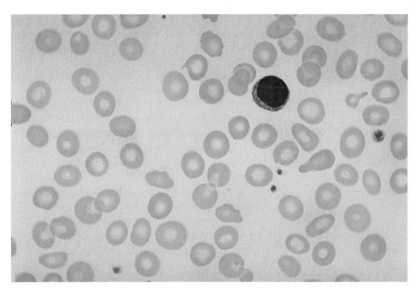

Figure 4-22 Hypochromic anemia, microscopic

The RBCs here are smaller than normal and have an increased zone of central pallor. This is indicative of a hypochromic (less hemoglobin in each RBC) and microcytic (smaller size of each RBC) anemia. Anisocytosis (variation in size) and poikilocytosis (variation in shape) are also increased. The most common cause of hypochromic microcytic anemia is iron deficiency. The most common nutritional deficiency is lack of dietary iron. Iron deficiency anemia is common, and individuals at greatest risk are children and women in their reproductive years (from menstrual blood loss and from pregnancy).

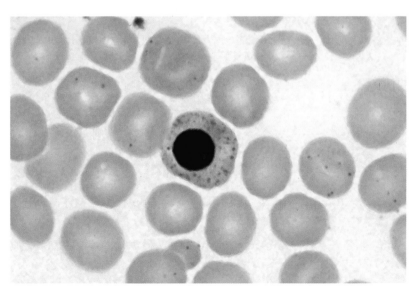

Figure 4-23 Basophilic stippling, microscopic

This peripheral blood smear shows a nucleated RBC in the center that contains basophilic stippling of the cytoplasm. The stippling is caused by inclusions of aggregated ribosomes. This suggests a toxic injury to the bone marrow, such as lead poisoning or drug effect. Such stippling may also appear with severe anemia, such as a megaloblastic anemia or thalassemia.

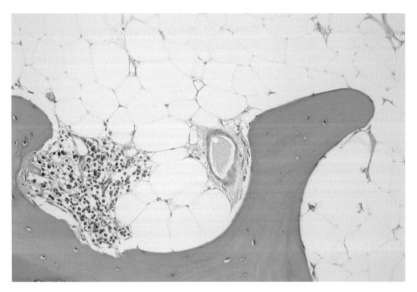

Figure 4-24 Aplastic anemia
The reduction of hematopoietic elements in the bone marrow here leaves mainly adipocytes remaining, with a residual focus at the lower left containing mainly lymphocytes. This leads to pancytopenia (anemia, neutropenia, thrombocytopenia). The most common cause is drugs known to be toxic to bone marrow, such as chemotherapy agents. Exposure to a drug such as a sulfonamide or to toxic substances such as benzene may precede development of an aplastic marrow. These agents may damage or suppress stem cells from which the erythroid, myeloid, and megakaryocytic cells are derived. Radiation exposure may damage the marrow. Some cases are idiopathic. If CD34+ hematopoietic stem cells remain, the marrow can become repopulated.

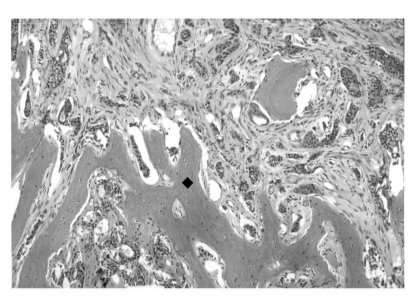

Figure 4-25 Myelophthisic anemia, microscopic
The marrow spaces between the reactive woven bone (◆) are filled with metastatic carcinoma replacing normal hematopoietic cells. The primary site in this case was breast. A bone scan can help to identify metastases. A bone marrow biopsy can confirm the diagnosis. A space-occupying process that destroys substantial marrow and reduces hematopoiesis is known as a *myelophthisic process*. Metastases, leukemias, lymphomas, and extensive infections can produce this effect. As a consequence, the peripheral blood shows a leukoerythroblastic appearance with immature white blood cells and nucleated RBCs.

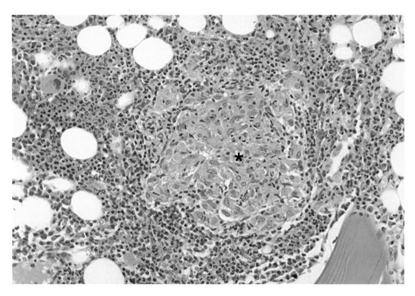

Figure 4-26 Marrow granuloma, microscopic
This granuloma (★) in this bone marrow biopsy can be part of a potential myelophthisic (space-occupying) process. Such marrow granulomas tend to be small and poorly formed. This one consists mainly of epithelioid macrophages. Multiple cultures and special stains are done to find an infectious cause, such as a mycobacterial or fungal infection. In this case, no organism was shown, and the clinical features fit with sarcoidosis. Patients with a fever of unknown origin may have such a finding. A myelophthisic process may lead to release of hematopoietic precursors, giving the peripheral blood a "leukoerythroblastic" picture with metamyelocytes, myelocytes, and nucleated RBCs.

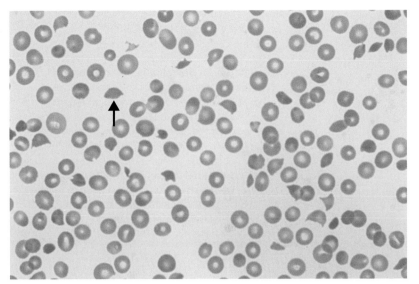

Figure 4-27 Microangiopathic hemolytic anemia, microscopic

The numerous fragmented RBCs seen in this peripheral blood smear include irregularly shaped cells, such as helmet cells (↑). These fragmented RBCs, known as *schistocytes,* are indicative of a microangiopathic hemolytic anemia or other cause for fragmentation such as trauma for intravascular hemolysis. Schistocytes can appear with thrombotic thrombocytopenic purpura (TTP) and with disseminated intravascular coagulation (DIC). In DIC, consumption of platelets and coagulation factors leads to hemorrhage. In DIC, the prothrombin time and the partial thromboplastin time are increased, platelets are decreased, and the D-dimer (indicative of fibrin degradation product formation) is increased.

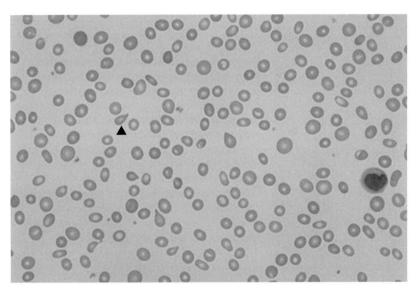

Figure 4-28 Myelofibrosis with teardrop cells, microscopic

This peripheral blood smear shows teardrop cells (▲). These characteristically shaped RBCs can be seen in patients with myelofibrosis, which can be the end result of a chronic myeloproliferative process. There is reticulin fibrosis filling the marrow spaces, reduction in hematopoiesis, and peripheral pancytopenia. A reticulocyte is present here, but the reticulocyte count would not be as increased as it should be, given that the marrow reserve is gone.

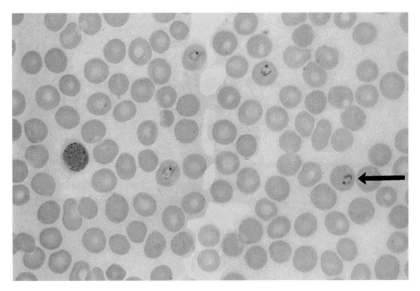

Figure 4-29 Malaria, microscopic

Malaria is a parasitic disease of erythrocytes caused by the parasitic genus *Plasmodium,* of which the following species affect humans: *Plasmodium vivax, Plasmodium falciparum, Plasmodium ovale, Plasmodium knowlesi*, and *Plasmodium malariae.* Shown here are ring forms (←) of *P. vivax* in RBCs. A large bluish gametocyte within an RBC is present at the left. After transmission via the *Anopheles* mosquito, initial replication occurs in the liver, followed by the erythrocytic phase producing recurrent fever with hemolysis and anemia.

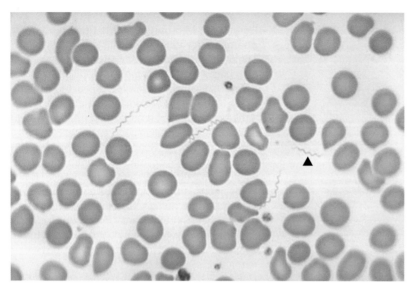

Figure 4-30 Borreliosis, microscopic
This peripheral blood smear shows multiple *Borrelia recurrentis* organisms (▲) among the RBCs of a peripheral blood smear. This organism produces the clinical picture of "relapsing fever" and is spread by lice and ticks. Variable expression of surface proteins helps these organisms evade immune destruction. Antibiotic therapy, especially with penicillin, can induce extensive cytokine release (Jarisch-Herxheimer reaction) with pronounced febrile reaction.

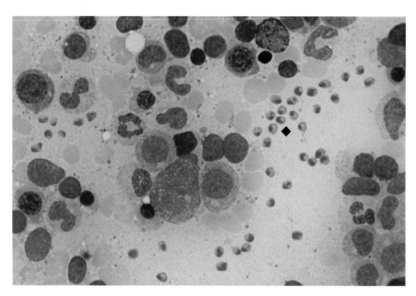

Figure 4-31 Leishmaniasis, microscopic
A myelophthisic anemia may result from infections involving the marrow, including fungal, mycobacterial, and parasitic infections. Seen here are multiple (◆) amastigotes of *Leishmania donovani infantum* in a bone marrow smear. The infiltrative process does not have to fill up much of the marrow to produce a characteristic peripheral blood leukoerythroblastic pattern. Leishmaniasis is spread by the sand fly vector. The visceral form of this disease, also involving liver and spleen, can cause fever, weight loss, hepatosplenomegaly, and pancytopenia.

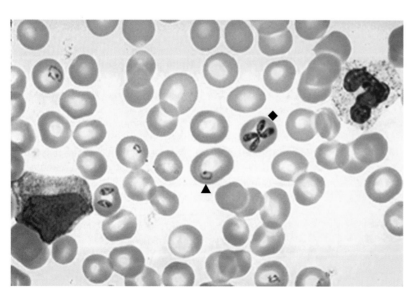

Figure 4-32 Babesiosis, microscopic
Babesiosis caused by infection with *Babesia microti* is a rare tick-borne disease endemic to the northeastern United States and parts of Europe. The organism proliferates within RBCs and can produce fever, hemolytic anemia, and hemoglobinuria. Shown here are a characteristic tetrad (◆) and ring forms (▲). Symptomatic patients are usually over the age of 50 years or lack a spleen.

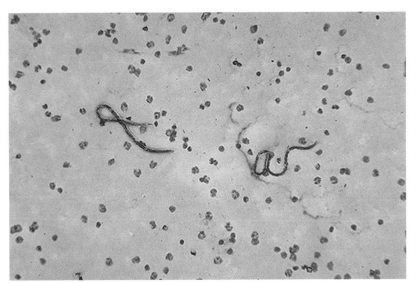

Figure 4-33 Filariasis, microscopic
Two microfilaria seen here are in lymph node aspirate fluid from a patient with peripheral eosinophilia. Infective larvae transmitted by mosquito bite migrate either to lymphatics *(Wuchereria bancrofti, Brugia malayi)* or to subcutaneous connective tissues *(Onchocerca volvulus)*. There they mature into adult worms that mate, and females release microfilaria. Varying host responses and repeated infections account for the manifestations. In lymphatic filariasis, the worms cause lymphedema of lower extremities, external genitalia, and sometimes upper extremities, called *elephantiasis* because of marked enlargement. Onchocerciasis can cause blindness, dermatitis with pruritus, depigmentation or hyperpigmentation, and fibrosis with nodularity.

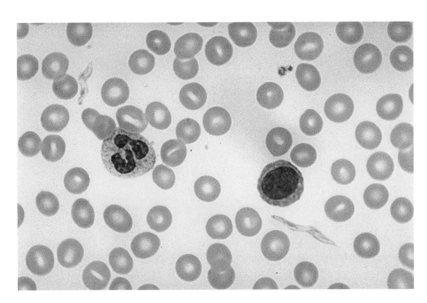

Figure 4-34 African trypanosomiasis, microscopic
Two trypomastigotes of *Trypanosoma brucei*, about two to three times as long and up to half as wide as an RBC, are present in this peripheral blood smear. The bite of the tsetse fly introduces infective trypomastigotes into the circulation, where they divide and multiply and spread to lymph nodes and spleen. Eventually they reach the central nervous system and proliferate in cerebrospinal fluid. Systemic manifestations include fever, lymphadenopathy, headache, and arthralgias. Central nervous system involvement follows and can manifest with convulsions, behavioral changes, and coma (hence the disease may be termed *sleeping sickness*).

The Lung

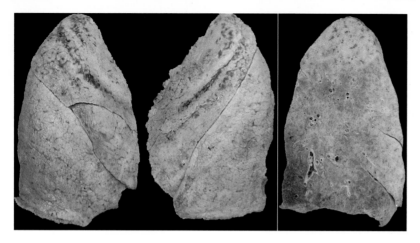

Figure 5-1 Normal lungs, gross
The external surfaces in radiologic orientation show upper, middle, and lower lobes on the right and upper and lower lobes on the left (right lung at left of *left panel*). In the *right panel* the cross-section of normal right lung shows minimal posterior and inferior congestion. There is minimal anthracotic pigment from dust in the air breathed in, scavenged by pulmonary macrophages, and transferred to pleural lymphatics to make them appear grayish black.

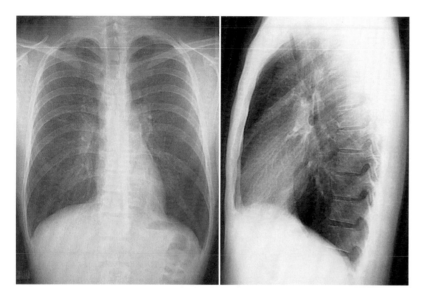

Figure 5-2 Normal lungs, radiographs
These chest radiographs reveal the normal posterior-anterior (PA) *(left)* and lateral *(right)* projection appearance of the lungs in a normal man. The darker air density represents the aerated lung parenchyma, with soft tissue and bone of the chest wall and hilum brighter. The normal PA heart shadow is about the width of the left lung.

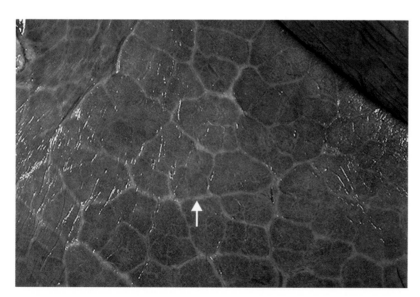

Figure 5-3 Normal lung, gross
The smooth, glistening pleural surface of a lung is shown here. This patient had marked pulmonary edema, which increased the amount of fluid in the lymphatics (↑) that run between lung lobules. The lung lobules are outlined here by the white markings. Anthracotic pigmentation derived from inhaled carbonaceous dusts is also carried by the lymphatics to the pleural surfaces and to hilar lymph nodes. Small amounts of anthracotic pigment are present in every adult lung. Smokers have more anthracosis.

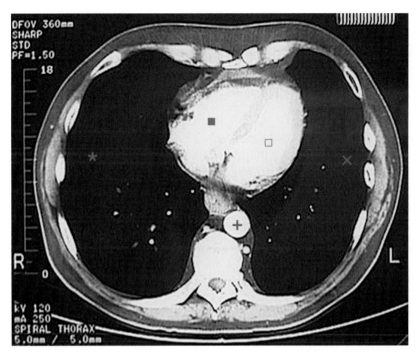

Figure 5-4 Normal lung, CT image
This chest CT scan at soft-tissue density reveals the normal appearance of the right (✱) and left (✖) lungs—essentially black from air density—in a normal man. Contrast material in the bloodstream gives the right (■) and left (□) chambers of the heart and the aorta (✚) a bright appearance. Bone of the vertebral body and ribs also appears bright. The AP diameter is normal.

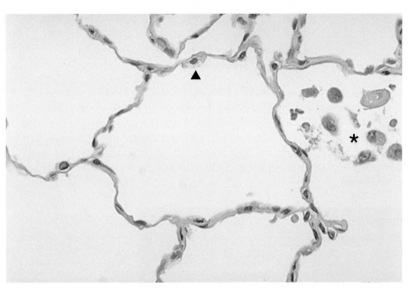

Figure 5-5 Normal adult lung, microscopic
The delicate alveolar walls of the lung are seen here at high magnification. The attenuated cytoplasm of the alveolar type I epithelial cells cannot easily be distinguished from the endothelial cells of the capillaries that are present within the alveolar walls. These thin alveolar walls provide for efficient gas exchange so that the alveolar-arterial (A-a) oxygen gradient is typically less than 15 mm Hg in young, healthy individuals, although the A-a gradient may increase to greater than 20 mm Hg in elderly individuals. Occasional alveolar macrophages (✱) can be found within the alveoli. The type II pneumocytes (▲) produce surfactant that reduces surface tension to increase lung compliance and help keep the alveoli expanded.

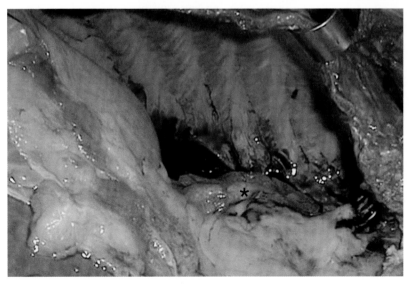

Figure 5-6 Atelectasis, gross
This right lung (✱) seen at autopsy is collapsed. In this case, blood filled the pleural cavity (hemothorax) after chest wall trauma. Such a compression atelectasis can also result from filling the potential pleural space of the chest with air (pneumothorax), transudate (hydrothorax), lymph (chylothorax), or purulent exudate (empyema). The collapsed lung is not aerated, creating a ventilation/perfusion ($\dot{V}/\dot{Q}$) mismatch, acting as a shunt similar to a cardiac right-to-left shunt that bypasses the lungs, with blood gas parameters similar to the mixed venous blood entering the right side of the heart.

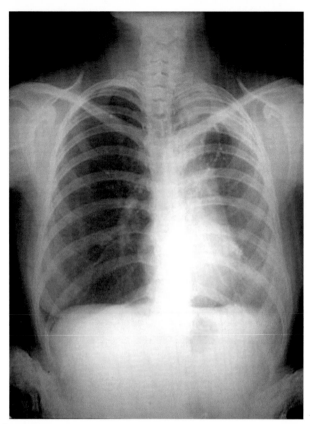

Figure 5-7 Atelectasis, radiograph

This chest radiograph reveals a right pneumothorax with expansion of the right chest cavity and displacement of the heart to the left. A pneumothorax occurs with a penetrating chest injury, inflammation with rupture of a bronchus to the pleura, rupture of an emphysematous bulla, or barotrauma from positive-pressure mechanical ventilation. The escape of air into the pleural space eliminates the negative pressure of the thoracic cavity and collapses the lung. The example seen here is a tension pneumothorax shifting the mediastinum because a ball-valve air leak is increasing the amount of air in the right chest cavity. A chest tube can be placed to re-expand the lung. In contrast, a resorption atelectasis from airway obstruction and resorption of air in the lung parenchyma leads to collapse with a shift of the mediastinum toward the involved lung.

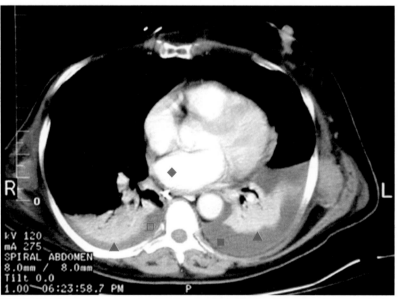

Figure 5-8 Atelectasis, CT image

This chest CT scan shows a large right pleural effusion (■) and a smaller left pleural effusion (□). The pleural effusions seen here resulted from right-sided heart failure as a consequence of rheumatic mitral stenosis with chronic pulmonary congestion and subsequent pulmonary hypertension. Note the enlargement of the right atrium (◆). This large effusion has produced bilateral atelectasis of the lower lobes, characterized by a small, dense crescent of lung tissue in the region of the effusion on each side (▲).

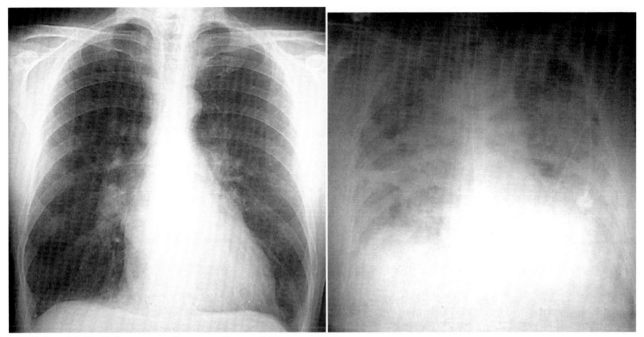

Figures 5-9 and 5-10 Pulmonary edema, radiographs

Pulmonary passive congestion from left-sided heart failure (cardiogenic edema) increases interstitial markings, and edema fluid spills into alveoli, creating infiltrates. This PA chest radiograph on the *left* shows pulmonary congestion and edema throughout all lung fields. The pulmonary veins are distended near the hilum. The left heart border is prominent because of left atrial enlargement. This patient had mitral stenosis. The PA chest radiograph on the *right* shows extensive congestion and edema throughout all lung fields from severe congestive heart failure from cardiomyopathy, and the edema obscures the cardiac silhouette.

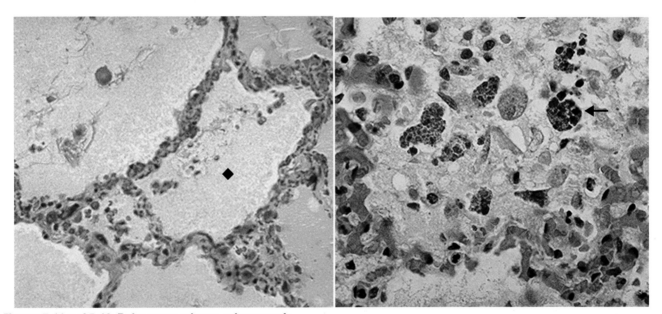

Figures 5-11 and 5-12 Pulmonary edema, microscopic

The alveoli on the *left* are filled with a smooth to slightly floccular pink material (◆) characteristic of pulmonary edema. Capillaries within alveolar walls are congested, filled with many red blood cells (RBCs). Pulmonary congestion with edema is common in patients with heart failure and in areas of inflammation of the lung. On the *right* is more marked pulmonary congestion with dilated capillaries and leakage of blood into alveolar spaces, leading to the appearance of hemosiderin-laden macrophages ("heart failure cells") containing brown cytoplasmic hemosiderin granules (←) from breakdown of RBCs.

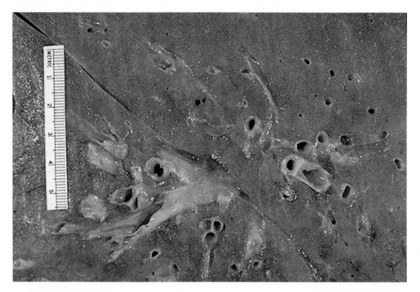

Figure 5-13 Diffuse alveolar damage, gross
This lung is virtually airless, diffusely firm, and rubbery with a glistening appearance on cut section. Clinically, this is known as *adult respiratory distress syndrome* (ARDS). Diffuse alveolar damage (DAD) is a form of acute restrictive lung disease resulting from capillary wall endothelial injury from multiple causes, including pulmonary infections, sepsis, inhaled noxious gases, microangiopathic hemolytic anemias, trauma, oxygen toxicity, aspiration, fat embolism, or opiate overdose. DAD causes severe hypoxemia. The lung diffusing capacity for carbon monoxide (DLCO) is reduced. Diseases that affect the alveolar walls (DAD or emphysema) or the pulmonary capillary bed (thromboembolism or vasculitis) decrease the DLCO.

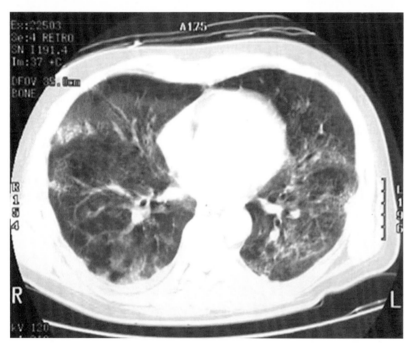

Figure 5-14 Diffuse alveolar damage, CT image
This chest CT scan with "lung window" setting reveals extensive brighter bilateral ground-glass opacifications of the lung parenchyma consistent with DAD. The acute phase of DAD can develop within hours of capillary injury, with increased vascular permeability and leakage of interstitial fluid into alveoli, forming diffuse ground-glass infiltrates. The exuded blood proteins can form hyaline membranes. Injury to type II pneumocytes diminishes surfactant production and reduces lung compliance. Release of interleukin-1 (IL-1), IL-8, and tumor necrosis factor promotes neutrophil chemotaxis and activation, which further potentiate parenchymal injury.

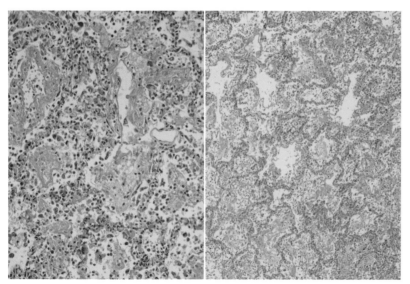

Figure 5-15 Diffuse alveolar damage, microscopic
At low magnification *(right panel)* all alveoli are filled with fibrin-rich edema fluid and inflammatory cells (noncardiogenic edema from alveolar injury) from damage to endothelial and epithelial cells. At medium magnification *(left panel)* the alveolar walls are congested and expanded from inflammation with acute DAD, a form of acute lung injury (ALI). Oxygenation is impaired from reduced alveolar ventilation and diffusion block. ALI and DAD may be part of multiorgan failure.

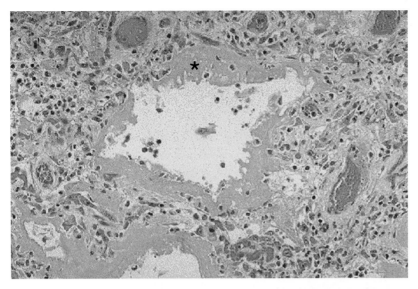

Figure 5-16 Diffuse alveolar damage, microscopic

DAD is the final common pathway for various severe lung injuries. In early DAD, hyaline membranes (★), as seen here, line the alveoli. Later in the first week after lung injury, the hyaline membranes resolve, and macrophage proliferation occurs. If the patient survives more than a week, interstitial inflammation and fibrosis become increasingly prominent, and lung compliance decreases. There are $\dot{V}/\dot{Q}$ mismatches. High oxygen tension is needed to treat the hypoxia resulting from DAD, and the oxygen toxicity from this therapy exacerbates DAD further.

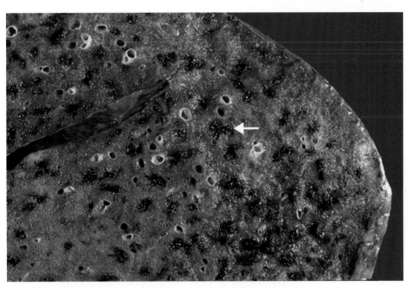

Figure 5-17 Pulmonary centrilobular emphysema, gross

The two major types of emphysema are centrilobular (centriacinar) and panlobular (panacinar). The former involves primarily the upper lobes, as shown here, whereas the latter involves all lung fields, particularly the bases. The central lobular loss of lung tissue with intense black anthracotic pigmentation (←) is apparent here. In contrast to increased risk for lung cancer, which diminishes when a smoker stops smoking, the lung tissue loss with emphysema is permanent. Centriacinar emphysema mainly involves loss of the respiratory bronchioles in the proximal portion of the acinus, with sparing of distal alveoli. This type is most typical for cigarette smokers.

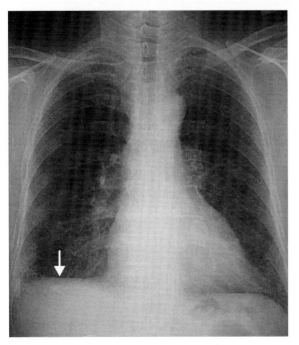

Figure 5-18 Pulmonary emphysema, radiograph

This PA chest radiograph shows increased interstitial markings with an irregular architecture, an increase in total lung volume, and bilateral flattening (↓) of the diaphragmatic leaves, consistent with centrilobular emphysema. The diaphragmatic flattening reduces the efficiency of muscular contraction and lung excursion, increasing the work of breathing. As the severity of emphysema increases, affected individuals begin to use accessory muscles of respiration, such as intercostal muscles and sternocleidomastoids. Affected individuals may also exhibit pursed lip breathing to increase central airway pressure to keep distal airways from collapsing as a consequence of the increased compliance. Most of the increase in total lung capacity seen with emphysema results from an increase in residual volume.

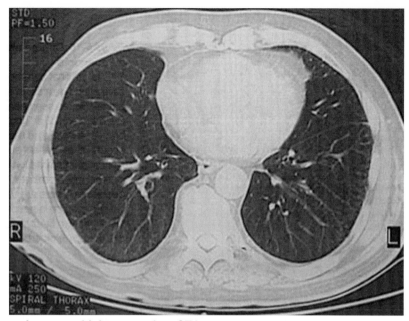

Figure 5-19 Pulmonary emphysema with hypertension, CT image

This chest CT scan in the lung window reveals an increase in bright vascular lung markings from pulmonary hypertension. There are parenchymal lucencies consistent with a pattern of centriacinar emphysema. The AP diameter of the chest is increased as a consequence of increased total lung volume, mainly the result of increased residual volume. When the pulmonary vascular bed is reduced, here from loss of lung tissue, then pulmonary arterial pressures increase.

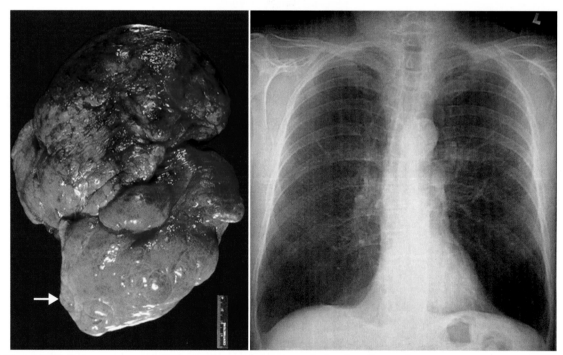

Figures 5-20 and 5-21 Pulmonary panacinar emphysema, gross and chest radiograph

Panacinar emphysema occurs with loss of all portions of the acinus from the respiratory bronchiole to the alveoli. This pattern is typical for α₁-antitrypsin deficiency. The bullae seen here are most prominent in the lower lobe (→) on the *left.* The typical chest radiographic appearance of panlobular emphysema, with increased lung volume and diaphragmatic flattening, is shown on the *right.*

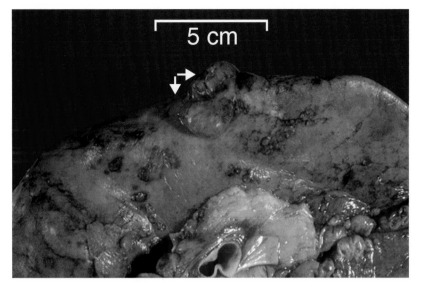

Figure 5-22 Distal acinar (paraseptal) emphysema, gross
This more localized form of emphysema can follow focal scarring of the peripheral lung parenchyma. Paraseptal emphysema is not related to smoking. Because this process is focal, pulmonary function is not seriously affected, but the peripheral location of the bullae, which can be 2 cm in size or more, along septa may lead to rupture into the pleural space, causing spontaneous pneumothorax. This is most likely to occur in young adults, with sudden onset of dyspnea. Two small bullae (↓ →) are seen here just beneath the pleural surface.

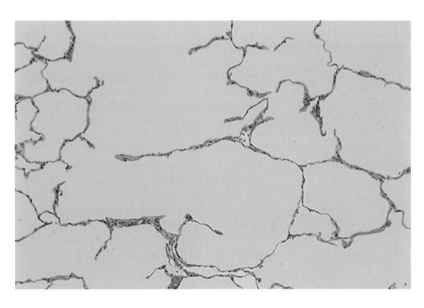

Figure 5-23 Pulmonary emphysema, microscopic
There is loss of distal airspaces: bronchioles, alveolar ducts, and alveoli. The remaining airspaces become dilated as shown here; overall, there is less surface area for gas exchange. Emphysema leads to loss of lung parenchyma, loss of elastic recoil with increased lung compliance, and increased pulmonary residual volume with increased total lung capacity. There is decreased diaphragmatic excursion and increased use of accessory muscles for breathing. Over time, with reduced ventilation and air trapping, the Pao_2 decreases, the $Paco_2$ increases, and respiratory acidosis ensues.

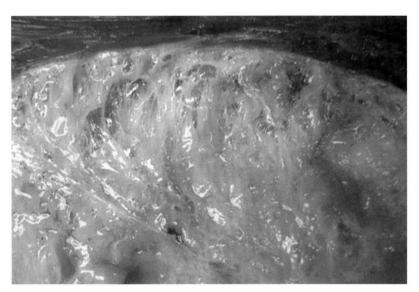

Figure 5-24 Interstitial emphysema, gross
Air leaking from the lung has produced clear bubbles of gas within subcutaneous adipose tissue of the chest wall, as shown here with skeletal muscle at the top. Entrance of air into the connective tissue of the lung, mediastinum, or subcutaneous tissue produces interstitial emphysema. The term *pulmonary interstitial emphysema* (PIE) is employed when air leaks within the lung into peribronchovascular sheaths, interlobular septa, and visceral pleura. Trauma and mechanical ventilation are risk factors for this condition.

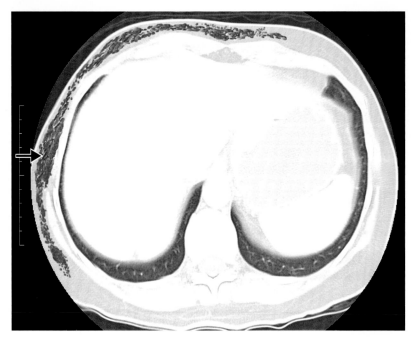

Figure 5-25 Interstitial emphysema, CT image
Note the decreased attenuation (→) of the sub-cutaneous fat on the right and anterior regions, essentially the same density as the posterior lung in this upper abdominal CT scan. An air leak from the lungs after trauma, particularly with tension pneumothorax, or around a chest tube, or positive pressure ventilation, may produce dissection of air into soft tissues. On examination there can be crepitus. It looks worse than it feels. If air dissects into the mediastinum or around large airways, pulmonary function can be compromised.

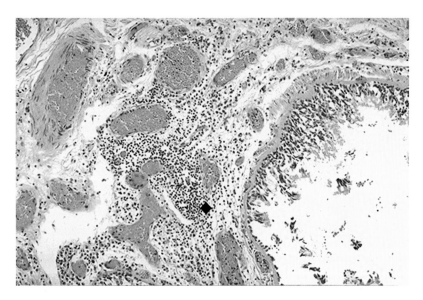

Figure 5-26 Chronic bronchitis, microscopic
Note increased numbers of chronic inflammatory cells (◆) in the submucosal region. Chronic bronchitis does not have characteristic pathologic findings but is defined clinically as a persistent productive cough for at least 3 consecutive months in at least 2 consecutive years. Most patients are smokers, but inhaled air pollutants can exacerbate chronic bronchitis. Often there is parenchymal destruction with features of emphysema as well, and there is often overlap between pulmonary emphysema and chronic bronchitis, with patients having elements of both. Secondary infections are common and worsen pulmonary function further.

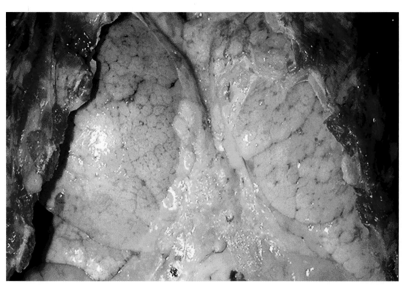

Figure 5-27 Bronchial asthma, gross
These are the hyperinflated lungs of a patient who died with status asthmaticus. The two major clinical forms of asthma can overlap and symptomatically present similarly. With *atopic (extrinsic) asthma* there is typically an association with atopy (allergies) IgE-mediated type I hypersensitivity; asthmatic attacks are precipitated by contact with inhaled allergens. This form begins most often in childhood. In *nonatopic (intrinsic) asthma,* more likely to occur in adults with hyper-reactive airways, asthmatic attacks are precipitated by a variety of stimuli such as respiratory infections and exposure to cold, exercise, stress, inhaled irritants, and drugs such as aspirin.

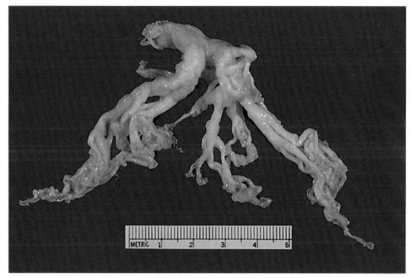

Figure 5-28 Bronchial asthma, gross
This cast of the bronchial tree is formed from inspissated mucus secretions and was coughed up during an acute asthmatic attack. The outpouring of mucus from hypertrophied bronchial submucosal glands, bronchoconstriction, and dehydration all contribute to the formation of mucus plugs that can block airways in asthmatic patients, exacerbating airflow obstruction. The result is sudden, severe dyspnea with wheezing and hypoxemia. A severe attack, known as *status asthmaticus,* can be life-threatening.

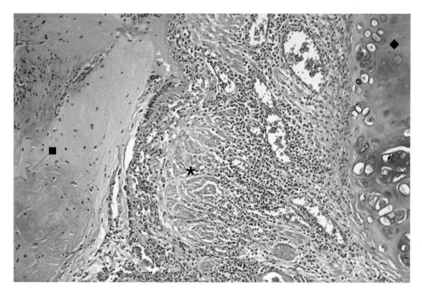

Figure 5-29 Bronchial asthma, microscopic
Between the bronchial cartilage (◆) on the right and the bronchial lumen (■) filled with mucus on the left is a submucosa widened by smooth muscle hypertrophy (★), edema, and an inflammatory infiltrate with many eosinophils. These are changes of bronchial asthma, more specifically, atopic asthma from type I hypersensitivity to allergens. Sensitization to inhaled allergens promotes a subtype 2 helper T-cell (T_H2) immune response with release of IL-4 and IL-5 promoting B-cell IgE production and eosinophil infiltration and activation. The peripheral blood eosinophil count and/or sputum eosinophils can be increased.

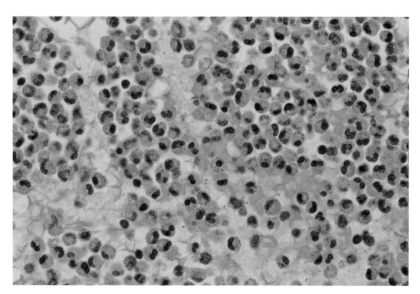

Figure 5-30 Bronchial asthma, microscopic
At high magnification, the numerous eosinophils are prominent from their bright-red cytoplasmic granules in this case of bronchial asthma. The two major clinical forms of asthma, atopic and nonatopic, can overlap in symptoms and pathologic findings. In the early phase of an acute atopic asthmatic attack, there is cross-linking by allergens of IgE bound to mast cells, causing degranulation with release of biogenic amines and cytokines producing an immediate response in minutes with bronchoconstriction, edema, and mucus production. A late phase develops over hours from leukocyte infiltration with continued edema and mucus production.

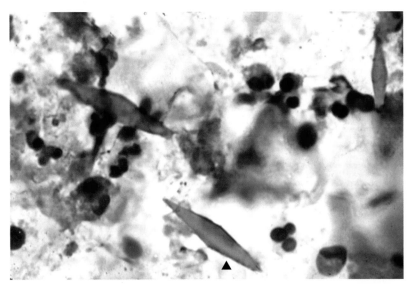

Figure 5-31 Bronchial asthma, microscopic
Sputum analysis with an acute asthmatic episode may reveal Charcot-Leiden crystals (▲) derived from breakdown of eosinophil granules. Pharmacologic therapies used emergently to treat asthma include short-acting β-adrenergic agonists, such as albuterol, and longer-acting agents such as salmeterol. Theophylline, a methylxanthine, promotes bronchodilation by increasing cyclic adenosine monophosphate (cAMP), whereas anticholinergics, such as tiotropium, also produce bronchodilation. Long-term asthma control includes use of glucocorticoids, leukotriene inhibitors such as zileuton, receptor antagonists such as montelukast, and mast cell–stabilizing agents such as cromolyn sodium.

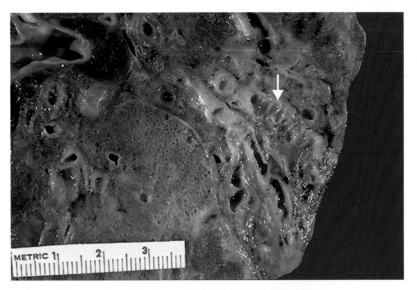

Figure 5-32 Bronchiectasis, gross
This focal area of dilated bronchi (↓) is typical of a less common form of obstructive lung disease. Bronchiectasis tends to be a localized process associated with diseases such as pulmonary neoplasms and aspirated foreign bodies that block a portion of the airways, leading to obstruction with distal airway distention mediated by inflammation and airway destruction. Widespread bronchiectasis is more typical in patients with cystic fibrosis, who have recurrent infections and obstruction of airways by mucus plugs throughout the lungs. A rare cause is primary ciliary dyskinesia, seen with Kartagener syndrome.

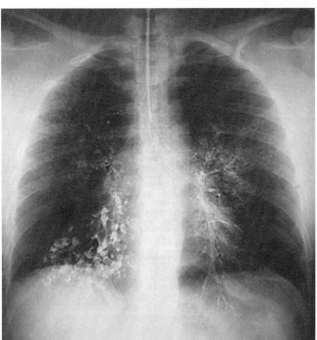

Figure 5-33 Bronchiectasis, chest radiograph
This bronchogram shows saccular bronchiectasis involving the right lower lobe. The bright contrast material fills dilated bronchi, giving them a saccular outline. Bronchiectasis occurs with ongoing obstruction or infection with inflammation and destruction of bronchi so that there is permanent bronchial dilation. When these dilated bronchi are present, the patient is predisposed to recurrent infections because of the stasis in these airways. Copious purulent sputum production with cough is a common clinical manifestation. There is a risk for sepsis and dissemination of the infection elsewhere. In patients with severe, widespread bronchiectasis, cor pulmonale can occur.

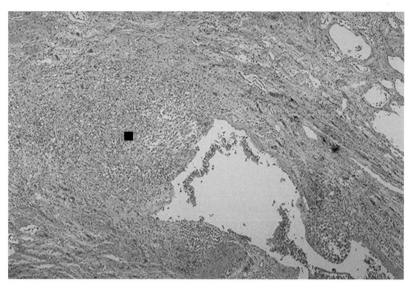

Figure 5-34 Bronchiectasis, microscopic

The mid and lower portion of this photomicrograph shows a dilated bronchus in which the mucosa and bronchial wall are not seen clearly because of the necrotizing inflammation (■) with tissue destruction. Bronchiectasis is not a specific disease, but a consequence of another disease process that destroys airways. Innate immune defense from normal structure and function is compromised.

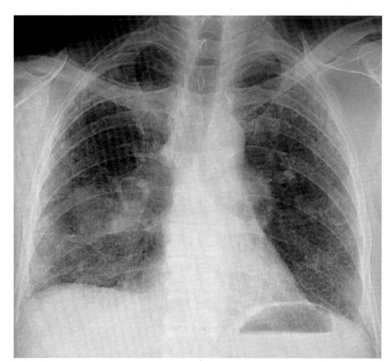

Figure 5-35 Idiopathic pulmonary fibrosis, radiograph

There are increased brighter interstitial markings in all lung fields as a consequence of idiopathic pulmonary fibrosis (IPF; usual interstitial pneumonitis [UIP]). Affected patients have continuing loss of lung volumes; pulmonary function studies show reduced forced vital capacity (FVC) and forced expiratory volume at 1 second (FEV$_1$). Because both are reduced, the FVC/FEV$_1$ ratio generally remains unchanged. These reductions are typically proportional with restrictive lung diseases such as IPF. This disease is probably mediated by an inflammatory response to alveolar wall injury, but the inciting event in IPF is unknown. Patients may survive weeks to years, depending on the severity, with eventual end-stage honeycomb fibrosis.

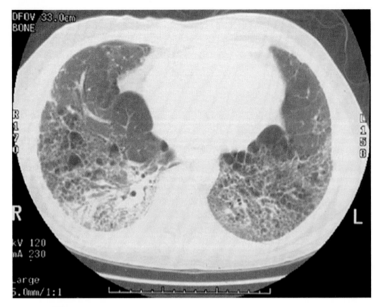

Figure 5-36 Idiopathic pulmonary fibrosis, CT image
This chest CT scan in lung window mode shows very prominent bright interstitial markings in the posterior lung bases. There are also smaller darker lucent areas that represent honeycomb change, a characteristic feature of *usual interstitial pneumonitis,* a descriptive term for an idiopathic and progressive restrictive lung disease that can affect middle-aged individuals with progressive dyspnea, hypoxemia, and cyanosis. Patients develop pulmonary hypertension and cor pulmonale as a result. Some familial forms of IPF are associated with telomerase gene defects. The term *nonspecific interstitial pneumonia* is reserved for cases with less severe restrictive disease and microscopic findings that include either more pronounced chronic inflammation or fibrosis at the same stage of development.

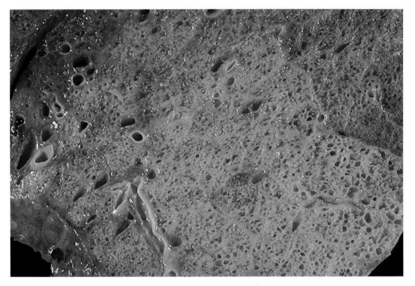

Figure 5-37 Honeycomb change, gross
Regardless of the cause of restrictive lung diseases, many eventually lead to extensive pulmonary interstitial fibrosis. The gross appearance shown here in a patient with organizing DAD is known as "honeycomb lung" because of the appearance of the irregular residual small dilated airspaces between bands of dense fibrous interstitial connective tissue. The lung compliance is markedly diminished so that patients receiving mechanical ventilation require increasing positive end-expiratory pressure (PEEP), predisposing them to airway rupture and development of interstitial emphysema.

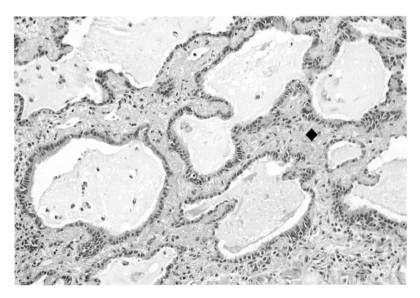

Figure 5-38 Honeycomb change, microscopic
There is dense fibrous connective tissue (◆) surrounding residual airspaces filled with pink proteinaceous fluid. These remaining airspaces have become dilated and lined with metaplastic bronchiolar epithelium as shown here. This produces marked diffusion block to gas exchange. Vital capacity as well as residual volume both become diminished with this restrictive, interstitial lung disease.

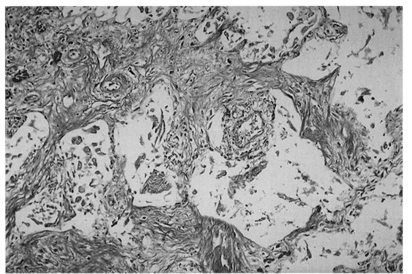

Figure 5-39 Interstitial fibrosis, microscopic
A trichrome stain highlights in blue the collagenous interstitial connective tissue of pulmonary fibrosis. The extent of the fibrosis determines the severity of disease, which is marked by progressively worsening dyspnea. The alveolitis that produces fibroblast proliferation and collagen deposition is progressive over time. If such patients are intubated and given mechanical ventilation, just as in the case of severe chronic obstructive pulmonary disease, it is unlikely that they can be extubated. It is crucial to determine patient advance directives for medical care.

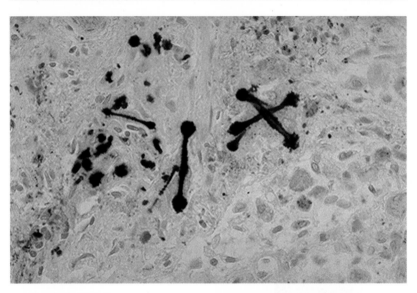

Figure 5-40 Ferruginous bodies, microscopic
The cause of interstitial lung disease is apparent here as asbestosis. The inhaled long, thin object known as an *asbestos fiber* becomes coated with iron and calcium, then is called a *ferruginous body,* several of which are seen here with a Prussian blue iron stain. Ingestion of these fibers by macrophages sets off a fibrogenic response through release of cytokine growth factors that promote continued collagen deposition by fibroblasts. Some houses, business locations, and ships still contain construction materials with asbestos, particularly insulation, so care must be taken to prevent inhalation of asbestos fibers during remodeling or reconstruction.

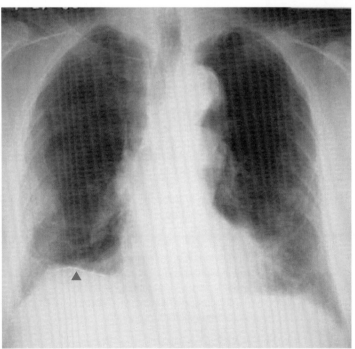

Figure 5-41 Pneumoconiosis, radiograph
This PA chest radiograph shows interstitial fibrosis with irregular infiltrates. A left and a right pleural plaque (▲) with calcification are present. Significant exposure to asbestos fibers in inhaled dusts has occurred. The fibers are phagocytized by macrophages, which secrete cytokines such as transforming growth factor–β (TGF-β), which can activate fibroblasts that produce collagenous fibrosis that increases over time. The amount of dust inhaled and the length of exposure determine the severity of disease. Patients may remain asymptomatic for years until progressive massive fibrosis reduces vital capacity, and there is onset of dyspnea.

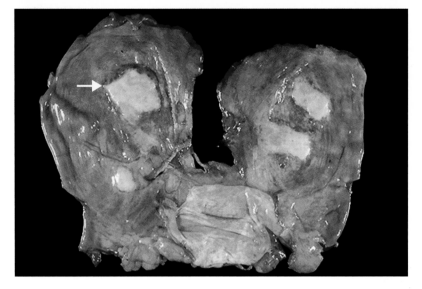

Figure 5-42 Pleural fibrous plaques, gross
Seen here on the pleural aspects of the diaphragmatic leaves are several tan-white pleural plaques (→) typical of pneumoconioses and of asbestosis in particular. Chronic inflammation induced by the inhaled dust particles results in fibrogenesis.

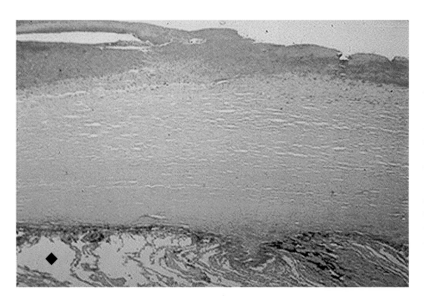

Figure 5-43 Pleural fibrous plaque, microscopic
This fibrous pleural plaque is composed of dense laminated layers of collagen that give a pink appearance with H&E staining and a white-to-tan appearance grossly. Adjacent lung tissue is seen below (◆). Progressive pulmonary fibrosis leads to restrictive lung disease. Reduction in pulmonary vasculature leads to pulmonary hypertension and cor pulmonale with subsequent right-sided congestive heart failure manifested by peripheral dependent edema, hepatic congestion, and body cavity effusions.

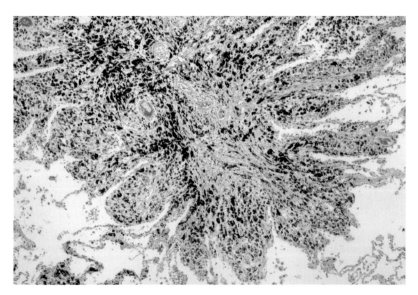

Figure 5-44 Coal worker's pneumoconiosis, microscopic
Anthracotic pigment deposition in the lung is common but ordinarily is not fibrogenic because the amount of inhaled carbonaceous dusts from environmental air pollution is not large. Smokers have more anthracotic pigmentation because of tobacco smoke tar but still do not have significant disease from the carbonaceous pigment. Massive amounts of inhaled particles (as in black lung disease in coal miners), elicit a fibrogenic response to produce coal worker's pneumoconiosis with the coal macule seen here, accompanied by progressive massive fibrosis. There is no increased risk for lung cancer.

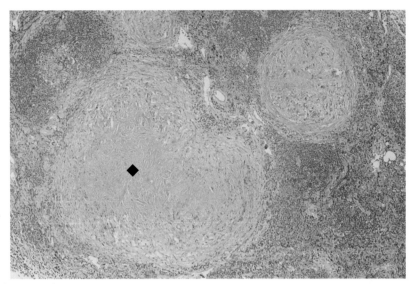

Figure 5-45 Silicosis, microscopic

The most common pneumoconiosis is silicosis. There is an interstitial pattern of disease with eventual development of larger silicotic nodules (◆) that can become confluent. The silicotic nodules shown here are composed mainly of bundles of interlacing pale pink collagen, and there is a surrounding inflammatory reaction. A greater degree of exposure to silica and an increasing length of exposure determine the amount of silicotic nodule formation and the degree of restrictive lung disease, which is progressive and irreversible. Silicosis increases the risk for lung carcinoma about twofold.

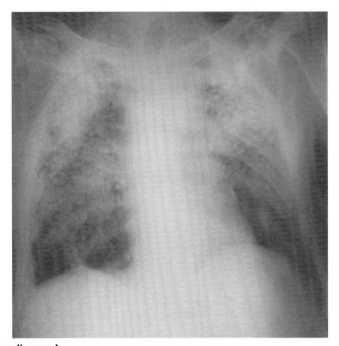

Figure 5-46 Pneumoconiosis, radiograph

This chest radiograph shows so many bright, irregularly shaped silicotic nodules, mainly in the upper lung fields, that have become confluent (progressive massive fibrosis) and have resulted in severe restrictive lung disease. This patient became severely dyspneic. All lung volumes are diminished on spirometry. Occupations such as mining and construction with dust exposure but without proper respiratory protection put workers at risk for pneumoconiosis. The most common form of pneumoconiosis is silicosis. Inhaled silica crystals are phagocytosed by macrophages and activate the inflammasome, leading to the release of inflammatory mediators, particularly IL-1 and IL-18.

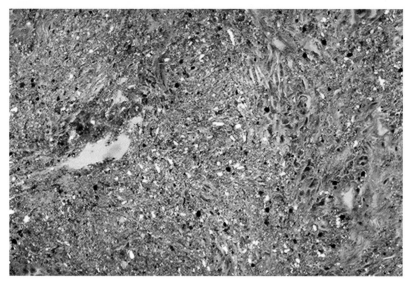

Figure 5-47 Silica crystals, microscopic
By polarized light microscopy, one can visualize one cause for pneumoconioses—silica crystals. Bright white polarizable crystals of varying sizes are shown here. The silica crystals that are inhaled and reach the alveoli are ingested by macrophages, which secrete cytokines to induce a predominantly fibrogenic response. Because the inorganic matrix of the crystals is never completely digested, this process continues indefinitely and is made worse by repeated exposure to dusts containing silicates. The result is the production of many scattered nodular foci of collagen deposition in the lung (silicotic nodules), and eventual restrictive lung disease leading to cor pulmonale.

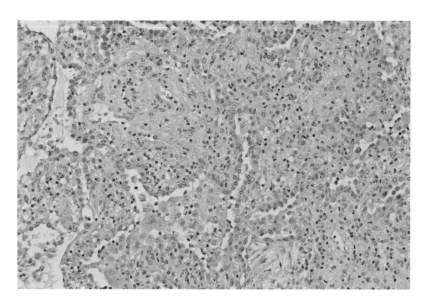

Figure 5-48 Eosinophilic granuloma, microscopic
Localized or multiple pulmonary nodules averaging 0.1 to 0.5 cm in size can occur with eosinophilic granuloma, which is an inflammatory process including a mixture of inflammatory cells with lymphocytes, plasma cells, macrophages, fibroblasts, and some eosinophils. These interstitial lesions appear in a bronchovascular distribution, often causing cough and dyspnea. More than 90% of cases occur in smokers, and the collection of Langerhans cells may be a response to cigarette smoke. Lesions may stabilize or regress with smoking cessation.

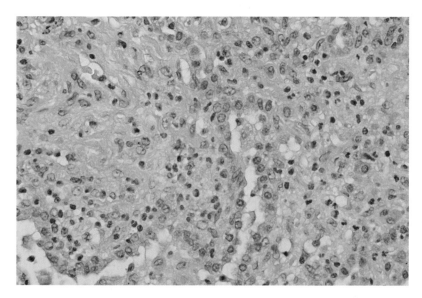

Figure 5-49 Eosinophilic granuloma, microscopic
Eosinophilic granuloma is a form of Langerhans cell histiocytosis (a more disseminated form in young children is called *Letterer-Siwe disease*). The most characteristic cell is a round to oval CD1a-positive macrophage that contains characteristic rod-shaped HX bodies (Birbeck granules) on electron microscopy. Note the prominent eosinophils with bright red cytoplasmic granules (but eosinophils are not always present). Late findings include bronchial wall destruction, cavitation, and stellate scar formation.

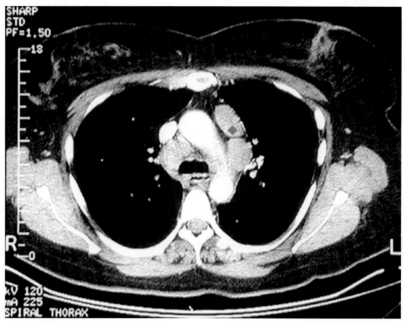

Figure 5-50 Sarcoidosis, CT image
Sarcoidosis is an idiopathic granulomatous disease that can affect many organs, but lymph node involvement is present in 100% of patients, and the hilar lymph nodes are most often involved. This chest CT scan with the bone window setting shows prominent hilar lymphadenopathy (◆) in a middle-aged woman with sarcoidosis. Patients often have fever, nonproductive cough, dyspnea, chest pain, night sweats, and weight loss. More severe cases can lead to restrictive lung disease, with increasing dyspnea along with nonproductive cough. Multiple organs may eventually become involved, particularly eyes, skin, skeletal muscle, and bone marrow.

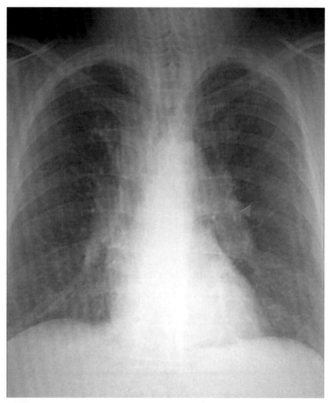

Figure 5-51 Sarcoidosis, radiograph
Pulmonary interstitial fibrosis may be a result of sarcoidosis. In addition to increased interstitial markings, this chest radiograph displays prominent hilar lymphadenopathy from noncaseating granulomatous inflammation (◀). Most patients have a benign course with minimal pulmonary disease that often resolves with corticosteroid therapy. Some patients have a relapsing and remitting course. About one fifth of patients, typically those in whom pulmonary parenchymal involvement is greater than lymph node involvement, go on to develop progressive restrictive lung disease.

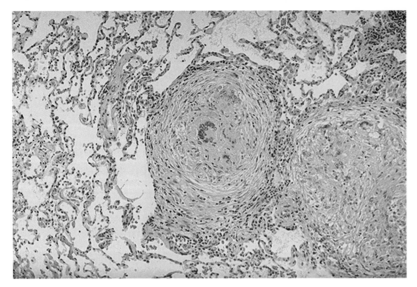

Figure 5-52 Sarcoidosis, microscopic
Interstitial granulomas can produce a restrictive lung disease. The granulomas tend to have a bronchovascular distribution. The small sarcoid granulomas shown here are noncaseating, but larger granulomas may have central caseation. The granulomatous inflammation is characterized by collections of epithelioid macrophages, Langhans giant cells, lymphocytes (particularly CD4 cells), and fibroblasts. The CD4 cells participate in a T_H1 immune response. However, immune dysregulation can occur along with anergy. Not seen here are inclusions within the giant cells, such as asteroid bodies and Schaumann bodies.

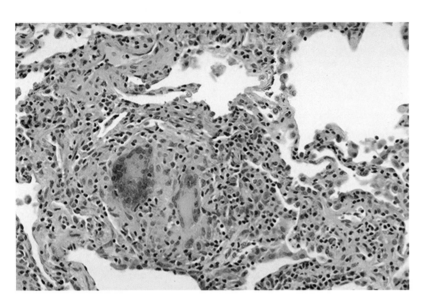

Figure 5-53 Hypersensitivity pneumonitis, microscopic
This type of interstitial pneumonitis is known as *extrinsic allergic alveolitis* because it occurs when inhaled organic dusts produce a localized form of type III hypersensitivity (Arthus) reaction from antigen-antibody complex formation. Symptoms of dyspnea, cough, and fever abate when the affected person leaves the environment with the offending antigen. The disease shown here has become a more chronic, granulomatous type of inflammation, indicative of type IV hypersensitivity. The diagnosis and the offending antigen are often difficult to determine. Radiographic imaging reveals reticulonodular infiltrates. Progression to fibrosis is uncommon.

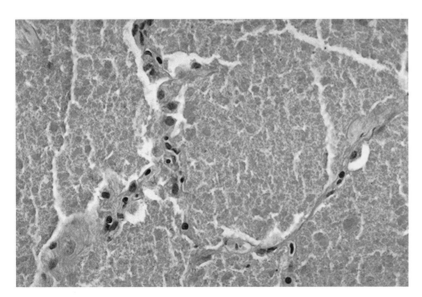

Figure 5-54 Pulmonary alveolar proteinosis, microscopic
Pulmonary alveolar proteinosis (PAP) is a rare disease in which the alveolar walls are normal histologically, but alveoli become filled with a PAS-positive granular exudate, as shown, containing abundant lipid and lamellar bodies (on electron microscopy). Patients coughing up copious amounts of gelatinous sputum are treated with lung lavage to try to remove the proteinaceous fluid. The rare inherited form of PAP results from gene defects leading to a deficiency of granulocyte-macrophage colony-stimulating factor (GM-CSF) receptor signaling involving alveolar macrophages. An autoimmune form has antibodies to GM-CSF.

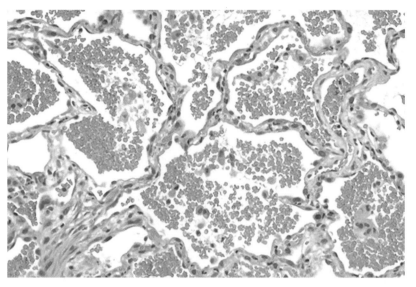

Figure 5-55 Diffuse pulmonary hemorrhage, microscopic
The acute intra-alveolar hemorrhage shown here is a consequence of capillary injury from basement membrane antibody in a patient with Goodpasture syndrome. The glomerular capillaries are targeted as well, leading to a rapidly progressive glomerulonephritis. The target antigen is a component of the noncollagenous (NCI) domain of the α_3 chain of type IV collagen, the α_3 chain being preferentially expressed in glomerular and pulmonary alveolar basement membrane. Circulating anti–glomerular basement membrane (anti-GBM) antibody can be detected. Plasmapheresis can be used as treatment.

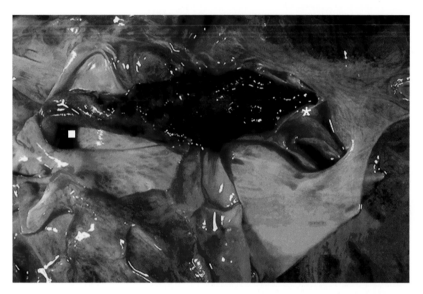

Figure 5-56 Pulmonary embolism, gross
Here is a saddle embolus that bridges the pulmonary artery trunk as it divides into right (■) and left (★) main pulmonary arteries. A saddle embolus can be a cause of sudden death from acute cor pulmonale. This thromboembolus displays an irregular surface, and there are pale tan areas admixed with dark-red areas. The embolus often has the outlines of the vein in which it originally formed as a thrombus. Most large pulmonary thromboemboli originate within large deep veins of the lower extremities.

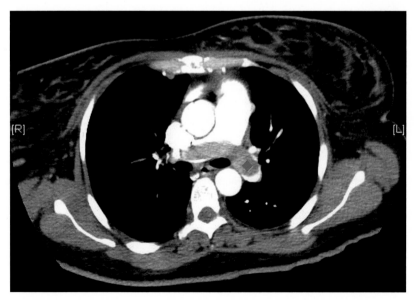

Figure 5-57 Pulmonary embolism, CT image
In many cases of suspected pulmonary embolism, the most definitive, readily available study in hospitalized patients is a chest CT scan. This CT scan shows a darkly attenuated saddle pulmonary embolus (♦) with extension into the right pulmonary artery. Brightly attenuated contrast fills the vasculature. A common laboratory finding is an increased plasma D-dimer, although this test is more useful as a negative predictor of pulmonary embolism when it is not elevated. Risks for pulmonary thromboembolism include prolonged immobilization, advanced age, and hypercoagulable states.

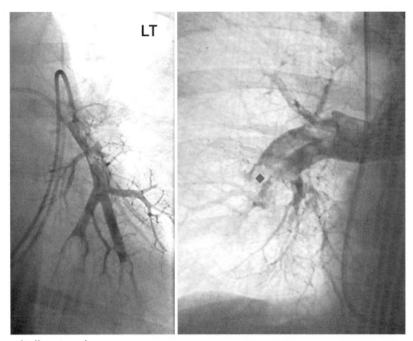

Figure 5-58 Pulmonary embolism, angiogram

These views from a thoracic CT angiogram show multiple pulmonary thromboemboli (◆). There should be contrast material filling pulmonary arteries into the periphery. This patient's risk factors included older age, history of smoking, and immobilization during prolonged hospitalization. Although the angiogram is the gold standard to show pulmonary thromboemboli, a standard CT scan has a high sensitivity for diagnosis. Clinical findings include dyspnea, tachypnea, tachycardia, cough, fever, and chest pain.

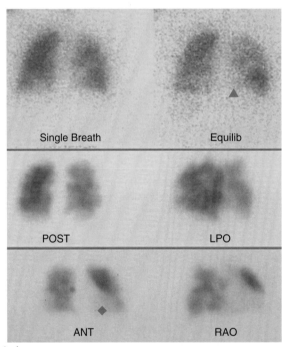

Figure 5-59 Pulmonary embolism, V̇/Q̇ scan

In the *top panel,* ventilation is assessed as the patient inhales a radiolabeled compound that becomes distributed throughout the lung. In this case, distribution appears uniform except for a portion of the left lower lobe in which there is lack of ventilation (▲). Perfusion is assessed after injection of a radiolabeled compound that is distributed through the pulmonary vasculature. In the *bottom two panels,* various views indicate multiple areas in which perfusion is diminished (◆), and these areas are different from the area of decreased ventilation. There is a V̇/Q̇ mismatch that gives a high probability for pulmonary embolism. Because most of these lungs are ventilated but not perfused, giving an affected patient oxygen therapy increases the Pao$_2$ minimally.

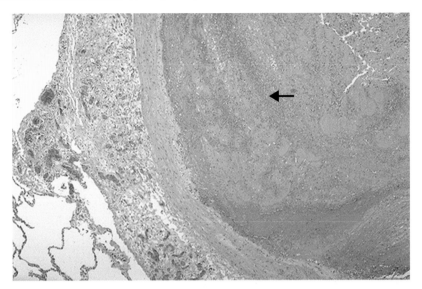

Figure 5-60 Pulmonary embolism, microscopic

Within this pulmonary artery are interdigitating areas of pale pink and red that form the lines of Zahn (◄-) characteristic of a thrombus. These lines represent layers of RBCs, platelets, and fibrin that are laid down as the thrombus forms within a vein. Here the thrombus has become a thromboembolus that has traveled up the inferior vena cava and the right side of the heart to become packed into a pulmonary artery branch. Over time, if the patient survives, the thromboembolus can undergo organization and dissolution.

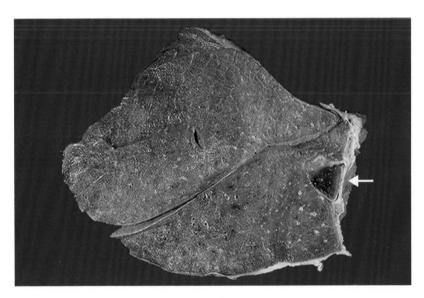

Figure 5-61 Pulmonary infarct, gross

Medium-sized thromboemboli (blocking a pulmonary artery to a lobule or set of lobules) can produce a hemorrhagic pulmonary infarction (◄-) because the patient survives. The infarct is wedge shaped and based on the pleura. These infarcts become hemorrhagic because, although the pulmonary artery carrying most of the blood is cut off, the bronchial arteries from the systemic circulation (supplying about 1% of the blood to the lungs) are not cut off. It is also possible to have multiple small pulmonary thromboemboli that do not cause sudden death and do not occlude a large enough branch of pulmonary artery to cause infarction. Clinical findings include chest pain and hemoptysis.

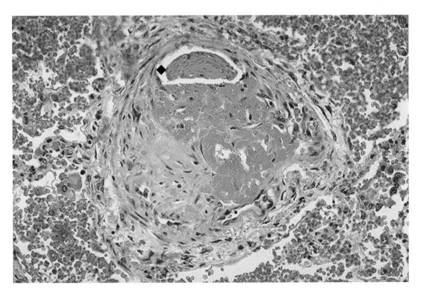

Figure 5-62 Pulmonary embolism, microscopic

Here is a small peripheral pulmonary artery thromboembolus in the region of a hemorrhagic infarct, marked by many RBCs within alveolar spaces. There is partial recanalization (◆) of this blocked artery. Such a small embolus probably would not cause dyspnea or pain, unless there were many emboli and they were showered into the lungs over time. They could collectively block enough small arteries to produce secondary pulmonary hypertension with cor pulmonale.

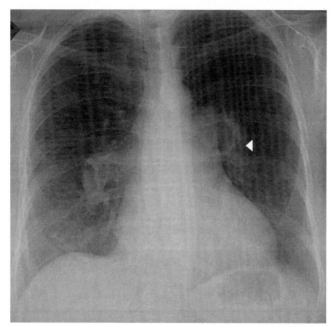

Figure 5-63 Pulmonary hypertension, radiograph

This PA chest radiograph shows prominent dilated pulmonary arteries (◀) that are branching from the hilar regions. The lung fields are clear. This patient had the rare condition of primary pulmonary hypertension, without an underlying restrictive or obstructive lung disease to account for the increased pulmonary arterial pressure. The pulmonary capillary wedge pressure tends to remain normal until late in the disease, when right-sided heart failure leads to left-sided heart failure and impaired left ventricular filling. This familial form of pulmonary hypertension results from mutations in the bone morphogenetic protein receptor type 2 (*BMPR2*) gene. *BMPR2* encodes a surface protein that binds TGF-β. A decrease of BMPR2 increases endothelial apoptosis leading to leakage of serum factors that promote smooth muscle proliferation. Inactivating mutations in the BMPR2 gene may be present in 75% of familial cases and in 25% of sporadic cases of primary pulmonary hypertension.

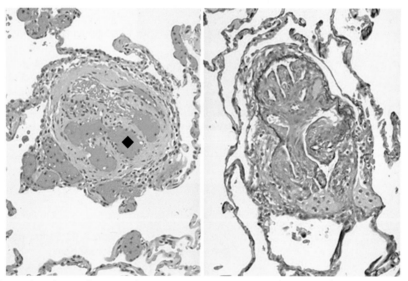

Figure 5-64 Pulmonary hypertension, microscopic

Restrictive and obstructive lung diseases can affect the pulmonary arterial circulation. The loss of normal lung parenchyma leads to pulmonary hypertension, resulting in thickening of the small pulmonary arteries along with reduplication to form a plexiform lesion, as shown here in thickened peripheral pulmonary arteries with multiple small channels (◆), in the *left panel* with H&E stain and in the *right panel* with elastic tissue stain. The ongoing pulmonary hypertension with mean pulmonary arterial pressure equal to or greater than 25 mmHg at rest leads to cor pulmonale and eventual right heart failure.

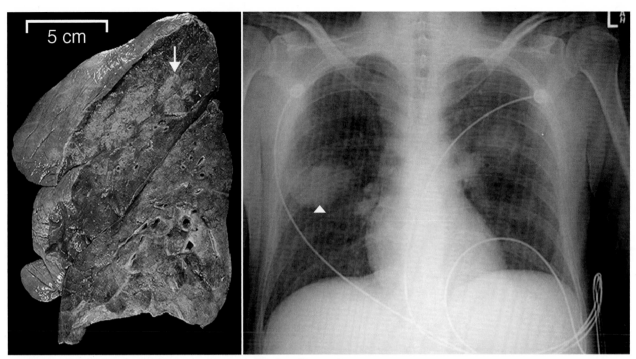

Figures 5-65 and 5-66 Bacterial pneumonia, gross and radiograph

On the *left* are lighter areas (↓) that appear to be raised on cut surfaces from the surrounding lung. Bronchopneumonia (lobular pneumonia) has patchy areas of pulmonary consolidation. The PA chest radiograph on the *right* shows extensive bilateral patchy brighter infiltrates (▲) that are composed primarily of alveolar exudates. The infiltrates seen here are made even denser through hemorrhage from vascular damage by infection with the bacterial organism *Pseudomonas aeruginosa.*

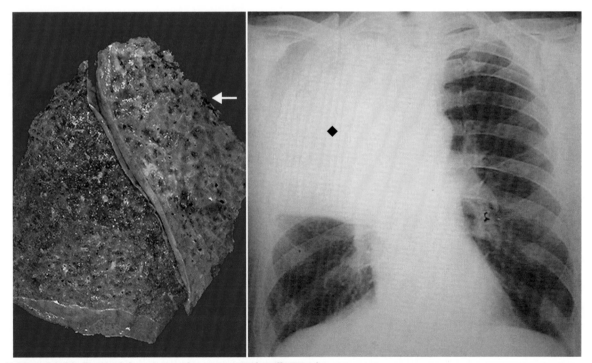

Figures 5-67 and 5-68 Bacterial pneumonia, gross and radiograph

This is a lobar pneumonia with consolidation of the entire left upper lobe (←), as seen on the *left.* This pattern is much less com-mon than the bronchopneumonia pattern. Most lobar pneumonias are caused by community-acquired *Streptococcus pneumoniae* (pneumococcus) infection. The PA chest radiograph on the *right* shows complete right upper lobe (◆) consolidation, consistent with a lobar pneumonia. The mediastinal and right heart borders are obscured by this process. Fever and cough productive of sputum are commonly present. Microscopic examination of the sputum shows numerous neutrophils, and a gram stain often shows a pre-dominance of one bacterial organism.

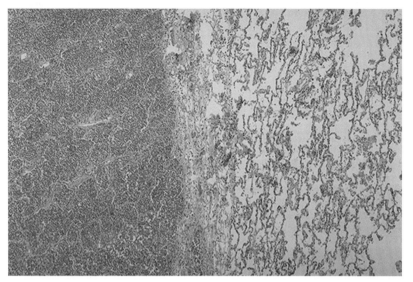

Figure 5-69 Bacterial pneumonia, microscopic

On the left, the alveoli are filled with a neutrophilic exudate that corresponds to the areas of grossly apparent consolidation with bronchopneumonia. This contrasts with the aerated lung on the right. The pattern matches the patchy radiographic distribution of bronchopneumonia. The consolidated areas may match the distribution pattern of lung lobules—hence the term *lobular pneumonia.* Bronchopneumonia is classically a hospital-acquired pneumonia seen in patients already ill. Typical causative bacterial organisms include *Staphylococcus aureus, Klebsiella pneumoniae, Haemophilus influenzae, Moraxella catarrhalis, Escherichia coli,* and *Pseudomonas aeruginosa.*

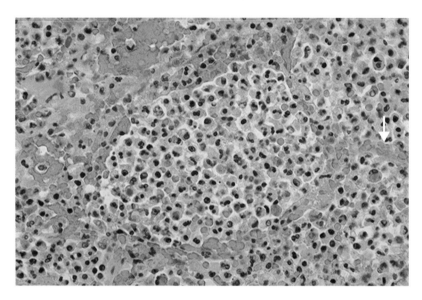

Figure 5-70 Bacterial pneumonia, microscopic

These alveolar exudates are composed mainly of neutrophils. The surrounding alveolar walls (↓) have congested capillaries (dilated and filled with RBCs). This exudative process is typical for bacterial infection. The exudate gives rise to a productive cough of purulent yellow sputum often seen with bacterial pneumonias. The alveolar architecture is still maintained, which is why even an extensive pneumonia often resolves with minimal residual destruction or damage to the pulmonary parenchyma. In patients with compromised lung function from underlying obstructive or restrictive lung disease or cardiac disease, however, even limited pneumonic consolidation can be life-threatening.

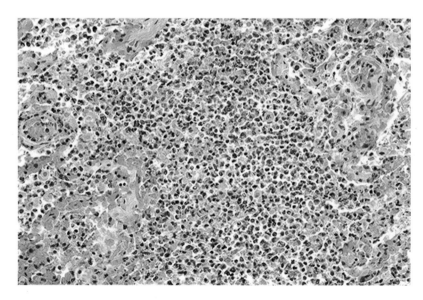

Figure 5-71 Bacterial pneumonia, microscopic

More virulent bacterial organisms or more severe inflammation with pneumonia can be associated with destruction of lung tissue and hemorrhage. Alveolar walls are no longer visible in the center here because there is early abscess formation with sheets of neutrophils and adjacent hemorrhage. Many bronchopneumonias follow an earlier viral pneumonia, particularly in older individuals in the colder months when infection with viral agents such as influenza is more common.

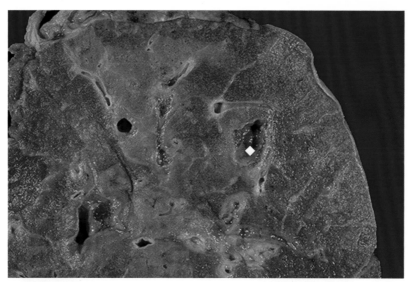

Figure 5-72 Lung abscesses, gross

This bronchopneumonia has several abscesses (◆) with irregular, rough-surfaced walls within areas of tan consolidation. If large enough, abscesses contain liquefied necrotic material and purulent exudate that often results in an air-fluid level on chest radiograph or CT scan. An abscess is typically a complication of severe pneumonia, most often from virulent organisms such as *Staphylococcus aureus,* some pneumococci, and *Klebsiella pneumoniae.* Abscesses often complicate aspiration, particularly in patients with neurologic diseases, in whom they appear more frequently in the right posterior lung. Abscesses can continue to be a source of septicemia and are difficult to treat.

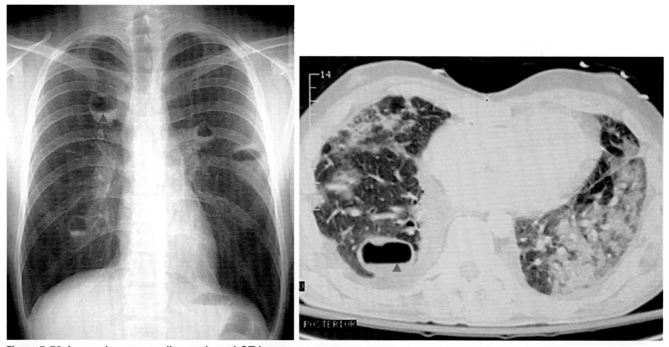

Figure 5-73 Lung abscess, radiograph and CT image

The chest radiograph *(left)* shows multiple rounded abscesses with an air-fluid level. The chest CT scan *(right)* in the lung window setting shows an air-fluid level (▲) within an abscess involving the right lower lobe. Note the adjacent areas of bright, patchy pneumonic infiltrates, which are bilateral and extensive. Also note the indentation of the anterior chest in the midline, a variation known as *pectus excavatum.* Abscesses may develop after aspiration, from antecedent bacterial infections, with septic embolization from venous sources or from right-sided infective endocarditis, and after bronchial obstruction. Affected patients can have fever with cough productive of copious purulent sputum. Spread of the infection with sepsis and septic emboli to other organs can complicate pulmonary abscesses.

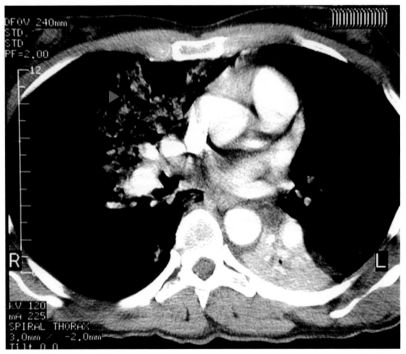

Figure 5-74 Aspiration, CT image

Aspiration of oropharyngeal contents, gastric contents, or ingested food and liquids may be the result of a mechanical disorder of the epiglottis. More likely there is an underlying neurologic impairment such as stroke, drug effect, or Alzheimer disease. Note here the spray of bright flecks (▶) representing aspirated material into the right lung. Because the aspirated material is typically nonsterile, a polymicrobial pneumonia, including abscess formation, may ensue. Anaerobic organisms from the oral cavity such as *Bacteroides, Fusobacterium,* and *Peptococcus* species, are found in many patients.

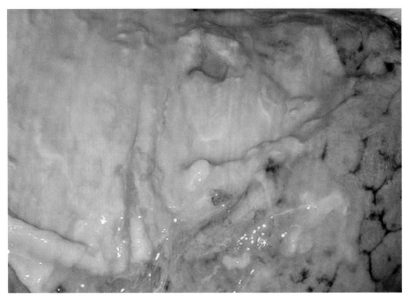

Figure 5-75 Empyema, gross

This pleural surface shows a thick, yellow-tan purulent exudate and adjacent unaffected lung at the far right. A collection of pus in the pleural space is an *empyema.* Pneumonia may spread within the lung and may be complicated by pleuritis with chest pain. Initially there may be only an effusion with a transudate into the pleural space. There may also be exudation of blood proteins to form a fibrinous pleuritis. Bacterial infections in the lung can spread to the pleura to produce a purulent pleuritis. A thoracentesis yields cloudy fluid characteristic of an exudate, with a high protein and a high white blood cell count, mainly neutrophils.

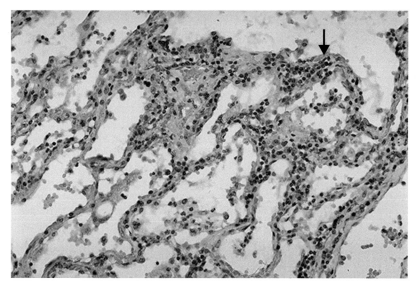

Figure 5-76 Viral pneumonia, microscopic

A viral pulmonary infection is characterized by interstitial lymphocytic infiltrates (↓) without an alveolar exudate and without a productive cough. The most common causes are influenza virus types A and B, parainfluenza virus, adenovirus, human metapneumovirus, and respiratory syncytial virus (RSV), which occurs mostly in children. Cytomegalovirus infection is most common in immunocompromised hosts. Some strains of coronavirus can cause severe acute respiratory syndrome. Viral cultures of sputum or bronchoalveolar lavage fluid may be performed. Alternatively, serologic testing may reveal the causative agent.

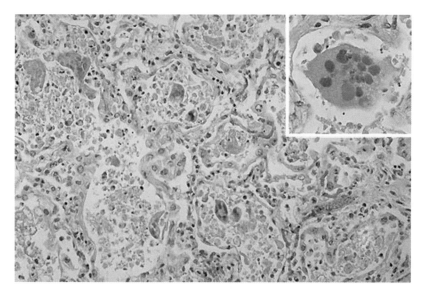

Figure 5-77 Respiratory syncytial virus pneumonia, microscopic

RSV pneumonia in a child is shown. Note the giant cells, which are a consequence of the viral cytopathic effect. The *inset* shows a typical multinucleated giant cell with a prominent round, pink intracytoplasmic inclusion. RSV accounts for many cases of pneumonia in children younger than 2 years and can be a cause of death in infants 1 to 6 months old or older. RSV often leads to bronchiolitis and manifests with low-grade fever, cough, and wheezing. If severe there can be retractions and cyanosis. Most patients recover with supportive care.

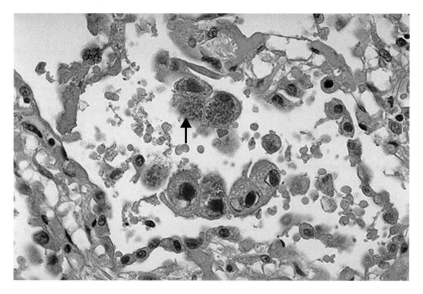

Figure 5-78 Cytomegalovirus pneumonia, microscopic

Note the very large cells that have large violet intranuclear inclusions surrounded by a small clear halo. Basophilic stippling (↑) can be seen in the cytoplasm of these cytomegalic cells. This is an infection typically seen in immunocompromised patients, such as patients with HIV infection. Endothelial and epithelial cells can become infected. There are no characteristic gross or microscopic features of cytomegalovirus pneumonia. Though infection may begin in the lungs, dissemination to other organs is common.

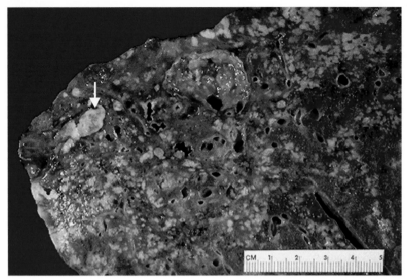

Figure 5-79 Secondary tuberculosis, gross
These scattered tan granulomas (↓) are present mostly in upper lung fields. Granulomatous lung disease grossly appears as irregularly sized, rounded nodules. Larger nodules may have central caseous necrosis that includes elements of liquefactive and coagulative necrosis. This upper lobe pattern of involvement is most characteristic of secondary (reactivation or reinfection) tuberculosis, typically seen in adults. Fungal granulomas (histoplasmosis, cryptococcosis, coccidioidomycosis, blastomycosis) can mimic this pattern as well. This propensity of granulomas to involve upper lobes is typical and helps distinguish this infection from metastatic disease with radiographic imaging studies.

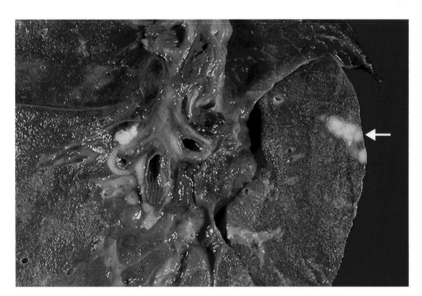

Figure 5-80 Primary tuberculosis, gross
There is a small, tan-yellow subpleural granuloma (←) in the mid lung field. In the hilum is a small yellow-tan granuloma in a hilar lymph node next to a large bronchus. This is the Ghon complex, which is the characteristic gross appearance with primary tuberculosis. In most individuals, this granulomatous disease is subclinical and does not progress further. Over time, the granulomas decrease in size and can calcify, leaving a focal bright spot on a chest radiograph that suggests remote granulomatous disease. Primary tuberculosis is seen with initial infection, most often in children. Diagnosis of tuberculosis can be aided by a positive interferon-gamma release assay, positive tuberculin skin test, and findings on chest radiograph.

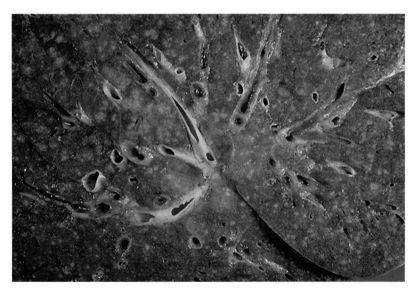

Figure 5-81 Miliary tuberculosis, gross
When the immune response is poor or is overwhelmed by an extensive infection, it is possible to see the gross pattern of granulomatous disease known as a *miliary* pattern because there are a multitude of small, pale tan granulomas, averaging 2 to 4 mm in size, scattered throughout the lung parenchyma. This pattern gets its name from the resemblance of the granulomas to millet seeds. Dissemination of the causative infectious agent (*Mycobacterium tuberculosis* or fungi) may produce a similar miliary pattern in other organs.

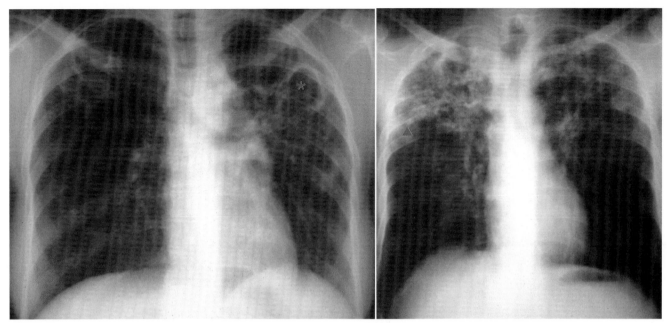

Figures 5-82 and 5-83 Secondary tuberculosis, radiographs

The PA chest radiograph on the *left* reveals upper lobe granulomatous disease marked by irregular reticular and nodular densities and upper lobe cavitation (✱) caused by the central caseous necrosis typical for tuberculosis. The PA chest radiograph on the *right* reveals extensive granulomatous disease of both lungs. The focal brighter calcifications are typical of healed tuberculosis. Other small white calcifications (▲) are scattered, mainly in mid to upper lung fields, seen here more prominently on the right. There can be reactivation or reinfection to produce this pattern in secondary tuberculosis.

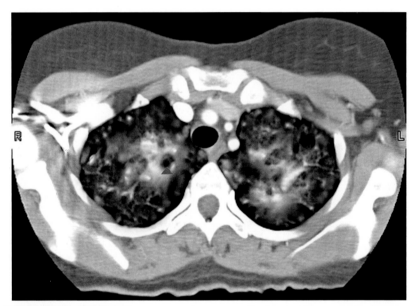

Figure 5-84 Secondary tuberculosis, CT image

The axial view of the upper chest shows cavitary lesions (▲) typical of the reactivation-reinfection pattern of secondary tuberculosis most common in adults. A third of the world's population has been infected with *Mycobacterium tuberculosis,* but just a subset of those persons have active disease. Persons who are able to mount a more rapid and robust TH1 immunologic response, with interferon-γ stimulated expression of inducible nitric oxide synthase in macrophages, are more likely to have a subclinical infection with minimal lung disease.

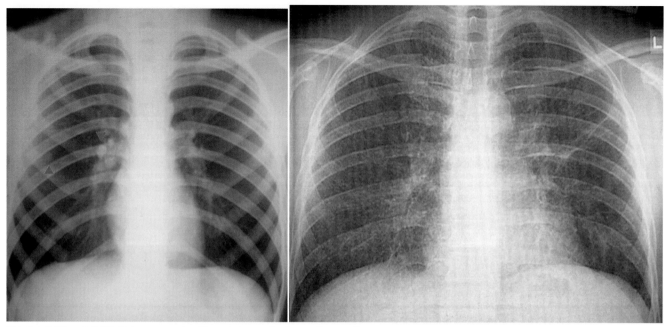

Figures 5-85 and 5-86 Primary and miliary tuberculosis, radiographs

The PA chest radiograph on the *left* is characteristic of primary tuberculosis with a subpleural granuloma (▲) and marked hilar lymphadenopathy (▼). These two findings together constitute the Ghon complex. Most cases of primary tuberculosis are asymptomatic, although marked adenopathy may obstruct proximal airways. The PA chest radiograph on the *right* reveals a miliary pattern in all lung fields. Note the stippled appearance throughout, an effect reminiscent of the pointillist style of art.

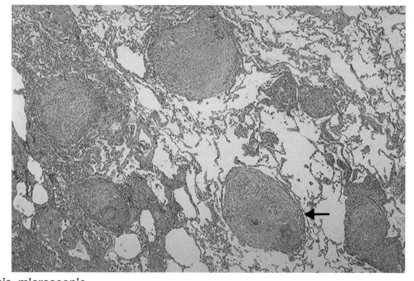

Figure 5-87 Tuberculosis, microscopic

Well-defined granulomas (←) have rounded outlines with discrete borders. Granulomas are composed of transformed macrophages called *epithelioid cells,* along with lymphocytes, occasional polymorphonuclear leukocytes, plasma cells, and fibroblasts. The macrophages stimulated by cytokines, such as interferon-γ secreted from nearby T lymphocytes, may group together to form Langhans giant cells. The localized, small appearance of these granulomas suggests that the immune response is good, and the infection is being contained. This would produce a reticulonodular radiographic pattern in the lungs.

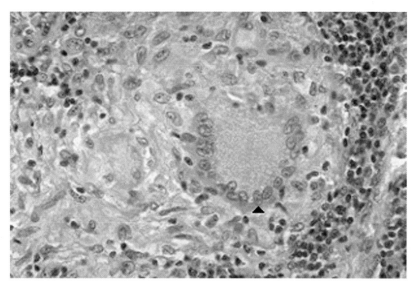

Figure 5-88 Tuberculosis, microscopic
A granulomatous inflammatory response to tuberculosis includes mainly epithelioid cells, lymphocytes, and fibroblasts. This granuloma shows that the epithelioid macrophages are elongated with long, pale nuclei and pink cytoplasm. The macrophages organize into committees called *giant cells.* The typical giant cell for infectious granulomas is called a *Langhans giant cell* and has the nuclei (▲) lined up along one edge of the cell. The process of granulomatous inflammation occurs over months to years (did you ever hear of a committee action that was completed in a short time?).

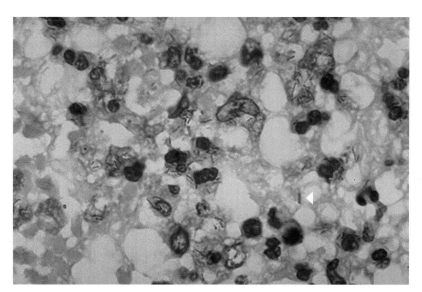

Figure 5-89 Acid-fast bacilli, microscopic
To identify the mycobacteria in a tissue section, a stain for acid-fast bacilli (AFB) is performed. The mycobacteria stain as red rods (◀), seen here at high magnification. The large amount of lipid in the form of mycolic acid imparts this acid-fast property to the mycobacteria and accounts for their resistance to immune cell destruction. Their destruction depends on a T_H1 immune response with CD4 cell elaboration of interferon-γ that recruits monocytes and transforms them into epithelioid macrophages, then stimulates upregulation of nitric oxide synthase within epithelioid cell and giant cell phagosomes. Microscopic identification of AFB in sputum aids in diagnosis; use of PCR amplification of mycobacterial DNA is a more sensitive diagnostic technique.

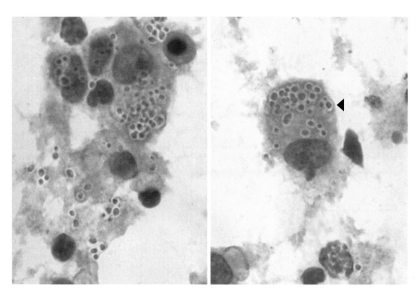

Figure 5-90 Histoplasmosis, microscopic
Inhalation of aerosols from soil with bird or bat droppings contaminated with spores of *Histoplasma capsulatum* can produce pulmonary granulomatous inflammation. Pulmonary infection can spread to other organs, particularly in immunocompromised individuals. Macrophages ingest the organisms, as shown here filled with numerous small 2- to 4-μm organisms (◀). The organisms have a clear zone around a central blue nucleus, which gives the cell membrane the appearance of a capsule—hence, the name of the organism. The macrophages elaborate interferon-γ to activate and recruit more macrophages to destroy these yeasts.

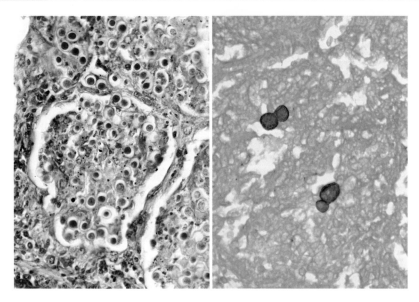

Figure 5-91 Blastomycosis, microscopic
Soil contaminated with the mycelial form of *Blastomyces dermatitidis* may be inhaled, producing pulmonary granulomatous inflammation. The pulmonary infection may become disseminated to other organs. A rare cutaneous form of disease occurs with direct skin inoculation. The 5- to 15-μm organisms exist in the yeast phase at body temperature. Note the broad-based budding, highlighted by the Gomori methenamine silver (GMS) stain in the *right panel*. This organism has a broad distribution in temperate to semitropical areas of North America, Africa, and India.

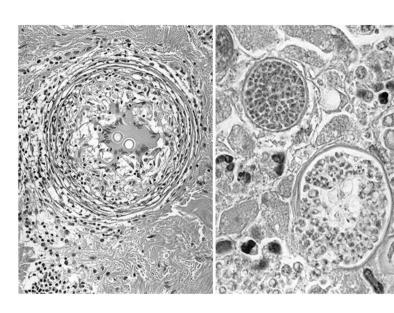

Figure 5-92 Coccidioidomycosis, microscopic
The well-formed granuloma seen in the *left panel* has a large Langhans giant cell at the center containing two small spherules of *Coccidioides immitis*. At much higher magnification in the *right panel*, with a disseminated infection to liver, the thick walls of two *C. immitis* spherules are seen. One spherule is bursting to expel its endospores, which grow in tissues and continue the infection. In the United States, *C. immitis* is endemic to the deserts and dry plains of North and South America. In nature, *C. immitis* exists in a hyphal form with characteristic alternating arthrospores that give rise to highly infectious airborne arthroconidia.

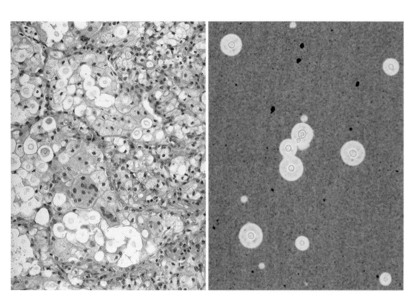

Figure 5-93 Cryptococcosis, microscopic
The *left panel* shows numerous *Cryptococcus neoformans* organisms that have a large polysaccharide capsule, giving the appearance of a clear zone around a faint, central round nucleus. The India ink preparation *(right panel)* highlights the clear capsule around the nucleus. This capsule inhibits inflammatory cell recruitment and macrophage phagocytosis. The India ink preparation is typically performed on cerebrospinal fluid when dissemination to the central nervous system occurs. This fungus is distributed worldwide. Immunocompetent persons may also be infected, more often by the species *C. gattii*.

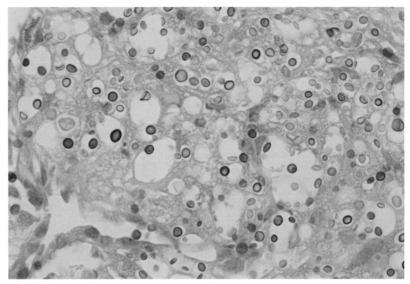

Figure 5-94 Cryptococcosis, microscopic

The bright red organisms and surrounding clear space that is the capsule are highlighted with this mucicarmine stain. Cryptococcal infection with pneumonia can occur after inhalation of aerosols from soils contaminated with bird droppings. These 5- to 10-μm yeasts can become disseminated to other organs, particularly the central nervous system, often producing meningitis in immunocompromised individuals. Immunocompetent persons may also be infected, but less severely and without wide dissemination. The inflammatory reaction can range from suppurative to granulomatous.

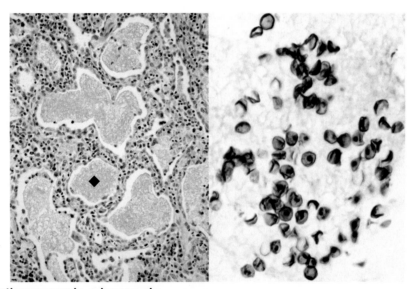

Figure 5-95 *Pneumocystis* pneumonia, microscopic

The granular pink alveolar exudate (◆) of *Pneumocystis jiroveci* pneumonia *(left panel)* consists of edema fluid, protein, *Pneumocystis* organisms, and dead inflammatory cells. Mononuclear cells infiltrate the interstitium. Gomori methenamine silver (GMS) stain on bronchoalveolar lavage fluid *(right panel)* shows the 4- to 8-μm dark cyst walls of organisms appearing as crushed Ping-Pong balls. This infection typically occurs in immunocompromised individuals but is uncommonly disseminated. Patients typically present with fever, nonproductive cough, and dyspnea. Radiographic studies show bilateral diffuse infiltrates, most pronounced in perihilar regions.

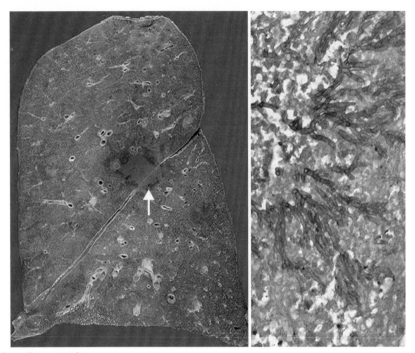

Figure 5-96 Aspergillosis, microscopic

In the *left panel,* a sagittal section of left lung shows a necrotizing fungal "target lesion" with a hemorrhagic border (⬆) invading across the major fissure and into vessels. The 5- to 10-μm thick branching septate hyphae of *Aspergillus* are seen in the *right panel.* Inhalation of airborne conidia of *Aspergillus* species may produce pulmonary infection, particularly in immunocompromised individuals, especially individuals with neutropenia or receiving corticosteroid therapy. Hematogenous dissemination to other organs can occur. *Aspergillus* may colonize preexisting cavitary lesions caused by tuberculosis, bronchiectasis, abscess, or infarct. An allergic reaction to this fungus with a T_H2 cell–mediated immune response can lead to allergic bronchopulmonary aspergillosis with acute features similar to those of asthma and chronic changes of obstructive lung disease.

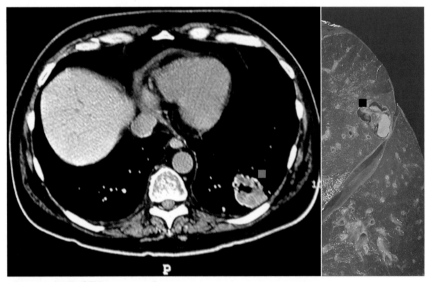

Figure 5-97 *Aspergillus* fungus ball, CT image and gross

A fungal granuloma (fungus ball) may have sharply demarcated borders (■) that give it a discrete, spherical appearance (■) on radiologic imaging. There can be cavitation (note the central dark attenuation within the nodule in the *left panel* corresponding to the air-filled space within the lesion in the *right panel*). Vascular invasion by fungal hyphae can produce surrounding hemorrhage that appears as bright attenuation on CT. Such nodular densities can appear in immunocompromised patients, particularly patients with neutropenia. Virulence factors for this organism include β-1, 3-glucan and galactomannan that can be detected in the serum of infected persons.

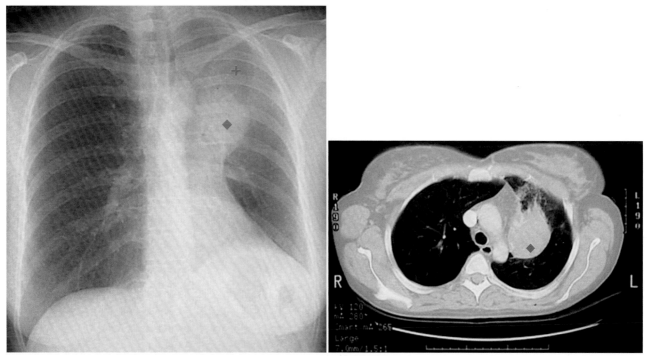

Figures 5-98 and 5-99 Bronchogenic carcinoma, radiograph and CT image
There is a carcinoma (◆) at the left hilum in the upper lobe that has caused postobstructive atelectasis (with mediastinal shift to the left) and a lipid pneumonia, marked by haziness (✛) and infiltrates distal to the mass. Primary lung neoplasms that arise centrally, such as small cell carcinoma, can produce these complications. The chest CT scan shows the same hilar mass (◆) and distal lipid pneumonia (✛), and the mediastinum is shifted to the left.

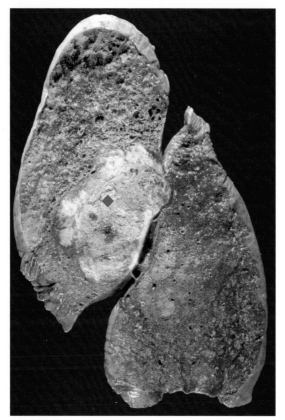

Figure 5-100 Bronchogenic carcinoma, gross
The large carcinoma (◆) in the upper lobe is arising in a lung with centriacinar emphysema, suggesting cigarette smoking as the risk factor. There are patchy infiltrates in the lower lobe representing pneumonia, likely from central airway obstruction by this large mass. There is inferior congestion, likely exacerbated by heart failure. Stepwise accumulation of mutations in genes such as *TP53* and *KRAS* predispose to carcinogenesis. Inhaled carcinogens, as well as radiation therapy, may induce mutagenesis.

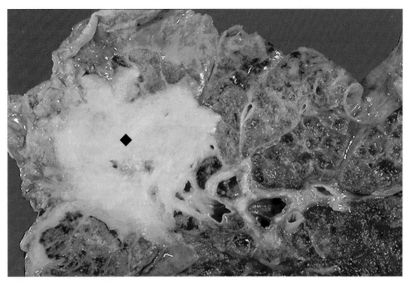

Figure 5-101 Squamous cell carcinoma, gross

This carcinoma (◆) is arising centrally in the lung (as most squamous cell carcinomas do) and is obstructing the right main bronchus. This neoplasm is very firm and has a pale white to tan cut surface. This is one of the most common primary malignancies of lung and is most often seen in smokers; emphysema is also seen here. The black areas represent anthracotic pigment trapped in the tumor and hilar lymph nodes. *TP53* mutations are frequently present in these tumors.

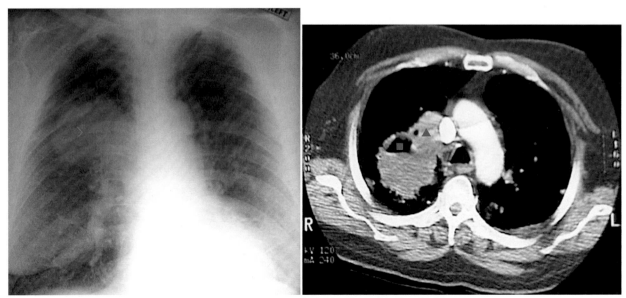

Figures 5-102 and 5-103 Squamous cell carcinoma, radiograph and CT image

Note the appearance of a large hilar mass (◆).Chest CT scan reveals the large squamous cell carcinoma involving the right upper lobe and extending around the right main bronchus (■), invading into the mediastinum and involving hilar lymph nodes (▲). The paraneoplastic syndrome most likely to occur with this type of lung cancer is hypercalcemia from parathormone-related peptide elaboration. This form of lung cancer is strongly associated with cigarette smoking. They can arise in either central or distal airways.

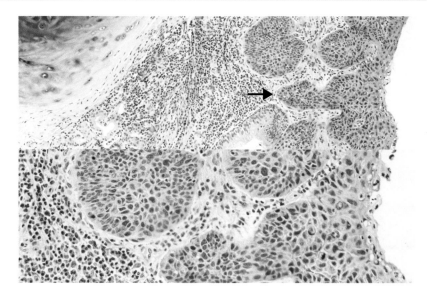

Figure 5-104 Squamous metaplasia, carcinoma in situ, microscopic
Although rarely diagnosed, carcinoma in situ (CIS) of the lower respiratory tract is the precursor to invasive squamous cell carcinoma. The bronchial epithelium shown here has squamoid features and full-thickness dysplasia but has not breached the basement membrane (→). The dysplastic cells extend into submucosal glands. Carcinogens, such as benzo(a)pyrene in cigarette smoke, induce mutational events in epithelial cells, driving carcinogenesis.

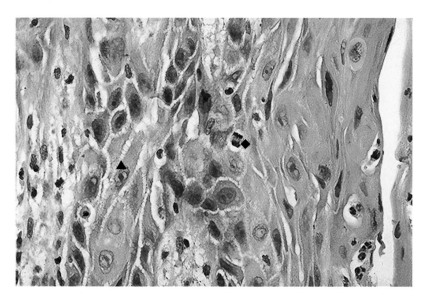

Figure 5-105 Squamous cell carcinoma, microscopic
The cells with their pink cytoplasm containing keratin along with distinct cell borders and intercellular bridges (▲) are characteristic of squamous cell carcinoma, shown here at high magnification. A mitotic figure (◆) is present. Such features are seen in well-differentiated tumors (tumors that more closely mimic the cell of origin). Most bronchogenic carcinomas are poorly differentiated, however. *RB, TP53,* and *p16* gene mutations are often present. The most common paraneoplastic syndrome seen with pulmonary squamous cell carcinoma is hypercalcemia from production of parathormone-related peptide. In 10% of cases there can be another histologic form of bronchogenic carcinoma present.

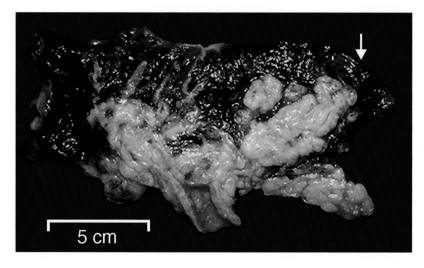

Figure 5-106 Small cell carcinoma, gross
Arising centrally in this lung and spreading extensively is a small cell anaplastic (oat cell) carcinoma. The cut surface of this tumor has a soft, lobulated, white to tan appearance. This tumor has caused obstruction of the left main bronchus so that the distal lung (↓) is collapsed (atelectatic). Oat cell carcinomas are very aggressive and often metastasize widely before the primary tumor mass in the lung reaches a large size. These neoplasms are more amenable to chemotherapy than radiation therapy or surgery, but the prognosis is still poor. Oat cell carcinomas occur almost exclusively in smokers.

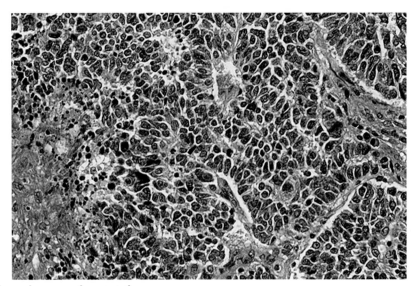

Figure 5-107 Small cell carcinoma, microscopic

The small dark-blue cells (resembling rolled oats; hence "oat cell") with minimal cytoplasm (high nuclear-to-cytoplasmic ratio) are packed together in sheets and irregular nests. The cells often show "crush artifact" from handling the specimen. Mutations in *TP53* and *RB* tumor suppressor genes and antiapoptotic *BCL2* gene are often present. This highly malignant form of neuroendocrine tumor expressing markers such as chromogranin and synaptophysin is often associated with paraneoplastic syndromes from hormonal effects. Ectopic adrenocorticotropic hormone produces Cushing syndrome, and the syndrome of inappropriate secretion of antidiuretic hormone leads to hyponatremia.

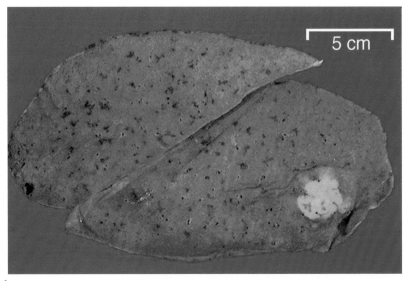

Figure 5-108 Adenocarcinoma, gross

Note the peripheral location of this mass in the left lung. Adenocarcinomas and large-cell anaplastic carcinomas tend to arise peripherally in lung. Adenocarcinoma is the one cell type of primary lung tumor that occurs more often in nonsmokers and in smokers who have quit. If this neoplasm were confined to the lung (a lower stage), resection would have a greater chance of cure. The solitary appearance of this neoplasm suggests that the tumor is primary rather than metastatic.

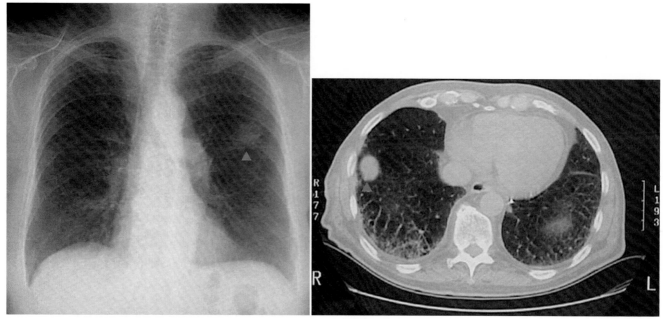

Figures 5-109 and 5-110 Adenocarcinoma, radiograph and CT image

A peripheral adenocarcinoma (▲) appears in this chest radiograph of a nonsmoker. Lung cancers in nonsmokers are rare, but if they occur, they are likely to be adenocarcinomas. The chest CT scan in lung window density shows a peripheral right lung adenocarcinoma that was removed easily with a wedge resection. Adenocarcinomas may have *TTF-1* mutations.

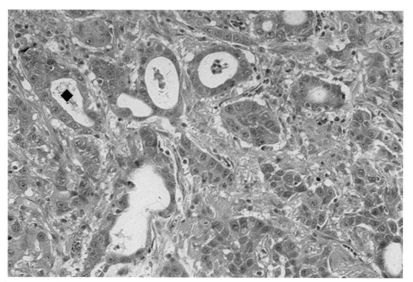

Figure 5-111 Adenocarcinoma, microscopic

The glandular structures (◆) formed by this neoplasm are consistent with a moderately differentiated adenocarcinoma. Droplets of mucin may be found within the tumor cell cytoplasm. Prominent nucleoli are often present. Many bronchogenic carcinomas, including adenocarcinomas, are poorly differentiated, however, making diagnosis of the cell type challenging. From a therapeutic standpoint, a designation of non–small cell carcinoma may be sufficient, depending on the tumor stage. *EGFR* mutations are characteristic in nonsmokers; *K-RAS* mutations are more likely to be present in smokers.

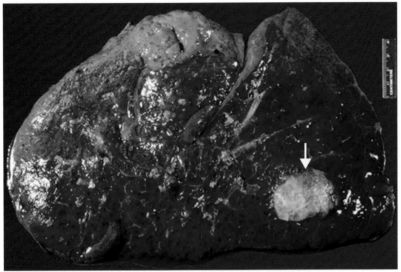

Figure 5-112 Large cell carcinoma, gross
The peripheral lung mass (↓) seen here in a smoker (note the centriacinar emphysema) proved to be a large cell anaplastic carcinoma. This particular type of bronchogenic carcinoma is poorly differentiated, without light microscopic features of either adenocarcinoma or squamous cell carcinoma. Thus, it is a diagnosis of exclusion, when features of other forms of lung carcinoma are lacking. From a treatment standpoint, it is still a non–small cell carcinoma (similar to adenocarcinoma and squamous cell carcinoma), for which the stage is the most important determinant of therapy and prognosis.

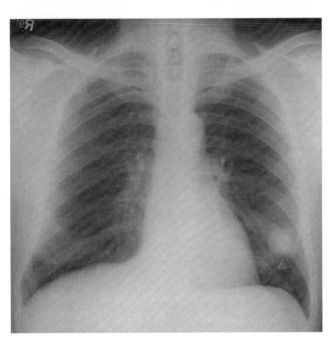

Figure 5-113 Large cell carcinoma, radiograph
This chest radiograph shows a mass lesion (▲) in the left lower lobe that proved to be a non–small cell carcinoma, which was best termed *large cell anaplastic carcinoma* on microscopic examination. Large cell carcinomas are seen with increased frequency in smokers.

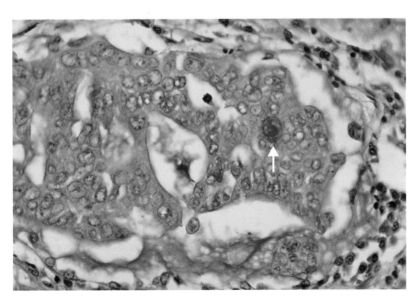

Figure 5-114 Poorly differentiated carcinoma, microscopic
A large cell carcinoma is distinguished by its distinct lack of glandular or squamous differentiation. Many large cell carcinomas are probably adenocarcinomas or squamous carcinomas that are so poorly differentiated that it is difficult to determine the cell of origin. Seen here with PAS stain are droplets (↑) of intracellular mucin that suggest adenocarcinoma. Non–small cell pulmonary carcinomas are less frequently associated with paraneoplastic syndromes than small cell carcinomas. Other extrapulmonary manifestations of bronchogenic carcinoma include Lambert-Eaton myasthenic syndrome, acanthosis nigricans, peripheral neuropathy, and hypertrophic pulmonary osteoarthropathy.

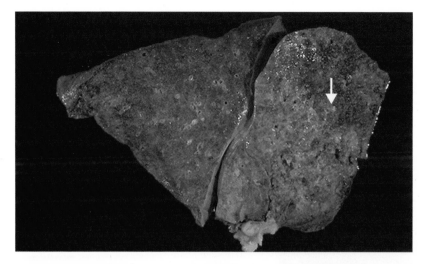

Figure 5-115 Adenocarcinoma in situ, gross
This less common variant of lung carcinoma appears grossly (and on chest radiograph) as a less well-defined area resembling pneumonic consolidation. A poorly defined mass involving the lung lobe toward the right here has a pale tan-to-gray appearance with an irregular border (↓).

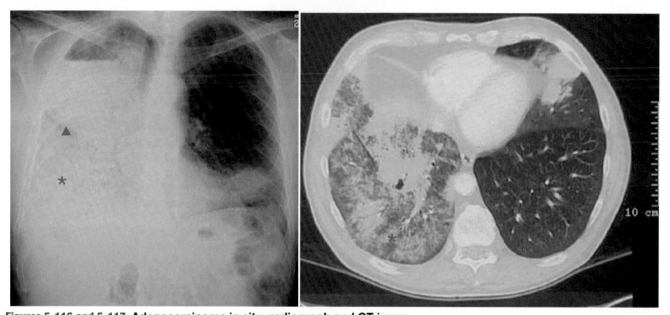

Figures 5-116 and 5-117 Adenocarcinoma in situ, radiograph and CT image
The PA chest radiograph on the *left* and the chest CT scan on the *right* show tumor involving most of the right lung. The extensive spread of the tumor within the lung leads to an appearance resembling areas of consolidation (✱) similar to those seen with pneumonia. There is a loculated pleural effusion (▲) above the neoplasm, as seen on the *left*.

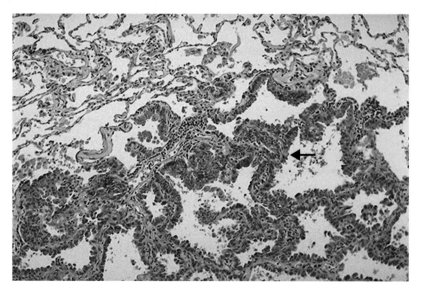

Figure 5-118 Adenocarcinoma in situ, microscopic
Formerly called *bronchioloalveolar carcinoma*, adenocarcinoma in situ is composed of well-differentiated columnar cells (←) that proliferate along the framework of alveolar septa, a so-called *lepidic* growth pattern. These neoplastic cells are well differentiated. This form of adenocarcinoma generally has a better prognosis than most other primary lung cancers, but it may not be detected at an early stage. Nonmucinous variants are usually solitary nodules that are amenable to resection. Mucinous variants tend to spread and form satellite tumors or pneumonia-like consolidation.

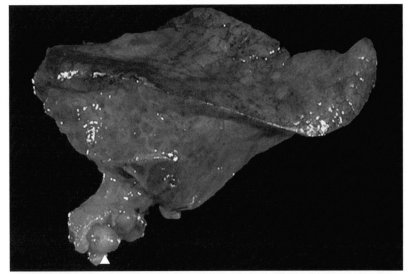

Figure 5-119 Bronchial carcinoid, gross
This lung resection was necessitated by the presence of a bronchial carcinoid tumor (▲) that caused hemoptysis and obstruction with distal atelectasis. These endobronchial, discrete, polypoid masses can occur in young to middle-aged adults. Their appearance is not related to smoking. They are uncommon; they are a form of neuroendocrine tumor that arises from neuroendocrine cells found within the mucosa of the airways.

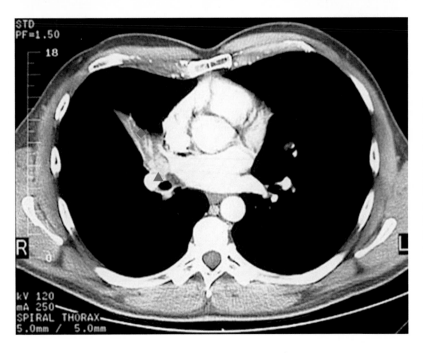

Figure 5-120 Bronchial carcinoid, CT image
Chest CT scan in bone window shows a bronchial carcinoid tumor (▲) that is causing obstruction with atelectasis (◆) of the right middle lobe. Typical clinical findings include cough and hemoptysis. These highly vascular lesions may bleed profusely when biopsied. Other bronchial adenomas are low-grade endobronchial neoplasms that can be locally invasive or even metastasize; these include adenoid cystic and mucoepidermoid tumors.

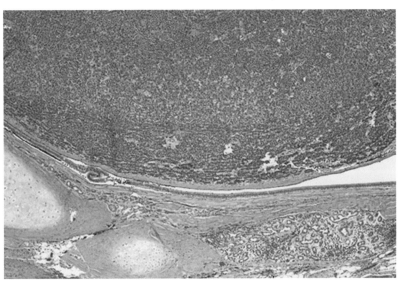

Figure 5-121 Bronchial carcinoid, microscopic
A well-circumscribed mass is shown arising from the bronchial wall and composed of uniform small blue cells in sheets and nests. Because these tumors are of neuroendocrine origin, immunohistochemical staining may be positive for compounds such as chromogranin, serotonin, and neuron-specific enolase. This carcinoid tumor is considered the benign counterpart of a small cell carcinoma, at opposite ends of the spectrum of neuroendocrine tumors of the lung. In between are atypical carcinoids. Bronchial carcinoids usually reach 1 to 2 cm in size before producing symptoms related to obstruction and bleeding. They are unlikely to produce hormonal effects.

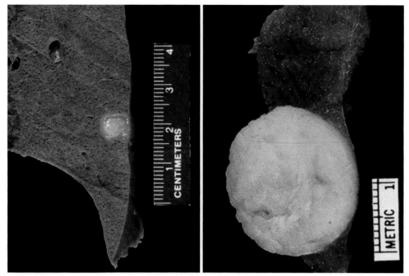

Figure 5-122 Hamartoma, gross

Two examples of a benign lung tumor known as a *pulmonary hamartoma* are shown. These uncommon lesions appear on chest radiograph as a "coin lesion"; the differential diagnosis includes granuloma and localized malignant neoplasm. They are firm and discrete and often have calcifications that also appear on radiography. Most are small (<2 cm). They are true neoplasms with clonal expansion of cells with 6p21 or 12q14-q15 chromosomal alterations.

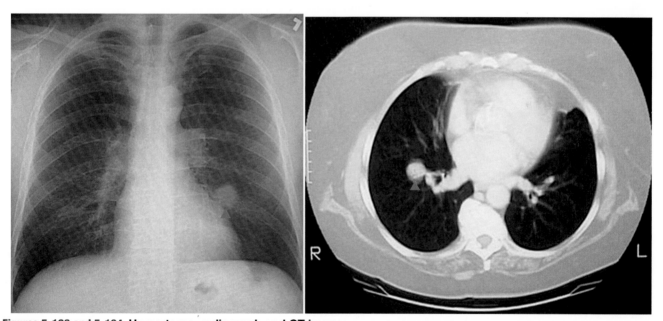

Figures 5-123 and 5-124 Hamartoma, radiograph and CT image

The PA chest radiograph on the *left* shows a discreet coin lesion (▲) that did not greatly increase in size over time. The chest CT scan in lung window density at the right reveals the presence of a small rounded mass (▲) in the right lung of this large individual. The differential diagnosis includes granuloma, peripheral carcinoma, solitary metastasis, or hamartoma. This mass lesion proved to be a hamartoma, a good diagnosis to have—but not a common one.

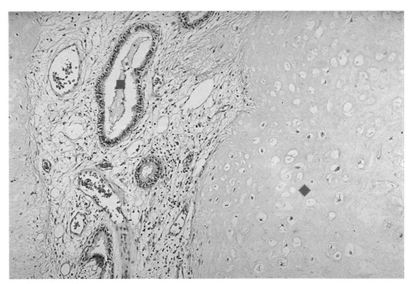

Figure 5-125 Hamartoma, microscopic
This pulmonary hamartoma microscopically is composed mostly of benign elements: cartilage (◆) on the right that is jumbled with a fibrovascular stroma and scattered bronchial glandular structures (■) on the left. The cartilaginous nature of this mass causes it to bounce off a biopsy needle like a Ping-Pong ball. A hamartoma is a neoplasm in an organ that is composed of tissue elements normally found at that site but growing in a haphazard mass.

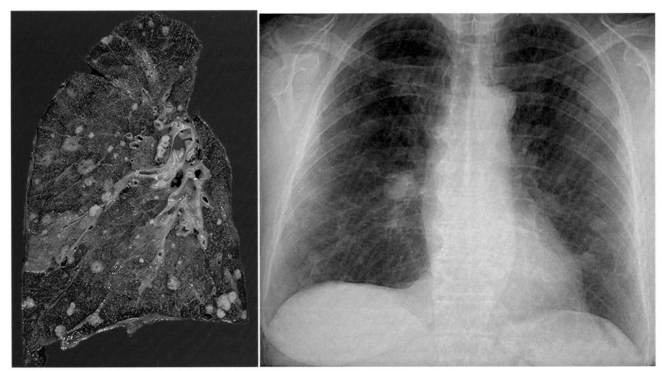

Figures 5-126 and 5-127 Metastases, gross and radiograph
Multiple, variable-sized masses (▲) are seen in all lung fields in the gross and PA chest radiographic images. These tan-white nodules are characteristic of metastatic carcinoma. Metastases to the lungs are more common even than primary lung neoplasms simply because so many other primary tumors can metastasize to the lungs. The hilar nodes also show nodules of metastatic carcinoma. Such nodules are often in the periphery and do not cause major airway obstruction.

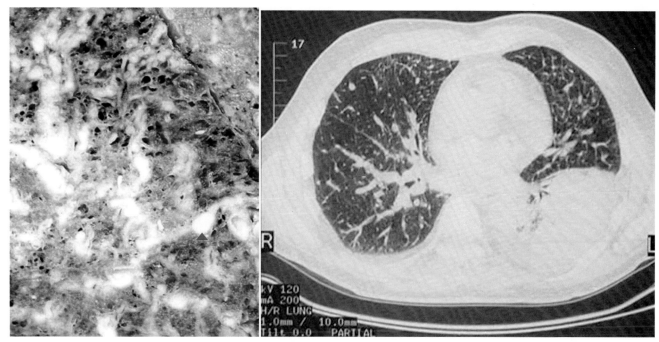

Figures 5-128 and 5-129 Metastases, gross and CT image

The cut surface of the lung reveals linear interstitial markings (▲) and nodules in a case of lymphangitic metastatic carcinoma, one of the less common patterns of metastasis. The chest CT scan shows a diffuse reticular and nodular pattern of involvement by metastatic carcinoma spreading into the lymphatic channels of the lung. There is also a large malignant pleural effusion at the lower left.

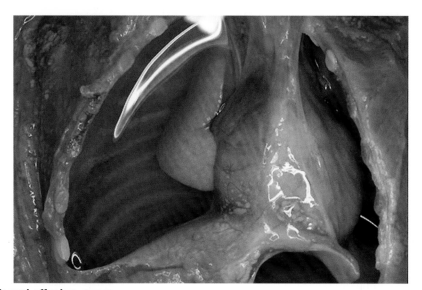

Figure 5-130 Serous pleural effusion, gross

This is fluid collection into a body cavity, or an effusion. This is a right pleural effusion (in an infant). Note the clear reflective, pale yellow appearance of the fluid, indicative of a serous effusion. A extravascular fluid collection can be classified as an exudate or transudate. An *exudate* is a fluid collection that is rich in protein, cells, or both. The fluid appears grossly cloudy. A *transudate* is an extravascular fluid collection that is basically an ultrafiltrate of plasma with little protein and few or no cells, so the fluid appears grossly clear.

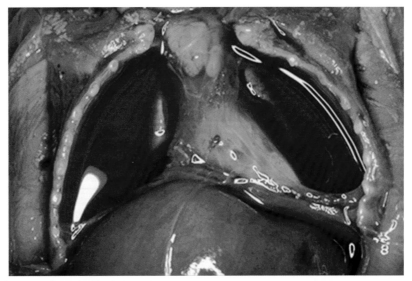

Figure 5-131 Serosanguineous pleural effusion, gross
The fluid within these pleural cavities appears reddish because of hemorrhage into the effusions. Effusions into body cavities can be further described in four different ways. A *serous* effusion is a transudate with mainly edema fluid and few cells. A *serosanguineous* effusion is an effusion with RBCs. A *fibrinous (serofibrinous)* effusion consists of fibrin strands that are derived from a protein-rich exudate. A *purulent* effusion contains numerous polymorphonuclear leukocytes (also called *empyema* when it occurs in the pleural space).

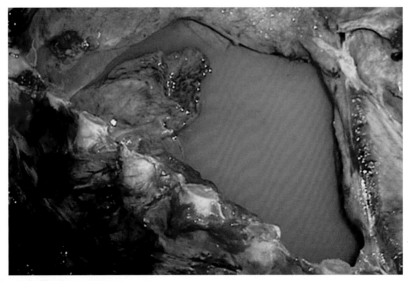

Figure 5-132 Chylous pleural effusion, gross
This right pleural cavity is filled with a cloudy, milky fluid, characteristic of a chylothorax, which is uncommon. The fluid has numerous fat globules and few cells, mainly lymphocytes. Penetrating trauma or obstruction of the thoracic duct, usually by a primary or metastatic neoplasm, may lead to chylothorax formation. In this patient, malignant lymphoma involving the lymphatics of the chest and abdomen led to the collection of chylous fluid. The right lung here is markedly atelectatic from external compression by the pleural fluid collection.

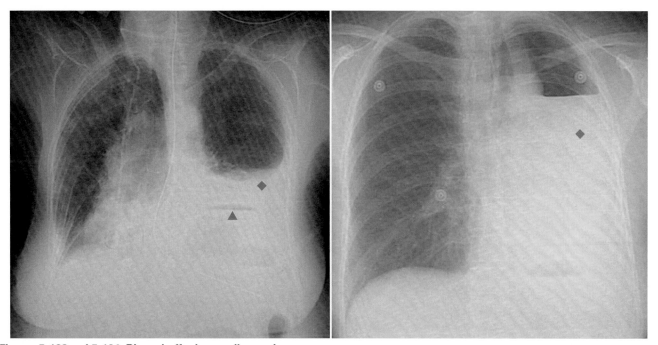

Figures 5-133 and 5-134 Pleural effusion, radiographs

The PA chest radiograph on the *left* shows fluid (◆) in the left pleural cavity in a patient with lung carcinoma causing obstruction and pneumonia. An air-fluid level (▲) is seen in the stomach below the dome of the left diaphragmatic leaf, which is much higher than the right, consistent with atelectasis on the left. The PA chest film on the *right* shows a large pleural effusion (◆) nearly filling the left chest cavity. This fluid collection occurred postoperatively after a left pneumonectomy.

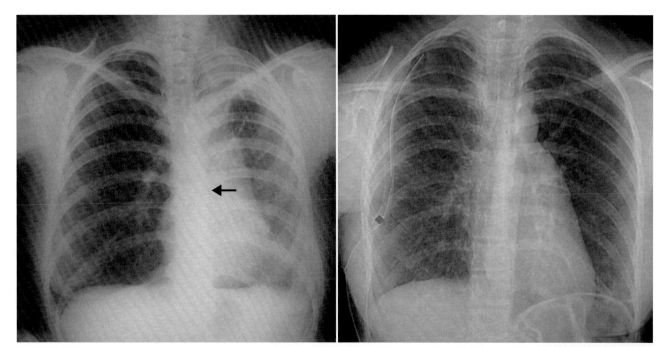

Figures 5-135 and 5-136 Pneumothorax, radiographs

These PA chest radiographs show pneumothorax. Note the displacement of the heart (◄-) to the left. Pneumothorax occurs with a penetrating chest injury, inflammation with rupture of a bronchus to the pleura, rupture of an emphysematous bulla, or positive-pressure mechanical ventilation. Escape of air into the pleural space collapses the lung. The examples show tension pneumothorax, shifting the mediastinum because a ball-valve air leak is increasing the air in the left chest cavity *(left panel).* The radiograph *(right panel)* shows a chest tube (◆) inserted to help re-expand the lung.

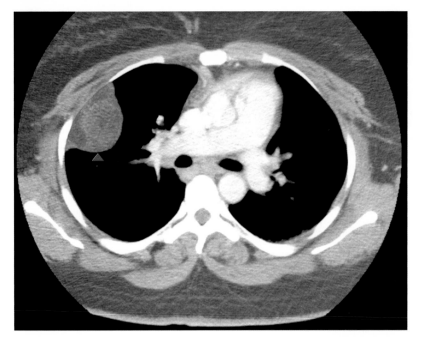

Figure 5-137 Solitary fibrous tumor, CT image
The mass (▲) here at the left pleural surface is localized. It often arises as a pedunculated mass, attached by a pedicle, from visceral pleura, but may originate within lung. These masses are not related to asbestos exposure or other environmental dust. The mass is composed of dense connective tissue and occasional cysts filled with fluid.

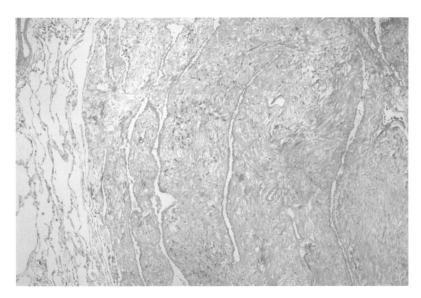

Figure 5-138 Solitary fibrous tumor, microscopic
Microscopically this tumor is typically low grade. The one shown here has a predominantly collagenous pink stroma with little cellularity. Compressed normal lung is at the left. Rarely, there are larger, more cellular tumors with malignant behavior. They are CD34 positive and cytokeratin negative, the opposite of malignant mesotheliomas. Cytogenetic analysis reveals an inversion of chromosome 12 with *NAB2-STAT6* fusion gene that encodes a chimeric transcription factor.

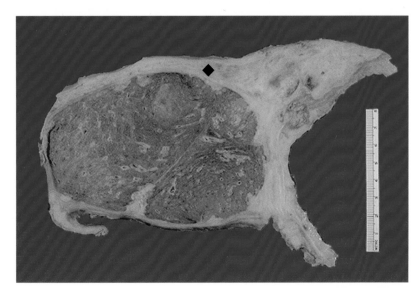

Figure 5-139 Malignant mesothelioma, gross
The dense, white encircling tumor mass (◆) is arising from the visceral pleura and is a malignant mesothelioma. These are big, bulky tumors that can fill the chest cavity. The risk factor for mesothelioma is asbestos exposure. Asbestosis more commonly predisposes to bronchogenic carcinomas, increasing the risk by a factor of five. Smoking increases the risk for lung cancer by a factor of 10. Smokers with a history of asbestos exposure have a 50-fold greater likelihood of developing bronchogenic lung cancer.

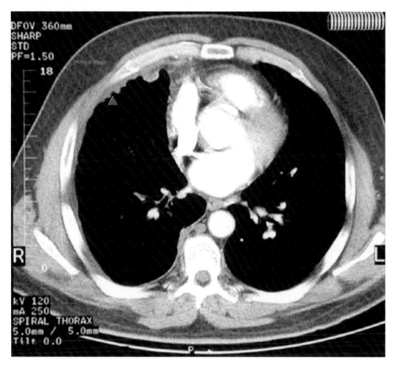

Figure 5-140 Malignant mesothelioma, CT image
Chest CT scan in the bone window setting shows a malignant mesothelioma involving the right pleura, with thickening (▲) and nodularity. This may obscure pleural plaques that may have been present. The neoplasm is seen near the base of the lung. The development of mesothelioma may follow the initial asbestos exposure by 25 to 45 years, and the amount and duration of the initial exposure may have been minimal. Adjacent lung, in cases of more significant asbestos exposure, may have interstitial fibrosis. Asbestos (ferruginous) bodies are increased in number within the lung parenchyma.

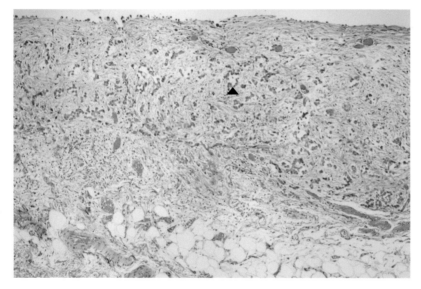

Figure 5-141 Malignant mesothelioma, microscopic
There are either spindle cells or plump, rounded cells forming glandlike configurations (▲) as shown here in the pleura. Cytogenetic abnormalities are often present, as are *p16* and *p53* mutations. Malignant mesotheliomas are very difficult to diagnose cytologically. They are rare, even in individuals with asbestos exposure, and are virtually never seen in individuals without a history of asbestos exposure. In addition to the pleura, other, less common sites of occurrence of this neoplasm are the peritoneum, pericardium, and testicular tunica.

Head and Neck

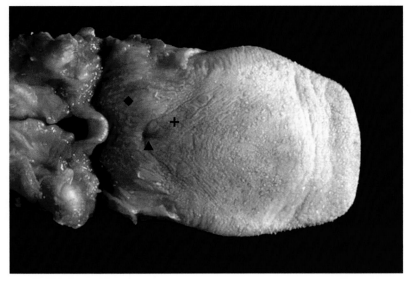

Figure 6-1 Normal tongue, gross
Viewed superiorly, the abundant submucosal lymphoid tissue (lingual tonsil) gives the posterior tongue (◆) a lobulated surface. The small indentation at the posterior tongue represents a vestigial foramen cecum (▲). The tongue surface has papillae. The filiform papillae impart a velvety texture to the upper surface and allow for a scraping function. Circumvallate papillae (✚) arranged in a V pattern toward the back of the tongue have associated taste buds. Foliate papillae at the posterolateral aspects have associated taste buds. Fungiform papillae have a rounded surface and are nonkeratinized to give the appearance of a red dot pattern on the dorsum of the tongue and have associated taste buds.

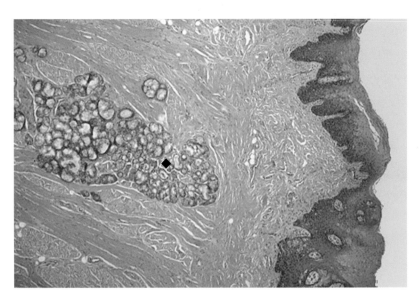

Figure 6-2 Normal tongue, microscopic
The tongue is covered with thick stratified squamous epithelium. The bulk of the tongue consists of the genioglossus muscle with the muscle bundles arranged in three planes to provide movement in any direction. The squamous mucosa extends across the floor of the oral cavity to become the gingiva at the base of the teeth. Scattered throughout the tongue, but more prominent toward the back of the tongue, are minor salivary glands (◆).

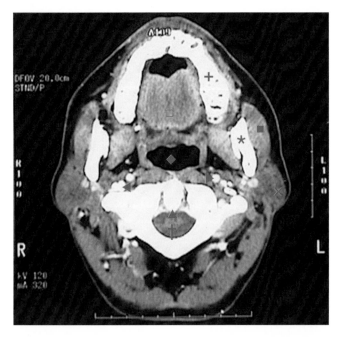

Figure 6-3 Normal head, CT image
This normal axial CT scan of the head and neck shows the relationships of the maxilla (✚) with teeth and nasopharynx (◆), tongue (□), ramus of mandible (✱), masseter muscle (■), C2 and dens (▲), spinal canal (†), internal jugular vein (◀), internal carotid artery (▶), and parotid gland (✖).

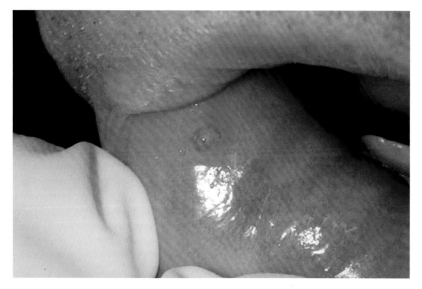

Figure 6-4 Cold sore, gross
The small cold sore shown here on the buccal mucosa just inside the lower lip is the result of herpes simplex virus type 1 (HSV-1) infection. Most adults have had past HSV-1 infection, but it remains latent, only to produce small sores during periods of stress, from local trauma, or with environmental changes such as exposure to cold. This vesicle may rupture to produce an ulcer, which can become secondarily infected. A similar lesion is the aphthous ulcer, or canker sore, which can appear under conditions of stress, local trauma, or hormonal changes, but does not have an infectious cause. Up to 40% of the population have had aphthous ulcers, particularly during the second decade of life. They spontaneously resolve.

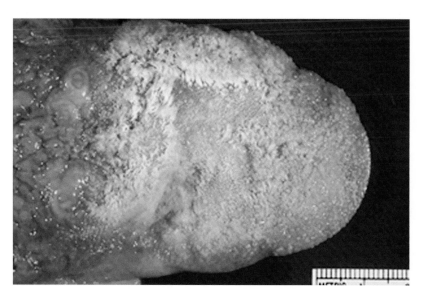

Figure 6-5 Oral candidiasis, gross
The tongue is covered with a tan, matted layer of *Candida* organisms enmeshed in a fibrinopurulent exudate, forming the pseudomembranous form of candidiasis. This can be scraped off to reveal an erythematous base. *Candida albicans* is a frequent oral commensal, present in half of the population; it is normally held in check by normal oral flora. Thrush, as shown here, is most likely to occur in immunocompromised individuals.

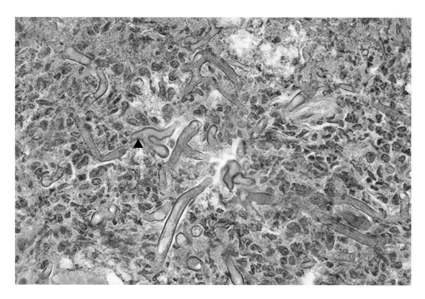

Figure 6-6 Mucormycosis (zygomycosis), microscopic
Note the broad, nonseptate hyphae (▲) (6 to 50 μm wide) with necrotizing inflammation. Infection with *Mucor circinelloides* and related genera *Rhizopus* and *Absidia* of the true sexual fungi (Zygomycetes) can produce extensive tissue invasion and necrosis. Inhalation of airborne spores by immunocompromised individuals, particularly patients with diabetes mellitus in ketoacidosis, corticosteroid therapy, and neutropenia, can lead to nasopharyngeal, pulmonary, and gastrointestinal infection. Spread of these organisms into the orbit and intracranial cavity (rhinocerebral mucormycosis) is a feared complication.

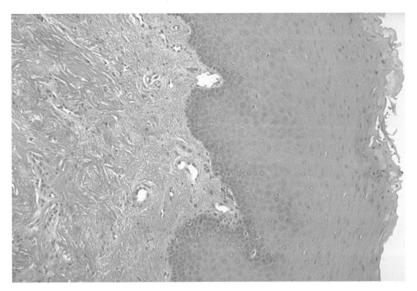

Figure 6-7 Leukoplakia, microscopic
In this excised lesion from the buccal mucosa, the overlying squamous epithelium is thickened (acanthotic), producing the gross appearance of a white plaque (leukoplakia) on the oral mucosa. In addition, the underlying submucosa has increased collagen deposition, leading to the diagnosis of irritation fibroma in this patient with ill-fitting dentures. Although no cellular atypia is shown here, persistent leukoplakia can be a precursor to squamous atypia and carcinoma. In addition to mechanical irritation, use of tobacco, alcohol, and betel nut can predispose to leukoplakia. Areas of grossly red and eroded epithelium denote erythroplakia, which carries a higher risk for malignant transformation.

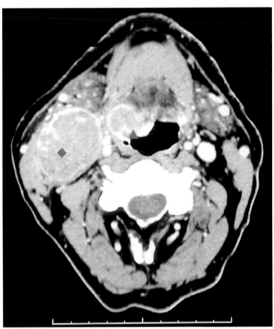

Figure 6-8 Squamous cell carcinoma, CT image
Shown is a prominent mass (▲) involving the right posterior base of the tongue in the region of the lingual tonsil. There is a large confluent mass of adjacent lymph nodes (◆) involved with metastatic squamous carcinoma. The oral cavity, floor of the mouth, tongue, and soft palate are the most common locations for squamous carcinoma to arise, but multiple lesions may occur. Distant metastases may involve lungs, liver, and bone marrow. The major risk factors are tobacco use (particularly the "smokeless" tobacco products) and alcohol abuse. In regions where chewing betel nut is popular, the incidence of oral cavity cancers is higher. Half of oropharyngeal cancers are associated with human papillomavirus (HPV) infection. Chronic mucosal irritation from trauma or infection may promote the neoplastic process. About 95% of head and neck primary carcinomas are squamous cell carcinomas, and these now constitute the sixth most common malignant neoplasm in the world. Mutations of *p16, p63,* and *TP53* tumor suppressor genes are common.

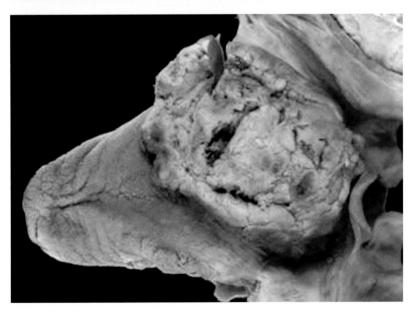

Figure 6-9 Squamous cell carcinoma of tongue, gross
The large fungating mass shown here involving the right posterior tongue has extensive surface ulceration. This large mass led to difficulty swallowing and progressive cachexia. Squamous cell carcinomas may progress from in situ lesions to invasive lesions over a variable time that can range from months to years. Smaller lesions discovered earlier have a less advanced stage, are more easily excised, and have a better prognosis, but most of these oropharyngeal cancers are discovered at a more advanced stage.

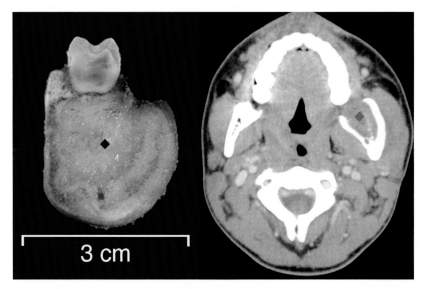

Figures 6-10 and 6-11 Ameloblastoma, gross and CT image
On the *left,* a coronal section through an excised portion of the mandible reveals a mass lesion (◆) that is below a molar tooth. This lesion is slow growing and locally invasive but has a benign course in most cases. The head CT scan in the "soft-tissue window" shows the mass lesion (◆) expanding the left mandibular ramus of a teenage boy. The histologic pattern of an ameloblastoma mimics the enamel organ of the tooth. Neoplasms of a related histologic appearance include craniopharyngiomas of the sella turcica and adamantinomas of long bone.

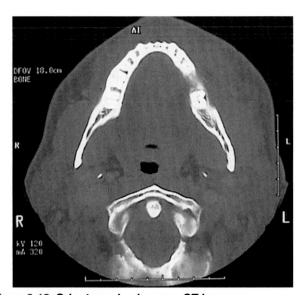

Figure 6-12 Odontogenic abscess, CT image
This head CT scan shows an abscess (◆) involving the first molar of the left mandible. Lack of dental care can lead to serious complications from dental caries. When the tooth enamel is breached, infection can reach the inner tooth pulp and extend down the tooth root to the tooth socket and the bone of the mandible or maxilla. The health of a society is directly proportional to the level of dental care.

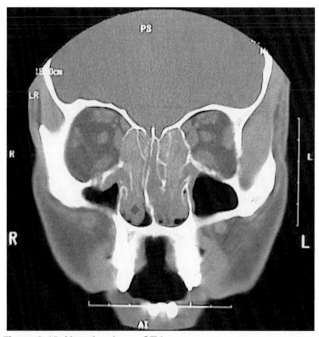

Figure 6-13 Nasal polyps, CT image
These lobulated soft-tissue densities (◆) in the nasal cavities are inflammatory, or allergic, nasal polyps extending into paranasal sinuses. Although benign, they can obstruct the nasal passages and cause discomfort from difficulty breathing and mass effect. The polyps start as local inflammation with areas of edema and enlargement of the turbinates. Patients with such polyps may have a history of allergic rhinitis, or hay fever, from increased inflammatory reactivity with type I hypersensitivity to allergens such as plant pollens. The allergens contact and cross-link IgE bound to mast cells, causing degranulation with immediate release of vasoactive amines such as histamine, which cause vasodilation and fluid exudation. There is also mast cell synthesis of arachidonic acid metabolites, such as prostaglandins, which produce more vasodilation. Mast cell cytokines, such as tumor necrosis factor and interleukin-4, attract neutrophils and eosinophils. Only about 0.5% of atopic individuals develop nasal polyps. The polyps can reach 3 to 4 cm in length and produce nasal airway obstruction.

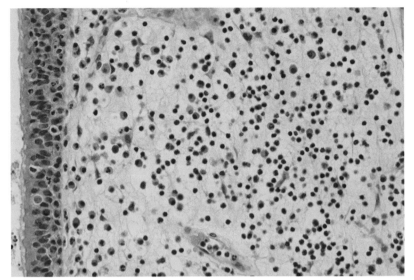

Figure 6-14 Allergic nasal polyp, microscopic
Recurrent attacks of rhinitis may lead to the development of nasal polyps, which may be multiple and measure a few millimeters to several centimeters in size. There is overlying respiratory mucosa at the left, an underlying edematous stroma with inflammatory cells, including the eosinophils, characteristic of an acute allergic response. Neutrophils, plasma cells, and occasional clusters of lymphocytes also can be seen here in the later inflammatory reaction. Such polyps are rare in children and are most often seen in individuals older than 30 years. Sometimes these polyps can become eroded and secondarily infected. Such polyps can be excised.

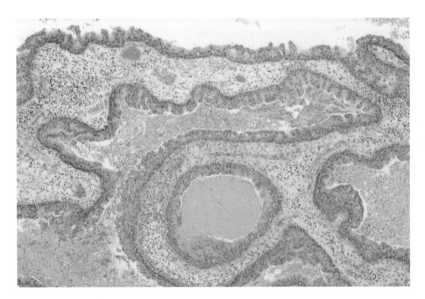

Figure 6-15 Sinonasal papilloma, microscopic
Note the respiratory pseudostratified epithelium overlying invaginations extending beneath the surface as an endophytic lesion. They may arise from HPV type 6 or 11 infection, typically in men aged 30 to 60 years. These benign but locally aggressive lesions arise in the nose and paranasal sinuses and may recur if not completely excised. The exophytic form of sinonasal papilloma is covered by squamous epithelium.

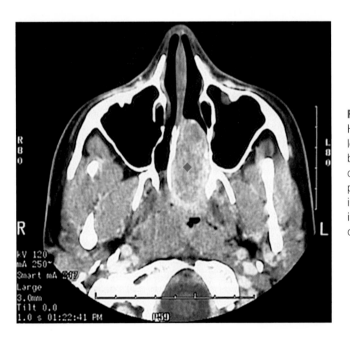

Figure 6-16 Nasopharyngeal angiofibroma, CT image
Here is a mass (◆) filling and expanding the nasal cavity on the left. The maxillary sinuses are not involved. It can cause nosebleeds and nasal obstruction, and sometimes proptosis or facial deformity. Angiofibromas arise in the posterior or lateral nasopharynx. This lesion, which is uncommon, is almost always seen in adolescent boys. Although circumscribed, it can slowly invade into surrounding bone, nasal cavities, paranasal sinuses, and orbits. Larger masses may extend intracranially.

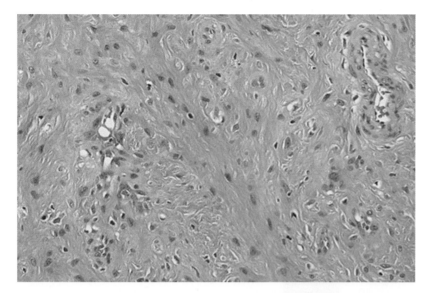

Figure 6-17 Nasopharyngeal angiofibroma, microscopic
The nasal angiofibroma is histologically benign but can block the nasal passages, erode adjacent structures, ulcerate, and bleed. The tumor is composed of a fibrous stroma with plump fibroblastic cells along with scattered capillaries. They can recur after excision.

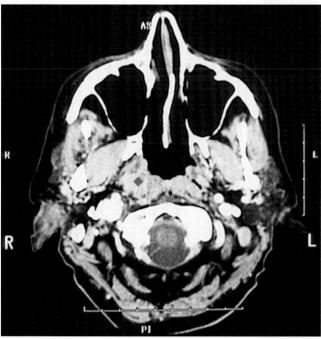

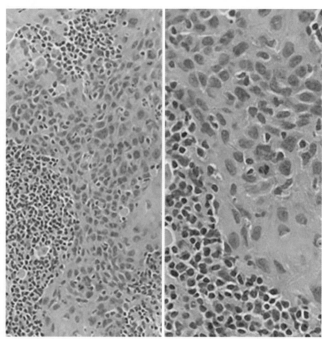

Figures 6-18 and 6-19 Nasopharyngeal carcinoma, CT image and microscopic
This head CT scan with contrast enhancement shows a 3-cm mass (◆) on the right between the pterygoid plate anteriorly and the prevertebral and right carotid space posteriorly. These carcinomas have features of squamous cell carcinoma along with a prominent lymphoid component. Many are associated with Epstein-Barr virus infection. The tumor often infiltrates locally into orbits and even the cranial cavity. Metastases occur most often to cervical lymph nodes.

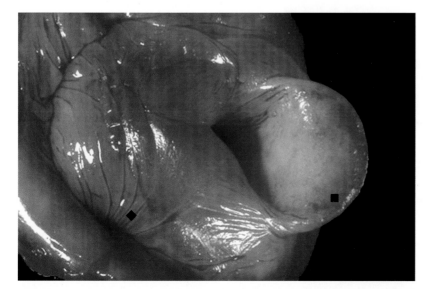

Figure 6-20 Laryngeal edema, gross
The epiglottis (■) and the larynx (◆) show marked enlargement from swelling with edema. This may occur with infection but can also be the result of a systemic anaphylactic (type I hypersensitivity) immune reaction, as with penicillin or bee sting allergy, and can occur within minutes of exposure to the antigen, resulting in life-threatening airway obstruction.

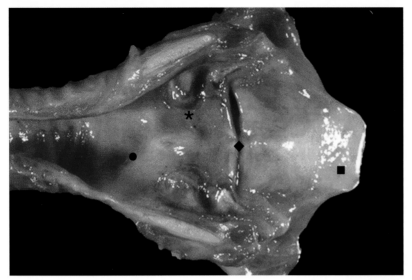

Figure 6-21 Laryngeal erosions, gross
The larynx is shown opened anteriorly at autopsy. Note the epiglottis (■), the vocal folds of the larynx (◆), and the upper trachea (●). The false vocal fold (cord) is to the right, and the true cord is to the left, with the recess of the ventricle in between. Note the bilateral subglottic erosions (★). These developed in a patient who had been intubated for weeks.

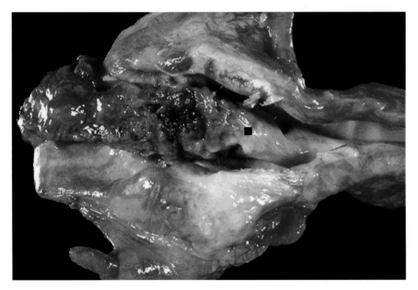

Figure 6-22 Aspiration, gross
The larynx opened here at autopsy reveals aspiration of gastric material, which appears as the large variegated bolus (■) filling the upper airway. Aspiration may occur accidentally while eating. Young children may aspirate objects they place in their mouths. Aspiration is often the terminal event in individuals with underlying neurologic disease, as in this patient with Alzheimer disease, and the manner of death is natural. In a healthy patient who dies suddenly and unexpectedly from aspiration, the medical examiner determines an accidental manner of death.

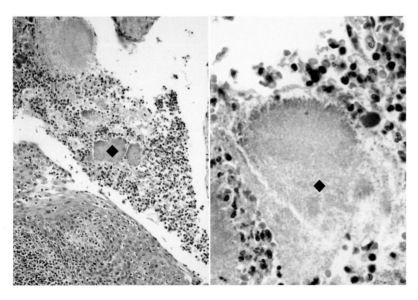

Figure 6-23 Tonsil, sulfur granule, microscopic
The oropharyngeal region is colonized by a variety of commensal microorganisms. In immunocompetent persons, *Actinomyces* species may produce superficial colonies large enough to appear grossly as yellow-to-orange granules, termed "sulfur" granules from their color, often in tonsillar crypts. At lower magnification *(left panel)* there is acute inflammation around the fuzzy blue granules (◆) lying above squamous epithelium. At high magnification *(right panel)* the matted filamentous gram-positive rodlike bacterial organisms are shown forming rounded clusters (◆). Actinomycetes may participate in polymicrobial infections.

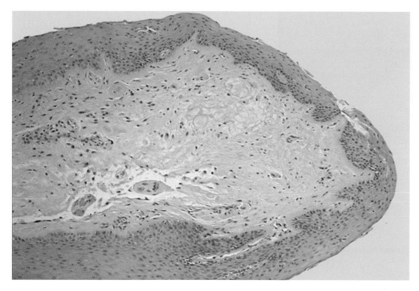

Figure 6-24 Laryngeal nodule, microscopic
Also known as a *reactive nodule* or *laryngeal polyp,* this lesion occurs most frequently in individuals who abuse their voice (e.g., a singer's nodule) or who smoke. Such polypoid lesions are typically found on the true vocal cord and are covered by nonkeratinizing stratified squamous epithelium surrounding an edematous submucosa. The overlying epithelium may become hyperkeratotic or hyperplastic. The nodule may impart a hoarse quality to the voice or a change in the character of the voice but is very unlikely to predispose to malignancy. Larger nodules (≤1 cm) may ulcerate.

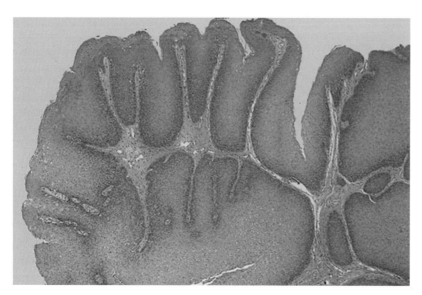

Figure 6-25 Laryngeal papilloma, microscopic
A squamous papilloma of the larynx is found on the true vocal fold. Note the long projections of orderly, benign squamous epithelium overlying fibrovascular cores. These uncommon lesions are solitary in adults and may cause some bleeding. Although rare in children, juvenile papillomas of the larynx tend to be multiple and continually recur after resection. With laryngeal papillomatosis, dozens of lesions may be resected over many years. Some may regress with onset of puberty. Infection with HPV types 6 and 11 typically drives this process. Such papillomas are unlikely to progress to carcinoma.

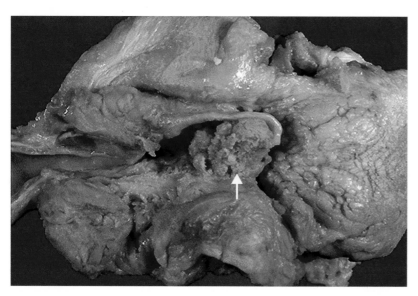

Figure 6-26 Laryngeal carcinoma, gross
The region from tongue at the right to the upper trachea at the left is shown with a large fungating squamous cell carcinoma (♠) extending from the larynx to the epiglottis, and a portion of the right epiglottis is eroded. Such large masses can have presenting symptoms including hoarseness, cough, and dysphagia. More advanced lesions may ulcerate and lead to hemoptysis. Metastases to local lymph nodes are often found, producing nontender lymphadenopathy. Most cases are related to tobacco and alcohol use. The precursor lesions begin with focal epithelial hyperplasia that progresses to dysplasia, but these early lesions are often clinically inapparent.

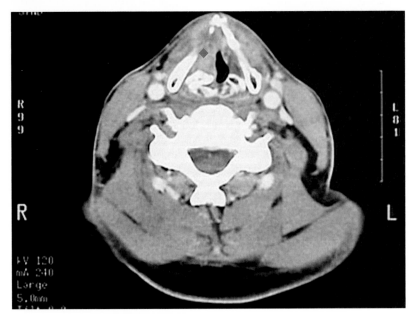

Figure 6-27 Laryngeal carcinoma, CT image
The region of the mid neck shows irregular thickening (♦) of the right vocal fold, representing a squamous cell carcinoma. This carcinoma is invading laterally into the region of the hyoid bone on the right, indicating a worse overall prognosis because it has become extrinsic to the larynx. Intrinsic lesions confined to the larynx would have a better prognosis. Resection can be accompanied by radiation therapy and chemotherapy to eradicate or to control the disease.

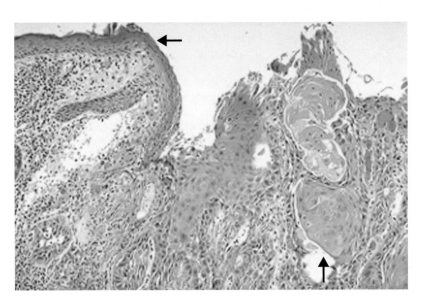

Figure 6-28 Laryngeal carcinoma, microscopic
The normal respiratory tract pseudostratified columnar epithelium has been replaced by the metaplastic squamous epithelium (◄) shown at the left. Arising at the center and extending to the right is a well-differentiated squamous cell carcinoma with overlying ulceration. This neoplasm infiltrates downward (↑) into the submucosa. Many of the cells are arranged in nests and infiltrate downward.

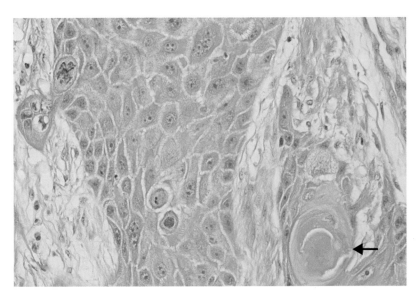

Figure 6-29 Laryngeal carcinoma, microscopic
This well-differentiated squamous cell carcinoma has large cells with abundant pink cytoplasm, distinct cell borders, and intercellular bridges. There is a keratin pearl (◄). Of laryngeal carcinomas, 95% have squamous differentiation. Most arise in cigarette smokers, particularly with the cofactor of alcohol abuse, and manifest with hoarseness, a change in voice, and/or difficulty swallowing.

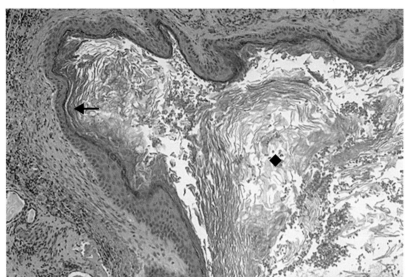

Figure 6-30 Cholesteatoma, microscopic

Severe inflammation from otitis media or rupture of the tympanic membrane of the middle ear may result in the trapping of squamous epithelium that starts to proliferate, expanding as a cystic mass lesion that can rupture and erode surrounding structures such as the mastoid. Shown here is the wall (◄) of such an excised non-neoplastic cyst. The center of the cyst is filled with keratinaceous debris (◆). The cholesteatoma can elicit an inflammatory reaction because the keratinaceous debris acts as a foreign body, with foreign body giant cells and mononuclear cells. Hemorrhage and necrosis lead to formation of cholesterol clefts. Cholesteatomas require surgical removal.

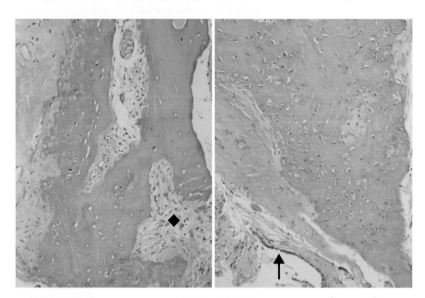

Figure 6-31 Otosclerosis, microscopic

Note the cellular, eosinophilic, woven bone along with areas of fibrosis and prominent vascularity (◆) in the *left panel*. This process is impinging on the stapedial footplate, with residual epithelium (↑) at the oval window *(right panel)*. More active lesions may have osteoblastic and osteoclastic activity. There is bony ankylosis of ossicles, and there can be extension to the cochlea. The result is diminished conductive hearing loss and tinnitus. The disease is more common in Caucasians, particularly with a family history, and bilateral in 75% of patients.

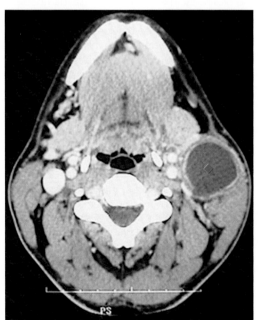

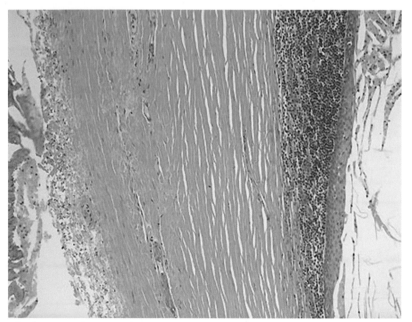

Figures 6-32 and 6-33 Branchial cyst, CT image and microscopic

CT scan in the region of the upper neck (with the inferior, anterior portion of the mandible shown here) shows a large but circumscribed branchial cyst (◆) in the neck. Such lesions typically occur in the anterolateral neck region and grossly have a cystic cavity filled with cellular debris formed from desquamation of the epithelial lining. A branchial cyst (lymphoepithelial cyst) enlarges slowly over time. Microscopically, branchial cleft cysts are lined by benign stratified squamous epithelium and are often surrounded by lymphoid tissue, as shown.

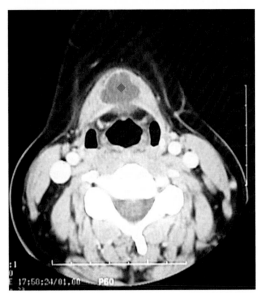

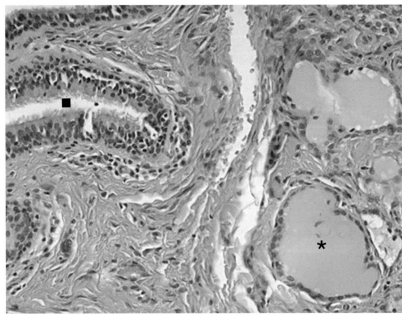

Figures 6-34 and 6-35 Thyroglossal duct cyst, CT image and microscopic

The region of the mid neck at the level of the hyoid bone shows a circumscribed midline thyroglossal duct cyst (◆). Such cysts are embryologic remnants within the migration route made by the primordial thyroid tissue from the foramen cecum of the tongue down to the final location of the thyroid anterior to the thyroid cartilage. Microscopically, there is typically a lining of respiratory epithelium (■), but there may also be squamous epithelium. Around the cyst there may be thyroid follicles (★) and lymphoid aggregates.

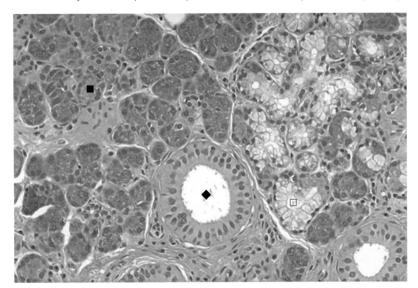

Figure 6-36 Normal salivary gland, microscopic

Major and minor salivary glands composed of tubuloalveolar glands produce serous and mucous secretions that aid in chewing and swallowing. Ducts from the major salivary glands drain into the oral cavity. The major salivary glands include the submandibular gland and the parotid gland. Salivary gland amylase provides some initial digestion of carbohydrates. The histologic appearance of normal submandibular gland with serous (■) and mucinous (□) acini and ducts (◆) is shown here.

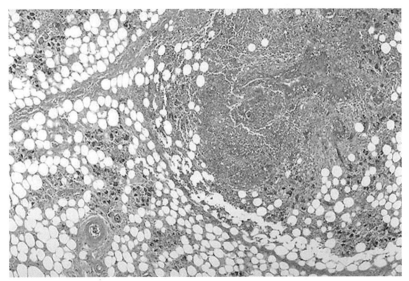

Figure 6-37 Sialadenitis, microscopic

Obstruction of salivary gland ducts from lithiasis or inspissated secretions predisposes to stasis and infection. An acute parotitis is shown here, with neutrophils infiltrating the parotid gland and formation of an abscess around a duct at the upper right. Elderly individuals are more prone to develop this problem. *Staphylococcus aureus* is the most common infectious agent isolated. Bilateral inflammation of salivary glands can also occur acutely with mumps virus infection, but the inflammatory infiltrates are mainly composed of macrophages and lymphocytes. Sialadenitis is often patchy and resolves with minimal scarring.

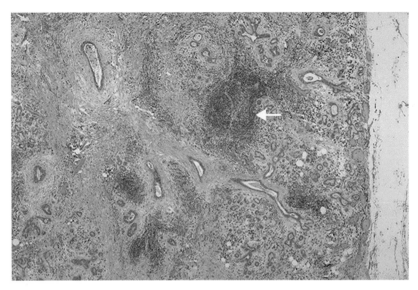

Figure 6-38 Sialadenitis, microscopic
Chronic obstruction of a salivary gland duct can lead to chronic inflammatory cell infiltrates (◄) along with fibrosis and acinar atrophy. The chronic sialadenitis shown here is caused by ductal obstruction. A similar appearance can occur with Sjögren syndrome, an autoimmune disease that involves salivary glands (with xerostomia) and lacrimal glands (with xerophthalmia). There can be extensive lymphoid infiltrates and even formation of lymphoid follicles with reactive germinal centers. Sjögren syndrome is often accompanied by serologic testing results that are positive for autoantibodies to the ribonucleoprotein antigens SS-A and SS-B, and there is an increased risk for subsequent development of non-Hodgkin lymphoma.

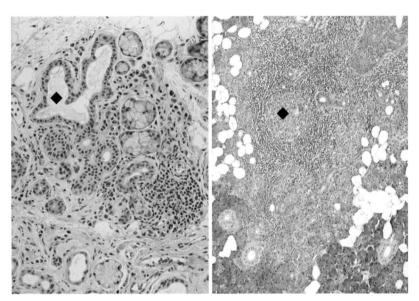

Figure 6-39 Sjögren syndrome, microscopic
This autoimmune disease affects salivary glands and lacrimal glands to produce sicca syndrome with dry mouth and dry eyes. Initially there is gland enlargement from extensive chronic inflammation, shown here with lymphoid follicle and germinal center (◆) in the parotid gland *(right panel).* Eventually the glands atrophy as inflammatory infiltrates are replaced by fibrous connective tissue with interspersed residual glandular acini (◆) as in the *left panel.* Serologic markers may include SS-A and SS-B autoantibodies, as well as antinuclear antibody (ANA) and rheumatoid factor (RF). SS can be part of overlap syndromes with other autoimmune diseases present. There is increased risk for non-Hodgkin lymphoma.

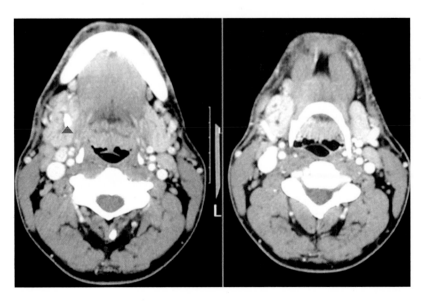

Figure 6-40 Sialolithiasis, CT images
This head CT scan reveals a calculus (▲) within the submandibular gland in the *left panel.* Obstruction has resulted in inflammation and duct dilation, producing more brightness in this gland compared with the normal left submandibular gland. The inflamed gland is enlarged, shown in the *right panel.* Salivary gland duct lithiasis leads to obstruction with localized pain and swelling of the gland with microscopic findings of acute or chronic inflammation.

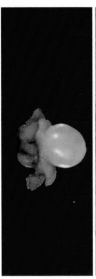
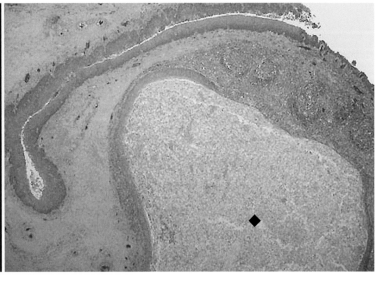

Figure 6-41 Mucocele, gross and microscopic

This mucocele (mucous retention cyst) involving a minor salivary gland of the oral cavity was removed surgically. The duct from the small gland became obstructed and led to the expansion of the gland with secretions to form the small, smooth-surfaced mass shown here. Sometimes the mucocele can rupture and produce a surrounding foreign body granulomatous response with pain and enlargement. In the *right panel,* microscopically, the mucocele is filled with pale blue mucinous material (◆).

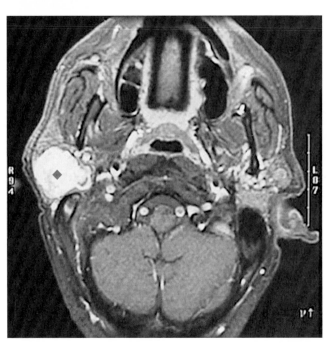

Figure 6-42 Pleomorphic adenoma, MRI

This axial MRI scan of the head shows a mass lesion (◆) involving the superficial aspect of the right parotid gland. This is a pleomorphic adenoma, or mixed tumor, of the salivary gland. Pleomorphic adenomas are the most common salivary gland tumor (65% of all salivary gland tumors), and the most common location for them is in the parotid gland (usually the superficial lobe). The highest incidence occurs in older adults. These neoplasms usually manifest as a painless, movable swelling that has often been present for a long time. They are solid and circumscribed, but not encapsulated. Most act in a benign manner, although they can recur after incomplete resection because they are not strictly encapsulated.

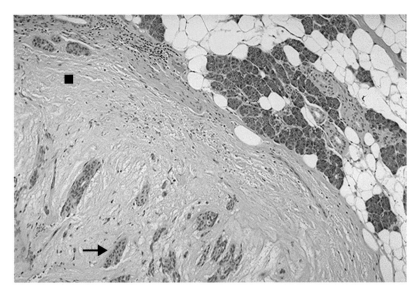

Figure 6-43 Pleomorphic adenoma, microscopic

At low magnification, this heterogeneous tumor borders the surrounding normal parotid gland. This neoplasm has a mixed proliferation of epithelial elements (→) resembling ductal cells or myoepithelial cells arranged in ducts and acini and dispersed within a mesenchyme-like background of loose myxoid tissue (■). There may also be islands of chondroid, hyaline, or a mesenchyme-like myxomatous stroma. The facial nerve nearby can be involved, making a nerve graft necessary with a wide tumor excision. If not removed, about 10% have malignant transformation after 15 years.

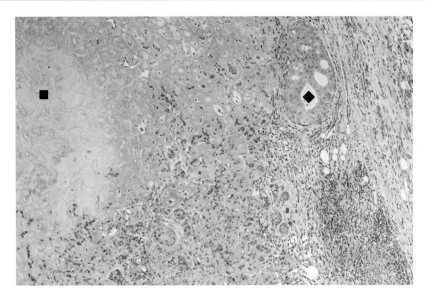

Figure 6-44 Pleomorphic adenoma, microscopic

Note the chondroid (cartilage-like) to hyaline stroma (■). There are elements of ductal epithelium with myoepithelial cells and a larger focus of epithelial proliferation (◆). Immunohistochemical staining for muscle specific actin helps identify myoepithelial components. Most of these neoplasms arise in the parotid gland and have a benign biologic behavior, although they may recur after excision. Multiple recurrences predict malignant behavior in 5% of cases.

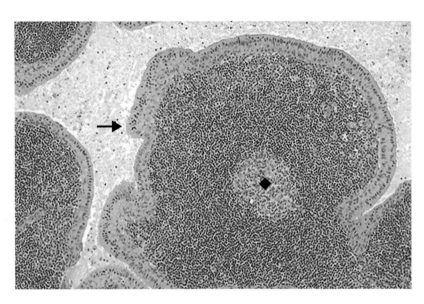

Figure 6-45 Warthin tumor, microscopic

Papillary fronds project into cystic to cleftlike spaces filled with pale pink mucinous to serous secretions. The papillary fronds are covered by a double layer of pink (oncocytic) cuboidal to columnar epithelial cells (→). Beneath the epithelium are lymphocytes, sometimes with germinal centers (◆). The oncocytic cells on electron microscopy are filled with mitochondria. This neoplasm, also known as *papillary cystadenoma lymphomatosum,* is the second most common salivary gland tumor. It is almost always found in the parotid gland and is much more common in men and in smokers. About 10% of cases are multifocal, and 10% are bilateral.

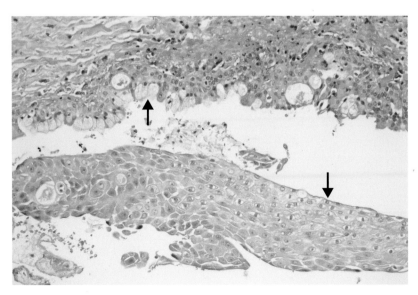

Figure 6-46 Mucoepidermoid tumor, microscopic

There are areas of both squamoid (↓) and mucinous (↑) differentiation. Parotid gland and minor salivary glands are often involved. If malignant elements are present, then the term *mucoepidermoid carcinoma* applies. Although circumscribed, they often have infiltrative borders. A t(11;19)(q21;p13) chromosomal translocation is found in most cases. This translocation leads to elaboration of a fusion protein that disrupts the Notch signaling pathway. Tumors with this translocation have a better prognosis. High-grade carcinomas tend to recur and metastasize.

The Gastrointestinal Tract

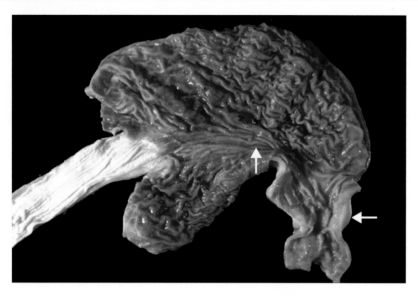

Figure 7-1 Normal esophagus and stomach, gross
The normal esophagus on the left has the usual white-to-tan mucosa. The gastroesophageal junction with the lower esophageal sphincter (LES), whose physiologic function is maintained by muscle tone, is in the center left, and the normal stomach is on the right, opened along the greater curvature. The lesser curvature (↑) can be seen in the fundus. Just beyond the antrum is the pylorus (←) with thick surrounding muscle that empties into the first portion of duodenum on the lower right. The rugal folds of the normal stomach are prominent.

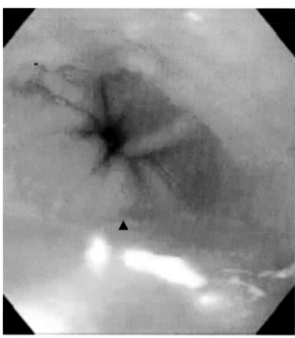

Figure 7-2 Normal esophagus, endoscopy
This normal upper gastrointestinal (GI) endoscopic view shows the transition from the pale pink-to-tan squamous mucosa of the esophagus to the darker pink columnar mucosa of the stomach at the gastroesophageal junction (▲). The LES is a physiologic sphincter maintained by normal muscle tone. Distention of the lower esophagus by food produces relaxation of the LES and receptive relaxation of the proximal stomach through a vasovagal reflex with release of vasoactive intestinal peptide from postganglionic peptidergic vagal nerve fibers. A loss of this tone allows reflux of acidic gastric contents into the lower esophagus that often produces a burning retrosternal or substernal chest pain (heartburn). An abnormality of the esophageal sphincter can also produce difficulty in swallowing (dysphagia). Lesions of the esophageal mucosa may cause pain on swallowing (odynophagia). Abnormalities in intrinsic or extrinsic esophageal innervation may lead to failure of LES relaxation, leading to achalasia and progressive dysphagia with esophageal dilation above the LES.

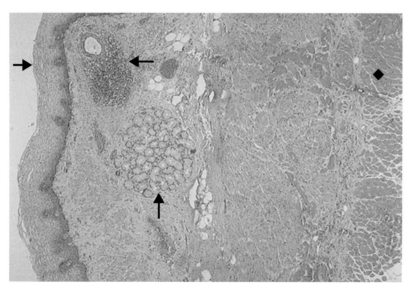

Figure 7-3 Normal esophagus, microscopic
The normal squamous mucosa (→) is on the left, with underlying submucosa containing minor mucous glands (↑) and a duct surrounded by lymphoid tissue (←). The muscularis (◆) is on the right. Predominantly voluntary striated muscle to initiate swallowing in the upper esophagus merges and changes to involuntary smooth muscle distally in the lower esophagus, which provides propulsive peristalsis of food and liquid boluses into the stomach. There is a physiologic LES of smooth muscle with muscle tone providing an effective barrier to regurgitation. At the gastroesophageal junction, the squamous epithelium interdigitates with the glandular epithelium of the stomach.

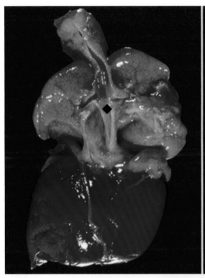
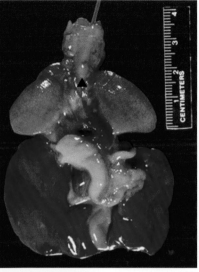

Figure 7-4 Tracheoesophageal fistula, gross
Congenital anomalies involving the esophagus include atresia and fistula with the trachea. Embryologically, the lung buds off the esophagus, an endodermal derivative, so both are intimately associated in development. The esophageal atresia (▲) shown here is present in the mid esophagus in the *right panel*. The tracheoesophageal fistula (◆) is located below the carina in the *left panel*. Depending on the location of the atretic portion or the fistula, an infant at birth may exhibit vomiting or aspiration. Additional congenital anomalies are often present. Agenesis (complete absence) of the esophagus is very rare.

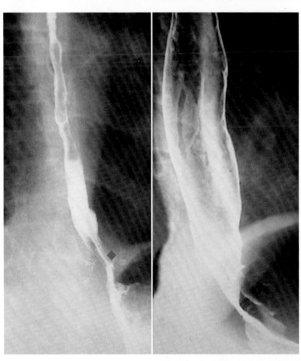
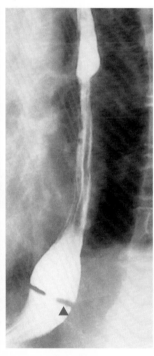

Figures 7-5 and 7-6 Esophageal stricture and Schatzki ring, barium swallow radiographs
The two panels on the *left* show stricture (◆) (stenosis) of the lower esophagus. This can occur from inflammation with reflux, scleroderma with submucosal fibrosis, radiation injury, or ingestion of caustic chemicals. The lateral view on the *right* reveals a Schatzki ring (▲) of the lower esophagus. There is an infolding of the muscular wall just above the diaphragm. With these conditions, there is progressive dysphagia, more marked for solid foods than liquids initially.

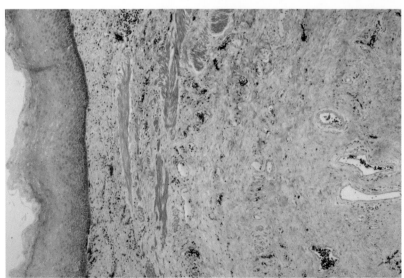

Figure 7-7 Esophageal fibrosis with scleroderma, microscopic
Beneath the stratified squamous epithelium at the left, this trichrome stain emphasizes the blue collagenous submucosal fibrosis of the esophagus, with a few remaining fascicles of red-appearing muscle. There is a minimal lymphocytic infiltrate. Systemic sclerosis is an autoimmune disease in which cytokines such as transforming growth factor–β (TGF-β) and interleukin-13 (IL-13) from CD4 cells lead to progressive interstitial and perivascular fibrosis and, with the diffuse form, multiple organ involvement, particularly GI tract, lungs, and kidneys. Esophageal dysmotility with dysphagia is common.

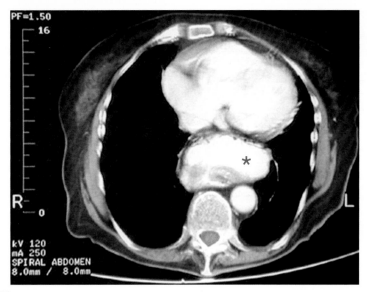

Figure 7-8 Hiatal hernia, CT image
Chest CT scan shows a dilated portion of gastric fundus (✱) sliding through a widened esophageal hiatus into the lower chest. About 95% of hiatal hernias are of this sliding type. About 9% of patients with hiatal hernias have associated symptoms of acid reflux with gastroesophageal reflux disease (GERD). Conversely, some cases of GERD are associated with a hiatal hernia. The widened esophageal hiatus interferes with maintenance of the normal LES function. Patients may have symptoms of "heartburn" from reflux of gastric contents into the lower esophagus, with retrosternal burning pain, particularly after eating, and exacerbated by lying down after a meal.

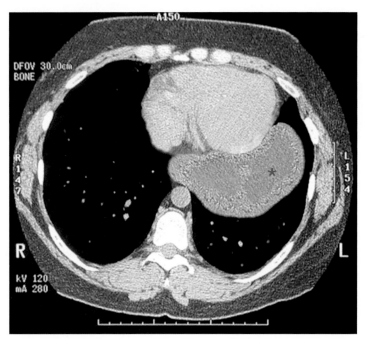

Figure 7-9 Paraesophageal hernia, CT image
Chest CT scan without contrast enhancement reveals that much of the stomach (✱) is present in the left chest cavity adjacent to the heart. This is a complication of a hiatal rolling hernia known as *paraesophageal hernia,* an uncommon but serious form of hernia. The vascular supply to the stomach becomes compromised when the stomach herniates upward through the small opening, leading to incarceration, then strangulation with ischemia and infarction.

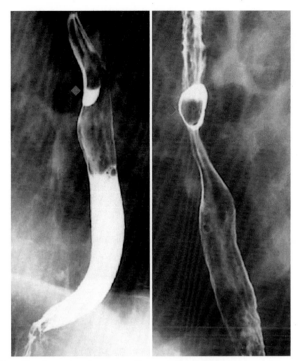

Figure 7-10 Esophageal pulsion diverticulum, barium swallow radiographs
These two views from an upper GI series with barium contrast material reveal a pulsion diverticulum (◆) in the upper esophagus. Note the contrast material that fills this small outpouching. Such a diverticulum represents enlargement and outpouching of esophagus through a weak point in the muscular wall, typically between the constrictor muscles in the upper esophagus or through the muscularis just above the diaphragm. Such a lesion is also known as a *Zenker diverticulum.* This lesion can produce a mass effect, interfere with swallowing, and collect food that decays and produces marked halitosis.

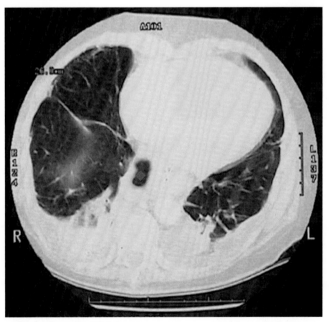

Figure 7-11 Mallory-Weiss syndrome, CT image
Longitudinal tears in the esophagus leading to hemorrhage may occur from bouts of severe or forceful vomiting. The rare complication of rupture (Boerhaave syndrome) is shown on this chest CT scan with contrast enhancement that shows a lucency (◆) representing an air leak from the esophageal rupture into the mediastinum. The point of rupture in the lower esophagus lies just above the gastroesophageal junction. Leakage of esophageal contents into the mediastinum leads to infection with inflammation that can quickly spread to other areas of the chest cavity.

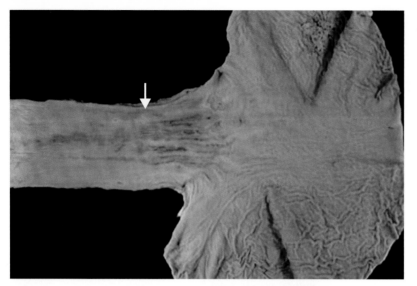

Figure 7-12 Esophageal varices, gross
These prominent purplish dilated veins (↓) near the gastroesophageal junction are a source of bleeding with hematemesis. Submucosal varices occur in patients with portal hypertension (usually from micronodular cirrhosis resulting from chronic alcoholism or schistosomiasis) because the submucosal esophageal plexus of veins is a collateral channel for portal venous drainage. This plexus of veins also drains part of the upper stomach, but it is generically called the *esophageal plexus of veins;* bleeding here is termed *esophageal variceal bleeding.*

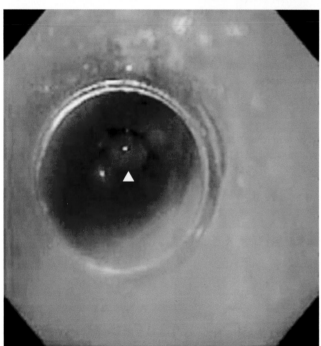

Figure 7-13 Esophageal varices, endoscopy
The dilated submucosal veins (▲) of the esophageal plexus bulge into the lower esophageal lumen as shown here on upper GI endoscopy. This venous dilation is most often a complication of portal hypertension with hepatic cirrhosis. Eventually about two thirds of patients with cirrhosis develop esophageal varices. With erosion and rupture of these delicate submucosal veins, there can be sudden, massive life-threatening hematemesis. Banding of the varices, octreotide infusion, and balloon tamponade have been employed as therapeutic measures to halt or prevent blood loss.

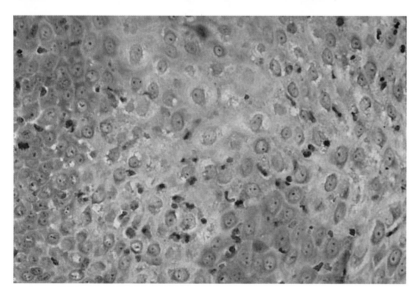

Figure 7-14 Esophagitis, microscopic
Reflux of acidic gastric contents into the lower esophagus from incompetence of the LES leads to GERD with esophagitis. Histologic findings in mild reflux esophagitis include epithelial hyperplasia with basal zone hyperplasia and lengthened papillae, and inflammation with neutrophils, eosinophils, and lymphocytes (eosinophils, especially in children, are a sensitive and specific indicator of reflux, as shown here with a Giemsa stain). Causes of GERD with esophagitis include hiatal hernia, neurologic disorders, scleroderma, lack of esophageal clearance, and delayed gastric emptying. Severe esophagitis can be complicated by ulceration and subsequent stricture.

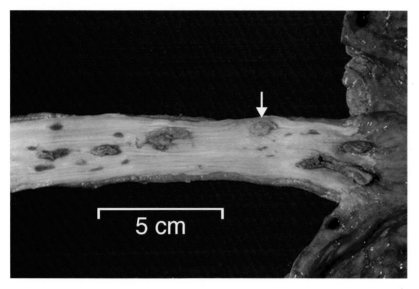

Figure 7-15 Herpes esophagitis, gross
The lower esophagus shows sharply demarcated, oblong ulcerations (⬇) that have a brown-red base, contrasted with the surrounding normal pale or white esophageal squamous mucosa. These ulcerations have a "punched-out" appearance suggestive of herpes simplex virus (HSV) infection. Opportunistic infections such as HSV are most often seen in immunocompromised patients. Odynophagia is a typical symptom. Herpetic esophagitis usually remains localized, rarely causes significant bleeding or obstruction, and is unlikely to become disseminated.

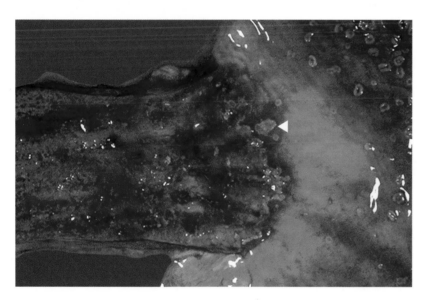

Figure 7-16 *Candida* esophagitis, gross
Tan-yellow plaques (◀) appear in the lower esophagus, along with mucosal hyperemia. The same lesions also appear at the upper right in the upper gastric fundus. *Candida* infections involving the oral cavity ("oral thrush") and upper GI tract tend to remain superficial, but invasion and dissemination occasionally occur in immunocompromised patients. A few *Candida* organisms can be part of the normal flora of the mouth. These lesions rarely cause significant hemorrhage or obstruction. These lesions may coalesce to form pseudomembranes.

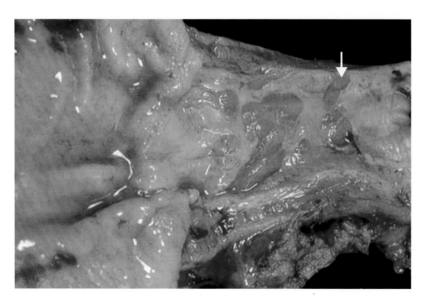

Figure 7-17 Barrett esophagus, gross
Islands of reddish metaplastic mucosa (⬇) are shown here in the lower esophagus, above the gastroesophageal junction, with remaining surrounding white squamous mucosa. Chronic GERD with esophageal mucosal injury can lead to metaplasia of the normal esophageal squamous mucosa into gastric-type columnar mucosa, but with intestinal-type goblet cells, known as *Barrett esophagus.* Ten percent of patients with chronic gastric reflux may develop Barrett esophagus. Ulceration leads to bleeding and pain; inflammation with stricture may ensue.

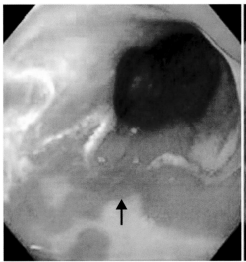
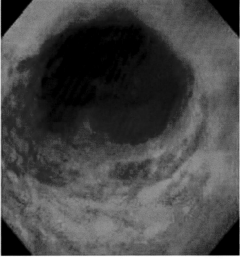

Figure 7-18 Barrett esophagus, endoscopy
These endoscopic views of the lower esophagus just above the LES show areas of red metaplastic mucosa (↑) typical of Barrett esophagus along with islands of normal pale esophageal squamous mucosa. If the area of Barrett mucosa extends less than 2 cm above the normal squamocolumnar junction, the condition is called *short-segment Barrett esophagus.*

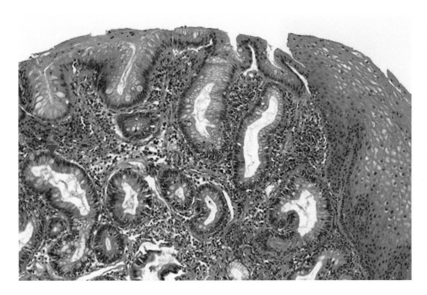

Figure 7-19 Barrett esophagus, microscopic
Note the abnormal columnar epithelium on the left of this image and the normal squamous epithelium on the right. This is "typical" Barrett mucosa on the left because there is intestinal metaplasia with goblet cells (▼) in the columnar mucosa. Chronic reflux of gastric contents into the lower esophagus over many years predisposes to development of this metaplasia. Barrett esophagus is mostly diagnosed on endoscopy with biopsy in persons 40 to 60 years old. There is a long-term risk (>30- to 40-fold compared with the general population) for development of esophageal adenocarcinoma when more than 3 cm of Barrett mucosa is present in the esophagus.

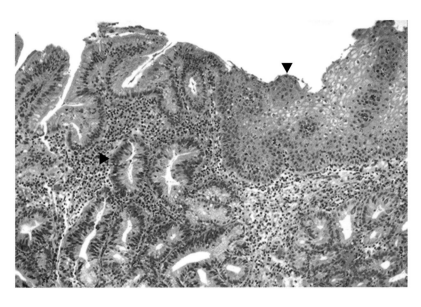

Figure 7-20 Barrett esophagus with dysplasia, microscopic
Adjacent to remaining squamous mucosa (▼) on the right is an area of high-grade dysplasia of the metaplastic columnar epithelium in the Barrett mucosa. Note the crowded, hyperchromatic nuclei (▶) in the columnar cells, a few remaining goblet cells at the upper surface on the left, and the glandular architectural irregularity. Because the columnar cell nuclei are basally oriented, this is a low-grade dysplasia; an apical orientation is part of high-grade dysplasia, which has a much greater likelihood of advancing to adenocarcinoma. Dysplasia may develop after years of untreated GERD with Barrett esophagus.

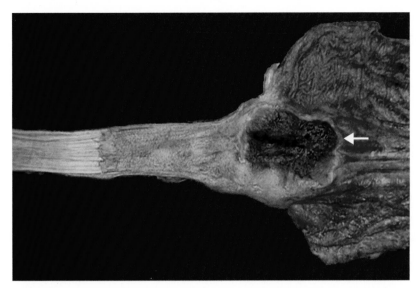

Figure 7-21 Adenocarcinoma, gross
Normal tan upper esophageal mucosa is at the far left. The distal esophagus is replaced by Barrett mucosa, producing a darker, slightly erythematous gross appearance. In the distal esophagus arising near the gastroesophageal junction is a large ulcerating adenocarcinoma with a dark center that extends (◀) into the upper stomach. Adenocarcinomas most often arise in Barrett esophagus, with frequent mutation of *TP53*, followed by *CDKN2A* gene downregulation, then by nuclear translocation of β-catenin and *ERBB2* amplification. As with squamous cell carcinoma, there are often no early symptoms, so the cancer is advanced at the time of diagnosis, with a poor prognosis.

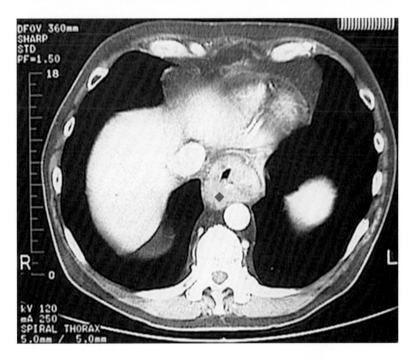

Figure 7-22 Adenocarcinoma, CT image
Abdominal CT scan with contrast enhancement shows a mass (◆) that surrounds the central esophageal lumen and extended into the upper stomach. This tumor arose in a Barrett mucosa that followed chronic GERD. Preexisting high-grade dysplasia arising in Barrett mucosa increases the risk for development of subsequent adenocarcinoma. By the time an adenocarcinoma arises, untreated GERD has been present for years, and the patient is older than 40 years. The increased epithelial cell turnover with increased proliferative activity in Barrett mucosa is the background for mutations to arise with subsequent loss of cell cycle control.

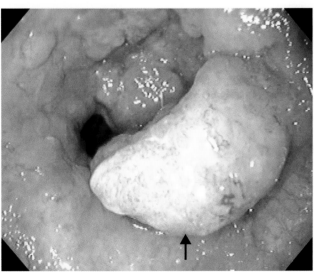

Figure 7-23 Adenocarcinoma, endoscopy
Endoscopy of the lower esophagus shows irregular reddish mucosa representing Barrett esophagus. A pale, polypoid, exophytic mass (↑) extends into the esophageal lumen, which on biopsy proved to be a moderately differentiated adenocarcinoma. This patient had a long history of poorly controlled GERD. Clinical findings with esophageal carcinomas include hematemesis, dysphagia (solids more than liquids), chest pain, and weight loss.

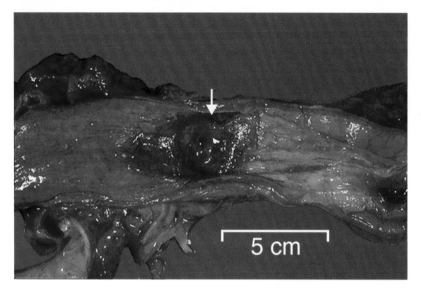

Figure 7-24 Squamous cell carcinoma, gross
An irregular reddish, ulcerated, exophytic mid-esophageal mass (↓) is visible here on the mucosal surface. The distensibility of the esophagus partly ameliorates the mass effect so that early symptoms are uncommon, and by the time a diagnosis is made there is often extensive mediastinal invasion that precludes a surgical cure. The overall prognosis for this tumor is poor. Risk factors for esophageal squamous carcinoma in the United States include smoking and alcohol abuse. In other parts of the world, dietary factors, such as a high nitrate or nitrosamine content, deficiency of zinc or molybdenum, and human papillomavirus (HPV) infection may play a role.

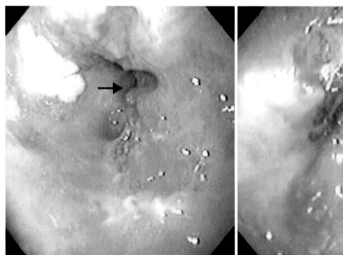
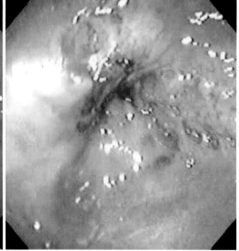

Figure 7-25 Squamous cell carcinoma, endoscopy
Endoscopy shows an ulcerated mid-esophageal squamous cell carcinoma causing luminal stenosis (→). Pain and dysphagia are typical presenting problems. Interference with swallowing leads to cachexia with weight loss. Most of these carcinomas have invaded and spread by the time of diagnosis.

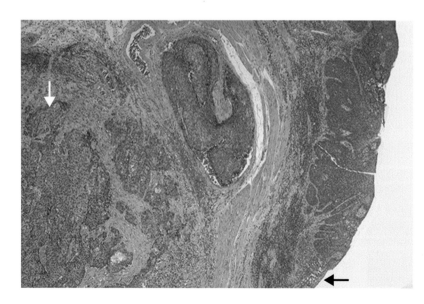

Figure 7-26 Squamous cell carcinoma, microscopic
At the lower right is a small remnant of normal squamous esophageal mucosa (←) that merges into abnormal, thick squamous cell carcinoma. Solid nests (↓) of neoplastic cells are infiltrating down through the submucosa on the left. These carcinomas often spread to surrounding structures, making surgical removal difficult. Half of these cancers have *p53* tumor suppressor gene mutations. The *p16/CDKN2A* tumor suppressor gene is abnormal in some cases, whereas cyclin D1 may be amplified in others. These mutations can arise in the setting of chronic inflammation with increased epithelial cell proliferation.

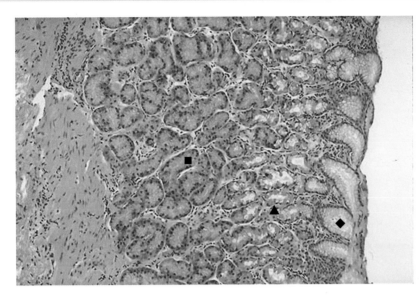

Figure 7-27 Normal gastric mucosa, microscopic

The mucosa of the fundus has short gastric pits (◆), beneath which are long glands (■). These fundic glands contain parietal cells (▲) secreting hydrochloric acid and intrinsic factor. Acid is secreted through the H^+,K^+-ATPase ("proton pump") in parietal cells under the influence of acetylcholine secreted from the vagus nerve acting on muscarinic receptors, histamine from mast cells acting on H_2 receptors, and gastrin. Fundic glands also have chief cells secreting pepsinogen, a proteolytic enzyme. Cuboidal mucous neck cells in the glands secrete mucus to protect the mucosa against the acid and enzyme secretions.

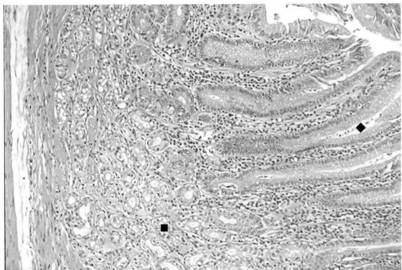

Figure 7-28 Normal gastric mucosa, microscopic

The gastric antral epithelium has long pits (◆) with shorter glands (■) than the fundus. In the antrum and pyloric regions distally in the stomach, there are columnar mucous cells in pits and glands. Mucosal cells produce prostaglandins that favor production of mucus and bicarbonate, and increase mucosal blood flow to protect the mucosa from the effects of gastric acid. Peristaltic movements in the stomach mix the chyme. The rate of gastric emptying is partially controlled by the amount of H^+ and fat entering the duodenum. Duodenal fat increases the secretion of cholecystokinin, which slows the rate of gastric emptying.

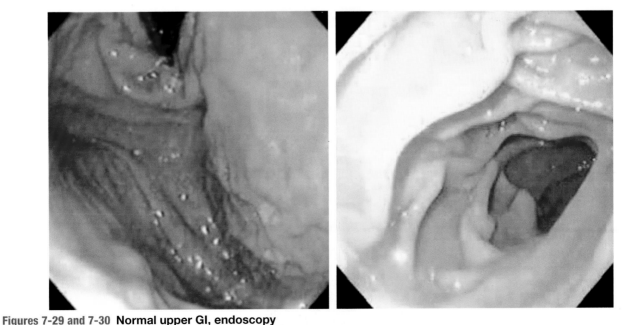

Figures 7-29 and 7-30 Normal upper GI, endoscopy

The normal appearance of the gastric fundus with rugal folds is shown on the *left,* and the normal duodenal appearance is shown on the *right.*

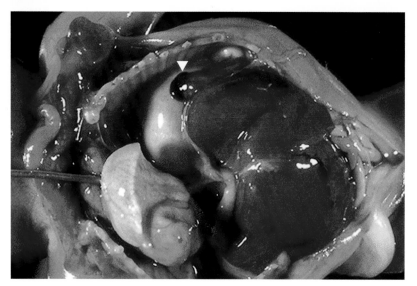

Figure 7-31 Congenital diaphragmatic hernia, gross
The left diaphragmatic dome is absent here, allowing herniation of abdominal contents into the chest cavity during fetal development. The metal probe is positioned behind the left lung, which has been displaced into the right chest by the herniated stomach. Visible below the stomach is a dark spleen (▼) that overlies the left lobe of the liver herniating upward. Incursion of abdominal contents into the chest during development results in pulmonary hypoplasia. Although diaphragmatic hernia may be an isolated congenital anomaly that is potentially reparable, most are associated with multiple anomalies and often with chromosomal abnormalities such as trisomy 18.

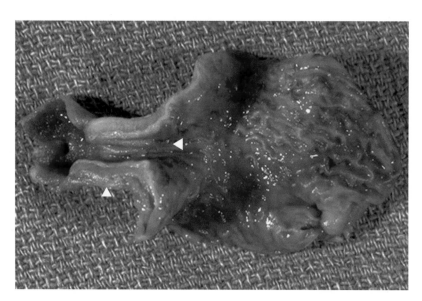

Figure 7-32 Pyloric stenosis, gross
Note the hypertrophied muscle (▲) at the gastric outlet (left pointing arrowhead). Pyloric stenosis is uncommon but is a cause of "projectile" nonbilious vomiting in infants 3 to 6 weeks old. The muscle hypertrophy may be so prominent that there is a palpable mass. Pyloric stenosis manifests the genetic phenomenon of "threshold of liability," above which the disease manifests when more genetic risks are present. The incidence is 1 in 300 to 900 live births, with boys affected more often than girls because more risks must be present in girls for the disease to occur. Myotomy is curative.

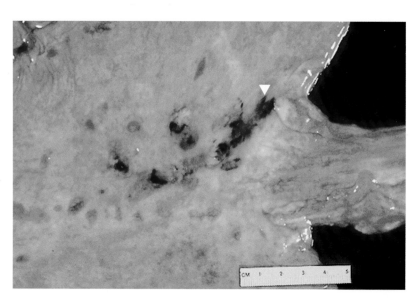

Figure 7-33 Gastropathy-gastritis, gross
Larger irregular areas of gastric hemorrhage (▼) are shown, which could best be termed *erosions* because the superficial mucosa is eroded away, but not completely gone. The clinical term *gastropathy* describes several different patterns of gastric mucosal epithelial or endothelial injury with mucosal damage without significant inflammation. Causes of gastropathy are similar to those of acute gastritis and include nonsteroidal anti-inflammatory drugs (NSAIDs), alcohol, stress, bile reflux, uremia, portal hypertension, radiation, and chemotherapy. The erosions here suggest gastritis with inflammation.

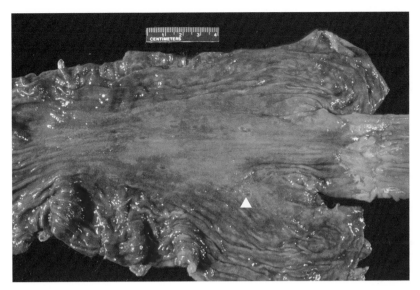

Figure 7-34 Acute gastritis, gross
The gastric mucosa of the fundus is diffusely hyperemic, with multiple petechiae, and with small erosions (▲) but no ulcerations. Acute gastritis (also called *hemorrhagic gastritis,* or *acute erosive gastritis* if mucosal erosions are present) can be caused by ischemia (from shock, burns, or trauma) or toxins (e.g., alcohol, salicylates, or NSAIDs). Damage to the mucosal barrier allows back-diffusion of acid. Patients may be asymptomatic or have massive hemorrhage. The lesions can progress to erosions or ulcerations. The stress of burn injuries (Curling ulcer) or central nervous system trauma (Cushing ulcer) can cause acid hypersecretion.

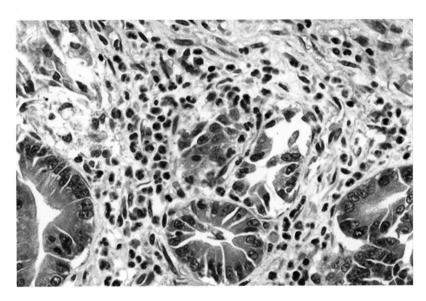

Figure 7-35 Acute gastritis, microscopic
Microscopic findings include hemorrhage, edema, and variable degrees of acute inflammation with neutrophilic infiltrates. The gastric mucosa here shows infiltration of glands and lamina propria by neutrophils. Typical clinical findings range from mild to severe epigastric pain, nausea, and vomiting. In severe cases there can be significant hematemesis, particularly in patients with a history of chronic alcohol abuse; this can be termed *acute hemorrhagic gastritis.* Although the presence of gastric acid is a necessary antecedent to ulceration, the amount of acid is not typically the determining factor for development of most gastric ulcerations.

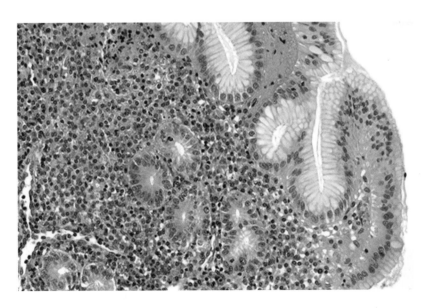

Figure 7-36 Chronic gastritis, microscopic
Chronic nonspecific (antral) gastritis is typically the result of *Helicobacter pylori* infection. Other causes include bile reflux and drugs (salicylates and alcohol). The inflammatory cell infiltrates are composed mainly of lymphocytes and plasma cells, and occasionally some neutrophils, shown here at the left. Mucosal atrophy and intestinal metaplasia are sequelae that can be the first step toward development of gastric adenocarcinoma. An autoimmune form of gastritis can occur when antiparietal or intrinsic factor antibodies are present, leading to atrophic gastritis and pernicious anemia. Fasting serum gastrin levels are inversely proportional to gastric acid production, and a high serum gastrin level suggests atrophic gastritis.

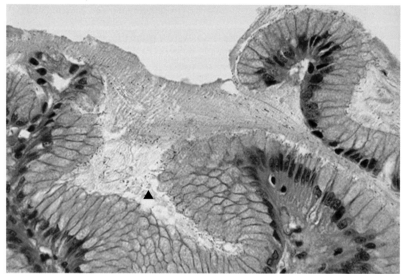

Figure 7-37 *Helicobacter pylori*, microscopic
H. pylori is a small, spiral, rod-shaped, gram-negative bacterium residing under microaerobic conditions in a neutral microenvironment between the mucus and the superficial columnar mucosal cells. The organisms here are pale pink rods (▲) with H&E staining. *H. pylori* strains that possess the *cagA* pathogenicity island induce more severe gastritis and augment the risk for developing peptic ulcer disease and gastric cancer. These organisms do not invade or directly damage the mucosa, but rather change the microenvironment of the stomach to promote mucosal damage. *H. pylori* organisms contain urease and produce a protective surrounding cloud of ammonia to resist gastric acid. The urea breath test is used to detect the presence of *H. pylori*.

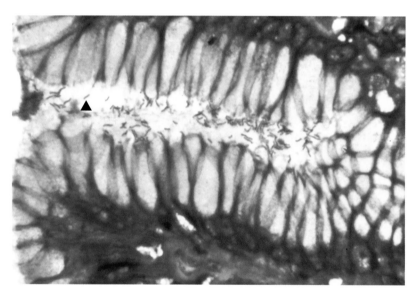

Figure 7-38 *Helicobacter pylori*, microscopic
H. pylori organisms (▲) stimulate cytokine production by epithelial cells that recruit and activate immune and inflammatory cells in the underlying lamina propria. This infection is thought to be acquired in childhood, but inflammatory changes progress throughout life. Colonization rates vary from 10% to 80% around the world. Only a few of the persons infected with *H. pylori* develop the complications of chronic gastritis, gastric ulcers, duodenal ulcers, mucosa-associated lymphoid tissue (MALT) lymphoma, or adenocarcinoma. *H. pylori* is found in the surface epithelial mucus of most patients with active gastritis. The organisms are shown here with methylene blue stain.

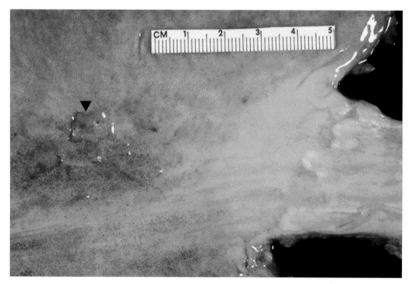

Figure 7-39 Acute gastric ulcer, gross
An ulcer (▼) is an area of full-thickness loss of the mucosa (an erosion is a partial-thickness loss). Ulcers can be complicated by hemorrhage, penetration (extension into an adjacent organ), perforation (communication with the peritoneal cavity), and stricture (as a result of scarring). A 1-cm, shallow, and sharply demarcated acute gastric ulcer with surrounding hyperemia is shown here in the upper fundus. This ulcer is probably benign. All gastric ulcers should undergo biopsy because of the risk for malignancy. Isolated gastric ulcers may be seen with chronic atrophic gastritis; they are usually located in the antrum and lesser curve or at the junction of the antrum and body. *H. pylori* is the most common cause, followed by NSAID use. Although acid is required for ulceration, most patients are normochlorhydric or hypochlorhydric.

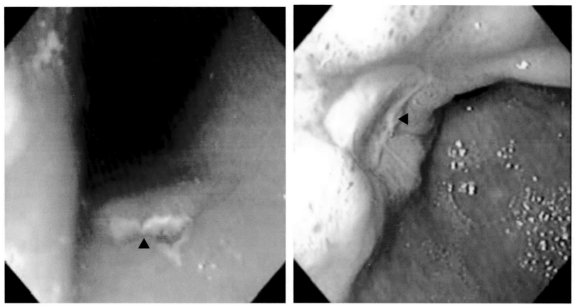

Figures 7-40 and 7-41 Acute gastric ulcers, endoscopy

The *left panel* shows a small prepyloric ulcer (▲), and the *right panel* shows a larger antral ulcer (◀). All gastric ulcers undergo biopsy because gross inspection alone cannot determine whether a malignancy is present. Smaller, more sharply demarcated gastric ulcerations are more likely to be benign.

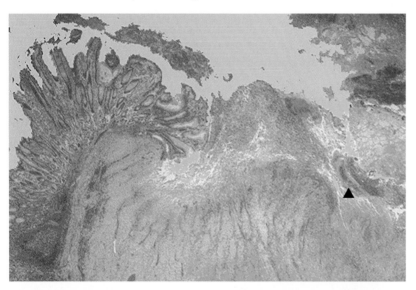

Figure 7-42 Acute gastric ulcer, microscopic

Note the loss of the epithelium and extension of the ulcer downward to the muscularis. This ulcer is sharply demarcated, with normal gastric mucosa on the left falling away into a deep ulcer crater whose base contains inflamed, necrotic debris. An arterial branch (▲) at the ulcer base is eroded and bleeding. Ulcers penetrate more deeply over time if they remain active and do not heal. Penetration leads to pain. If the ulcer penetrates through the muscularis and through adventitia, the ulcer is said to "perforate," leading to an acute abdomen with peritonitis, and an abdominal radiograph may show free air.

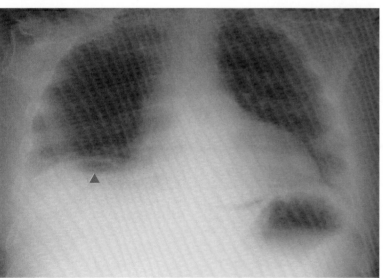

Figure 7-43 Perforated gastric ulcer, radiograph

This AP portable upright chest radiograph shows free air (▲) under the right diaphragmatic dome. This patient had a perforation of a duodenal peptic ulcer. The intraluminal air released from a perforated viscus can be detected as free peritoneal air, and a good place to detect it is under a diaphragmatic leaf on an upright abdominal plain film radiograph. Such patients have an acute abdomen with pain and sepsis. The pathogenesis of duodenal ulcers is hyperacidity. These ulcers occur in the proximal duodenum and are associated with peptic duodenitis. Almost all duodenal ulcers are associated with *H. pylori* infection in the stomach.

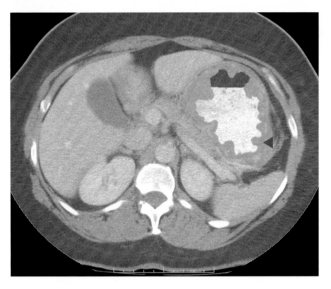

Figure 7-44 Ménétrier disease, CT image
The gastric rugal folds (◀) are markedly thickened and irregular from excessive secretion of TGF-α. There is diffuse hyperplasia of the foveolar epithelium of the body and fundus, but not the antrum. There is loss of protein from the epithelium, leading to diarrhea and weight loss. Hypoproteinemia is indicative of this form of protein-losing enteropathy. In children this condition is usually self-limited. In adults it can persist, and there is increased risk for adenocarcinoma. If the condition is severe, gastrectomy may be performed.

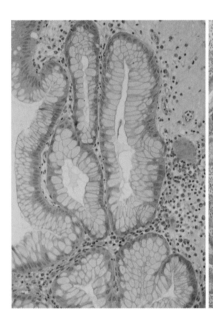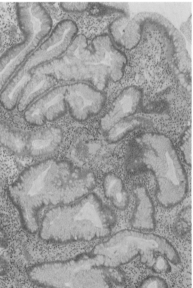

Figure 7-45 Hyperplastic polyp, microscopic
H. pylori infection in the stomach may predispose to development of chronic gastritis with reactive hyperplasia and growth of inflammatory and hyperplastic polyps. Treatment of *H. pylori* may lead to their regression, whereas growth above 1.5 cm increases risk for dysplasia and carcinoma. Their smooth surfaces may become eroded. Microscopically there are irregular, cystically dilated, and elongated glands with edematous lamina propria containing acute and chronic inflammation *(right panel)*. There is foveolar hyperplasia with tall columnar mucinous epithelium *(left panel)*.

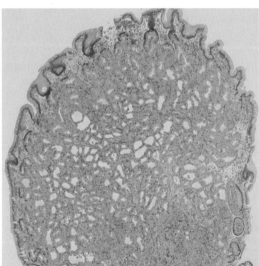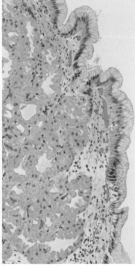

Figure 7-46 Fundic gland polyp, microscopic
Proton pump inhibitor therapy to reduce acid secretion may increase gastrin secretion, leading to gastric glandular hyperplasia. These polyps are more common in women, occurring at an average age of 50 years; they may be asymptomatic or associated with nausea, vomiting, or epigastric pain. Grossly they are circumscribed and smooth. When sporadic they are single; when multiple they are often associated with familial polyposis. Microscopically there are dilated, irregular glands *(left panel)* lined by pink parietal and chief cells *(right panel)* with minimal to absent inflammation.

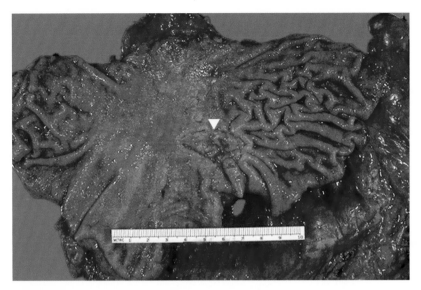

Figure 7-47 Adenocarcinoma, gross
The shallow gastric ulcer (▼) shown is about 2 to 4 cm in size. This ulcer on biopsy proved to be malignant, so the stomach was resected. In the United States, most gastric cancers are discovered at a late stage when the neoplasm has invaded or metastasized, whereas in Japan screening programs detect early gastric cancers. *All* gastric ulcers and *all* gastric masses must undergo biopsy because it is impossible to determine malignancy from their gross appearance. In contrast, virtually all duodenal peptic ulcers are benign. Worldwide, gastric carcinoma is the second most common cancer, but the incidence has been declining for decades in the United States.

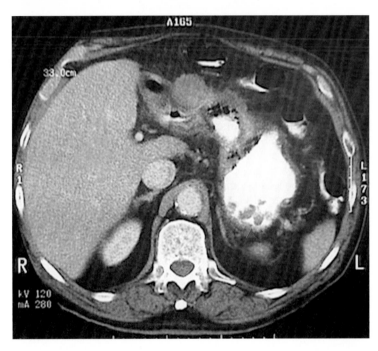

Figure 7-48 Adenocarcinoma, CT image
Abdominal CT scan with contrast enhancement reveals an exophytic mass (▲) lesion distorting the gastric antrum. This patient had *H. pylori* infection with chronic gastritis for many years. Few individuals with *H. pylori* infection develop gastric cancer, however. Risks, including dietary factors such as ingestion of pickled or smoked foods, nitrosamines derived from ingested nitrites, and excessive salt intake, predispose to development of the intestinal type of gastric cancer; changes in dietary patterns have led to a steady decrease in the incidence of this form of cancer. Risk factors for the diffuse form of gastric cancer are less well defined. Clinical manifestations include nausea, vomiting, abdominal pain, hematemesis, weight loss, altered bowel habits, and dysphagia. Early gastric cancers confined to the mucosa are usually asymptomatic and detected by endoscopic screening.

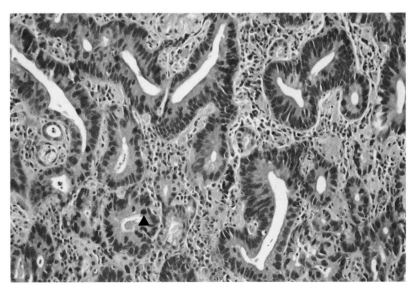

Figure 7-49 Adenocarcinoma, microscopic
This intestinal type of gastric adenocarcinoma has irregular shapes and sizes of neoplastic glands infiltrating into the submucosa. Some of the cells show mitoses (▲). The cells have an increased nuclear-to-cytoplasmic ratio and nuclear hyperchromatism. There is a desmoplastic stromal reaction to these infiltrating glands. Genetic abnormalities in the intestinal type of gastric cancer include *p53* mutation, abnormal E-cadherin expression, and instability of *TGFβ* and *BAX* genes.

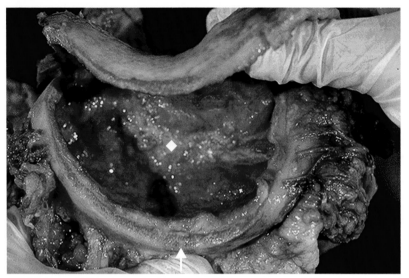

Figure 7-50 Adenocarcinoma, gross
This is an example of linitis plastica, a diffuse infiltrative gastric adenocarcinoma that gives the stomach a shrunken "leather bottle" appearance with extensive mucosal erosion, ulceration (◆), and a markedly thickened gastric wall (↑). This type of gastric carcinoma has a very poor prognosis. More localized gastric cancers are most likely to arise on the lesser curvature and show ulceration. The intestinal type of gastric cancer is more likely to arise from precursor lesions and to be related to *H. pylori* infection. The declining incidence of intestinal-type gastric cancers in the United States is probably related to diminishing prevalence of *H. pylori* infection. The incidence of the diffuse type of gastric cancer shown here has remained constant over time.

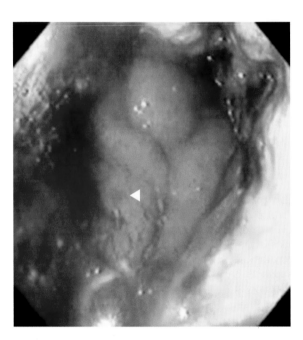

Figure 7-51 Adenocarcinoma, endoscopy
The endoscopic view of the linitis plastica appearance of the diffuse type of gastric adenocarcinoma reveals extensive mucosal erosion (◄). Exposure to ingested carcinogens may play a role in the development of diffuse gastric adenocarcinomas. Some of them are related to hereditary diffuse gastric cancer (HDGC) syndrome with mutations in the E-cadherin (*CDH1*) gene, with high risk for stomach and lobular breast carcinoma. Diets rich in fruits and vegetables reduce the risk for carcinoma.

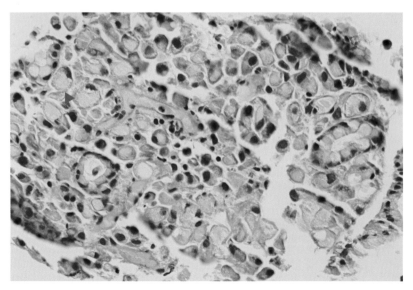

Figure 7-52 Adenocarcinoma, microscopic
This diffuse type of gastric adenocarcinoma is so poorly differentiated that mostly infiltrating neoplastic cells with marked pleomorphism are seen. Many of the neoplastic cells have cytoplasm filled with clear vacuoles of mucin (▶), displacing the cell nucleus to the periphery. This is the "signet ring" cell pattern that is typical of the diffuse type of gastric adenocarcinoma, which tends to be highly infiltrative and has a poor prognosis. Mutations in *CDH1* that encode E-cadherin involved in epithelial intercellular adhesion are found with some diffuse gastric carcinomas, including familial forms.

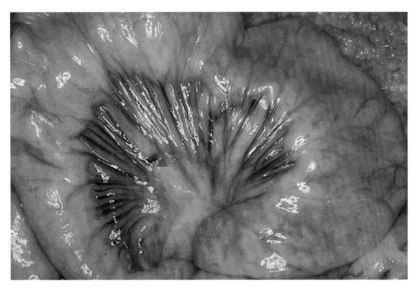

Figure 7-53 Normal small intestine and mesentery, gross

A loop of bowel attached through the mesentery is shown here. Note the extensive venous drainage (▲), which flows into the portal venous system draining into the liver. Arcades of arteries supplying blood to the bowel run in the same mesenteric location. The bowel is supplied by branches and collaterals from the celiac axis, superior mesenteric artery, and inferior mesenteric artery, providing an extensive anastomosing arterial blood supply to the bowel, making it more difficult to infarct. Note the smooth, glistening peritoneal surfaces of the small intestine.

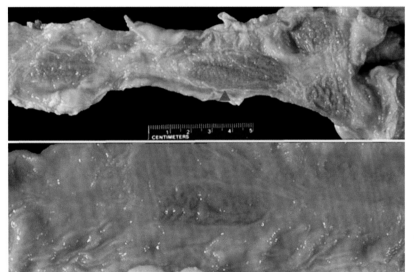

Figure 7-54 Normal small intestine, gross

This is the normal appearance of terminal ileum. In the *upper panel,* note the ileocecal valve; several darker oval Peyer patches (▲) are present on the mucosa. In the *lower panel,* note the prominent oval Peyer patch, which is a concentration of submucosal lymphoid tissue. In the duodenum, the lamina propria and the submucosa have proportionately more lymphoid tissue than the rest of the GI tract. The ileum has more prominent submucosal lymphoid tissue, which appears as small nodules or as elongated ovoid Peyer patches. Gut-associated lymphoid tissue (GALT) is present from the back of the tongue all the way to the rectum and is collectively the largest lymphoid organ of the body.

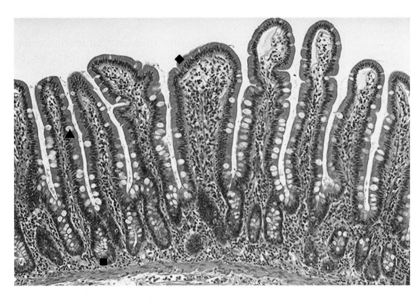

Figure 7-55 Normal small intestine, microscopic

The small intestinal mucosa has surface villi lined by columnar cells (◆) and scattered goblet cells (▲). The villi terminate in the lamina propria as glandular lumina known as *crypts of Lieberkühn* (■). The villi greatly increase the surface absorptive area. The jejunum has more prominent folds (plicae) of the mucosa to increase absorptive area. Each intestinal villus contains a blind-ended lymphatic channel known as a *lacteal.* The major immunoglobulin secreted by plasma cells of the GI tract (and respiratory tract) is IgA, so-called *secretory IgA.* This IgA is bound to protein on the glycocalyx overlying the microvilli of the brush border to neutralize harmful agents such as infectious organisms.

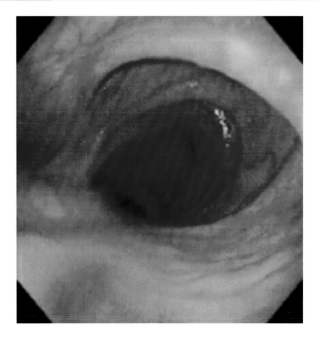

Figure 7-56 Normal transverse colon, endoscopy

Note the mucosal haustral folds typical of the colon. The function of the colon is primarily to absorb most of the remaining water and electrolytes passed from the small intestine to concentrate the volume of stool, so that only about 100 mL of water is lost per day in the stool. There are about 7 to 10 L of gas traversing the colon each day, primarily as a result of growth of normal bacterial flora, although only about 0.5 L is passed as flatus. The gaseous components include swallowed air (nitrogen and oxygen) and methane and hydrogen from digestive processes and bacterial growth. Irritable bowel disease has no gross or microscopic findings but results from abnormally exaggerated sensory responses to physiologic stimuli from gas in the bowel, which are worsened by stress. Anticholinergic drugs may provide temporary relief.

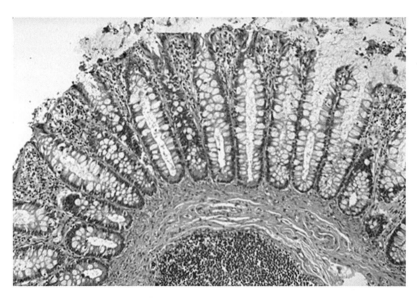

Figure 7-57 Normal colon, microscopic

The colon has a mucosal architecture of long tubular glands (crypts of Lieberkühn) lined by columnar mucous cells. Goblet cells are numerous and provide lubrication for transit of stool. Lymphoid nodules are in the lamina propria and submucosa. The outer longitudinal layer of muscle is coalesced into long bands known as *taeniae coli*. At the anorectal junction, there is a mucosal transition from columnar cells lining crypts to stratified squamous mucosa. Above and below this junction are prominent submucosal veins (internal and external hemorrhoidal veins) that when dilated form hemorrhoids with itching and bleeding. A layer of skeletal muscle at the anus provides a sphincter under voluntary control.

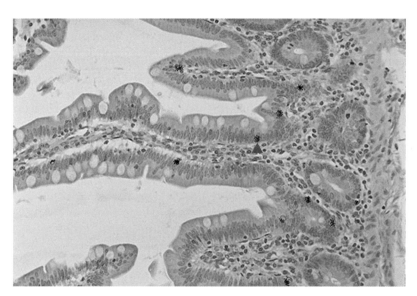

Figure 7-58 Normal intestinal endocrine cells, microscopic

The areas of black, stippled staining (▲) identify the scattered enteroendocrine (neuroendocrine) cells in the mucosal crypts of the small intestine (Kulchitsky cells). These cells are scattered within the glands and become more numerous distally in the small intestine. A variety of enteroendocrine cells are present in the mucosa of the gut. When food passes into the small intestine, some of it releases cholecystokinin, which delays gastric emptying while promoting digestion by causing the gallbladder to contract and release bile, which aids in digestion of lipids. Cholecystokinin also causes release of various enzymes from pancreatic acinar cells.

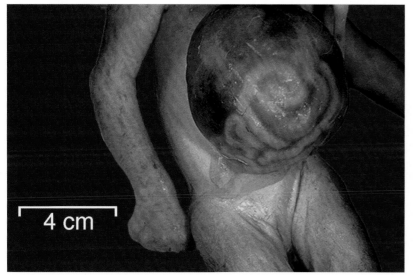

Figure 7-59 Omphalocele, gross
This ventral midline abdominal wall defect in a newborn girl involves the region of the umbilical cord, so it is called an *omphalocele*. There is a thin membrane covering the herniated abdominal contents (including loops of bowel and liver). Because this bowel has mainly developed outside of the abdominal cavity during fetal life, it is malrotated, and the abdominal cavity is not properly formed (too small). Such a defect would have to be repaired in several stages. An omphalocele may occur sporadically, but most are associated with other congenital malformations and may be the result of a genetic abnormality, such as trisomy 18.

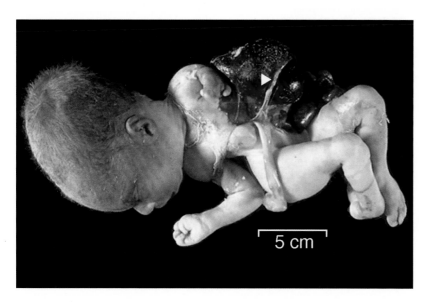

Figure 7-60 Gastroschisis, gross
This large lateral abdominal wall defect does not involve the cord and is not covered by a membrane. Much of the bowel, stomach, and liver have developed outside the abdominal cavity in utero. This gastroschisis is associated with limb–body wall (LBW) complex, sometimes called *amnionic band syndrome*, but such fibrous bands (▶) may be present in only half of cases of LBW complex. It results from early amnion disruption, which occurs sporadically in embryonic development and is not part of a defined genetic abnormality. Shown here in association with LBW complex are reductions of the extremities, particularly the left upper extremity, and scoliosis. Not seen here are craniofacial clefts and defects that can also occur with LBW complex.

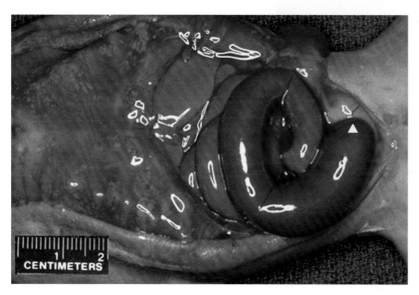

Figure 7-61 Intestinal atresia, gross
The meconium-filled intestine shown here ends in a blind pouch (▲). This is complete obstruction, or atresia. Partial or incomplete obstruction is called *stenosis.* Such a defect, similar to many anomalies, often occurs in conjunction with other anomalies. Bowel atresias in utero are accompanied by polyhydramnios because the swallowing and absorption of amniotic fluid by the fetal GI tract is impaired. Atresia is uncommon, but one place it can be seen is the duodenum; half of all duodenal atresias occur with Down syndrome, although conversely, few cases of Down syndrome have duodenal atresia. On ultrasound, there is a "double-bubble" sign from duodenal enlargement proximal to the atresia accompanying the normal stomach bubble.

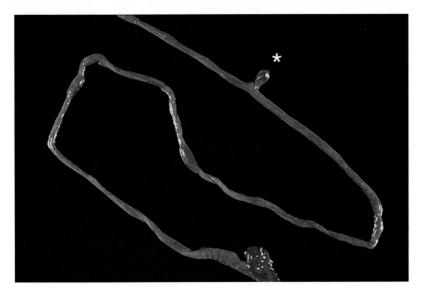

Figure 7-62 Meckel diverticulum, gross
Congenital anomalies of bowel consist mainly of diverticula or atresias, which often occur in association with other congenital anomalies. Shown here is the most common congenital anomaly of the GI tract—a Meckel diverticulum (★). It occurs from failed involution of the omphalomesenteric (vitelline) duct and thus extends from the antimesenteric side of the bowel wall. Remember the number *2:* about 2% of people have them; they are usually located 2 feet from the ileocecal valve, are 2 inches long, are twice as common in males, and may become symptomatic by age 2.

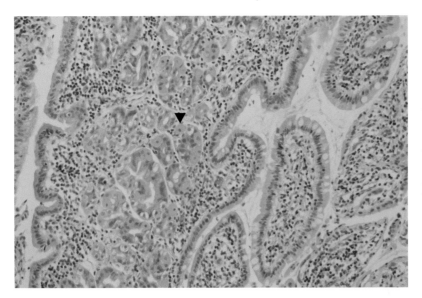

Figure 7-63 Meckel diverticulum, microscopic
Present is intestinal-type epithelium with goblet cells, intermixed with gastric glands containing pink parietal cells (▼). There may be pain from ulceration of surrounding mucosa unprotected from the acid secretion. Iron deficiency anemia is also possible. This "true" diverticulum with all three bowel wall layers is usually an incidental finding in an adult. It may contain ectopic pancreas, which is of little consequence unless it forms a mass large enough to predispose to intussusception.

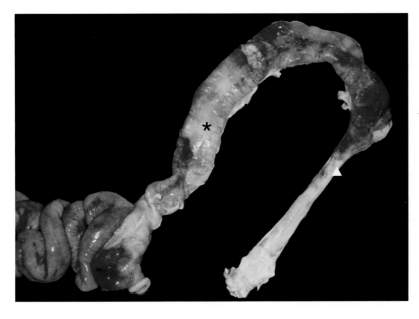

Figure 7-64 Hirschsprung disease, gross
Shown here is dilation of bowel (megacolon) caused by failure of migration of neuroblasts that form the myenteric plexus in the lower bowel wall. This dilation (★) is proximal to the affected aganglionic region (▲) at the lower left center in the sigmoid colon. The result is intestinal obstruction, marked by delayed passage of meconium after birth, caused by lack of normal peristalsis in affected neonates. The incidence is 1 per 5000 live births, mostly males. Various genetic defects can cause Hirschsprung disease, but about half of familial cases and one sixth of sporadic cases result from *RET* gene mutations. Mucosal damage and secondary infection may follow.

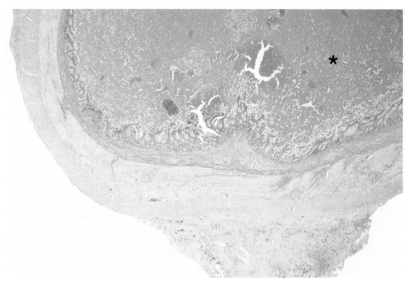

Figure 7-65 Meconium ileus, microscopic

This form of bowel obstruction most often occurs in neonates with cystic fibrosis but can rarely occur in normal infants. In cystic fibrosis the abnormal pancreatic secretions lead to inspissated meconium with intestinal obstruction. The dilated ileum is shown filled with meconium (★). The gross appearance is dark green; meconium may also be tarry or gritty. Little or none of this highly viscid meconium is passed per rectum after birth. A potential complication is meconium peritonitis with bowel rupture. Calcifications in the spilled meconium may be visible radiographically. Another complication of meconium ileus is volvulus.

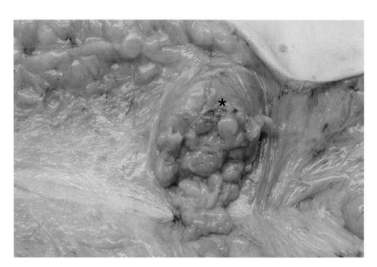

Figure 7-66 Hernia, gross

External hernias represent an outpouching of peritoneum through a defect or weakness in the abdominal wall. This outpouching most often occurs in the inguinal region, but it also can occur in the umbilical region, as shown here. An "internal" herniation of bowel can result from an abnormal opening formed by adhesions. The defect may be large enough to admit a portion of omentum or bowel. In this abdominal incision, a small hernia sac (★) can be seen that contains adipose tissue from omentum.

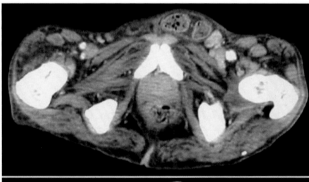

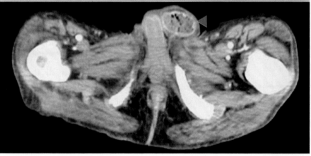

Figure 7-67 Hernia, CT image

A left inguinal hernia is present, identified here because a portion of bowel (◀) has herniated down the inguinal canal and into the scrotum, leading to the remarkable physical examination finding of bowel sounds on auscultation of the scrotum. This is an "indirect" hernia; direct hernias are medial to the femoral artery. A persistent embryologic processus vaginalis may predispose to an indirect inguinal hernia; weakening of lower abdominal transversalis fascia predisposes to a direct hernia. A reducible hernia contains bowel that can slip in and out of the opening; bowel can become trapped, or incarcerated, within the hernia, which predisposes to strangulation of the bowel, with ischemia from a compromised blood supply.

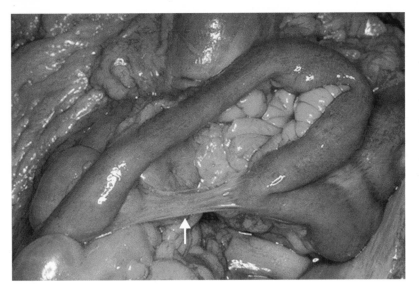

Figure 7-68 Adhesion, gross
A bandlike adhesion (↑) between loops of small intestine is shown. Such adhesions are most likely to form after abdominal surgery. More diffuse adhesions may also form after peritonitis. Adhesions may predispose to bowel obstruction when loops of bowel become trapped in the abnormal opening created by adhesions. In populations in which prior abdominal surgery for various conditions, such as acute appendicitis, has been performed, adhesions are often the most common cause of bowel obstruction. The presence of abdominal scars on physical examination of a patient with acute abdominal pain, distention, and ileus is a clue to this diagnosis.

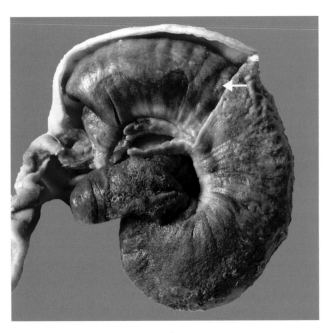

Figure 7-69 Intussusception, gross
One rare form of bowel obstruction occurs when a segment of small intestine telescopes on itself, a process called *intussusception*. The blood supply to that segment becomes compromised, predisposing to infarction. A portion of this infarcted bowel is opened superiorly to reveal the telescoped segment within (←), giving the "bowel within a bowel" appearance. When this condition occurs in children, it is typically idiopathic. In adults, a mass lesion such as a polyp, or diverticulum, driven by peristalsis may lead to intussusception.

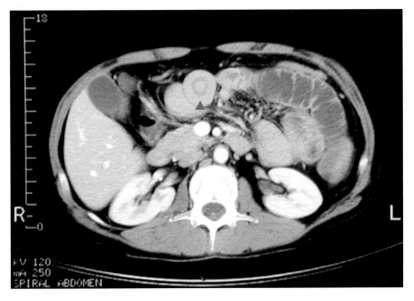

Figure 7-70 Intussusception, CT image
Abdominal CT scan shows a thickened portion of small intestine that has a target appearance (▲) because of the presence of an intussuscepted portion of bowel, a "bowel within a bowel" characteristic of intussusception. An abdominal plain film radiograph typically shows loops of small bowel dilated with air, or air-fluid levels from ileus, as a consequence of bowel obstruction. Patients have abdominal pain, abdominal distention, obstipation, and diminished or abnormal bowel sounds on physical examination.

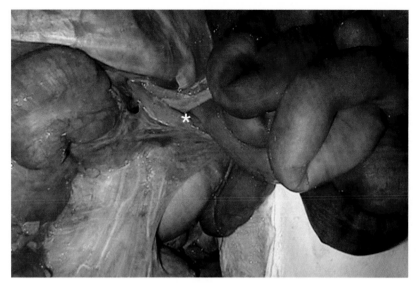

Figure 7-71 Volvulus, gross
Torsion, or twisting, of the bowel so that the blood supply and the bowel itself become obstructed, leads to ischemia with infarction. Obstruction of venous outflow can produce marked congestion. If caught early, the bowel can be untwisted to restore blood supply, but this is often not the case. Visible here is twisting (★) of the mesentery so that the entire small intestine from jejunum through ileum has become ischemic and is dark red from infarction. Volvulus is rare and most often is seen in adults, in whom it occurs with equal frequency in small intestine (around a twisted mesentery) and colon (in either sigmoid or cecum, which are more mobile). In very young children, volvulus almost always involves the small intestine.

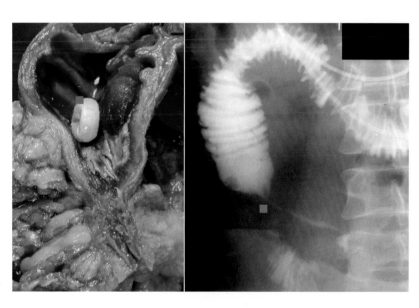

Figure 7-72 Intestinal stricture, gross and radiograph
A radiograph from a small bowel series *(right panel)* reveals a stricture (■) resulting from inflammation produced from irritation by a foreign body (■) found at surgery *(left panel)* that did not pass through the lumen, but did not perforate either. Sharp foreign bodies may perforate bowel wall and lead to peritonitis. A foreign body may cause inflammation that progressively narrows the bowel lumen. In the past, enteric-coated capsules of medications were known to produce this finding. Ulceration from NSAIDs may lead to perforation or stricture.

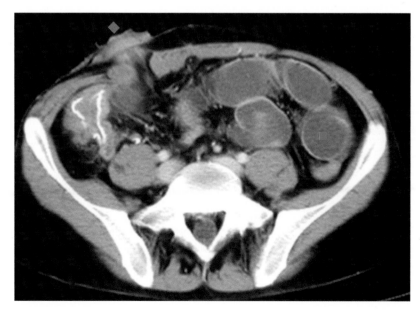

Figure 7-73 Ileus, CT image
Note the dilated loops (■) of small bowel. Ileus is hypomotility or absence of peristalsis, with lack of movement of intestinal contents, and it may be mechanical or paralytic (adynamic). Mechanical obstruction most often results from adhesions, hernias, and neoplasms. Paralytic ileus may be the result of inflammation, drugs, and electrolyte disturbances. In this case, postoperatively there are dilated loops of small bowel in this abdominal CT scan. Contrast material was administered, but it has not made its way to the small intestine. An ileostomy stoma (◆) also is present, from the surgery that led to resection of bowel with removal of the colon.

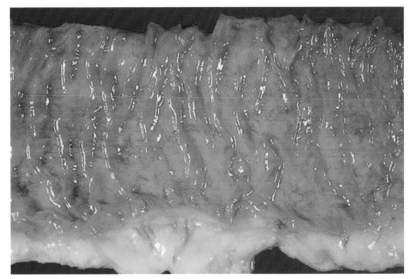

Figure 7-74　Ischemic bowel disease, gross
This small intestinal mucosa shows marked red hyperemia of the tips of the villi as a result of early ischemic enteritis. Ischemia most often results from hypotension (shock) secondary to cardiac failure, marked blood loss, or loss of blood supply from mechanical obstruction (as with the bowel incarcerated in a hernia or with volvulus or intussusception). Less frequently, thrombosis or embolization with occlusion of one or more mesenteric arterial branches can produce acute intestinal ischemia. Venous thrombosis from hypercoagulable states is less frequent. If the blood supply is not quickly restored, the bowel becomes infarcted.

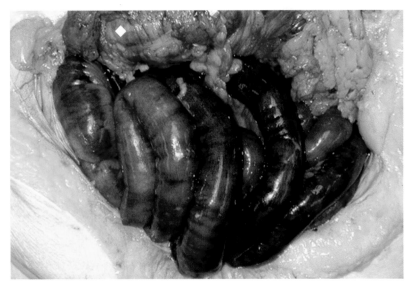

Figure 7-75　Ischemic enteritis, gross
The dark-red to gray infarcted small intestinal loops contrasts with the pale pink normal transverse colon (◆) at the top. In some organs, such as bowel with anastomosing blood supplies or liver with a dual blood supply, infarction is more difficult. This bowel was caught in a hernia created by internal adhesions from prior surgery. A similar finding could result from incarceration of bowel in an inguinal hernia sac. The mesenteric blood supply was constricted here. Bowel ischemia often produces acute abdominal pain with distention. Lack of peristalsis, marked by absence of bowel sounds, is known as *ileus.*

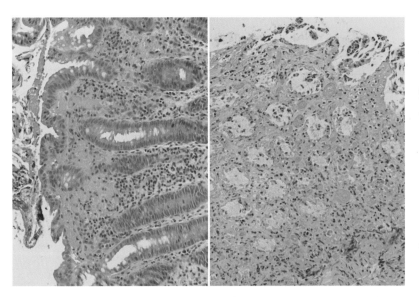

Figure 7-76　Ischemic enteritis, microscopic
The mucosal surface of the bowel shows early red hyperemia *(left panel)* and necrosis *(right panel)* with hyperemia extending all the way from mucosa to submucosal and muscular wall vessels. The submucosa and muscularis are still intact, however. With more advanced ischemia and necrosis, the small intestinal mucosa can show hemorrhage with acute inflammation. Progression of ischemia produces transmural necrosis extending into submucosa and muscularis. Patients can have abdominal pain, vomiting, and bloody or melanotic stools. With ischemic necrosis, intestinal bacterial organisms can gain access to blood, producing septicemia, or to peritoneal cavity, producing peritonitis and leading to shock.

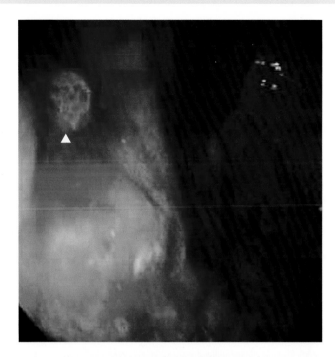

Figure 7-77 Angiodysplasia, endoscopy

On upper GI endoscopy, an area of malformed vasculature (▲) is shown; this condition is more common in older individuals and is a cause for GI tract bleeding. This bleeding is often intermittent and rarely severe. One or more foci of irregular, tortuous, thin-walled, dilated venous or capillary channels are present in the mucosa or submucosa, typically the colon but occasionally elsewhere. The lesions are often quite small (<0.5 cm), making them hard to find. Colonoscopy and mesenteric angiography can be performed for diagnosis, and affected areas can be resected. Some cases are associated with the uncommon systemic disorder known as *hereditary hemorrhagic telangiectasia* (Osler-Weber-Rendu syndrome). A similar Dieulafoy lesion is a focal submucosal arterial or arteriovenous malformation of the gut submucosa with overlying mucosal disruption, most often found in the stomach, that can produce bleeding.

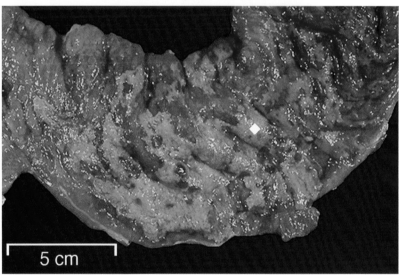

Figure 7-78 Pseudomembranous colitis, gross

The colonic mucosal surface shown is partially covered by yellow-green exudate (◆). The mucosa is erythematous and superficially denuded, but not eroded. It may cause an acute or chronic diarrheal illness associated with fever, leukocytosis, abdominal pain, and cramps. Broad-spectrum antibiotic usage (e.g., clindamycin) or immunosuppression allows overgrowth of normally suppressed intestinal bacterial flora, such as *Clostridium difficile,* or other organisms such as *Staphylococcus aureus, Salmonella,* or fungi such as *Candida,* to cause this antibiotic-associated colitis. Exotoxins elaborated by the bacteria damage the mucosa by inducing cytokine production to cause cellular apoptosis.

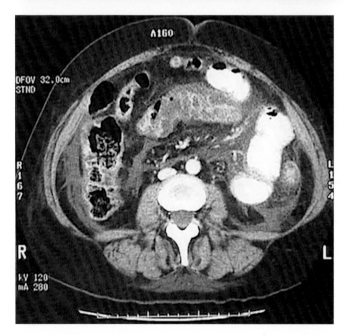

Figure 7-79 Pseudomembranous colitis, CT image

Abdominal CT scan reveals a narrowed lumen with thickened, edematous transverse colon (▲) and colonic splenic flexure as a consequence of antibiotic-associated (pseudomembranous) colitis. This appearance can also be present with ischemic colitis and neutropenic colitis (typhlitis). Typhlitis typically involves the cecum, where blood flow is most likely to be diminished, in an immunocompromised patient with neutropenia.

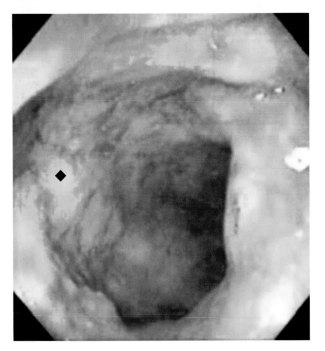

Figure 7-80 Pseudomembranous colitis, endoscopy
On colonoscopy, there is a tan-to-green exudate (◆) overlying the surface of the colonic mucosa. This appearance may also be seen with ischemia and with severe acute infectious colitis. Diagnosis is aided by detection of the organism, or in most cases *C. difficile* toxin. Patients with this disorder may have abdominal pain and develop a severe diarrhea, typically nonbloody. With progression of disease, there can be sepsis and shock. The affected bowel may need to be resected.

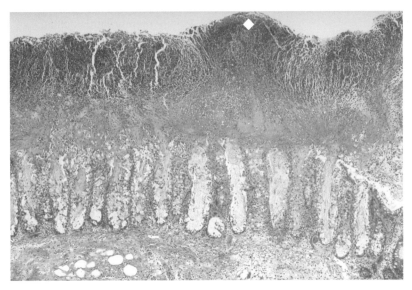

Figure 7-81 Pseudomembranous colitis, microscopic
The underlying colonic mucosa is intact, so grossly bloody diarrhea is unlikely, but there is a marked overlying exudate with necrotic epithelial cells admixed with inflammatory cells. The exudate within crypts may be so extensive that it erupts (◆) from the surface in volcano-like fashion (more like Mauna Loa, as shown here). *C. difficile* toxins disrupt the epithelial cytoskeleton, with loss of tight junction barrier function, and promote cytokine release and apoptosis. Recurrent infection may occur.

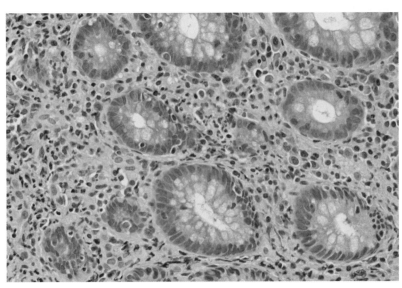

Figure 7-82 Infectious colitis, microscopic
Infectious agents such as *Shigella, Salmonella,* and *Campylobacter* can produce an acute self-limited colitis with cryptitis, crypt ulcers, and extensive infiltrates of neutrophils and lymphocytes between crypts, as shown here. Additional findings can include edema, abscesses, and small granulomas. The crypt architecture and goblet cells are preserved, unlike in inflammatory bowel disease. Resolution typically occurs within 2 to 3 weeks.

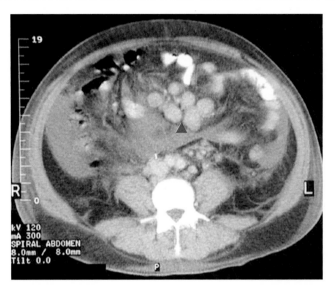

Figure 7-83 Mesenteric lymphadenitis, CT image

Note the enlarged mesenteric lymph nodes (▲). There can be abrupt or more insidious onset of abdominal pain accompanied by fever. Nausea and vomiting may precede the pain (opposite from appendicitis), but the pain may be mainly in the right lower quadrant, as well as diffuse. *Yersinia enterocolitica* enteritis may occur first, from a fecal-oral route of infection. Swallowed organisms from respiratory tract infection may precede the adenitis. Mild cases typically resolve; severe cases may require antibiotic therapy, guided by results from blood culture.

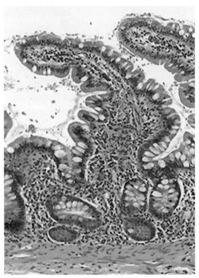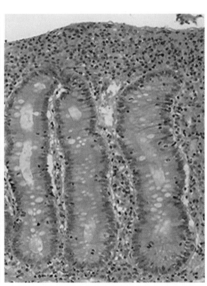

Figure 7-84 Celiac disease (sprue), microscopic

Compare normal small intestinal mucosa *(left panel)* and mucosa involved by celiac disease *(right panel)* with blunting and flattening of villi (in severe cases, loss of villi with flattening of the mucosa, as shown here), loss of crypts, increased mitotic activity, loss of the brush border, and infiltration with CD4 cells producing cytokines. There is sensitivity to gluten, which contains gliadin protein, found in wheat, oats, barley, and rye. Gliadin induces IL-15 expression from enterocytes that attracts cytotoxic CD8 cells. It has a prevalence of 0.6% to 1% worldwide. More than 95% of affected patients have the HLA DQ2 or HLA DQ8 antigen. Removing the offending grains from the diet results in subsidence of enteropathy.

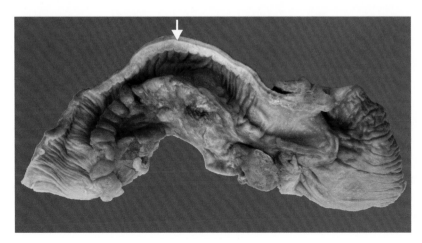

Figure 7-85 Crohn disease (CD), gross

The center portion of terminal ileum shown here has a thickened wall (↓), and the mucosa has lost the regular folds and contains deep fissures. The serosal surface shows reddish indurated adipose tissue that creeps over the surface. The areas of inflammation tend to be discontinuous throughout the bowel ("skip" lesions). Although any portion of the GI tract may be involved with CD, the small intestine—and the terminal ileum in particular—is most likely to be affected. CD is more common in the United States and Western Europe; women are affected more often than men. A genetic susceptibility may be related to the presence of certain HLA types and to *NOD2* gene mutations that may be related to the microbe receptor triggering NF-κB transcription factor production, which promotes cytokine release driving inflammation.

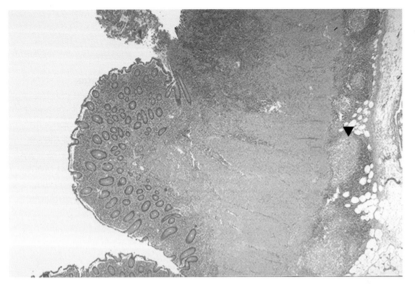

Figure 7-86 Crohn disease (CD), microscopic
Note the transmural inflammation with inflammatory cells (bluish infiltrates) extending from the ulcerated mucosa through submucosa and muscularis to the serosa, appearing as nodular granulomatous infiltrates (▼) on the serosal surface. This transmural inflammation predisposes to formation of adhesions and fistulas with adjacent intra-abdominal structures from serosal involvement. Enteroenteric fistulas between loops of bowel and perirectal fistulas are common complications. Mucosal injury predisposes to malabsorption, particularly of vitamin B_{12}, and steatorrhea from loss of bile salt recirculation, because of terminal ileal involvement.

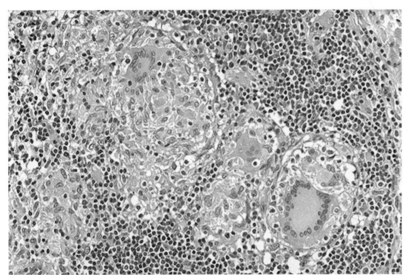

Figure 7-87 Crohn disease (CD), microscopic
The granulomatous inflammation of CD is shown here with epithelioid cells, giant cells, and many lymphocytes. Both T_H1 and T_H17 immune responses participate. Most patients have a relapsing course over decades, some have quiescent disease for many years, and others have continuously active disease after onset. *Saccharomyces cerevisiae* IgG antibodies are found in 80% of CD patients, but only 20% of patients with ulcerative colitis (UC). *S. cerevisiae* IgA antibodies are found in 35% of CD patients, but less than 1% of UC patients. Perinuclear antineutrophil cytoplasmic antibodies (p-ANCA) are found in 75% of UC patients, but in only 20% of CD patients.

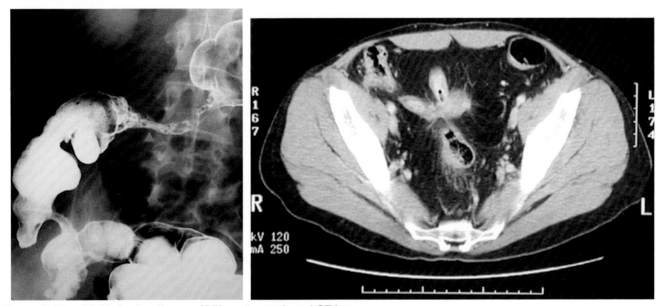

Figures 7-88 and 7-89 Crohn disease (CD), radiograph and CT image
The upper GI series on the *left* with bright barium contrast medium filling the bowel lumen reveals a long area of narrowing (▲) involving nearly the entire terminal ileum, a favorite site of involvement of CD, but the remaining small bowel and the colon may also be involved. The stomach is rarely involved. The abdominal CT scan without contrast enhancement on the *right* shows enteroenteric fistula formation. Loops of small bowel converge (▲) because of the adhesions resulting from the transmural inflammation.

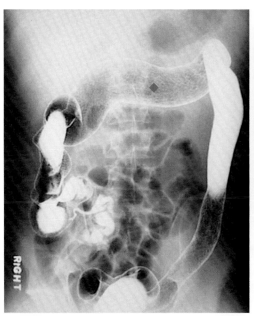
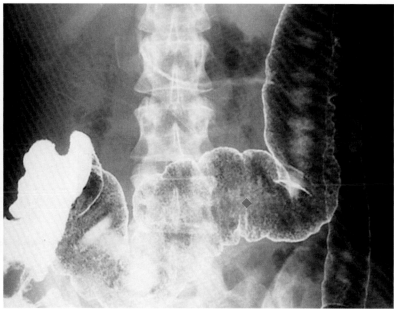

Figures 7-90 and 7-91 Ulcerative colitis (UC), radiographs

The barium enema on the *left* has fine granularity (◆) of the mucosa from the rectum to the transverse colon, typical of earlier involvement of the mucosa with UC. UC, along with CD, is a form of idiopathic inflammatory bowel disease. The barium enema on the *right* shows a closer view of an area of coarse granularity (◆) of the mucosa from the rectum to the transverse colon, typical of a more severe involvement of the mucosa with UC. UC typically involves the colonic mucosa in a continuous pattern, starting from the rectum and extending a variable distance proximally.

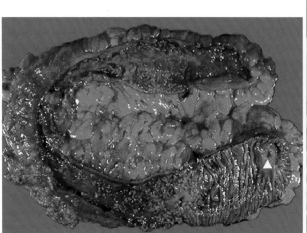
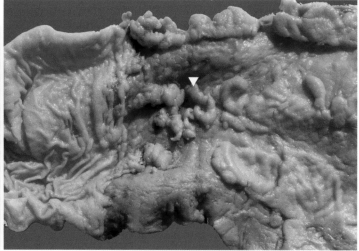

Figures 7-92 and 7-93 Ulcerative colitis (UC), gross

On the *left* is a colectomy specimen with extensive UC beginning in the rectum and extending all the way to the ileocecal valve (▲). There is diffuse mucosal inflammation with focal ulceration, erythema, and granularity. As the disease progresses, the mucosal erosions coalesce to linear ulcers that undermine remaining mucosa, leaving islands of residual mucosa (▼) called *pseudopolyps.* On the *right,* these pseudopolyps occur in a case of severe UC. The remaining mucosa has been ulcerated away, leaving only hyperemic submucosa and muscularis.

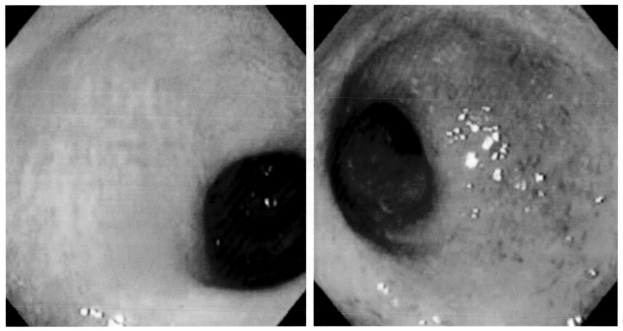

Figures 7-94 and 7-95 Ulcerative colitis (UC), endoscopy

On the *left,* a colonoscopic view of less severe UC shows friable, erythematous mucosa and reduction in haustral folds. On the *right* is shown a view of active UC, but not so eroded as to produce pseudopolyps. UC is idiopathic and occurs more frequently in the United States and Europe than in other areas of the world. UC is a chronic disease with a relapsing course in most patients, although a few patients have only one or two bouts; some patients may have continuous active disease. The onset of active UC is marked by low-volume but bloody, mucoid diarrhea along with abdominal cramping pain, tenesmus, and fever. Extraintestinal manifestations often develop over the course of an inflammatory bowel disease, including sclerosing cholangitis, migratory polyarthritis, sacroiliitis, uveitis, and acanthosis nigricans. There is a long-term risk for development of colonic adenocarcinoma. Extraintestinal manifestations occur with CD as well, although the risk for adenocarcinoma is not as great for CD as for UC.

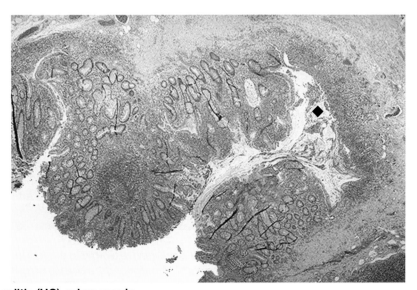

Figure 7-96 Ulcerative colitis (UC), microscopic

The inflammation of UC is confined primarily to the mucosa, shown here as an inflammatory process that undermines the surrounding mucosa to produce a flask-shaped (◆) ulceration. An exudate is present over the surface. Acute and chronic inflammatory cells can be present. The stools are typically of low volume but may contain blood and mucus. A relapsing but mild course is most common, seen in 60% of patients, although some patients may have a single episode, and others have almost continuous attacks. One third of patients may undergo colectomy within 3 years of onset because of uncontrolled colitis. In about 10% of inflammatory bowel disease cases, a clear distinction between CD and UC cannot be made, and the term applied is indeterminate colitis.

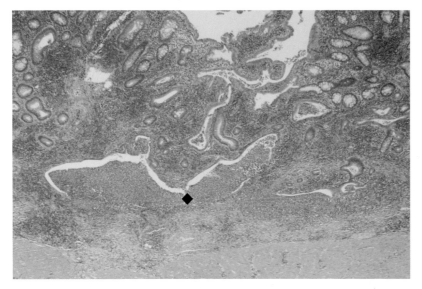

Figure 7-97 Ulcerative colitis (UC), microscopic

The muscularis is intact, but there is intense chronic inflammation throughout the mucosa. A broad-based flask-shaped ulcer (◆) along the long axis of the colon is filled with neutrophils. Irregularly shaped crypts of Lieberkühn, called *crypt distortion,* are a hallmark. The rectum is always involved, but more proximal colonic involvement can occur. Toxic megacolon with marked dilation and thinning of the bowel is a feared complication because of risk for rupture. Extraintestinal manifestations overlap those of CD and may include migratory polyarthritis, sacroiliitis, ankylosing spondylitis, uveitis, pericholangitis, and primary sclerosing cholangitis.

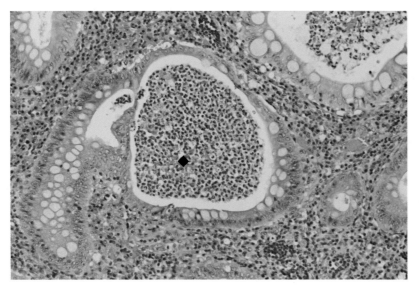

Figure 7-98 Ulcerative colitis (UC), microscopic

The colonic mucosa of active UC shows "crypt abscesses," in which a neutrophilic exudate (◆) is found within the glandular lumina of the crypts of Lieberkühn. The submucosa also shows intense inflammation. Inflamed crypts with architectural distortion show loss of goblet cells and hyperchromatic nuclei with inflammatory atypia. Crypt abscesses are a histologic finding more typical of UC than CD, but there is overlap between these two forms of idiopathic inflammatory bowel disease, and not all cases can be classified completely in all patients.

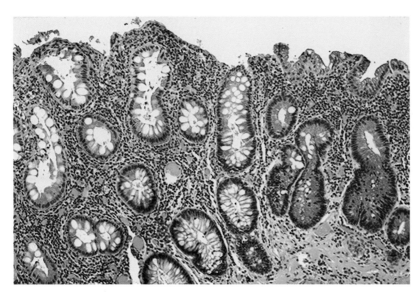

Figure 7-99 Ulcerative colitis (UC), microscopic

More normal colonic crypts with goblet cells are shown on the left, but the crypts on the right show distortion with dysplasia, the first indication that there is increasing risk for development of carcinoma. Chronic UC leads to DNA damage with microsatellite instability. Over time, after 10 to 20 years of pancolitis, there is such a significant risk for adenocarcinoma that total colectomy may be performed. Patients with long-standing UC may undergo screening colonoscopies to detect development of dysplasia.

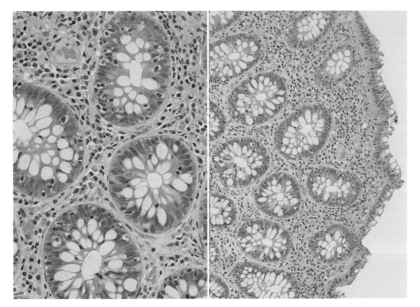

Figure 7-100 Lymphocytic colitis, microscopic
The colonic mucosa and surface epithelium *(right panel)* is intact but contains increased numbers of submucosal lymphocytes that are infiltrating into the crypts *(left panel)*. Some cases are found in association with celiac disease or other autoimmune diseases. Patients often have a mild chronic watery diarrhea. This is one form of microscopic colitis; the other is collagenous colitis with a dense subepithelial collagen layer not seen here.

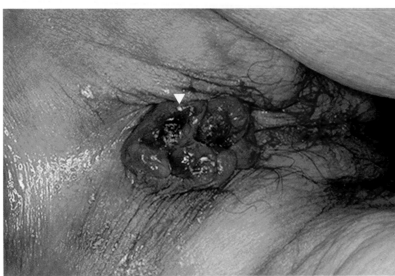

Figure 7-101 Hemorrhoids, gross
Shown here is the anus and perianal region with prominent prolapsed true (internal) hemorrhoids (▼), which consist of dilated submucosal veins predisposed to thrombose and rupture with hematoma formation. External hemorrhoids form beyond the intersphincteric groove to produce an "acute pile" at the anal verge. Chronically increased venous pressure leads to venous dilation. Hemorrhoids can itch and bleed (usually bright red blood, during defecation). Rectal prolapse is another complication. Hemorrhoids may become ulcerated. Healing of a thrombosed hemorrhoid results in a fibrous polyp, or anal tag.

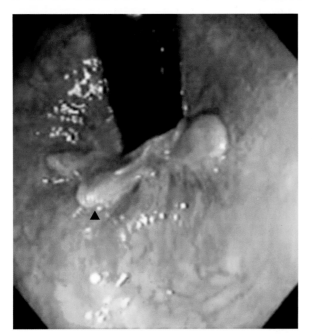

Figure 7-102 Hemorrhoids, endoscopy
These polypoid lesions (▲) are hemorrhoids at the anorectal junction. The vessels forming them have undergone at least partial thrombosis and have become shrunken, with a whitened appearance. Chronic constipation, low-fiber diet, chronic diarrhea, pregnancy, and portal hypertension enhance hemorrhoid formation. They are rarely present in individuals younger than 30 years.

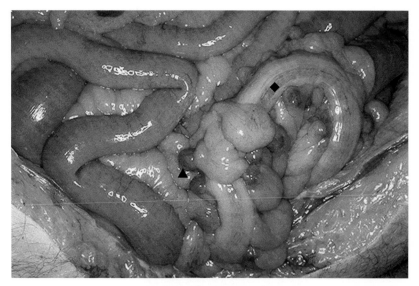

Figure 7-103 Colonic diverticular disease, gross
The sigmoid colon on the right has a band of taeniae coli (◆) muscle running longitudinally and appears lighter in color than the adjacent small intestine. Protruding from the sigmoid colon are multiple, rounded, bluish gray outpouchings (▲) known as *diverticula.* Diverticula average 0.5 to 1 cm in diameter, are much more common in the colon than in small intestine, and are more common in the left colon. Diverticula are more common in individuals living in developed nations and may be related to the usual diet, which has less fiber, leading to diminished motility and increased intraluminal pressure. The number of diverticula increases with age.

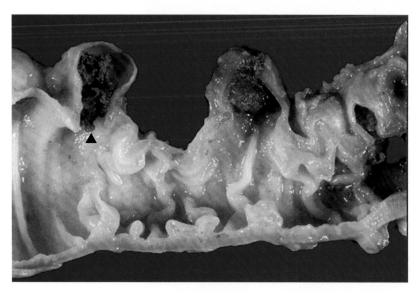

Figure 7-104 Colonic diverticular disease, gross
Sectioning the colon longitudinally reveals that the diverticula have an opening to the colonic lumen through a narrow neck (▲). Colonic diverticula are rarely larger than 1 cm in diameter. These are not true diverticula because only the submucosa and mucosa are herniated through an acquired focal weakness in the muscularis. Peristalsis does not empty them, so they become filled with stool. Focal weaknesses in the bowel wall and increased luminal pressure contribute to the formation of multiple diverticula, collectively termed *diverticulosis.* They rarely occur in individuals younger than 30 years of age, but are common past age 60, although most remain asymptomatic.

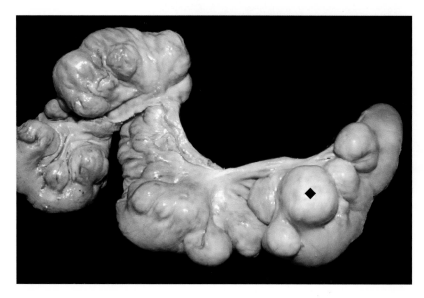

Figure 7-105 Jejunal diverticular disease, gross
Diverticula involving the small bowel are far less common than those in the colon. They may result from abnormal motility with increased segmental intraluminal pressure. They tend to arise in persons over age 50 and have wider mouths than colonic diverticula and therefore are less prone to inflammation, hemorrhage, and rupture, so most persons are asymptomatic. The diverticula (◆) shown are acquired, extraluminal, and arising on the mesenteric border.

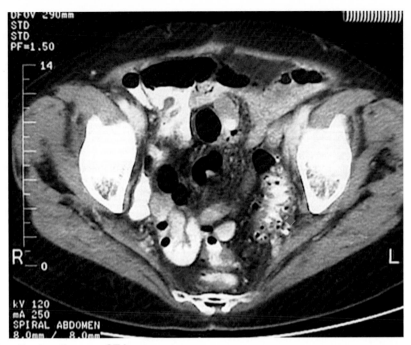

Figure 7-106 Colonic diverticular disease, CT image
Abdominal CT scan with contrast enhancement in the pelvic region shows diverticulosis (◆) most pronounced in the sigmoid colon in the pelvis. The small, rounded outpouchings are dark because they are filled with stool and air, not contrast material. Most diverticula are asymptomatic. Complications can develop in about 20% of patients with diverticulosis, including abdominal pain, constipation, intermittent bleeding, and inflammation (diverticulitis). Rarely, more extensive inflammation extending through the diverticular wall leads to rupture of a diverticulum with peritonitis.

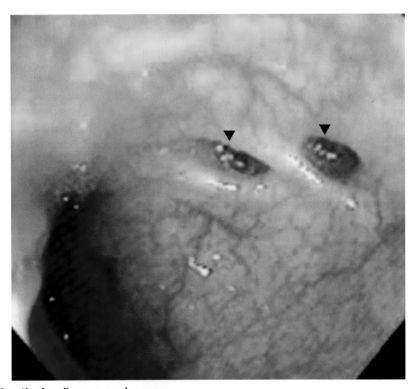

Figure 7-107 Colonic diverticular disease, endoscopy
This colonoscopic view of sigmoid colon shows two diverticula (▼), which proved to be incidental findings. The presence of multiple diverticula, or diverticulosis, may become complicated by inflammation, typically initiated at the narrow neck of a diverticulum, with mucosal erosion and irritation. The inflammation causes diverticulitis. Lower abdominal cramping pain, constipation (or, less commonly, diarrhea), and occasional intermittent bleeding are possible problems. Diverticulosis and diverticulitis can be causes of iron deficiency anemia. Diets higher in fiber prevent or mitigate colonic diverticular disease.

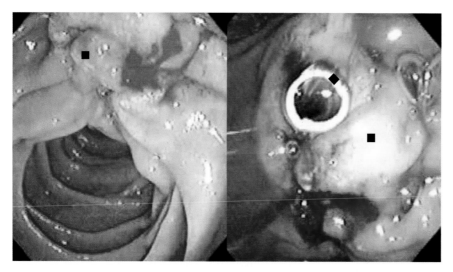

Figure 7-108 Primary small intestinal adenocarcinoma, gross

These mass lesions (■) visible on endoscopy are adenocarcinomas arising in the ampulla of Vater. Primary small intestinal carcinomas are very rare, but most that do occur arise in the region of the ampulla, where they may become symptomatic through biliary or pancreatic duct obstruction. In the *right panel,* placement of a stent (◆) for drainage is shown. Adenocarcinomas may arise in association with underlying conditions such as CD and with polyposis syndromes such as Plenk-Gardner syndrome.

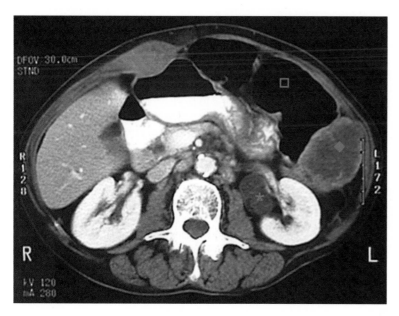

Figure 7-109 Metastases, CT image

This abdominal CT scan reveals metastases in the abdominal wall (■), left pericolic gutter (◆), liver hilum adjacent to the gallbladder (●), and retroperitoneum (✱) next to the left kidney. The colon is dilated (□) as a consequence of partial obstruction. Metastases are a common cause of mechanical bowel obstruction from extrinsic mass effect. The most likely primary sites are within nearby organs: colon, ovary, pancreas, or stomach.

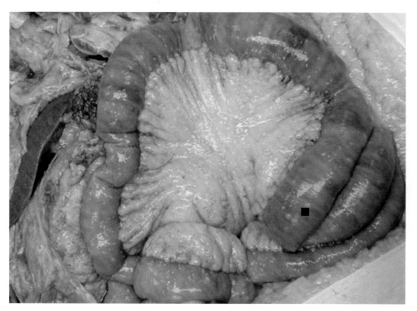

Figure 7-110 Seeding of metastases, gross

The most common malignant neoplasm involving the small bowel is a metastasis. One pattern of intra-abdominal metastases is so-called *seeding* of small pale tumor nodules (■) onto peritoneal surfaces. The nodules are usually quite small, but larger masses can cause obstruction; either form may produce ileus. There is often an ascitic fluid collection within the peritoneal cavity associated with metastases, and paracentesis can yield fluid with characteristics of an exudate (increased protein, cells, and lactate dehydrogenase) that shows the malignant cells on cytologic examination.

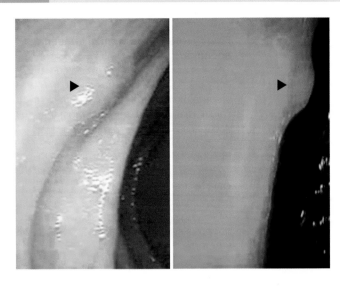

Figure 7-111 Hyperplastic polyp, microscopic

In each of these panels, a small flat mucosal polyp (▶) is present, about 0.5 cm in diameter. These are excrescences that represent mucosal crypt enlargement. They are most frequent in the rectum. They increase in number with age, and overall half of all people have at least one of them. They are non-neoplastic, carry no risk for development of cancer within them, and are unlikely to be a cause of an occult blood–positive stool. They occur more frequently in patients with tubular adenomas and may gradually enlarge. Hyperplastic polyps are typically incidental findings observed on colonoscopy.

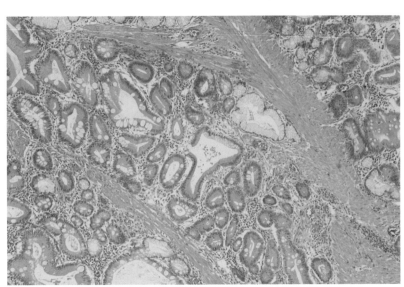

Figure 7-112 Juvenile polyp, microscopic

Juvenile polyposis syndrome (JPS), a rare autosomal dominant disorder, typically manifests during the first or second decade of life with more than three to five juvenile polyps in the colorectum; juvenile polyps throughout the intestinal tract; or any number of juvenile polyps along with a positive family history of JPS. There is an increased risk for colorectal carcinoma. However, the more common sporadic juvenile polyp carries no such risk. The spherical polyps often have surface erosion, an increased stroma, inflammation with reactive epithelial changes, and distorted and dilated crypts. Mutations in *SMAD4* or the TGF-β/BMP signaling pathway are often present.

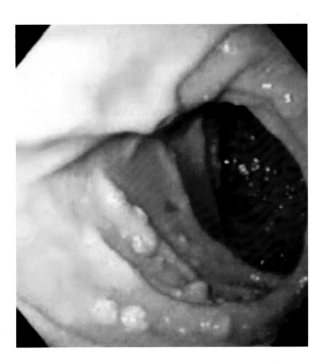

Figure 7-113 Peutz-Jeghers polyps, endoscopy

This syndrome includes mucocutaneous pigmentation with GI hamartomatous polyps. Polyps can occur in all parts of the GI tract, but mostly in the small intestine. Appearing on upper endoscopy are multiple small hamartomatous polyps in the duodenum. This rare autosomal dominant condition can be associated with heterozygous loss-of-function mutations in the *LKB1/STK11* gene in half of familial and some sporadic cases. Patients are at increased risk for developing malignant neoplasms in various organs, such as breast, ovary, testis, or pancreas, but malignancies do not directly arise within the polyps. Mucocutaneous freckle-like pigmentation is often seen on the buccal mucosa, genital region, hands, and feet. These polyps can be large enough to cause obstruction or intussusception.

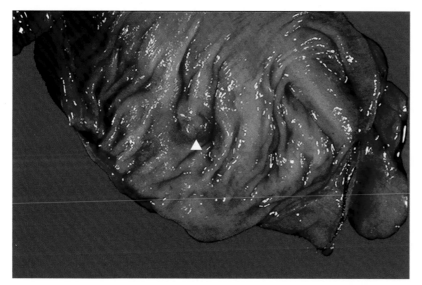

Figure 7-114 Adenoma, gross
A small adenomatous polyp (▲) is shown here in the left colon. A polyp is a structure that protrudes above the surrounding mucosa. It may be pedunculated or sessile. This lesion is histologically a tubular adenoma because of the rounded nature of the neoplastic glands that form it. It has smooth surfaces and is circumscribed. Such lesions are common, found in half of adults older than age 50. An adenoma is the benign precursor to adenocarcinomas. Small ones are virtually always benign. Adenomas larger than 2 cm carry a much greater risk for development of a carcinoma. These adenomas can collect mutations in *APC, SMAD4, K-RAS, p53,* and DNA mismatch repair genes over the years.

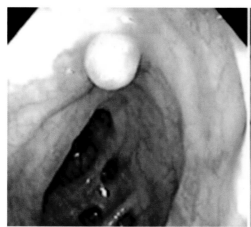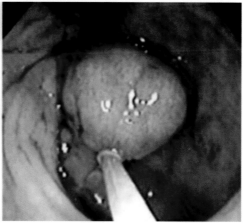

Figure 7-115 Adenoma, endoscopy
Colonoscopic appearance of rectal polyps; these proved to be tubular adenomas. Note the smooth, rounded appearance and slight pedunculating of the polyp in the *left panel.* The adenoma in the *right panel* is larger and has prominent vasculature, explaining the common appearance of stool occult blood in association with polyps.

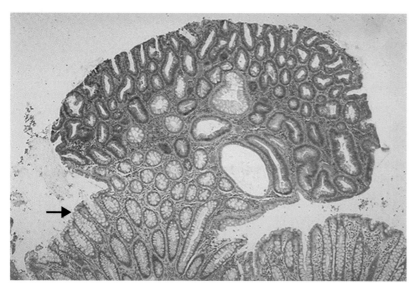

Figure 7-116 Adenoma, microscopic
This benign neoplasm is formed of new glandular or villous architecture with dysplastic epithelium. This small pedunculated adenomatous polyp on a small stalk is shown to have more crowded, disorganized but rounded glands (a tubular pattern) than the normal underlying colonic mucosa (→). Goblet cells are less numerous in the polyp, and the crowded cells lining the glands of the polyp have hyperchromatic nuclei. This small benign neoplasm is still well differentiated and circumscribed, without invasion of the stalk. Accumulation of additional mutations over time and with continued growth of the polyp could give rise to malignant transformation.

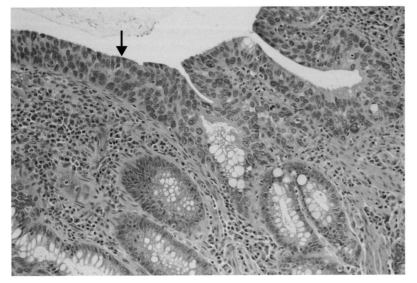

Figure 7-117 Anal intraepithelial neoplasia (AIN), microscopic
Note the disorderly hyperchromatic epithelial nuclei and lack of goblet cells in the overlying epithelium (↓) at the top. Underlying crypts retain goblet cells. AIN is the result of HPV infection and is most likely to occur in men who have sex with men and who are also HIV positive. There is a risk for progression of AIN to invasive carcinoma. AIN does not appear to diminish with antiretroviral therapy. Anogenital warts (condylomata acuminata) caused by HPV may also be present.

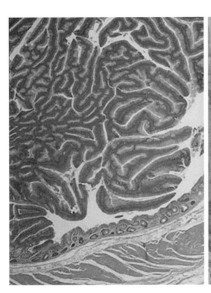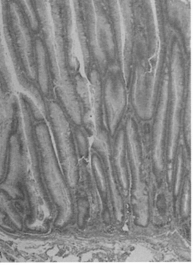

Figure 7-118 Villous adenoma, gross
The cauliflower-like gross appearance of a villous adenoma is shown from above the surface in the *left panel* and in cross-section through the bowel wall in the *right panel.* This type of adenoma is broad based and sessile, rather than pedunculated, and much larger than the typical tubular adenoma (adenomatous polyp). A villous adenoma averages several centimeters in diameter and may be as large as 10 cm. The risk for adenocarcinoma arising in larger villous adenomas is high. Polyps with both tubular and villous features may be termed *tubulovillous adenomas.*

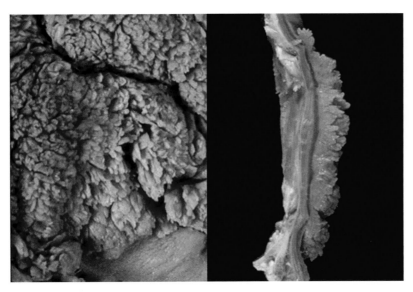

Figure 7-119 Villous adenoma, microscopic
A villous adenoma is shown at its edge in the *left panel* and projecting above the basement membrane in the *right panel.* The cauliflower-like appearance is caused by the elongated glandular structures covered by dysplastic epithelium. Although villous adenomas are less common than adenomatous polyps, they are much more likely to harbor invasive carcinoma (about 40% of villous adenomas). Their surfaces may exude potassium and protein to cause hypoproteinemic hypokalemia.

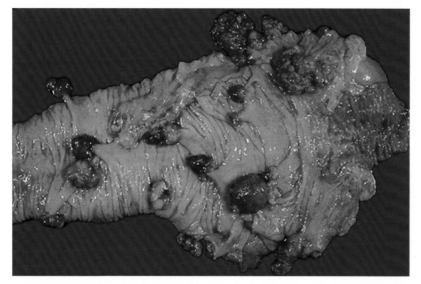

Figure 7-120 Hereditary nonpolyposis colon carcinoma (HNPCC), gross
Multiple adenomatous polyps of the cecum are shown here (there is a terminal ileum at the right). HNPCC (or Lynch syndrome when a genetic basis is defined) leads to right-sided colon cancer in young individuals. HNPCC is associated with extraintestinal malignancies (endometrium, urinary tract) resulting from germline mutations in mismatch repair genes with abnormal expression levels of hMLH1 and hMSH2 proteins. Tumors associated with HNPCC exhibit microsatellite instability (seen in 10% to 15% of sporadic cancers). There are far fewer polyps than in familial adenomatous polyposis with *APC* mutations, but the HNPCC polyps are aggressive.

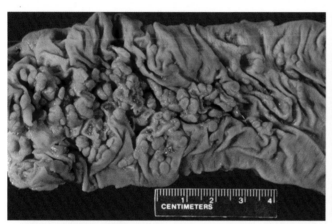
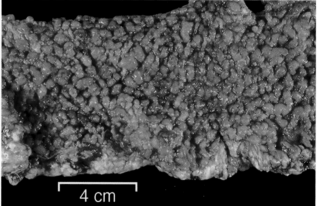

Figures 7-121 and 7-122 Familial adenomatous polyposis, gross
Faulty *APC* genes in familial adenomatous polyposis lead to accumulation of β-catenin translocating to the nucleus and activating transcription of genes, such as *MYH* and cyclin D1. This autosomal dominant condition leads to development by adolescence of more than 100 colonic adenomas that carpet the mucosa *(right panel)*. If untreated by total colectomy, nearly all individuals develop adenocarcinoma. An "attenuated" form of familial adenomatous polyposis *(left panel)* has fewer, more variable numbers of polyps, with older age at onset of colon cancer. Gardner syndrome, also with mutated *APC* gene, has in addition osteomas, periampullary adenocarcinoma, thyroid cancer, fibromatosis, dental abnormalities, and epidermal inclusion cysts.

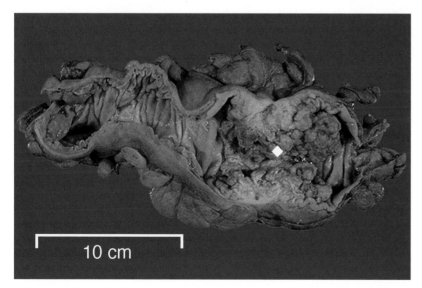

Figure 7-123 Adenocarcinoma, gross
The exophytic growth pattern of the carcinoma (◆) shown can obstruct the colonic lumen. One of the complications of a carcinoma is obstruction (usually partial). A change in stool or bowel habits can be created by the mass effect. A diet low in fiber and high in refined foods and fats predisposes to colon cancer. NSAIDs promote adenoma regression to protect against carcinogenesis.

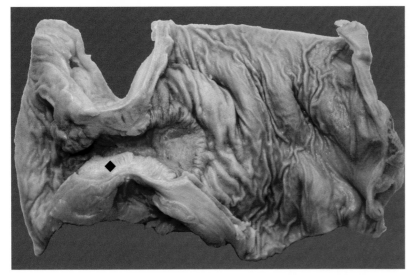

Figure 7-124 Adenocarcinoma, gross

This adenocarcinoma is encircling (◆) and narrowing the lumen. Hemorrhage from the surface of the tumor creates a guaiac-positive stool. This neoplasm was located in the sigmoid colon, just out of reach of digital examination, but easily visualized with colonoscopy. Various genetic abnormalities precede development of colonic carcinogenesis, including the APC/β-catenin pathway, *KRAS* mutations, loss of SMADs, loss of *TP53*, activation of telomerase, and the microsatellite instability pathway.

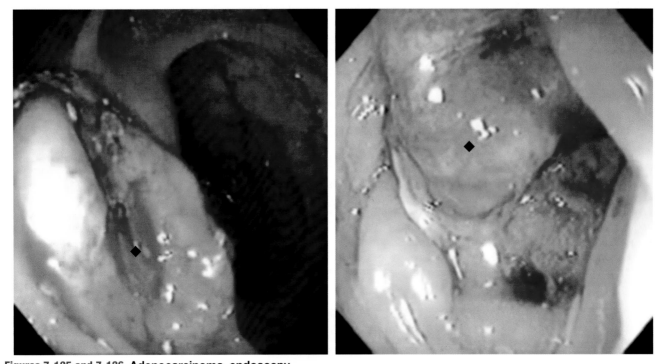

Figures 7-125 and 7-126 Adenocarcinoma, endoscopy

Here are colonoscopic views of colonic adenocarcinoma. The mass in the *left panel* has a central ulcerated crater (◆) with hemorrhage, explaining why testing for occult blood in the stool provides a good screening tool for detection of this lesion. In the *right panel* is another bulky mass (◆) that produces partial intraluminal obstruction.

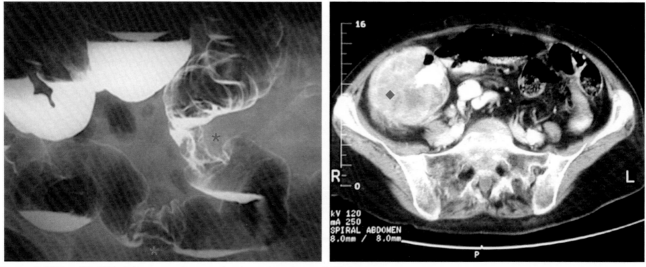

Figures 7-127 and 7-128 Adenocarcinoma, barium enema and CT image

The barium enema technique instills radiopaque barium sulfate into the colon, producing contrast with the surface of the colonic mucosa that highlights any masses present. In the *left panel* the procedure was performed in a lateral position (patient's head toward the right of the image), and the image shows two encircling masses (✱), one in the transverse colon and one in the descending colon, representing an adenocarcinoma that constricts the lumen. In the *right panel,* the large mass lesion (◆) visible on the abdominal CT scan with contrast enhancement is a large adenocarcinoma distending the cecum. Cecal carcinomas often become bulky masses and may first manifested with iron deficiency anemia from blood loss.

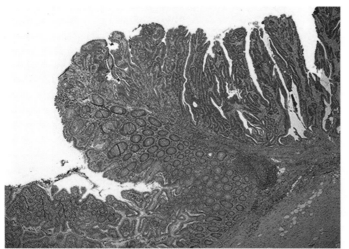

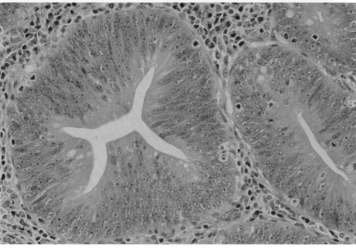

Figures 7-129 and 7-130 Adenocarcinoma, microscopic

In the *left panel* the edge of an adenocarcinoma can be seen. The neoplastic glands are long and frondlike, similar to the glands seen in a villous adenoma, but more disorganized. The growth is primarily exophytic (outward into the lumen), and invasion is not present at this point. Grading and staging of the tumor are done by the surgical pathologist, who examines multiple histologic sections of the tumor. In the *right panel* at high magnification, the neoplastic glands of adenocarcinoma have crowded nuclei with hyperchromatism, pleomorphism, prominent nucleoli, and mitoses. No normal goblet cells are visible. A series of genetic mutations may precede development of colon cancer. The *APC* gene may be mutated, followed by mutation of *KRAS, SMAD4,* and *p53.* Epidermal growth factor receptor (EGFR) is a surface membrane receptor that has been shown to occur in various solid malignancies, including colonic adenocarcinoma. The monoclonal antibody cetuximab directed against EGFR can be used for treatment for colonic adenocarcinomas expressing EGFR.

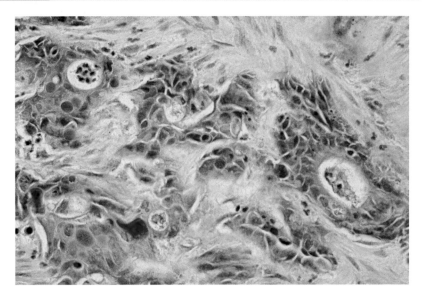

Figure 7-131 Adenocarcinoma, microscopic
This periodic acid–Schiff (PAS) stain highlights the red mucin globules found in the cytoplasm of the malignant glandular cells. This moderately differentiated adenocarcinoma retains some features of the normal colonic epithelium, with glandular configurations and mucin production. Poor differentiation and mucinous appearance on microscopy are associated with poor prognosis, but the most important prognostic factors are depth of invasion and lymph node metastases.

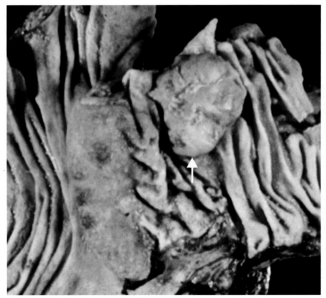 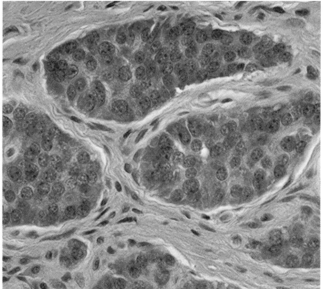

Figures 7-132 and 7-133 Carcinoid tumor, gross and microscopic
Neoplasms of the small intestine are uncommon. Benign tumors include leiomyomas, fibromas, neurofibromas, and lipomas. In the *left panel* a carcinoid tumor (↑) that has a faint yellowish color is present at the ileocecal valve. Most benign tumors are incidental submucosal lesions, although rarely they can be large enough to obstruct the bowel lumen. In the *right panel* at high magnification the nests of carcinoid tumor have a typical endocrine appearance, with small round cells having small round nuclei and purple-to-pale blue cytoplasm. Rarely, a malignant carcinoid tumor can occur as a large bulky mass. Metastatic carcinoid tumor to the liver can rarely result in the carcinoid syndrome.

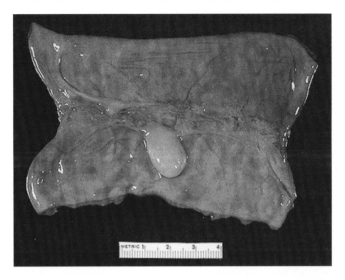

Figure 7-134 Lipoma, gross
The small, discrete yellow subserosal mass is a lipoma of the small intestine found incidentally at autopsy; it is composed of cells essentially resembling mature adipose tissue. Benign neoplasms closely resemble the cell of origin, are circumscribed, and are slow growing. If they do not impinge on a critical structure with mass effect, then they are unlikely to cause a problem.

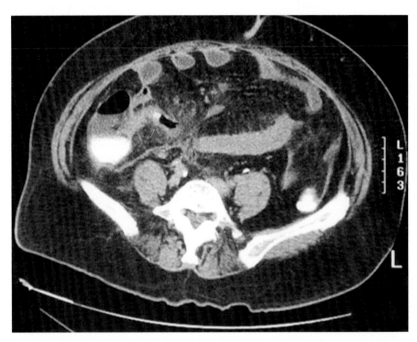

Figure 7-135 Acute appendicitis, CT image
Shown is an enlarged appendix with a fecalith (▲) that appears bright because it is partly calcified. The cecum to the left is partially filled with bright contrast material. Distal to the fecalith, the appendiceal lumen is dark because it is full of air. There is stranding of more brightly attenuated areas from inflammation extending to surrounding adipose tissue. Patients with acute appendicitis typically have a sudden onset of abdominal pain that localizes to the right lower quadrant, and on physical examination there is often rebound tenderness. Leukocytosis is often present. This patient presents an increased operative risk because of obesity (note the large amount of dark adipose tissue beneath the skin).

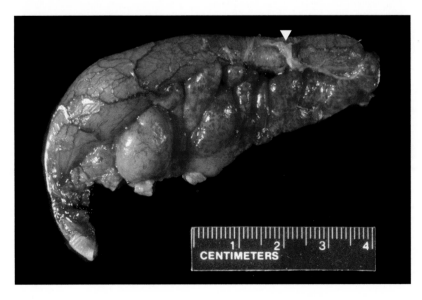

Figure 7-136 Acute appendicitis, gross
This is a resected appendix from abdominal laparoscopic surgery. There is a serosal tan-yellow exudate (▼), but the main features of this early acute appendicitis are edema and hyperemia. This patient had a fever and an elevated total white blood cell count with a left shift (increased band neutrophils) noted on the peripheral blood smear. The patient had minimal abdominal pain, but had flank pain because the appendix had a retrocecal orientation.

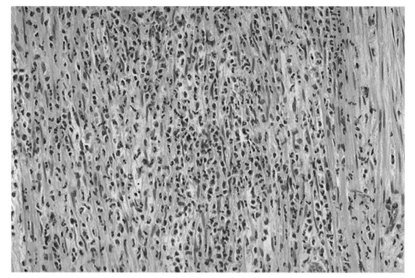

Figure 7-137 Acute appendicitis, microscopic
Acute appendicitis is marked by mucosal inflammation and necrosis. As shown here, numerous neutrophils extend into and through the wall of the appendix. A peripheral neutrophilia with bandemia is often present as well. This condition is treated surgically by removal of the inflamed appendix before potential complications of rupture or sepsis occur. If the inflammation is limited to the serosa (periappendicitis), it is likely that the instigating process is somewhere else in the abdomen and that the appendix is just an "innocent bystander."

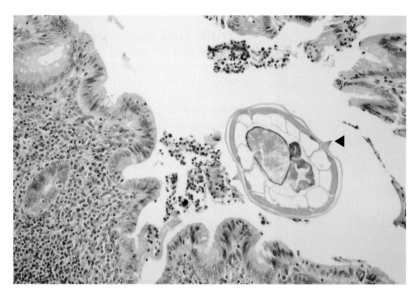

Figure 7-138 Pinworm in appendicitis, microscopic
Acute appendicitis has no identifiable cause in most cases. Rarely, mobile parasites lose their way and get into places they should not go. Pinworm infection (oxyuriasis) from *Enterobius vermicularis* infestation is usually an annoyance, more common in children, with larvae maturing into adult worms in the cecum then migrating to the perianal region to deposit eggs. Shown here are the lateral spines (◄) on a pinworm in the appendix. Multiple worms could obstruct the lumen.

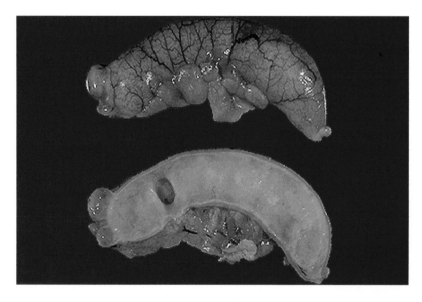

Figure 7-139 Mucocele, gross
The lumen of the appendix shown here is markedly dilated. It was filled with a clear, viscous mucoid material. Mucoceles that persist probably represent true neoplasms, most often a mucinous cystadenoma, rather than just an obstructed appendix. Rupture of a mucocele can fill and distend the peritoneal cavity with mucin. Mucinous cystadenocarcinomas of the appendix, colon, and ovary can also spread throughout the abdominal cavity and produce a similar pattern except that malignant cells are present; this condition is known as *pseudomyxoma peritonei*.

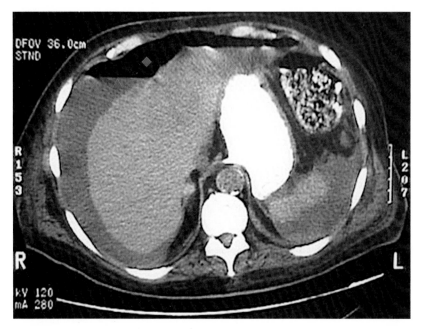

Figure 7-140 Perforation with free air, CT image
Abdominal CT scan reveals free air (◆) from perforation of a viscus. Inflammation or ulceration of the bowel, stomach, or gallbladder can be complicated by perforation. The presence of free air is a good indication that some viscus has ruptured or perforated within the peritoneal cavity. Also shown here is ascitic fluid adjacent to the liver on the right and forming an air-fluid level (▲). Peritonitis may occur in the absence of perforation, a condition known as *spontaneous bacterial peritonitis,* which usually occurs when there is ascites, most often in children with nephrotic syndrome or adults with chronic liver disease.

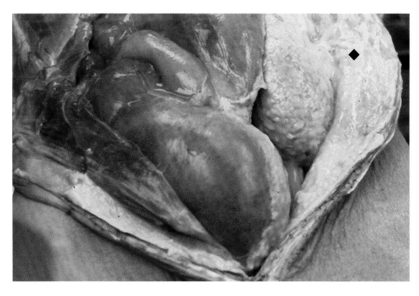

Figure 7-141 Peritonitis, gross
Perforation of the GI tract within the peritoneal cavity (anywhere from the lower esophagus to the colon) can result in peritonitis, as shown here at autopsy. A thick yellow purulent exudate (◆) covers peritoneal surfaces. Various bacterial organisms can contaminate the peritoneal cavity, including Enterobacteriaceae, streptococci, and *Clostridium* species. An ovarian carcinoma caused sigmoid colonic obstruction (the sigmoid is the markedly dilated gray-black bowel in the pelvis shown here) with perforation. Peritonitis can cause functional bowel obstruction from paralytic ileus, visible on abdominal plain film radiographs as dilated loops of bowel with air-fluid levels.

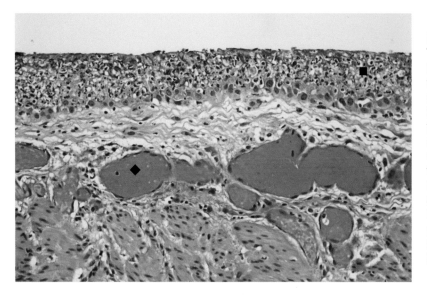

Figure 7-142 Peritonitis, microscopic
There is a thick layer of acute inflammatory cells (■) forming an exudate on the peritoneal surface, which ordinarily should be just a single layer of mesothelium. Note the dilated subserosal vessels (◆) from this inflammatory process. Paracentesis yields cloudy fluid with increased protein, lactate dehydrogenase, and inflammatory cells, mainly neutrophils. Peritonitis can lead to visceral pain from visceral sensory afferent nerves but is poorly localized, is perceived as midline, fluctuating, dull cramping, and is relieved by change of position. Inflammation involving the abdominal wall and parietal peritoneum may produce pain from somatic sensory afferents, which is more constant, boring, and localized.

CHAPTER

8

The Liver and Biliary Tract

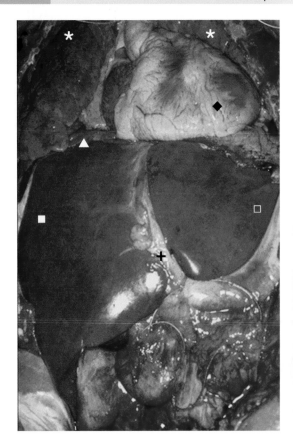

Figure 8-1 Normal liver in situ, gross
Here is the normal liver in situ in the upper abdomen, as seen at autopsy. The liver lies below the diaphragm (▲), and the chest cavity is above with the heart (◆) and lungs (✷). As can be seen, the liver is the largest parenchymal organ. The right lobe (■) (on the left) is larger than the left lobe (□). The falciform ligament (✚) is the rough dividing line between the two lobes. Embryologically, the liver is derived from an endodermal bud of foregut.

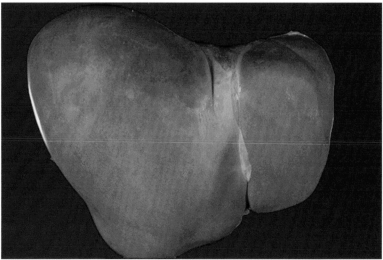

Figure 8-2 Normal liver, gross
The external surface of a normal liver is shown. The color is brown, and the surface is smooth. The normal liver in adults weighs 1400 to 1600 g. There is a dual blood supply, with one third of the blood flow but most of the oxygenated blood supplied by the hepatic artery, and two thirds of the blood flow coming through the portal venous system draining from the intestines. Bile formed in the liver drains from the canaliculi of hepatic lobules through increasing diameters of branching ducts to coalesce into right and left hepatic ducts, which join at the hilum just outside the inferior hepatic surface to form the common bile duct.

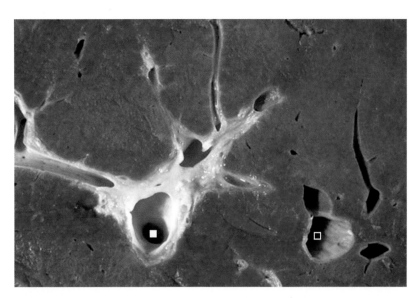

Figure 8-3 Normal liver, gross
The cut surface of a normal liver has a uniform brown color. Near the hilum, note the portal vein (■) carrying blood to the liver, which branches at center left, with accompanying hepatic artery and bile ducts. At the lower right is a branch of hepatic vein (□) draining blood from the liver to the inferior vena cava. The liver performs numerous metabolic functions, including the processing of dietary amino acids, carbohydrates, and lipids. It detoxifies and excretes waste products through the bile and synthesizes many plasma proteins.

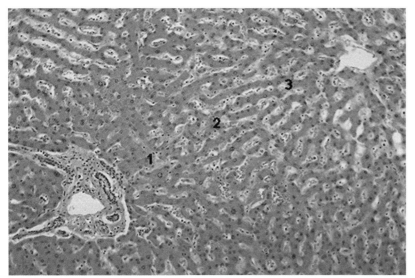

Figure 8-4 Normal liver zones, microscopic
The liver is functionally divided into lobules with a central vein and peripheral triads. Hepatic cords radiate from the central vein as single plates of one hepatocyte thickness sandwiching a bile canaliculus flowing toward the triad. Hepatocytes adjacent to the triad form a "limiting plate." The lobule has three zones, defined by their relationship to the portal triad at the upper right and the central vein at the lower left. *Zone 1* is periportal and receives blood with the highest oxygen concentration. *Zone 2* encompasses the central portion of a liver lobule (midzonal). *Zone 3* is centrilobular. Within the triad are branches of bile ducts, hepatic artery, and portal vein.

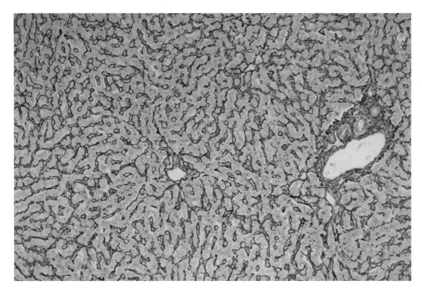

Figure 8-5 Normal liver, microscopic
The normal liver is shown at low power with a reticulin stain to outline the connective tissue support by the dark reticulin fibers. The hepatic cord architecture, with plates of hepatocytes staining pink, and sinusoids between, is outlined. A portal triad appears at the right, and a central vein is in the center. Hepatocytes are in the resting phase of the cell cycle, and in response to injury can re-enter the cycle and proliferate to regenerate hepatic parenchyma. Perisinusoidal stellate cells in the space of Disse can be transformed into myofibroblasts in response to hepatic inflammation.

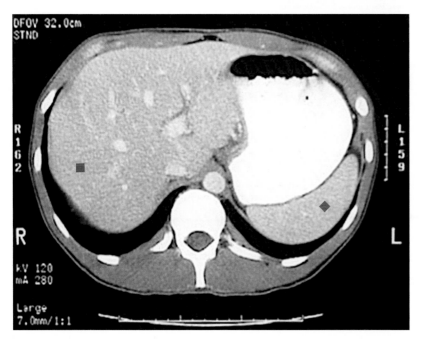

Figure 8-6 Normal liver, CT image
Abdominal CT scan with contrast enhancement shows the appearance of the normal liver. The attenuation (brightness) of the liver (■) and spleen (◆) is similar. Bright orally administered contrast material fills the stomach, shown here between the liver and spleen. Intravenous contrast material in the hepatic veins is brighter than the surrounding hepatic parenchyma. The right lobe of the liver is much larger than the left lobe, which extends across the midline. Because the liver is the largest abdominal organ, it may be injured with blunt abdominal trauma, producing surface lacerations through the thin Glisson capsule, leading to hemoperitoneum.

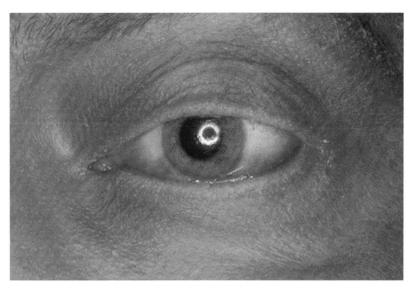

Figure 8-7 Jaundice, gross
The end product of heme degradation is bilirubin. The hepatocytes take up unconjugated bilirubin and conjugate it with glucuronic acid and excrete it into bile. Increased bilirubin production, decreased hepatic conjugation and excretion, or biliary tract obstruction leads to increasing bilirubin levels in the blood. This is observed as the physical examination finding of jaundice, or icterus. The normally white sclera of the eye is yellow here because of jaundice. Transient neonatal jaundice results from β-glucuronidases in maternal milk that deconjugate bilirubin diglucuronides in the gut, which are reabsorbed.

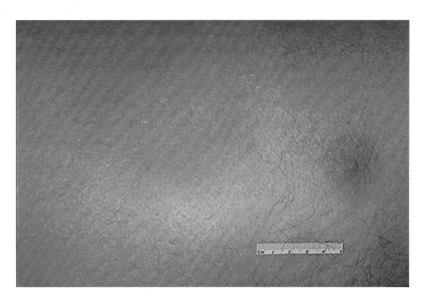

Figure 8-8 Jaundice, gross
Increased amounts of circulating bilirubin in the blood can lead to the physical examination finding of icterus, or jaundice, as shown here with the yellowish hue of the skin. With hemolysis of erythrocytes, there is an increase in unconjugated (indirect) bilirubin to produce icterus. An increase in the conjugated (direct) fraction of bilirubin suggests intrahepatic disease, such as hepatitis, or biliary tract obstruction. Direct and indirect bilirubin concentrations in serum add to the total serum bilirubin. An elevation in serum alkaline phosphatase suggests biliary tract obstruction because an isoenzyme of alkaline phosphatase is produced in bile ductular epithelium and in hepatocyte canalicular membranes.

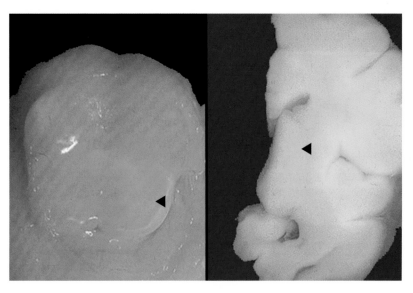

Figure 8-9 Kernicterus, gross
Unconjugated bilirubin is tightly bound to circulating albumin and is not excreted in urine; in premature newborns without the mature hepatic capacity to clear bilirubin, blood levels increase, and bilirubin accumulates in the brain to cause neurologic damage. The yellow staining (◄) in the brain of a neonate is known as *kernicterus*. Coronal sections of medulla in the *left panel* and cerebral hemisphere in the *right panel* show kernicterus in deep gray matter. Increased unconjugated bilirubin, which accounts for the kernicterus, is toxic to brain tissue. Kernicterus is more likely to occur with prematurity, low birth weight, and increased bilirubin levels.

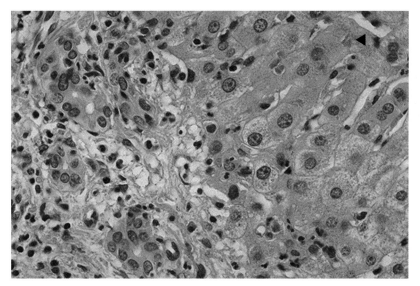

Figure 8-10 Cholestasis, microscopic
The yellowish pigmentation (◀) visible in the hepatocyte cytoplasm on the right is caused by the accumulation of bile pigments. Intrahepatic cholestasis can result from hepatocyte dysfunction or biliary tract obstruction. In addition to intrahepatic bile stasis, intracanalicular bile stasis is present, shown here. The continuing biliary obstruction can also lead to bile duct proliferation, shown on the left. The catabolism of heme derived from developing, damaged, and senescent erythrocytes produces bilirubin loosely bound to albumin in the blood. Bilirubin is taken up into hepatocytes, bound to cytosolic glutathione-*S*-transferases, conjugated with glucuronic acid by uridine diphosphate-glucuronyl transferase, and excreted into the bile canaliculus.

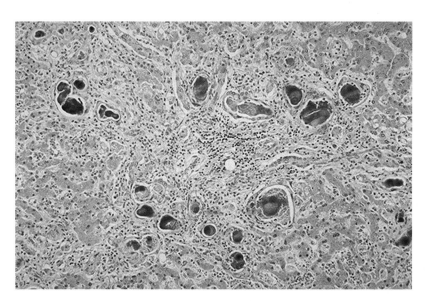

Figure 8-11 Cholestasis, microscopic
The yellowish green accumulations of pigment shown here in liver are bile. Obstruction of the biliary tree leads to intrahepatic biliary stasis and formation of bile lakes. Proliferation of bile ducts may occur in response to chronic obstruction. If prolonged, there can be portal fibrosis with biliary cirrhosis. Bile acts as an emulsifier and is an important component of lipid digestion in the small intestine. Lack of bile secretion into the duodenum leads to acholic (clay-colored) stools and possible steatorrhea with increased stool fat. Malabsorption of the fat-soluble vitamins A, D, E, and K can occur. Some vitamin D and K can be made endogenously.

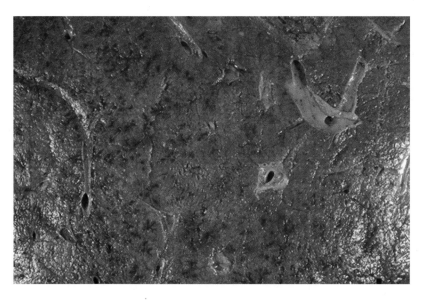

Figure 8-12 Hepatic necrosis, gross
Necrosis and hepatic lobular collapse are visible here as areas of hemorrhage with irregular furrows and granularity on the cut surface. Extensive necrosis can follow hepatocyte injury from toxins, infections (e.g., fulminant viral hepatitis), and ischemia. Alanine aminotransferase (ALT) and aspartate aminotransferase (AST) enzymes are released into the blood (the former more specific for liver injury). Extensive loss of hepatocyte function can lead to decreased protein synthetic function, with hypoalbuminemia and decreased production of clotting factors II, VII, IX, and X (initially manifested by an elevated prothrombin time), and decreased metabolic function, as in the urea cycle, with hyperammonemia.

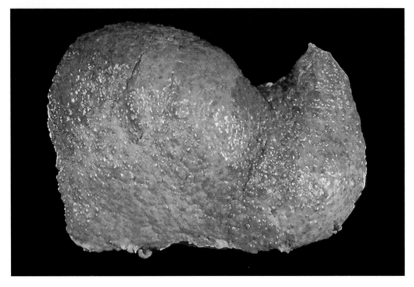

Figure 8-13 Cirrhosis, gross

Cirrhosis occurs when diffuse chronic hepatic injury leads to formation of fibrous septa that extend between portal tracts, disrupting the normal hepatic architecture, along with formation of regenerative nodules of parenchyma. The normal vascular inflow and outflow patterns are disrupted, with development of portal hypertension. The external appearance of the liver capsule is markedly bumpy. Fibrous septa surround regenerative hepatocyte nodules averaging less than 3 mm in size. Cirrhosis requires at least a decade to develop from chronic liver injury, and a cirrhotic lever tends to decrease in size. Cirrhosis regresses slowly but is potentially reversible to some extent. Here, hepatic failure is marked by hyperbilirubinemia with green-tinged appearance of some nodules after formalin fixation (with oxidation of bilirubin to biliverdin).

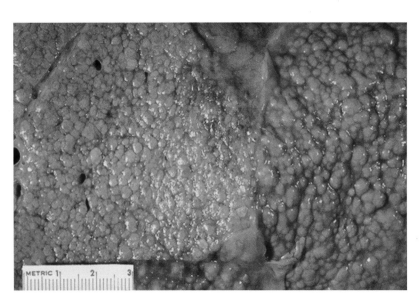

Figure 8-14 Cirrhosis, gross

In micronodular cirrhosis, the regenerative nodules average 3 mm or less in size. The yellow-brown appearance of these nodules is caused by concomitant hepatic steatosis. The most common cause of micronodular cirrhosis and steatosis is chronic alcohol abuse. A fine reticulin network of type IV collagen is normally present in the liver, but with cirrhosis there is extensive deposition of type I and III collagen generated from activated perisinusoidal stellate cells. Cirrhosis may remain clinically silent for many years until complications of portal hypertension, such as esophageal varices or ascites, develop or there is significant loss of liver parenchyma with diminished metabolic function.

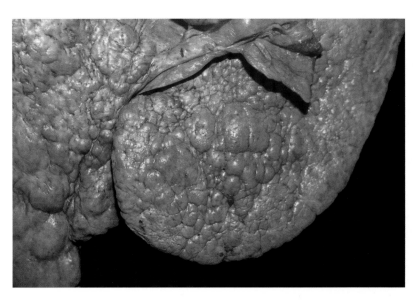

Figure 8-15 Cirrhosis, gross

Macronodular cirrhosis shown here from the inferior hepatic surface has multiple nodules greater than 3 mm in size with extensive deposition of tan-appearing collagen surrounding these regenerative nodules. This is end-stage decompensated cirrhosis; some cases remain well-compensated (no metabolic derangements) or partially compensated. The most common cause of macronodular cirrhosis is viral hepatitis. Most causes of cirrhosis can produce both patterns and a mixed micronodular and macronodular cirrhosis; the nodular pattern provides no reliable clue to the underlying cause.

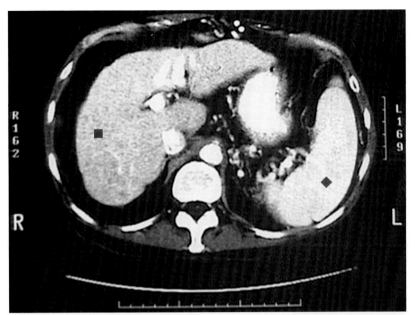

Figure 8-16 Cirrhosis, CT image
Abdominal CT scan shows a small, nodular cirrhotic liver (■) with more parenchymal heterogeneity (light and dark areas) than a normal liver. The abnormal blood flow through cirrhotic liver leads to an elevation in portal venous pressure. Portal hypertension leads to splenomegaly (◆), as shown here. Increased collateral venous blood flow may also lead to formation of esophageal varices, dilated superficial abdominal veins (caput medusae), and hemorrhoids. Chronic alcohol abuse, nonalcoholic fatty liver disease, viral hepatitis B and C, biliary tract disease, hereditary hemochromatosis (HH), Wilson disease, and α_1-antitrypsin (α_1-AT) deficiency can lead to cirrhosis. When no identifiable cause is found, the term *cryptogenic cirrhosis* is used.

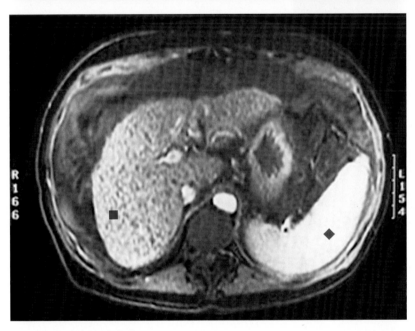

Figure 8-17 Cirrhosis, MRI
This abdominal T2-weighted MRI image in axial view shows a small, shrunken cirrhotic liver (■). The spleen (◆) is larger than normal from portal hypertension and can reach 1 kg in size. Transudation from the intravascular compartment producing an ascites often accompanies cirrhosis. This ascites results from multiple mechanisms, including hepatic sinusoidal hypertension, hypoalbuminemia, increased lymph drainage into the peritoneal cavity, leakage from intestinal capillaries, and secondary hyperaldosteronism with renal sodium and water retention. In addition, "hepatorenal syndrome" occurs with decreased renal function caused by diminished renal perfusion coupled with renal afferent arteriolar vasoconstriction.

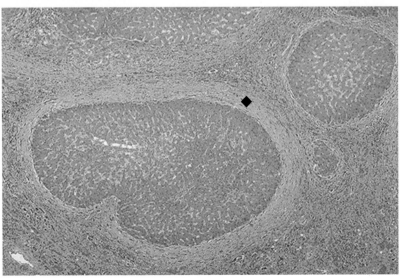

Figure 8-18 Cirrhosis, microscopic
Micronodular hepatic cirrhosis is shown at low power, with regenerative nodules of hepatocytes ringed by thick bands (◆) of collagenous fibrosis. Within the fibrous bands are lymphocytic infiltrates and a proliferation of bile ductules. The increased hepatocyte proliferation from nodular regeneration increases the risk for hepatocellular and (to a lesser extent) cholangiolar carcinoma. Liver injury leads to Kupffer cell activation with release of cytokines, such as platelet-derived growth factor and tumor necrosis factor (TNF), which stimulate stellate cells in the space of Disse to proliferate into myofibroblastic cells that contribute to the fibrogenesis.

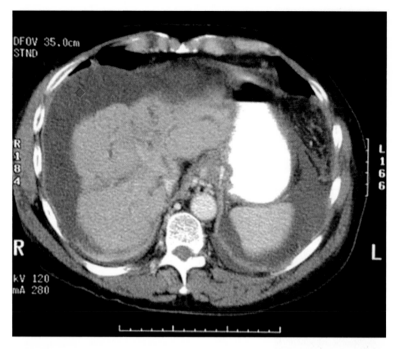

Figure 8-19 Cirrhosis and ascites, CT image
This abdominal CT scan shows ascites with extensive fluid collections (◆) in the peritoneal cavity, a complication of cirrhosis of the liver with portal hypertension. The cirrhotic liver has diminished protein synthetic function, leading to hypoalbuminemia and diminished intravascular oncotic pressure. This is combined with increased sodium and water retention by the kidneys and increased hydrostatic pressure in veins and capillaries to promote this extravascular fluid collection. The patient may note increasing abdominal girth, and a fluid wave may be observed on physical examination.

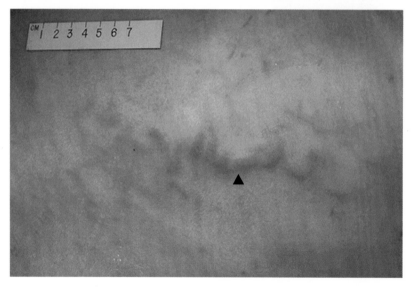

Figure 8-20 Caput medusae, gross
Portal hypertension results from the abnormal hepatic blood flow pattern created by cirrhosis. The increased pressure is transmitted to collateral venous channels that may become dilated. *Caput medusae* consists of dilated veins (▲) radiating from the umbilicus toward the rib margins, as shown here on the abdomen of a patient with cirrhosis of the liver. Other venous collaterals affected by portal hypertension include the esophageal plexus and the hemorrhoidal veins. In addition to cirrhosis, portal hypertension may result from infiltrative granulomatous diseases, schistosomiasis, and marked steatosis.

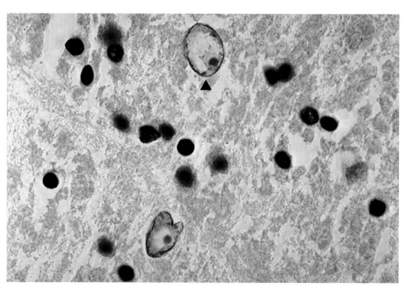

Figure 8-21 Hepatic encephalopathy, microscopic
On microscopic examination of the brain in hepatic encephalopathy, Alzheimer type 2 cells (▲) are found in the lower layers of the cortex and in the basal ganglia. These are enlarged protoplasmic astrocytes that are responding to the toxins (primarily ammonia) that are not cleared by the urea cycle in the failing liver. These cells as shown here have an enlarged watery nucleus with no visible cytoplasm and prominent nucleoli. Patients may exhibit muscular rigidity, hyperreflexia, and asterixis before onset of confusion progressing to stupor and coma.

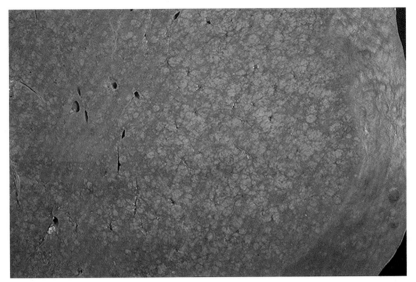

Figure 8-22 Viral hepatitis, gross
This liver involved with acute viral hepatitis has areas of necrosis with collapse of the liver lobules. The necrosis is shown here as ill-defined, pale yellow areas between more viable areas of light brown hepatic parenchyma. Note the irregularity of the capsular surface on the right from lobular collapse. If a significant portion of the parenchyma becomes necrotic, the liver becomes pale and shrunken—diffuse massive necrosis—a rare complication most likely to occur with the ordinarily subclinical hepatitis A infection or in some cases of hepatitis B virus (HBV) infection. Patients with acute viral hepatitis may have nausea, anorexia, malaise, and fever, then icterus, and progress to hepatic encephalopathy.

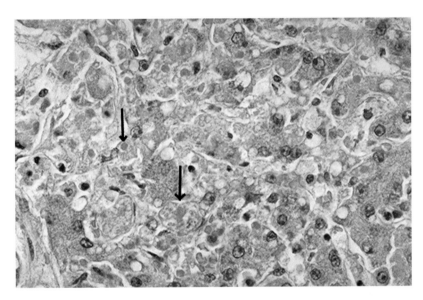

Figure 8-23 Viral hepatitis, microscopic
There is ballooning degeneration of many hepatocytes (↓) in this case of acute fulminant hepatitis. This ballooning is a manifestation of apoptosis (single cell necrosis). Hepatitis A virus, a picornavirus with single-stranded RNA in a capsid; HBV, an enveloped virus with double-stranded DNA; or hepatitis C virus (HCV), an enveloped virus with a single-stranded RNA genome, may induce cytotoxic CD8 lymphocytes to attack the virally infected hepatocytes. Drugs and toxins that produce hepatic necrosis, such as halothane or isoniazid, may be directly cytotoxic to hepatocytes. There are vaccines for hepatitis A and B.

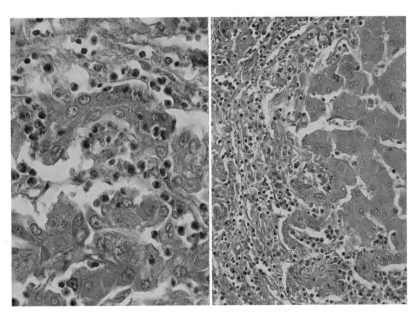

Figure 8-24 Viral hepatitis E, microscopic
In this acute viral hepatitis, note the presence of both lymphocytes (mainly in the portal tract—*left panel*) and neutrophils (mainly at the interface with adjacent hepatocytes—*right panel*) representative of hepatitis E virus (HEV) infection. Hepatitis E viral infection is more common in developing nations, where it is most often sporadic and epidemic in men, causes acute icteric hepatitis, and rarely leads to chronic hepatitis. Mortality is low except in pregnant women. It is most often spread through contaminated water. A less common form of endemic HEV infection occurs in developed nations with foodborne contamination (pigs as a vector).

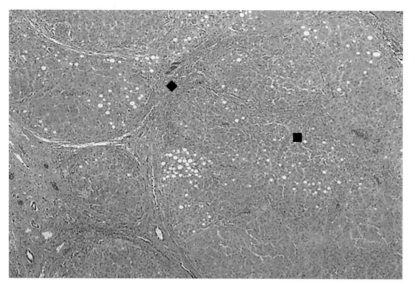

Figure 8-25 Viral hepatitis, microscopic
With chronic hepatitis there is lobular irregularity with fibrosis and inflammation (◆) between the lobules. In this case of hepatitis C viral infection, there is a minimal degree of steatosis as well. This case is at a high stage, with extensive fibrosis and beginning progression to macronodular cirrhosis, as evidenced by the large regenerative nodule (■) at the center right. Serologic testing for diagnosis of this form of viral hepatitis includes the HCV antibody test. Polymerase chain reaction testing for HCV RNA can identify HCV subtypes. HCV accounts for most (but not all) cases formerly called *non-A, non-B hepatitis*. About 85% of HCV cases proceed to chronic hepatitis, which remains stable in 80%, but leads to cirrhosis in 20%.

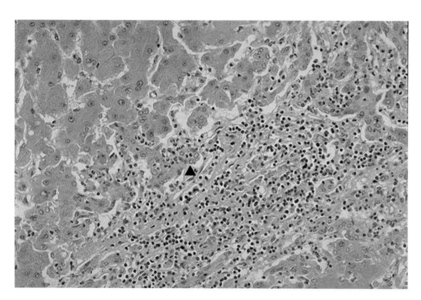

Figure 8-26 Viral hepatitis, microscopic
This portal triad is expanded by mainly mononuclear inflammatory cell infiltrates, and the limiting plate of hepatocytes around the triad has been breached, with extension of the inflammation into adjacent hepatic parenchyma, along with focal interface necrosis (▲) of the hepatocytes. This is typical of a chronic active form of hepatitis. The AST and ALT enzymes would be expected to remain elevated in the patient's serum. In this case, the hepatitis B surface antigen (HBsAg) and hepatitis B core antibody (HBcAb) were positive, along with hepatitis B e antigen (HBeAg) from continued viral proliferation. Chronic hepatitis C viral infection appears similarly.

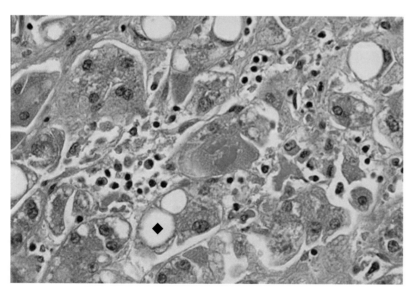

Figure 8-27 Viral hepatitis, microscopic
The extent of chronic hepatitis can be graded by the degree of activity (necrosis and inflammation) and staged by the degree of fibrosis. In this case, HCV has progressed to chronic hepatitis, and necrosis and inflammation are prominent, and there is some steatosis (◆). Regardless of the grade or stage, the cause of the hepatitis must be sought because the treatment may depend on knowing the cause, and chronic liver diseases of different causes may appear microscopically and grossly similar. Treatment with α-interferon and ribavirin can be effective for HCV infection. Antiretroviral drugs may be useful for HBV infection.

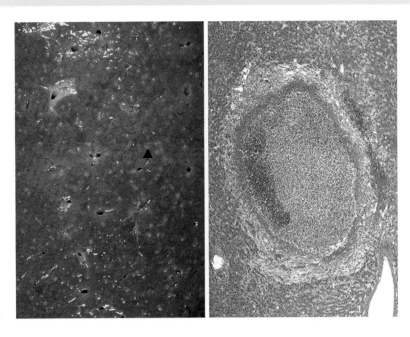

Figure 8-28 Hepatic abscesses, gross and microscopic

Pyogenic abscesses in liver are often bacterial and result from spread of infection to hepatic parenchyma with septicemia through the arterial supply; or abdominal infection through the portal vein, through an ascending biliary tract infection (cholangitis), with direct spread from an adjacent intra-abdominal infection; or direct introduction of organisms with penetrating trauma. The *left panel* shows multiple microabscesses (▲) in a patient with septicemia. The *right panel* shows a microabscess containing numerous neutrophils producing focal liquefactive necrosis, along with the beginning of an organizing abscess wall with some pink fibrin. Patients with abscesses can have fever, right upper quadrant pain, and hepatomegaly. Parasitic and helminthic infections may also cause hepatic abscesses.

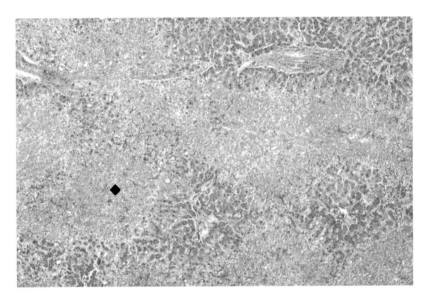

Figure 8-29 Acetaminophen toxicity, microscopic

Pale pink areas (◆) represent necrotic hepatocytes. The rate of serum AST and ALT increase indicates the extent of hepatic necrosis. Acetaminophen toxicity may be more severe with accidental overdose in many cases because of an additional risk factor of chronic alcohol abuse. Therapeutic drug levels are metabolized by hepatic conjugation with glucuronidation and sulfation, but acute ingestion of more than 140 mg/kg overwhelms normal metabolic pathways, so more acetaminophen is metabolized to the toxin *N*-acetyl-*p*-benzoquinone imine (NAPQI) by cytochrome P-450. NAPQI is normally detoxified by glutathione, but chronic alcoholism and malnutrition can deplete glutathione and induce P-450, increasing toxicity.

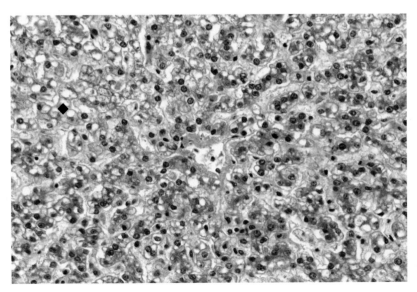

Figure 8-30 Reye syndrome, microscopic

The numerous small lipid droplets (◆) appear as clear vacuoles within these hepatocytes (microvesicular steatosis). Reye syndrome is a rare disease that may result from mitochondrial dysfunction associated with drug ingestion, particularly aspirin given to children for a febrile illness. Laboratory findings include hypoglycemia, elevated transaminases, hypoprothrombinemia, and hyperammonemia. The serum bilirubin is usually not elevated. A similar appearance can occur with acute fatty liver of pregnancy, a rare complication associated with preeclampsia and a defect in intramitochondrial fatty acid oxidation.

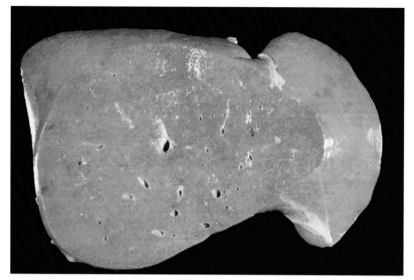

Figure 8-31 Hepatic steatosis, gross
This fatty liver is pale yellow-brown because of the increased lipid content within hepatocytes. The capsule is smooth, and the cut surface has a uniform texture. It is two to three times normal size—hepatomegaly. Steatosis is a consequence of increased lipid biosynthesis from generation of more NADH by alcohol dehydrogenase and acetaldehyde dehydrogenase, impaired assembly and secretion of lipoproteins, and increased peripheral fat catabolism. The most common cause is excessive alcohol consumption. Toxic injury from drugs and chronic liver injury produce steatosis, diminishing hepatocyte function, detected through hypoalbuminemia and hypoprothrombinemia.

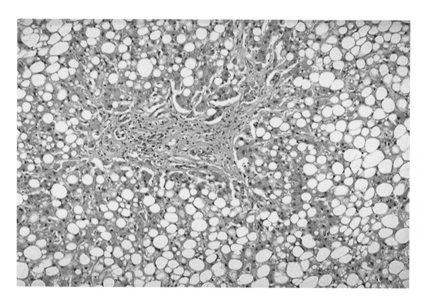

Figure 8-32 Hepatic steatosis, microscopic
Many hepatocytes have cytoplasm filled with large, clear lipid droplets. This is severe macrovesicular steatosis. This process is potentially reversible in weeks to months with cessation of alcohol abuse or discontinuation of a toxic drug. Chronic injury may be accompanied by varying degrees of portal fibrosis. Some degree of steatosis accompanies all cases of chronic alcohol abuse, but only about 10% to 15% of these patients go on to develop cirrhosis.

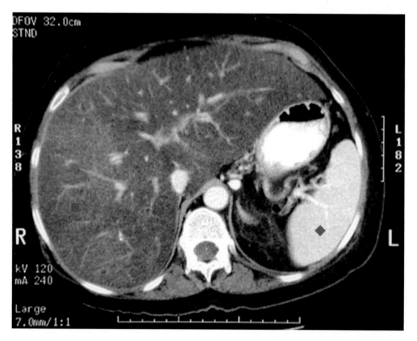

Figure 8-33 Hepatic steatosis, CT image
This abdominal CT scan illustrates a fatty liver (■) with hepatomegaly and decreased attenuation (brightness) from the increased lipid content (compare the brightness of the normal spleen [♦] with that of the fatty liver). A form of steatosis similar to that seen with alcohol-induced injury is known as *nonalcoholic fatty liver disease* (NAFLD), which most often accompanies obesity and diabetes mellitus type 2. More extensive injury may lead to nonalcoholic steatohepatitis (NASH). Progression to cirrhosis may occur. Lifestyle modification with cessation of alcohol abuse or weight reduction can lead to reversal of hepatic steatosis.

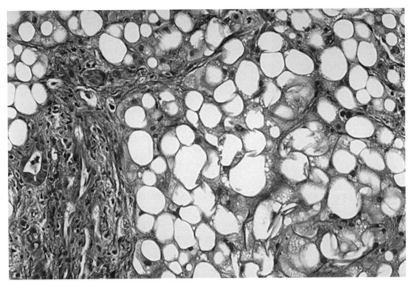

Figure 8-34 Nonalcoholic steatohepatitis, microscopic

This liver with trichrome stain shows blue-staining collagenous fibrosis within the liver parenchyma. Virtually every hepatocyte is filled with a clear lipid droplet (macrovesicular steatosis). This patient had a body mass index (BMI) of 30, in the obese range, a risk factor for NAFLD. A BMI of more than 25 is in the overweight range. Obesity diminishes homeostatic adiponectin production and increases inflammatory cytokines such as TNF-α and interleukin-6 (IL-6). These changes promote hepatocyte apoptosis. Patients may be asymptomatic for many years, with only mild elevations of serum ALT and AST.

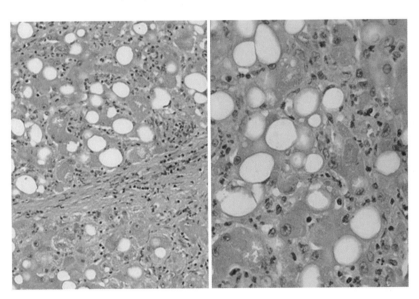

Figure 8-35 Alcoholic hepatitis, microscopic

Acute alcoholic hepatitis is a complication of heavy ethanol consumption superimposed on alcoholic liver disease in patients with a history of alcohol abuse. Mallory bodies, neutrophils, necrosis of hepatocytes, collagen deposition, and fatty change (steatosis) are shown here. Such inflammation can occur in a person with a history of alcohol abuse who goes on a drinking binge and consumes large quantities of alcohol over a short time. In this case, note a band of fibrosis in the *left panel,* with inflammatory cell infiltrates identified as neutrophilic in the *right panel.* The serum AST and ALT are markedly increased in these patients.

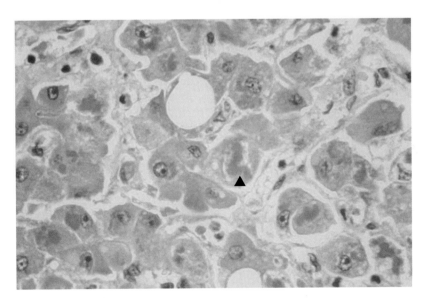

Figure 8-36 Alcoholic hepatitis, microscopic

This case of acute alcoholic hepatitis has prominent intracellular deposits of red globular (▲) Mallory-Denk bodies (alcoholic hyalin). This hyalin represents an intracellular accumulation of cytoskeletal elements, including cytokeratins, with the toxic hepatocellular injury. Mallory-Denk bodies are also known as *alcoholic hyalin* because they are most often seen in conjunction with liver injury from chronic alcohol abuse. Alcoholic hyalin may also be seen in cases of Wilson disease, primary biliary cirrhosis (PBC), and chronic cholestasis, and within hepatocellular neoplasms.

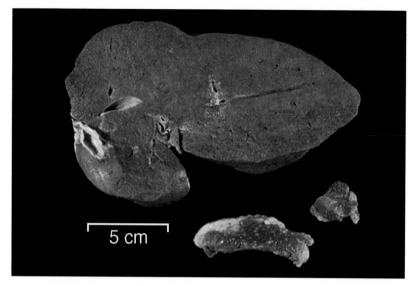

Figure 8-37 Hemochromatosis, gross
The dark brown color of this liver and the pancreas and lymph nodes on cross-sectioning is a result of extensive iron deposition with HH. HH results from a mutation involving the hemochromatosis gene *(HFE)* that leads to increased iron absorption from the gut. The prevalence is 1 in 200 to 1 in 500 people in the United States. About 1 in 10 individuals of northern European ancestry carries an abnormal recessive *HFE* gene, and most of these are the result of a single missense C282Y mutation, although some are the H63D or S65C mutations associated with a milder phenotype. Excessive iron deposition in tissues generates free radicals producing lipid peroxidation, fibrosis, and DNA damage.

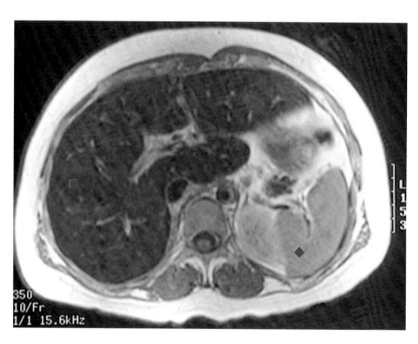

Figure 8-38 Hemochromatosis, MRI
On this T1-weighted axial MRI image of the abdomen, there is markedly decreased signal intensity within the liver (■) as a result of marked iron deposition in a patient with HH. Compare the attenuation (brightness) of the liver with that of the normally equivalent spleen (◆). Total body iron stores normally average 3 to 6 g, but in HH these stores can exceed 20 g by age 40 in men or age 60 in women, with onset of organ dysfunction from excessive iron stores. The normal HFE protein forms a complex with β_2-microglobulin and transferrin, and a mutation eliminates this interaction so that the mutant HFE protein remains trapped intracellularly, reducing transferrin receptor–mediated iron uptake by the intestinal crypt cell. This may upregulate divalent metal transporter 1 (DMT-1) on the intestinal brush border, leading to inappropriate iron absorption.

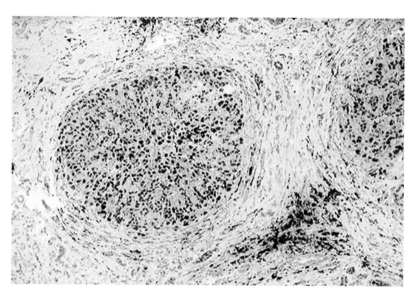

Figure 8-39 Hemochromatosis, microscopic
Prussian blue iron stain reveals extensive hepatic hemosiderin deposition in this case of HH with cirrhosis. Excessive iron deposition is toxic to tissues in many organs, but heart (congestive failure), pancreas (diabetes mellitus), liver (cirrhosis and hepatic failure), joints (pseudogout with polyarthropathy), skin (dark pigmentation), and pituitary and gonads (loss of libido, impotence, amenorrhea, testicular atrophy, gynecomastia) are the most severely affected. Treatment consists of periodic phlebotomy to remove 250 mg of iron with each unit of blood. Screening for *HFE* gene mutations in family members of affected patients should be done.

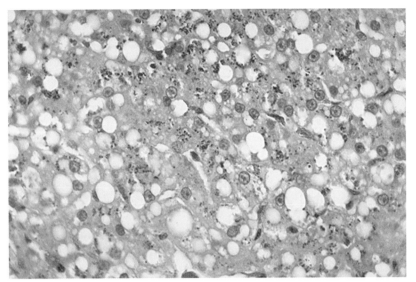

Figure 8-40 Wilson disease, microscopic
The red-brown granular material shown here with a copper stain is excessive lysosomal copper resulting from the rare autosomal-recessive disorder Wilson disease from mutation of the *ATP7B* gene encoding a copper-transporting ATPase. Decreased hepatic copper excretion into bile leads to copper accumulation in brain, eye, and liver. There is neuronal degeneration of basal ganglia, especially putamen. Corneal Kayser-Fleischer rings are seen on slit-lamp examination. Hepatic copper accumulation results in steatosis (shown here), cholestasis, acute or chronic hepatitis, and eventual cirrhosis. Urinary copper excretion is increased, and serum ceruloplasmin is decreased. Chelation therapy is used to remove the excess copper.

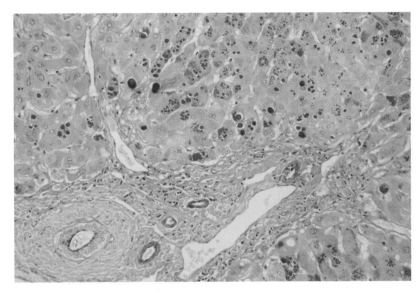

Figure 8-41 α_1-Antitrypsin deficiency, microscopic
The periportal red hyaline globules shown here with PAS stain are characteristic of α_1-AT deficiency. The globules are collections of abnormally folded and polymerized α_1-AT not excreted from hepatocytes, resulting in chronic hepatitis, cirrhosis, and hepatocellular carcinoma (HCC). The serum α_1-AT is low. α_1-AT deficiency sometimes leads to neonatal hepatitis, which may progress to cirrhosis. The normal allele is PiM, and a single gene mutation leads to PiZ or PiS. One in 10 individuals of European ancestry may have an abnormal phenotype (PiMM is normal). Homozygotes PiSS and PiZZ and the heterozygote PiSZ are more likely to develop panlobular emphysema or chronic liver disease, or both, than heterozygotes PiMS and PiMZ.

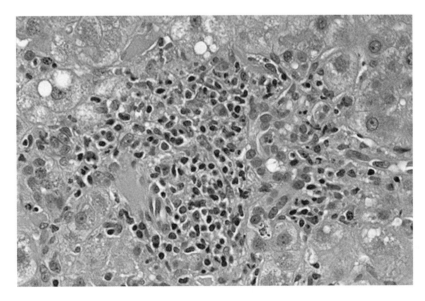

Figure 8-42 Primary biliary cirrhosis, microscopic
PBC is a rare autoimmune disease seen mostly in middle-aged women that causes intense pruritus along with hepatomegaly and xanthomas. Destruction of bile ductules within hepatic triads is shown here with intense mononuclear infiltrates and occasional granulomatous inflammation. Serum antimitochondrial antibody is often detectable, and it targets the E2 component of the pyruvate dehydrogenase complex (PDC-E2). Additional findings include elevations in serum alkaline phosphatase, cholesterol, and globulins. Either cirrhosis or nodular regeneration with hepatomegaly ensues. Jaundice is a late finding that suggests incipient liver failure.

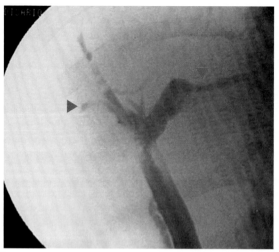
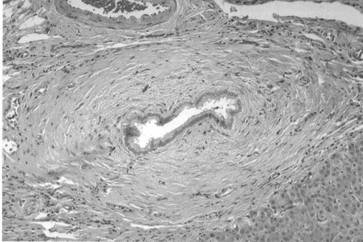

Figures 8-43 and 8-44 Primary sclerosing cholangitis, radiograph and microscopic

The cholangiogram shows a beaded pattern with bile ductular narrowing (▼) and pruning (▶) from irregular segmental strictures. This leads to fibrous obliteration of extrahepatic and intrahepatic bile ducts. Microscopic examination shows a bile duct surrounded by marked collagenous connective tissue deposition with epithelial atrophy and luminal narrowing. Patients can have marked alkaline phosphatase elevation along with icterus and pruritus. Idiopathic cases most often affect men 20 to 50 years old. About 70% of cases occur with idiopathic inflammatory bowel disease, particularly ulcerative colitis.

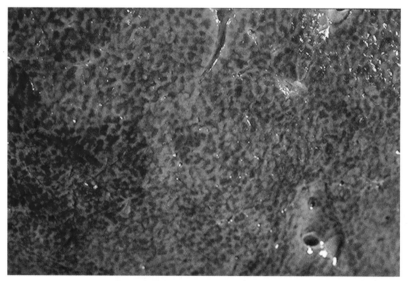

Figure 8-45 Centrilobular congestion, gross

This is a nutmeg liver with chronic passive congestion. Note the dark-red congested regions that represent accumulation of red blood cells within centrilobular regions. The nutmeg pattern results from congestion around the central veins, usually from right-sided heart failure. If the passive congestion is pronounced and heart failure leads to ischemia, there can be centrilobular necrosis because the oxygenation in zone 3 of the hepatic lobule is diminished, and the AST and ALT increase. Rarely, chronic passive congestion leads to fibrosis extending between central veins—a "cardiac cirrhosis." Extensive hepatic congestion can accompany disseminated intravascular coagulation and hemoglobinopathies such as sickle cell disease.

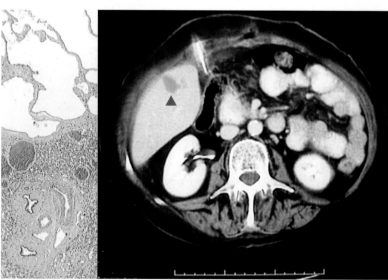

Figure 8-46 Hemangioma, CT image and microscopic

The discrete, darkly attenuated mass (▲) in the *right panel* lies just beneath the Glisson capsule, surrounded by normal, uniform hepatic parenchyma. Large, irregular, dilated vascular channels make up this mass *(left panel)*. About 1 individual in 50 has such a neoplasm, which is typically an incidental finding on abdominal CT scan because most are 2 cm or smaller, unless one puts a percutaneous biopsy needle into it. They can sometimes be multiple. Hemangiomas can be subcapsular, as shown here, or periportal. Most have a cavernous pattern of vascular spaces on microscopic examination.

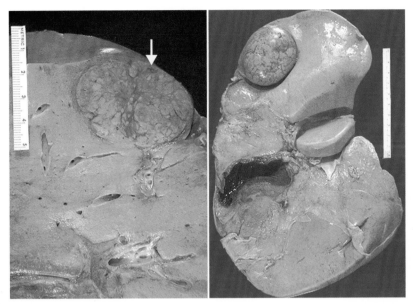

Figure 8-47 Hepatic adenoma, gross

This benign circumscribed neoplasm arises from a proliferation of cells resembling hepatocytes. There is an association with oral contraceptive use in women and anabolic steroid use in men, often in association with inactivating mutations in *HNF1-α*. Some are related to NAFLD. A subcapsular adenoma such as the one shown here *(right panel)* may rupture, producing a hemoperitoneum. These neoplasms are composed of cells resembling normal hepatocytes, but without a lobular pattern, so that normal triads and central veins are not recognized cells; they can produce bile, with the green appearance (↓) with formalin fixation shown here *(left panel)*.

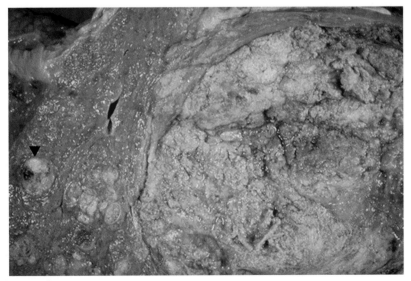

Figure 8-48 Hepatocellular carcinoma, gross

These large, bulky tumors have a greenish cast because bile is present. In addition to the main mass, there are smaller satellite nodules (▼) that represent either intrahepatic spread or multicentric origin of the tumor. There may be an elevated serum α-fetoprotein (AFP). Such masses can focally obstruct the biliary tract to increase the serum alkaline phosphatase. Primary liver cancers typically arise in the setting of chronic hepatitis and cirrhosis from increased hepatocellular proliferative activity. Worldwide, viral hepatitis B and C are the most common causes, but chronic alcohol abuse is a common cause. Other causes of HCC include aflatoxin exposure, hemochromatosis, α_1-AT deficiency, and NAFLD.

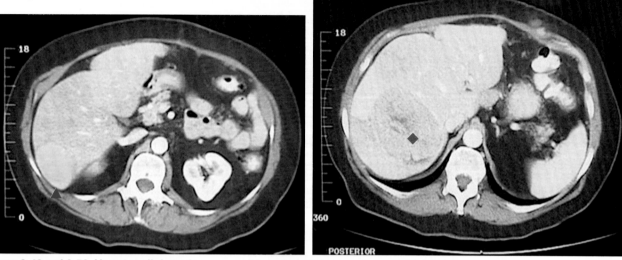

Figures 8-49 and 8-50 Hepatocellular adenoma and hepatocellular carcinoma, CT images
Compare the smaller homogenous mass (▲) in the *left panel* with the larger, more irregular heterogeneous mass (◆) in the *right panel.* Hepatic adenomas are typically not related to the risk factors seen with HCC, which most often arises in liver with chronic hepatitis or cirrhosis. These cancers can appear as one large mass, or there may be small surrounding satellite nodules, or multi-focal masses. Epigenetic signaling through the IL-6/JAK/STAT pathway may underlie their development. HCCs are very prone to undergo necrosis and hemorrhage. Hemorrhage from HCC at the liver capsule may lead to a hemoperitoneum. Intrahepatic mass lesions are unlikely to obstruct the biliary tract completely, so hyperbilirubinemia is infrequent. Clinical findings include malaise, fatigue, weight loss, abdominal pain, and abdominal enlargement.

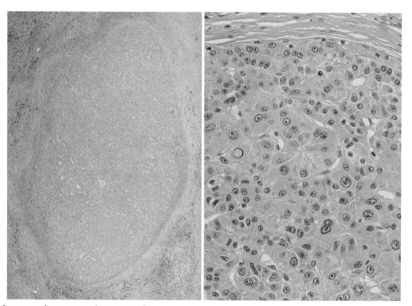

Figure 8-51 Hepatocellular carcinoma, microscopic
The precursor to HCC can be a dysplastic nodule, with loss of architecture and atypia. Note the nodule in the *left panel* that is architecturally different from and more cellular than the surrounding cirrhotic liver. The malignant cells of HCC in the *right panel* are well differentiated and resemble larger bur irregular hepatocytes. An HCC can form cords that are much wider and irregular than the normal liver plates, and there is no discernible normal lobular architecture, so triads and central veins are absent. Larger neoplasms may have areas of necrosis. Invasion of vascular channels, particularly portal vein branches, is frequent. Most patients with HCC survive less than 1 year because it is unlikely to be discovered at an early stage.

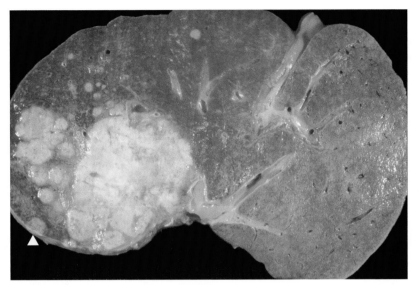

Figure 8-52 Cholangiocarcinoma, gross
This white mass has a few satellite nodules
(▲) but lacks bile staining. Cholangiocarcinoma is
less common than HCC, but identifiable risk
factors can be similar, although viral hepatitis
B and C infections are more strongly associated
with HCC. Chronic alcoholism has been reported
as a risk factor in both. The most common risk
factor in the United States is primary sclerosing
cholangitis, although cholangiocarcinoma is more
common in parts of the world where infection
with trematodes (liver flukes), such as *Clonorchis
sinensis,* occurs. Premalignant biliary intraepithelial neoplasia (BilIN) may precede its development.
Most cases are detected at an advanced stage
and thus have a poor prognosis. Clinically, the
presentation and course of cholangiocarcinomas
resembles that of HCCs.

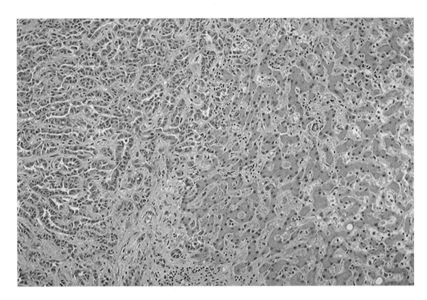

**Figure 8-53 Cholangiocarcinoma,
microscopic**
The carcinoma shown on the left is composed
of small, irregular glandular structures consistent
with a cholangiocarcinoma, although HCCs
occasionally can have such areas within them. A
primary liver cancer may have hepatocellular and
cholangiolar differentiation. Cholangiocarcinomas
do not make bile, but the cells do make mucin,
and they can be almost impossible to distinguish
from metastatic adenocarcinoma. Immunohistochemical staining in cholangiocarcinoma is positive for CK-7 and negative for CK-20 and AFP.
Metastases are more likely to be CK-20 positive.
HCCs are often AFP positive.

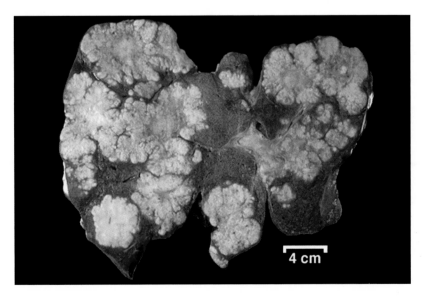

Figure 8-54 Hepatic metastases, gross
Note the numerous mass lesions of variable size.
Some of the larger masses show central
necrosis, producing a grossly umbilicated
appearance when seen beneath the hepatic
capsule. These masses are metastases to the
liver. The obstruction from such masses generally
elevates the serum alkaline phosphatase, but not
all bile ducts are obstructed, so that hyperbilirubinemia is typically not present. Also, the transaminases are usually not greatly elevated. Of all
neoplasms involving the liver, metastases are the
most common because the liver is a good place
for circulating neoplastic cells to settle down and
grow. Metastases usually occur as multiple mass
lesions throughout the liver.

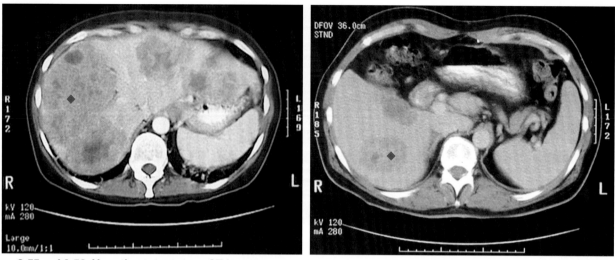

Figures 8-55 and 8-56 Hepatic metastases, CT images
These abdominal CT scans without intravenous contrast administration show multiple mass lesions (◆) with focal darker areas of necrosis, resulting in a markedly enlarged liver in the *left panel* that extends from the right side to nearly the left side of the upper abdomen. These are metastases from a primary colonic adenocarcinoma. A normal-sized spleen is shown at the lower left in *both panels*.

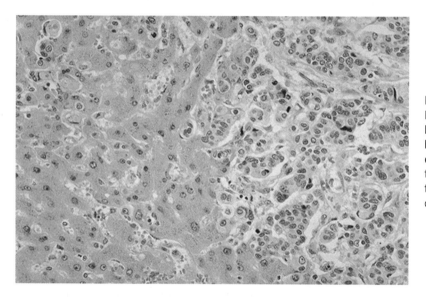

Figure 8-57 Hepatic metastases, microscopic
Metastatic infiltrating ductal carcinoma from a breast primary is shown on the right, with normal liver parenchyma on the left. As the metastases enlarge, they outgrow their blood supply, leading to central necrosis. Sufficient hepatic function is typically retained, so liver failure is unlikely to occur from metastases.

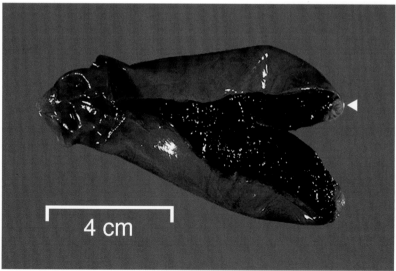

Figure 8-58 Normal gallbladder, gross
A normal gallbladder has a velvety dark green mucosa and a thin wall. One minor variation is the small yellowish bulbous projection (◀) on the right—a *phrygian cap*—resulting from a folded fundus. The gallbladder serves as a storage organ for bile secreted by the liver. The muscularis of the gallbladder contracts under the influence of cholecystokinin secreted by enteroendocrine cells of the small intestine with passage of food from the stomach into the duodenum, particularly fatty food. Modern gallbladders work harder than ancient gallbladders because of increasing dietary fat from such sources as fast food and ice cream.

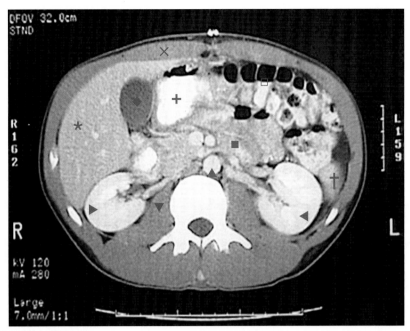

Figure 8-59 Normal gallbladder, CT image
This abdominal CT scan with contrast enhancement at the L2-L3 level shows normal structures, including the liver (✱), gallbladder (◆), gastric antrum (✚), jejunum (■), colon (□), right kidney (▶), left kidney (◀), spleen (✝), aorta (▲), psoas muscle (▼), and rectus abdominis muscle (✖). The gallbladder normally stores about 50 mL of concentrated bile. The location of the gallbladder on the inferior surface of the hepatic right lobe varies among 5% to 10% of the population, but congenital gallbladder anomalies, such as agenesis, are rare. Hypoplasia of all or part of the biliary tract may lead to biliary atresia.

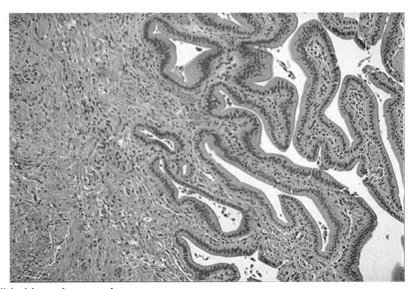

Figure 8-60 Normal gallbladder, microscopic
The columnar mucosa is arranged in folds over the lamina propria, allowing expansion as bile fills the gallbladder. Beneath the lamina propria is a muscularis, and not seen here surrounding the gallbladder are a connective tissue layer and serosa. The gallbladder mucosa transports sodium out of the bile, passively followed by chloride and water, leading to bile concentration. Bile excreted by the liver and stored in the gallbladder becomes more concentrated. The bile includes bile salts such as cholic and chenodeoxycholic acid, lecithin, calcium bilirubinate, and cholesterol. An imbalance in the relative concentrations of these bile components predisposes to precipitation and stone formation.

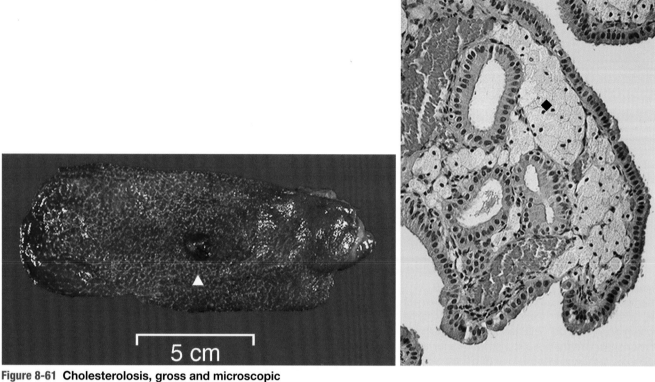

Figure 8-61 Cholesterolosis, gross and microscopic
The mucosa contains many foamy macrophages (◆) in the lamina propria, shown in the *right panel,* which produce the grossly visible strawberry-like appearance shown in the *left panel,* along with a solitary gallstone (▲). Genes encoding proteins that transport biliary lipids, including the *D19H* variant, may contribute 10% of the risk for cholesterol gallstones.

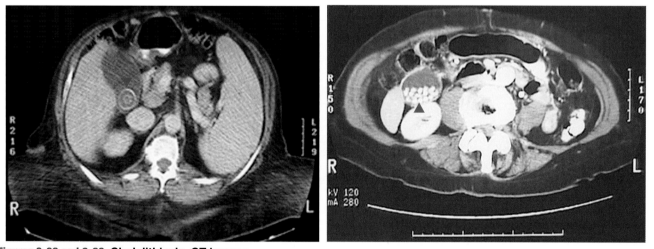

Figures 8-62 and 8-63 Cholelithiasis, CT images
The *left panel* shows a solitary gallstone (▼) within a dilated gallbladder. Gallstones may contain varying portions of cholesterol, calcium, and bilirubin. They are often built through apposition of layers, leading to the laminated appearance shown here. The *right panel* shows multiple small gallstones (▲) within the gallbladder. A small stone or a portion of a stone broken off may pass into the neck of the gallbladder and become impacted, or may pass down the cystic duct and impact at the ampulla.

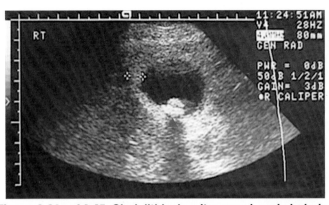
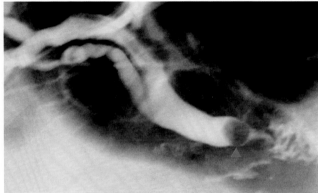

Figures 8-64 and 8-65 Cholelithiasis, ultrasound, and choledocholithiasis, radiograph

Note the gallstones (▲) in the gallbladder lumen on abdominal ultrasound *(left panel)*. The cursors mark the thickened wall of the gall-bladder, a finding consistent with chronic cholecystitis. The cholangiogram *(right panel)* reveals the outline of a gallstone (▲) occluding the distal dilated common bile duct near the ampulla.

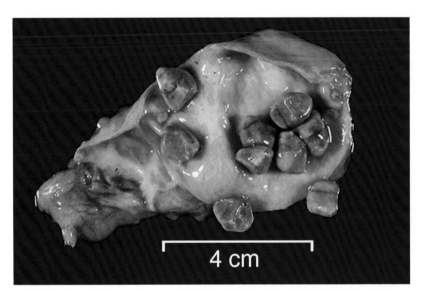

4 cm

Figure 8-66 Cholelithiasis, gross

Yellow-tan faceted gallstones are present in this gallbladder, which shows evidence of chronic cholecystitis because the mucosa is tan and the wall and surface are pale, suggesting collagenization as a result of scarring from chronic inflammation. Repeated bouts of acute cholecystitis can lead to chronic cholecystitis. About 10% to 20% of adults have gallstones, and most of them are asymptomatic. Most gallstones have a preponderance of cholesterol, giving them a yellow gross appearance. Some calcium bilirubinate is often present, however, and these are termed *mixed* stones. Stones mainly composed of calcium bilirubinate are dark-green to black and are known as *pigment* stones.

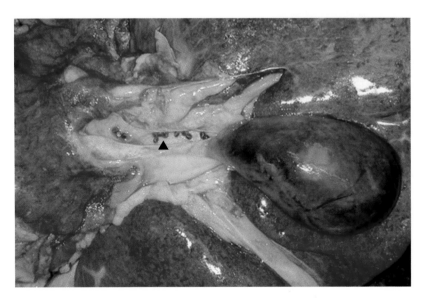

Figure 8-67 Choledocholithiasis, gross

The common bile duct emptying into the duodenum on the left is opened to reveal several small calculi (▲) within the lumen. The gallbladder on the right is dilated from obstruction by calculi at the gallbladder neck. Stones from the gallbladder, if small enough, can pass through (or impact within) the neck of the gallbladder and gain access to the common bile duct, a condition termed *choledocholithiasis*. Biliary tract obstruction can produce colicky right upper quadrant pain. In about two thirds of the population, the common bile duct joins the main pancreatic duct before emptying through the ampulla of Vater, and this allows a stone to obstruct the pancreatic duct, causing pancreatitis.

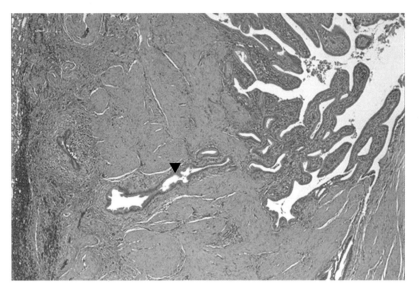

Figure 8-68 Chronic cholecystitis, microscopic
Chronic cholecystitis is almost always seen in association with gallstones, although precipitation of bile alone may be sufficient to produce inflammation. The term *acalculous cholecystitis* applies when inflammation is present, but cholelithiasis is absent. There may not be a history of bouts of acute cholecystitis. A thickened gallbladder wall is shown here beneath the mucosa with chronic inflammatory infiltrates and containing outpouchings (▼) of the mucosa, termed *Rokitansky-Aschoff sinuses*. In contrast, acute cholecystitis has neutrophilic infiltrates. Bacterial infection is typically absent from cases of acute and chronic cholecystitis.

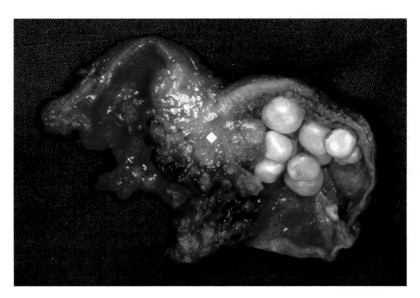

Figure 8-69 Adenocarcinoma, gross
This gallbladder has been opened, and to the left of the pale porcelain gallstones (averaging 1 cm in size) is a fungating mass (◆) that extends into the gallbladder lumen and into the gallbladder wall. This is a primary adenocarcinoma of gallbladder. Gallstones accompany such carcinomas in 60% to 90% of cases. Adenocarcinomas of the biliary tract are uncommon and typically occur in elderly patients. Larger tumors, or tumors arising in the extrahepatic bile ducts, may lead to biliary tract obstruction, with laboratory findings including direct hyperbilirubinemia and elevated serum alkaline phosphatase.

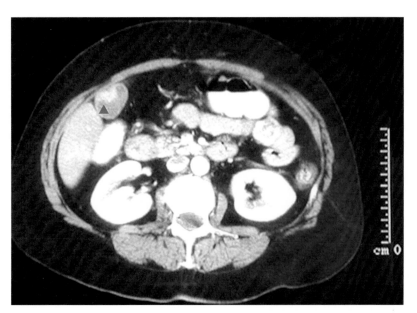

Figure 8-70 Adenocarcinoma, CT image
In this abdominal CT scan, there is an irregular bright mass (▲) within the lower portion of the gallbladder, with the inferior tip of the right lobe of liver adjacent to it. This mass proved to be an adenocarcinoma of the gallbladder. There often are no early signs or symptoms; most adenocarcinomas of the gallbladder are nonresectable at diagnosis, and the prognosis is poor. There may be clinical signs and symptoms similar to those of cholelithiasis with cholecystitis.

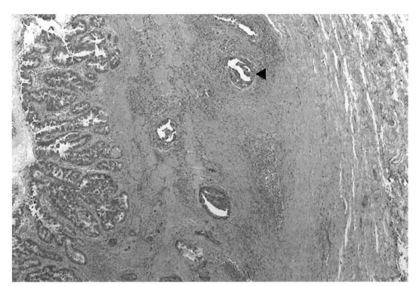

Figure 8-71 Adenocarcinoma, microscopic
The dysplastic epithelium can be seen on the left, and neoplastic glandular structures are invading (◀) into the muscular wall. Adenocarcinoma of the gallbladder is more common in elderly patients and more frequently seen in women. Carcinomas can arise in the rest of the biliary tree, but these are associated with gallstones in only one third of cases and are slightly more common in men.

The Pancreas

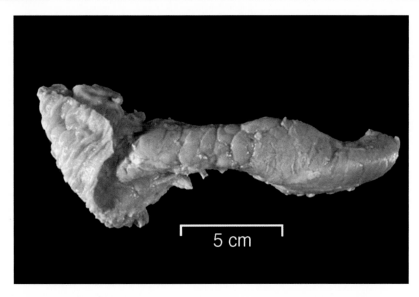

Figure 9-1 Normal pancreas, gross
The normal adult pancreas weighs 85 to 90 g and has indistinct regions, including a head adjacent to the duodenum (a small portion of duodenum appears here on the left), a body, and a tail (on the right) with a tan color and lobular architecture. Adjacent adipose tissue and lymph nodes are closely apposed. Of the pancreatic mass, 99% is acinar parenchyma producing digestive enzymes and bicarbonate, with the remainder being islets of Langerhans. The pancreas forms embryologically from a larger dorsal and smaller ventral endodermal bud from the duodenum; the buds fuse along with their respective developing ducts of Wirsung and Santorini. The pancreatic duct runs the length of the pancreas to empty into the duodenum at the ampulla of Vater.

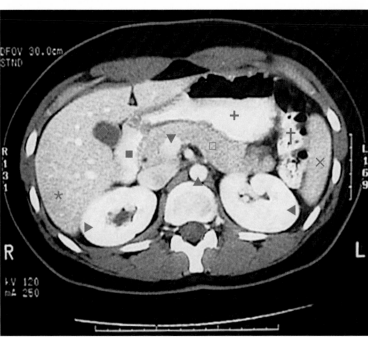

Figure 9-2 Normal pancreas, CT image
This is a normal abdominal CT scan with contrast enhancement at the L1 level showing the upper abdomen with the liver (✱), gallbladder (◆), stomach (✚), duodenum (■), pancreas (□), colon (†), spleen (✖), portal vein, inferior vena cava (▼), right kidney (▶), left kidney (◀), and aorta (▲). The pancreas forms embryologically from dorsal and ventral buds that form from gut outpouchings; these fuse to form the pancreas. Failure of fusion may produce pancreas divisum, with exocrine pancreatic tissue draining into the duodenum through a larger duct of Santorini and a smaller duct of Wirsung that normally forms the papilla of Vater. Much rarer is abnormal fusion of dorsal and ventral buds to form an annular pancreas that encircles the duodenum and can produce bowel obstruction. Pancreatic ectopia in gastrointestinal tract mucosa is common (2% of the population), but it is an incidental finding because the mass of tissue is typically less than 1 cm in diameter.

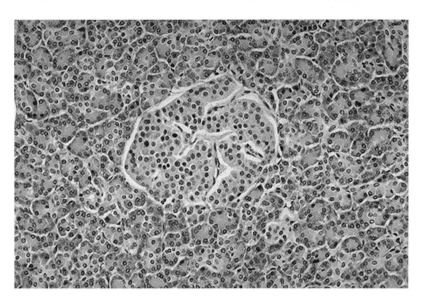

Figure 9-3 Normal pancreas, microscopic
Normal exocrine pancreas is composed of acini that secrete enzymes, including the proenzymes phospholipases A and B, trypsin, chymotrypsin, and elastase, under the influence of cholecystokinin. These proenzymes require activation in the gut. Amylase and lipase are secreted as active enzymes. Secretin triggers release of bicarbonate and water from ductal cells. The pancreas produces about 2 L of fluid per day, which flows into the duodenum. Interspersed within the exocrine acini are the islets of Langerhans with endocrine function, one of which is shown here in the center. Small capillaries within the islet receive the hormonal secretions of islet α cells (glucagon), β cells (insulin), and δ cells (somatostatin).

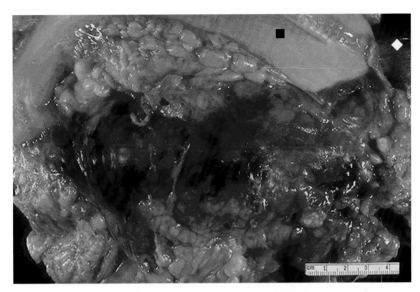

Figure 9-4 Acute pancreatitis, gross
At autopsy, the stomach (■) is reflected superiorly, and the spleen (◆) can be seen at the far upper right. The pancreas is swollen and does not show the typical tan color or lobulated architecture. Instead, hemorrhagic necrosis appears as blotchy black-to-red areas. Serum amylase and lipase are typically elevated. Several mechanisms are implicated in triggering intrapancreatic activation of trypsin and other proenzymes causing the inflammation. Mechanisms include pancreatic duct obstruction (the most common cause, typically from gallstone impaction), acinar cell injury (typical of viral infections), and defective intracellular transport of acinar cell proenzymes. Alcohol-induced pancreatitis can develop through all three of these.

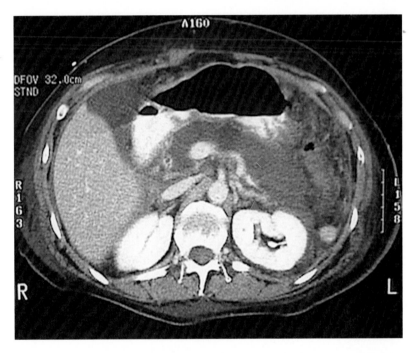

Figure 9-5 Acute pancreatitis, CT image
This abdominal CT scan with contrast enhancement reveals decreased attenuation of a swollen pancreas (◆) from edema, hemorrhage, and fat necrosis. In this case a consequence of the inflammation, splenic vein thrombosis (▲), can be seen. Pancreatitis is an emergency marked by an acute abdomen. Patients have severe abdominal pain and paralytic ileus. The clinical course can be complicated by disseminated intravascular coagulation, shock, and secondary bacterial infection with sepsis. Chalky deposits of fat necrosis can involve the pancreas and adipose tissue within the abdomen and lead to hypocalcemia. An intraperitoneal fluid collection (ascites) can be present.

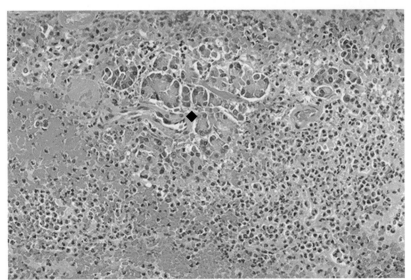

Figure 9-6 Acute pancreatitis, microscopic
Acute inflammation with necrosis and hemorrhage is seen here along with residual pancreatic acini (◆). The damage involves primarily the acinar cells, but the vasculature is also affected, and if severe and extensive, even the islets of Langerhans may be destroyed. Less common causes of pancreatitis include hypertriglyceridemia (typically >500 mg/dL); hypercalcemia; trauma; and drugs such as azathioprine, didanosine, pentamidine, valproic acid, opiates, and thiazides. In 10% to 20% of cases, an underlying cause cannot be identified.

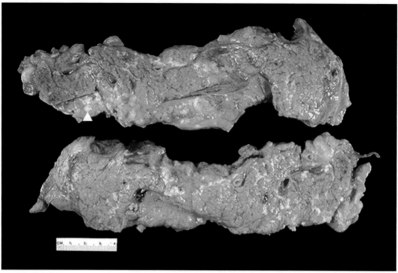

Figure 9-7 Fat necrosis, gross
Yellow-tan foci of fat necrosis (▲) are visible throughout the pancreas, seen here sectioned in half. There is some edema, but no hemorrhage, in this case of mild acute pancreatitis. Enzymatic release from the exocrine pancreas leads to autodestruction. Trypsin activation triggers a cascade of additional proenzyme activation, including proelastase and prophospholipase, which disintegrate adipocytes and pancreatic parenchyma. Trypsin release also activates prekallikrein to bring the kinin system into play, with vascular thrombosis and damage.

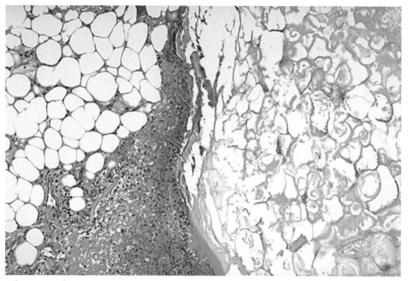

Figure 9-8 Fat necrosis, microscopic
The adipocytes here have lost their nuclei and their cytoplasm has a granular pink appearance, most pronounced on the right. The rare autosomal dominant condition of hereditary pancreatitis results from gain of function mutations in the *PRSS1* gene that lead to abnormal activation of trypsin. Another rare inherited autosomal recessive *SPINK1* gene mutation reduces inhibition of trypsin activity and leads to pancreatitis. These inherited forms of pancreatitis often have a chronic, relapsing course and increased risk for pancreatic adenocarcinoma.

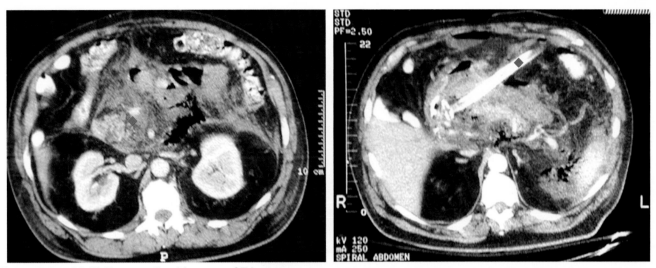

Figures 9-9 and 9-10 Pancreatic phlegmon, CT images

In these abdominal CT scans without contrast enhancement, there is a phlegmon that represents a swollen, inflamed mass (◆) in the region of the pancreas. This complication may occur if acute pancreatitis persists. Infection of a phlegmon results in a pancreatic abscess. In the *right panel,* a drain (◆) is in place after laparotomy with débridement of the abscess.

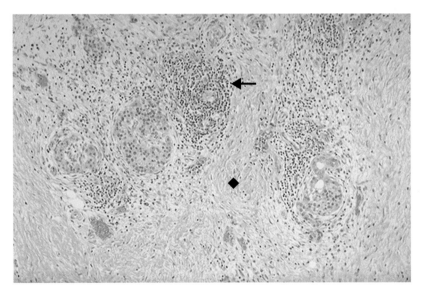

Figure 9-11 Chronic pancreatitis, microscopic

Seen here are scattered chronic inflammatory cells (←) in a collagenous stroma (◆) with absence of acini, but a few remaining islets of Langerhans. Chronic alcohol abuse is a common cause of this condition, which typically occurs after repeated bouts of mild to moderate acute pancreatitis. About 40% of the time, no specific cause is identified. Depending on the amount of remaining functional parenchyma, pancreatic insufficiency with malabsorption and steatorrhea may occur, and diabetes mellitus may eventually occur from loss of islets of Langerhans, although most of the islets are typically spared. Compound heterozygotes with variant *CFTR* gene mutations may develop chronic pancreatitis.

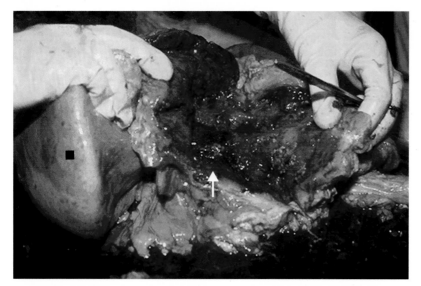

Figure 9-12 Pancreatic pseudocyst, gross
This structure at autopsy is hardly recognizable as pancreas because a large pseudocyst (↑) has formed and is shown opened here. The yellowish liver (■) with blunted edge at the left is consistent with steatosis from alcohol abuse. This pseudocyst has an irregular red-to-brown-to-black inner surface. A pseudocyst is a localized area of liquefactive necrosis bounded by granulation tissue. It appears grossly and radiographically as a cystic structure, and similar to a pancreatic phlegmon (which appears as a mass), it can become secondarily infected to form a pancreatic abscess.

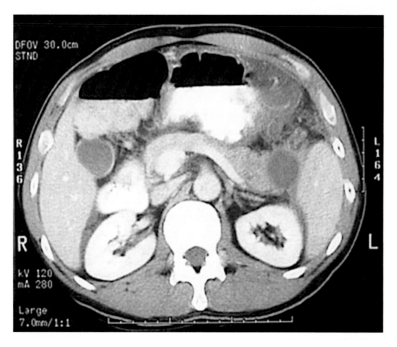

Figure 9-13 Pancreatic pseudocyst, CT image
This pseudocyst (▲) shows low attenuation in its liquefied center on CT scan with contrast. This lesion is located in the tail of the pancreas next to the spleen. Most pseudocysts involve the lesser sac. This one is small, but some may reach 30 cm in diameter. Inflammation with fluid collection here extends to the adjacent omentum near the stomach, in the region of the lesser omental sac. A pseudocyst is a serious complication of pancreatitis because hemorrhage, peritonitis, and sepsis may occur. Some pseudocysts may resolve; those that persist may be treated by drainage.

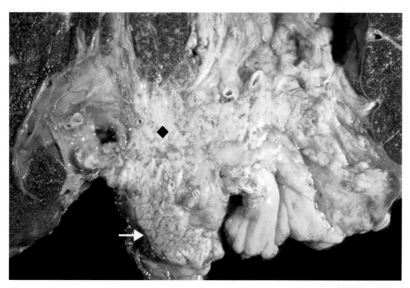

Figure 9-14 Adenocarcinoma, gross
This irregular mass lesion (◆) arising in the pancreas is very extensive, sparing only the uncinate process (→) at the lower left center. About 60% of cases involve the pancreatic head, with icterus, marked by the green color of the liver at the left after formalin fixation, and caused by biliary tract obstruction with jaundice and direct hyperbilirubinemia. Tumor invades into the hilum of the liver, and small parenchymal tan metastases to liver are present. Pancreatic cancer is the fourth most frequent cause of cancer death in the United States. Few cases are diagnosed early, so the typical prognosis is poor, with a 5-year survival rate of less than 5%. Constant, boring pain may be the initial presenting complaint when the cancer arises in the body or tail region.

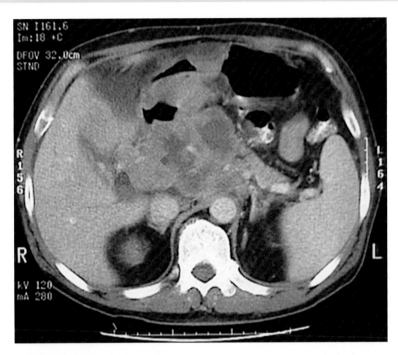

Figure 9-15 Adenocarcinoma, CT image
This large irregular mass (◆) involves the head and body of the pancreas, and it infiltrates into the hilum of the liver. Most pancreatic adenocarcinomas have infiltrated surrounding structures or have metastasized at the time of diagnosis. The *KRAS* oncogene and the *CDKN2A, TP53,* and *SMAD4* tumor suppressor genes are frequently found to have mutations in this condition. More than 80% of cases occur in individuals older than 60 years. Cigarette smoking is a risk factor, as are chronic pancreatitis and diabetes mellitus. Less common risk factors include Peutz-Jeghers syndrome and hereditary pancreatitis. Regardless of the cause, clinical findings include abdominal pain, anorexia, jaundice, and weight loss. Trousseau syndrome, a hypercoagulable state with arterial or venous thromboses, occurs in 10% of cases.

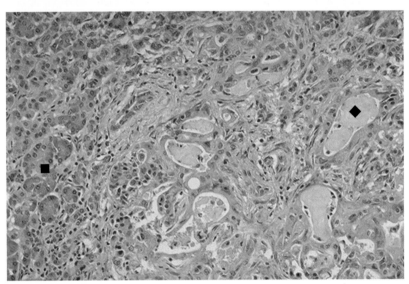

Figure 9-16 Adenocarcinoma, microscopic
This pancreatic malignancy is moderately differentiated, showing some irregular gland formation (◆) with intracytoplasmic mucin production and gland luminal mucin accumulation. These neoplasms often have significant desmoplasia (elaboration of a collagenous connective tissue stroma). Some residual normal pancreas (■) is seen at the upper left. They infiltrate locally and are difficult to resect because they are invariably diagnosed at a late stage. Perineural invasion is common and accounts for the constant pain typical of cancer. A serum marker, not specific for pancreatic cancer, is the CA19-9 antigen.

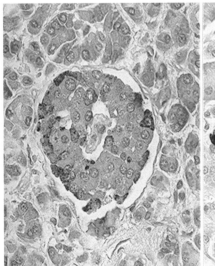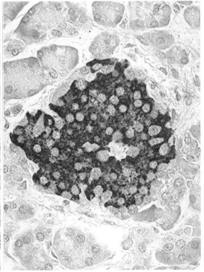

Figure 9-17 Normal islet of Langerhans, microscopic
The endocrine function of the pancreas resides in the islets of Langerhans scattered within the parenchyma, but concentrated more in the tail. With the immunohistochemical staining seen here, an islet contains β cells that secrete insulin (*left panel*), α cells secreting glucagon (*right panel*), and unstained δ cells producing somatostatin. The hormones are secreted directly into the bloodstream. Because there are multiple hormones that oppose insulin, loss of glucagon or somatostatin production from islets has minimal clinical consequence.

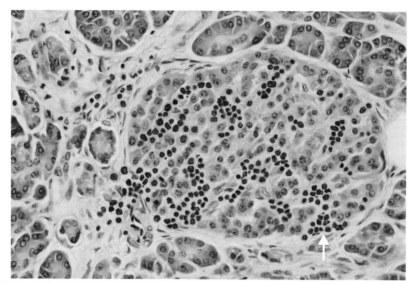

Figure 9-18 Insulitis, microscopic

The rarely seen hallmark of type 1 diabetes mellitus is inflammation of the islets, which occurs before the onset of clinical findings. Note the lymphocytic infiltrates (↑) in this islet. A genetic susceptibility, coupled with viral or toxic agents that damage the islet cells, culminates in an autoimmune reaction with islet destruction that underlies type 1 diabetes. The autoimmune nature of type 1 diabetes is shown by insulin autoantibody, glutamic acid decarboxylase (GAD65), and islet cell antigen (IA-2). Islets are nearly absent by the onset of overt diabetes with hyperglycemia, polyuria, polydipsia, and polyphagia, and there is an absolute lack of circulating insulin. Lack of insulin results in catabolism of adipose tissue and muscle, leading to metabolic acidosis (ketoacidosis) and muscle wasting.

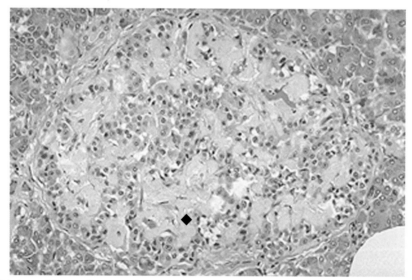

Figure 9-19 Islet amyloid deposition, microscopic

This islet of Langerhans shows pink hyaline (◆) material (with deposition of amyloid) around many of the islet cells. This is a form of localized amyloidosis. The amyloid is derived from amylin, a protein secreted along with insulin. This finding is typical in patients with type 2 diabetes mellitus, who have a relative lack of insulin, but in whom islets are still present. There may be deranged secretion of insulin by β cells or peripheral insulin resistance. Islet β-cell dysfunction leads to decreased insulin and islet amyloid polypeptide (amylin) secretion. Most patients with type 2 diabetes are obese. Not all type 2 diabetic patients have amyloid in islets; its role in the pathogenesis of the disease is unclear.

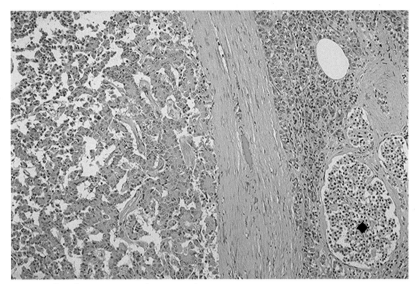

Figure 9-20 Pancreatic neuroendocrine tumor, microscopic

The pancreatic neuroendocrine tumor (PanNET), formerly termed *islet cell adenoma,* on the left contrasts with the normal pancreas with islets (◆) on the right, separated by a capsule of collagenous connective tissue. Similar to carcinoid tumors seen in the gastrointestinal tract, PanNETs are endocrine neoplasms that can potentially secrete a variety of hormonal products. β-Cell (insulin-producing) neoplasms are the most common, and excess circulating insulin causes hypoglycemia with resulting mental confusion, weakness, or even convulsions. However, symptoms can occur episodically, and the tumor can be quite small, making diagnosis difficult. G-cell (gastrin-producing) tumors are the second most common and may give rise to the Zollinger-Ellison syndrome (gastric hypersecretion leading to gastric, duodenal, and jejunal peptic ulcers). The serum gastrin levels in such patients are generally at least five times normal.

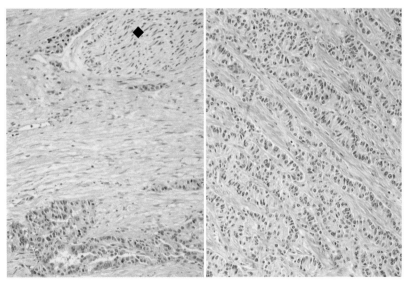

Figure 9-21 Pancreatic neuroendocrine tumor, microscopic

In the *right panel* are nests and ribbons of cells with intervening stroma, but atypical features are not marked. In the left panel the tumor cells are infiltrating a peripheral nerve (◆) and the stroma, evidence of malignancy. Most α-cell (glucagon-producing) PanNETs are malignant, but uncommon, and manifest with a clinical syndrome of mild diabetes mellitus and a peculiar widespread dermatitis known as *necrolytic migratory erythema.* Most of the cases have distant metastases, particularly to the liver.

δ-Cell (somatostatin-producing) tumors are very rare and produce diabetes mellitus, steatorrhea, and diarrhea. Most are malignant. Less commonly, PanNETs may produce adrenocorticotropic hormone, causing Cushing syndrome, or serotonin, producing the carcinoid syndrome. Vasoactive intestinal polypeptide may also be produced and probably gives rise to the Verner-Morrison syndrome of watery diarrhea, hypokalemia, and achlorhydria. PanNETs may be part of an autosomal dominant disorder known as *multiple endocrine neoplasia syndrome type I.* In addition to PanNETs, these patients may have hyperplasia or adenomas of the pituitary and parathyroid glands and may have various presenting problems depending on the hyperfunctioning tissue. Islet cell tumors usually produce either insulin or gastrin.

The Kidney

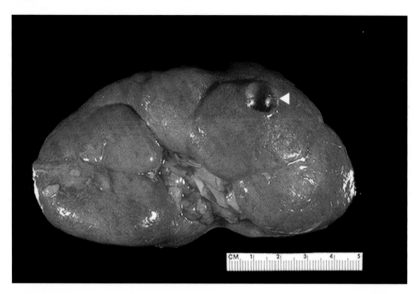

Figure 10-1 Normal kidney, gross

This normal adult kidney with the capsule removed has a pattern of fetal lobulations that still persists, as it sometimes does in adults. The hilum at the center contains some adipose tissue. An adult kidney ranges from 11 to 15 cm in length and weighs 125 to 200 g, depending on the size of the person. There is ordinarily enough renal reserve function that it is possible to survive with just half of one normal kidney. On the right is a smooth-surfaced, small, clear fluid–filled simple renal cyst (◄). Such cysts occur either singly or scattered around the renal parenchyma and are common in adults. The amount of renal reserve capacity is remarkable, and it is possible to survive with only half of one kidney.

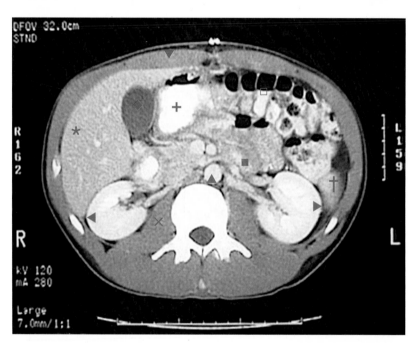

Figure 10-2 Normal kidneys, CT image

This normal abdominal CT scan with contrast enhancement at the L2-L3 level shows the right (▶) and left (◄) kidneys, liver (✶), gallbladder (◆), gastric antrum (✛), jejunum (■), colon (□), spleen (†), aorta (▲), psoas muscle (✗), and rectus abdominis muscle (▼). The kidneys are located in the retroperitoneum and are well protected by surrounding connective tissues with fat and skeletal muscle. Normal renal blood flow, which is about 25% of the cardiac output, is indicated here by the bright attenuation of the kidneys from the inflow of the injected intravenous contrast material. Branches of renal artery within each kidney have no anastomoses; branch arterial occlusion leads to focal infarction. Also, because renal tubular capillary beds derive from efferent arterioles, glomerular disease leads to parenchymal ischemia, and glomerular loss with aging results in diminution of renal size.

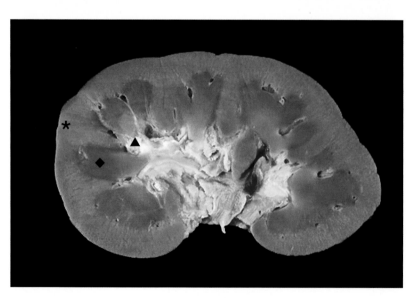

Figure 10-3 Normal kidney, gross

In cross-section, this normal adult kidney shows the lighter outer renal cortex (★), normally 5 to 10 mm in thickness, and darker inner medulla (◆) with central pelvis containing adipose tissue. Note the renal papillae (▲) projecting into the calyces, through which collecting ducts drain the excreted urine into the renal pelvis. The amount of renal reserve capacity is remarkable, and it is possible to survive with only half of one kidney. This explains why renal failure is not associated with aging. In addition to excretion of waste products, the kidney contributes to acid-base balance, salt and water volume with regulation of blood pressure, and maintenance of red blood cell (RBC) mass through elaboration of erythropoietin.

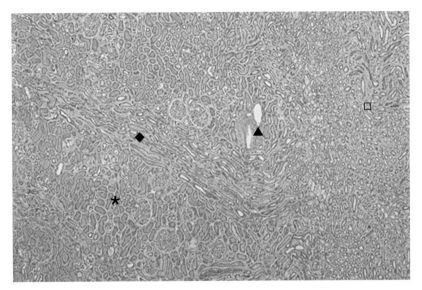

Figure 10-4 Normal kidney, microscopic
The corticomedullary junction of the kidney is shown. The cortex contains a medullary ray—a renal column (◆) extending to the medulla (□). Within the cortex (★) are glomeruli and tubules. Arcuate arteries (▲) arising from interlobar arteries course along the corticomedullary junction, giving rise to interlobular arteries from which the afferent arterioles originate to supply blood to individual glomeruli.

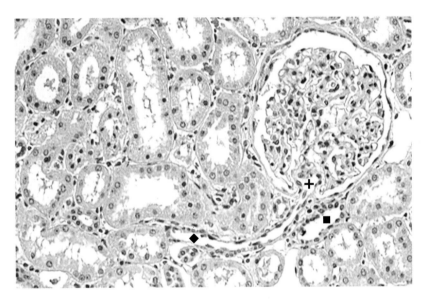

Figure 10-5 Normal kidney, microscopic
The afferent arteriole (◆) enters the glomerulus at the vascular pole (✛). The juxtaglomerular apparatus is a region of specialized smooth muscle cells called *JG cells* located in the afferent arteriole, which, along with a set of columnar cells called the *macula densa* in the adjacent segment of distal convoluted tubule (■), sense changes in blood pressure and sodium concentration. The JG cells secrete renin, which catalyzes conversion of angiotensinogen to angiotensin I. Angiotensin I is biologically inactive and converted to angiotensin II by angiotensin-converting enzyme (ACE). Angiotensin II is a potent vasoconstrictor and regulator of aldosterone secretion, which promotes sodium reabsorption and potassium excretion by the kidneys.

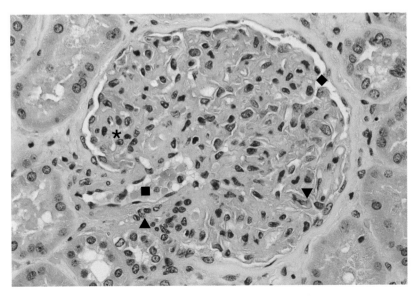

Figure 10-6 Normal kidney, microscopic
The normal glomerulus of the kidney at high power with PAS stain has thin, delicate capillary loops around the mesangial regions (★), which are not prominent, containing two to four mesangial cells. Most glomerular filtration occurs through the capillary loops into the Bowman space (◆). The mesangium accounts for about 16% of filtration and serves a macrophage-like function and a reparative function. The visceral epithelial cells (podocytes) that surround the capillary loops (▼) are not easily recognized by light microscopy; parietal epithelial cells line the external surface of the Bowman space. The afferent arteriole (■) in autoregulation and JG apparatus (▲) in tubuloglomerular feedback aid in maintaining homeostasis.

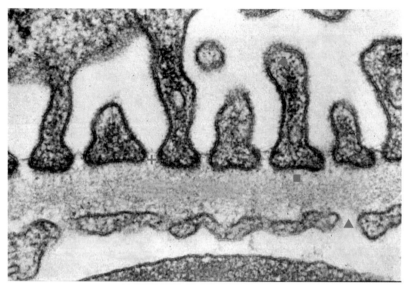

Figure 10-7 Normal kidney, electron microscopy
A glomerular capillary loop at high magnification has a visceral epithelial cell (podocyte) with interdigitating foot processes (◆) embedded in and adherent to the lamina rara externa (■) of the basement membrane. Adjacent foot processes (pedicels) are separated by 20- to 30-nm-wide filtration slits (✛). The basement membrane of uniform thickness (composed mainly of type IV collagen) has thin endothelial cell cytoplasm with fenestrations (▲) on the opposite surface. The exclusion of molecules such as albumin from the glomerular filtrate is a function of anionic charges from polyanionic proteoglycans and the anatomic size of the slit pores.

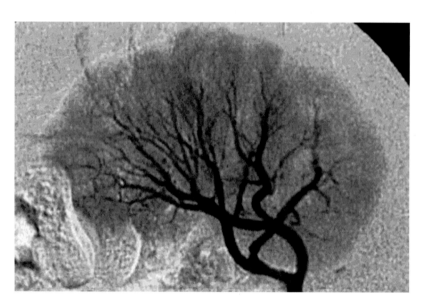

Figure 10-8 Normal kidney, angiogram
The normal distribution of blood flow in the kidney is shown here, extending distally from the main renal artery and branches to arcuate branches at the corticomedullary junction. The kidneys receive about 25% of the cardiac output, and the renal cortex receives 90% of this renal blood flow. Decreasing renal blood flow triggers release of renin, which triggers generation of angiotensin I converted to angiotensin II, elevating blood pressure through vasoconstriction to increase peripheral vascular resistance and through stimulation of aldosterone secretion from adrenal cortical glomerulosa cells, which promotes distal tubular sodium reabsorption to increase blood volume.

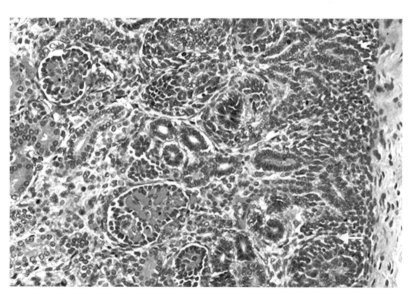

Figure 10-9 Normal fetal kidney, microscopic
Beneath the capsule of the developing fetal kidney is a nephrogenic zone (←) composed of primitive dark-blue cells in which development of glomeruli and tubules is taking place and from which the new cortex forms. At the time of birth, most of this formative process has occurred, with just a small remnant of the nephrogenic zone persisting for 3 months. At birth the infant's urine is quite dilute because the solute concentration of the medulla has not yet increased to the point that the countercurrent mechanism is fully operational.

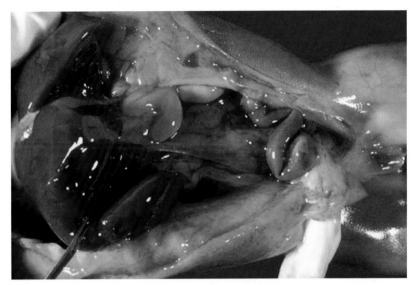

Figure 10-10 Renal agenesis, gross

Agenesis refers to absence of formation of a body part during embryogenesis. Here the kidneys are absent from the retroperitoneum; no ureteric bud induced metanephros. This results in oligohydramnios in utero because amniotic fluid is mainly derived from fetal urine. Bilateral renal agenesis is rare, present in about 1 in 4500 births, and incompatible with life. At birth, there is severe pulmonary hypoplasia from the oligohydramnios sequence. Unilateral renal agenesis is still rare but survivable; the opposite kidney develops to about twice the size of a normal kidney from compensatory hyperplasia.

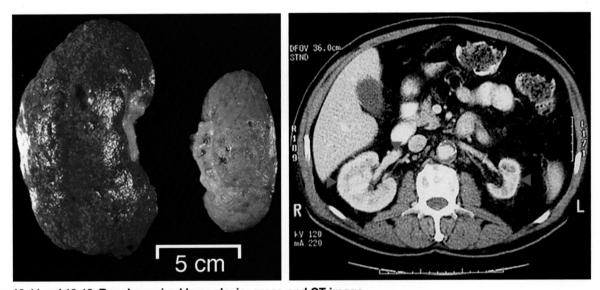

Figures 10-11 and 10-12 Renal acquired hypoplasia, gross and CT image

There is one normal-sized right kidney (▶) with a granular surface and a few scattered, shallow cortical scars as a result of left renal arterial occlusion from severe atherosclerosis. The renal veins (▼) here are highlighted by contrast material. The increased renin secretion from the smaller left kidney (◀) led to hypertension (Goldblatt kidney), which eventually damaged the opposite kidney. The atherosclerosis is marked by prominent aortic mural thrombus (darkly attenuated) contrasted with a rim of brightly attenuated calcification in the CT scan. True congenital hypoplasia is quite rare and without scars, and renal lobes and pyramids are reduced in number and size.

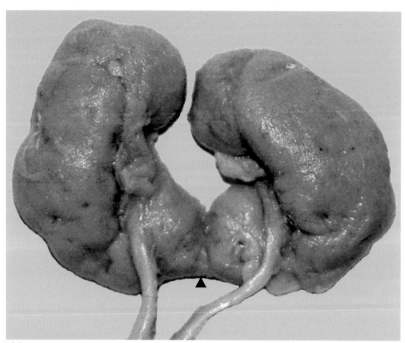

Figure 10-13 Horseshoe kidney, gross

Horseshoe kidney is a congenital anomaly that most often occurs in association with other anomalies or syndromes or with specific genetic defects, such as trisomy 18. Horseshoe kidney occurs as an isolated anomaly in about 1 in 500 people, however. Because the ureters take an abnormal course across the "bridge" (▲) of renal tissue, there is a potential for partial ureteral obstruction with resultant hydronephrosis. In many cases this is just an incidental finding because renal filtration function is not affected, and the total mass of renal tissue is normal. Abnormal fusion usually occurs at the lower renal poles.

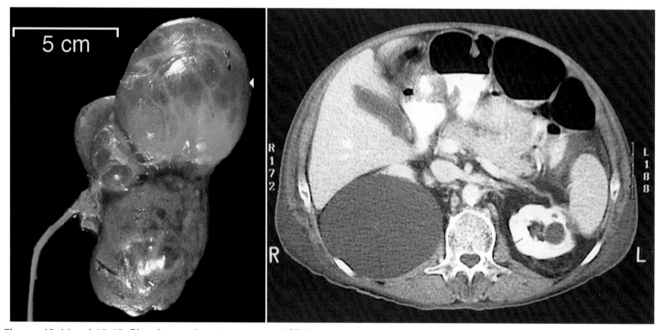

Figures 10-14 and 10-15 Simple renal cyst, gross and CT image

Note the large simple cyst of the right upper pole (◄). Other smaller cysts are also scattered within the renal cortex in the *left panel*. Simple renal cysts are a common incidental finding in adults. A large renal cyst (◆) can be seen in this CT scan, but it can be distinguished from a neoplasm by its fluid density and thin wall. In the CT scan, a smaller simple cyst on the left has the characteristic features of low fluid attenuation and discrete, round borders. There is sufficient remaining functional renal cortex to provide adequate renal function in nearly all individuals with simple renal cysts. An uncommon complication is cyst hemorrhage with pain.

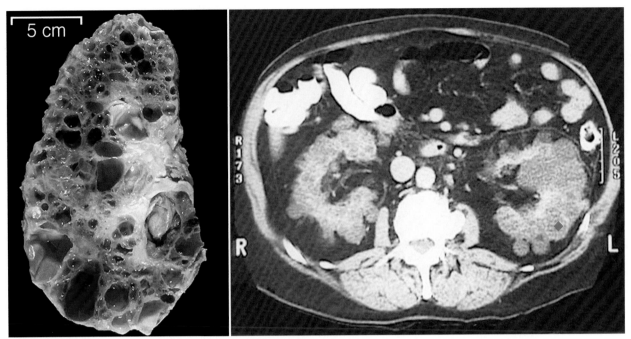

Figures 10-16 and 10-17 Autosomal dominant polycystic kidney disease (ADPKD), gross and CT image
The right kidney shown here grossly weighed 3 kg, as did the left kidney. ADPKD is a bilateral process. Mutations in the *PKD1* gene encoding polycystin-1 account for 85% of cases, and mutations in *PKD2* encoding polycystin-2 for most of the rest; these proteins are part of ciliated tubular epithelium regulating intracellular calcium. The cysts (◆) are not typically present at birth but develop slowly over time, so that onset of renal failure occurs in middle age to later adult life. An initial laboratory finding is often hematuria, followed by proteinuria (rarely >2 g/day). Patients often have polyuria and hypertension. Cysts may appear in other organs, such as liver, pancreas, and spleen. About 4% to 10% of patients with ADPKD have an intracranial berry aneurysm.

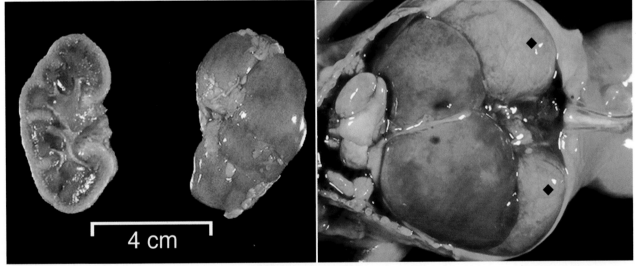

Figures 10-18 and 10-19 Normal fetal kidney and autosomal recessive polycystic kidney disease (ARPKD), gross
The normal term infant kidneys in the *left panel* reveal typical fetal lobulations and smooth cortical surfaces with some attached adipose tissue. Note the well-defined corticomedullary junctions on cut section. In the *right panel,* note the bilaterally massively enlarged kidneys (◆) that nearly fill the abdomen below the liver, consistent with ARPKD in this fetus at 23 weeks' gestation who died from pulmonary hypoplasia as a result of oligohydramnios. There are perinatal, neonatal, infantile, and juvenile subcategories depending on the nature of the *PKHD1* gene mutation (encoding a large novel protein, fibrocystin, that is part of tubular cell cilia), the time of presentation, and the presence of associated hepatic lesions. The first two are the most common; serious manifestations are usually present at birth, typically with renal failure from birth. The latter two are compatible with longer survival, but patients often develop congenital hepatic fibrosis leading to complications from portal hypertension. There are many *PKHD1* mutations, and cases of ARPKD are often compound heterozygotes, accounting for differences in severity.

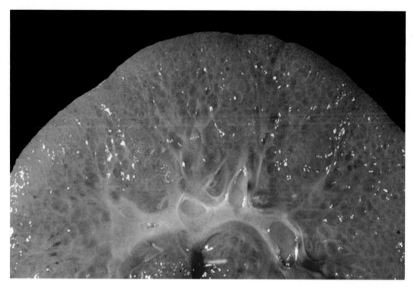

Figure 10-20 Autosomal-recessive polycystic kidney disease (ARPKD), gross
A bilaterally and symmetrically enlarged kidney with ARPKD is shown here on cut surface. The numerous glistening cysts are small, about 1 to 2 mm in diameter, but uniformly distributed throughout the parenchyma to produce a spongy appearance, and there is no distinguishable cortex or medulla. This condition is most often present from birth (hence the synonym *infantile polycystic kidney disease*). In utero this condition results in reduced production of fetal urine, which forms amniotic fluid. Fetal ultrasound shows oligohydramnios, or anhydramnios if severe.

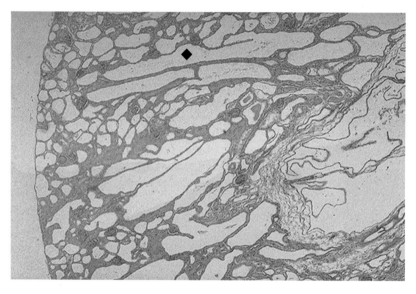

Figure 10-21 Autosomal-recessive polycystic kidney disease, microscopic
The microscopic appearance of ARPKD is characterized by many cysts (◆) involving the collecting ducts, often elongated and radially arranged or saccular. A few scattered glomeruli are within the residual renal cortex. The cysts have a uniform lining of cuboidal cells. Consequent oligohydramnios leads to a deformation sequence from constriction of the fetus in utero. In addition to pulmonary hypoplasia, there can be varus deformities of the lower extremities, glovelike redundant skin on hands, and flattened (Potter) facies.

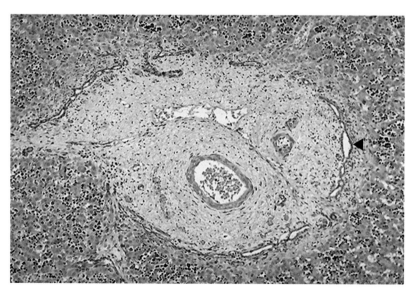

Figure 10-22 Autosomal recessive polycystic kidney disease (ARPKD), microscopic
Characteristic of ARPKD is the appearance in the liver shown here of congenital hepatic fibrosis, seen as expanded portal regions with collagenous fibrosis and a surrounding proliferation of radially arranged portal bile ducts (◄). The adjacent normal hepatic parenchyma contains islands of extramedullary hematopoiesis, mainly clusters of erythroid precursors, typical for second-trimester and third-trimester fetal liver. In cases where survival into childhood occurs, portal hypertension with splenomegaly may result.

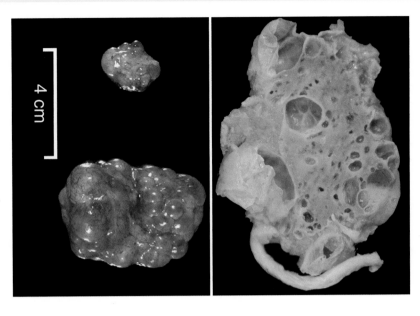

Figure 10-23 Multicystic renal dysplasia, gross

The fetal kidneys *(left panel)* are composed of cysts and are asymmetrical in size. The cut surface *(right panel)* of one kidney shows irregularly sized cysts separated by dense stroma. Multicystic renal dysplasia (or multicystic dysplastic kidney) is more common than ARPKD, has larger cysts, and occurs sporadically without a defined inheritance pattern. It may be part of a malformation complex, such as Meckel-Gruber syndrome. Many cases are associated with additional urinary tract anomalies, such as ureteropelvic obstruction, ureteral agenesis, or atresia. Often, multicystic dysplastic kidney is unilateral. If bilateral, it is often asymmetrical, as seen here, and oligohydramnios and its complications can ensue, just as with ARPKD.

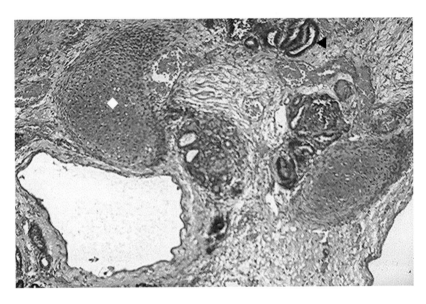

Figure 10-24 Multicystic renal dysplasia, microscopic

Dysplasia in pediatric terms implies disordered organ development (not an epithelial precursor to neoplasia). The dysplasia is evident here in the renal parenchyma composed of irregular vascular channels, islands of cartilage (◆), undifferentiated mesenchyme, and scattered immature collecting ductules (◀) in a fibrous stroma with cysts. There is also abnormal lobar organization. If the process is unilateral or involves just a part of a kidney, there is enough renal reserve capacity with compensatory hyperplasia of the remaining renal tissue for adequate renal function to live a normal life. A person may survive with just half of one normal kidney.

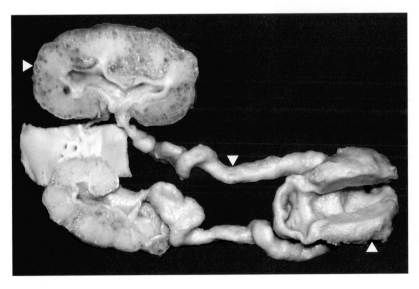

Figure 10-25 Congenital urinary obstruction with cystic change, gross

Urinary tract obstruction in utero can lead to renal cystic changes in addition to hydronephrosis. Obstruction below the bladder (▲) in this case (either urethral atresia or posterior urethral valves may be suspected) has led to bladder dilation and hypertrophy, bilateral hydroureter (▼), and numerous small cysts (▶) in the renal cortices. Oligohydramnios also accompanies this obstruction to urine flow.

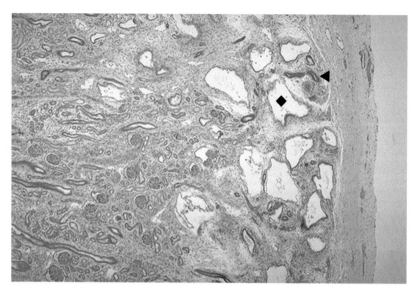

Figure 10-26 Congenital urinary obstruction with cystic changes, microscopic
The cysts (◆) appear near the nephrogenic zone (◀) because the developing glomeruli are most sensitive to the increased pressure. Cortical microcysts develop as shown here. Causes of congenital urinary tract obstruction include posterior urethral valves (in males) or urethral atresia (in both sexes). Obstruction below the bladder is detected via bladder enlargement on ultrasound scans; diminished (or absent) fetal urine production leads to oligohydramnios (or anhydramnios) with a diminished amniotic fluid index.

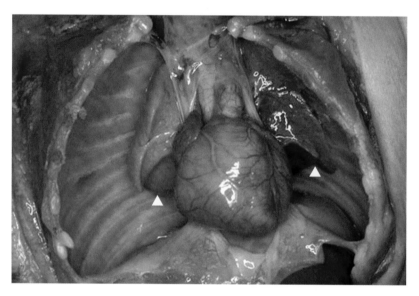

Figure 10-27 Pulmonary hypoplasia, gross
Congenital renal diseases or urinary tract outflow anomalies lead to the oligohydramnios sequence, which constricts lung development in utero, causing pulmonary hypoplasia. An ultrasound scan shows marked oligohydramnios when fetal urine that forms the bulk of the amniotic fluid volume is reduced. The chest cavity opened here at autopsy reveals a normal-sized heart but very small lungs (▲), which become the rate-limiting step for survival after birth. Additional features of the oligohydramnios sequence include Potter facies with flattened nose and prominent infraorbital creases. Deformations of the extremities are common, with talipes equinovarus and joint contractures.

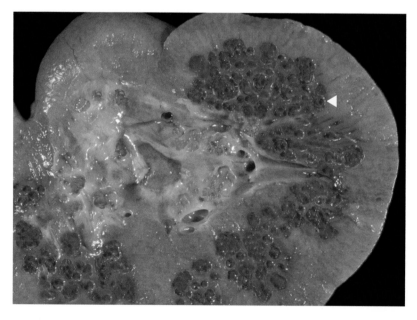

Figure 10-28 Medullary sponge kidney (MSK), gross
Note the 1- to 7-mm cysts (◀) involving the medulla of this kidney that resulted from nonprogressive dilation of the distal portion of the collecting ducts and tubules in the renal papillae. Most cases are bilateral and are discovered incidentally with radiologic imaging studies. Renal function is usually normal because the cortex is not involved. In 20% of cases of MSK there may be formation of renal calculi, which predispose to obstruction and infection (pyelonephritis) and hematuria in middle-aged individuals. Some cases appear in conjunction with Marfan syndrome, Ehlers-Danlos syndrome, and Caroli disease.

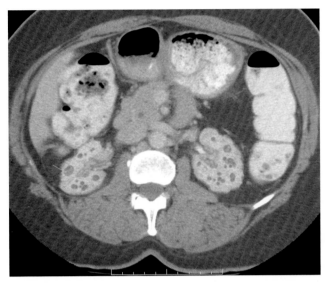

Figure 10-29 Nephronophthisis, CT image

Note medullary cysts (▶), which may be up to 2 cm, concentrated at the corticomedullary junctions in this abdominal CT with contrast. There is ongoing tubulointerstitial injury from tubular basement membrane disruption. Glomeruli are usually spared. Cases can occur sporadically, associated with retinal lesions, and most commonly as an autosomal recessive familial form with onset in childhood or adolescence, with multiple possible mutations, including *NPHP* genes. Patients have polyuria from lack of concentrating ability, sodium wasting, and tubular acidosis. There is progression to end-stage renal disease.

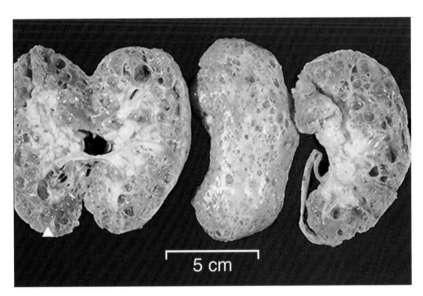

Figure 10-30 Acquired renal cystic disease, gross

Patients with chronic renal failure (CRF) who undergo hemodialysis for many years may develop multiple cortical cysts (▲). This is probably the result of obstruction with progressive interstitial fibrosis and/or oxalate crystal deposition in end-stage renal disease. When such cysts develop, they are more numerous than the common simple renal cysts, but usually less numerous than the cysts with ADPKD, and the size of the kidneys with dialysis-induced cystic disease is usually not markedly increased as it is with ADPKD, because it is superimposed on chronic renal disease. There may be hemorrhage into the cysts. There is an increased risk for development of renal cell carcinoma.

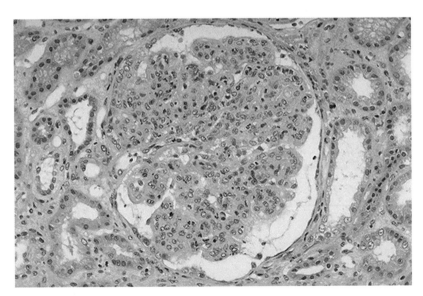

Figure 10-31 Postinfectious glomerulonephritis, microscopic

Postinfectious glomerulonephritis (GN) is hypercellular with increased inflammatory cells, and capillary loops are poorly defined. This type of acute proliferative GN is termed postinfectious glomerulonephritis, but is better known as *poststreptococcal glomerulonephritis* because historically most cases followed streptococcal pharyngitis (a different bacterial strain than that producing acute rheumatic fever). Other infections include staphylococcal endocarditis, pneumococcal pneumonia, hepatitis B or C, HIV, or malaria. The infectious agent induces an immune response with antibodies that cross-react with glomerular antigens or lead to antigen-antibody complex formation with glomerular deposition.

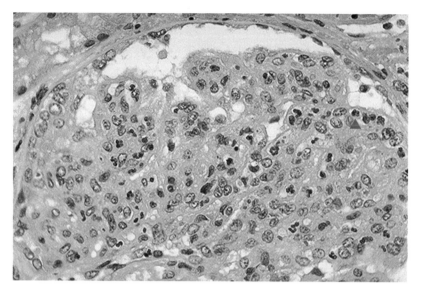

Figure 10-32 Postinfectious glomerulonephritis, microscopic
At higher magnification, the hypercellularity of postinfectious GN is caused by increased numbers of epithelial, endothelial, and mesangial cells and neutrophils (▲) infiltrating in and around the capillary loops. This disease may occur 1 to 4 weeks after recovery from infection with certain (nephritogenic) strains of group A β-hemolytic streptococci that involve the pharynx ("strep throat") or skin (impetigo). These patients typically have elevated antistreptolysin O (ASO), anti-DNase B, or antihyaluronidase titers. Patients may have microscopic hematuria, mild protein-uria, and mild to moderate hypertension.

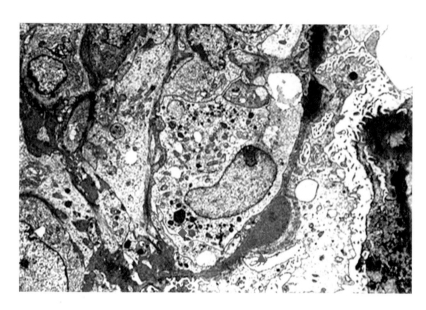

Figure 10-33 Postinfectious glomerulonephritis, electron microscopy
The immune deposits that appear in a bumpy granular pattern consist mainly of IgG, IgM, and C3, as shown by immunofluorescence, and shown here on electron microscopy to be predominantly subepithelial. There are electron-dense subepithelial "humps" (✱) above the basement membrane and below the epithelial cell (podocyte) foot processes (▲). The capillary lumen is filled with a leukocyte having multiple cytoplasmic granules (◆). More than 95% of children with this disease recover quickly, but <1% may evolve to rapidly progressive glomeru-lonephritis (RPGN). About 40% of adults with this condition go on to develop chronic renal disease.

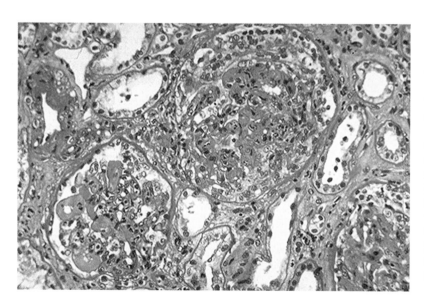

Figure 10-34 Rapidly progressive glomerulonephritis, microscopic
Seen here within three glomeruli are crescents (✱) composed of proliferating epithelial cells. Crescentic GN is known as *rapidly progres-sive glomerulonephritis* because this disease has a fulminant course. RPGN may be idiopathic or may result from anti–glomerular basement membrane (anti-GBM) antibody disease, such as Goodpasture syndrome (type 1); from im-mune complex deposition with diseases such as systemic lupus erythematosus (SLE) or postin-fectious GN (type 2); and from various types of vasculitis (type 3), often "pauci-immune" forms. In the lower left glomerulus, the capillary loops are markedly thickened (the so-called *wire-loop lesion* of lupus nephritis).

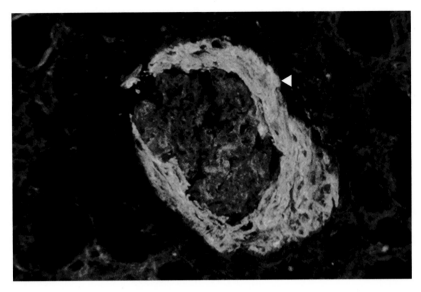

Figure 10-35 Rapidly progressive glomerulo-nephritis, immunofluorescence

This glomerulus shows bright green immunofluorescence (◄) with antibody to fibrinogen. With RPGN, the glomerular damage is so severe that fibrinogen leaks into the Bowman space, leading to proliferation of the epithelial cells and formation of a crescent. Patients typically develop RPGN over a few days. Clinical manifestations include hematuria, moderate to severe proteinuria with edema, and hypertension. Hemoptysis characterizes patients with Goodpasture syndrome, who also have detectable circulating anti-GBM antibody. Patients with systemic vasculitis, such as microscopic polyangiitis (MPA), may have circulating antineutrophil cytoplasmic antibody.

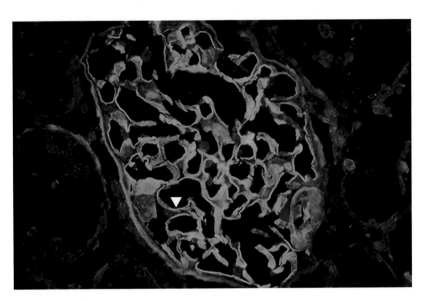

Figure 10-36 Rapidly progressive glomerulo-nephritis, immunofluorescence

There is bright green positivity with antibody to IgG with a smooth, diffuse, linear (▼) pattern that is characteristic of RPGN caused by circulating anti-GBM antibody with Goodpasture syndrome. The antibody is directed at the noncollagenous domain of the α_3 chain of type IV collagen. This leads to a form of type II hypersensitivity reaction. Patients with RPGN have rapidly increasing serum urea nitrogen and creatinine, decreasing urine output, and urinary sediment that may contain RBCs and RBC casts. The presence of the urinary dysmorphic RBCs and RBC casts along with oliguria and hypertension characterizes a nephritic syndrome.

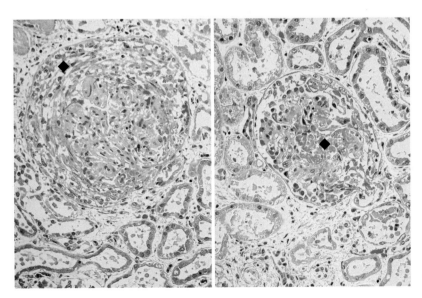

Figure 10-37 Microscopic polyangiitis, microscopic

Note the focal segmental necrotizing GN (◆) in the *right panel* and a glomerular crescent (◆) in the *left panel* in this case of an antineutrophil cytoplasmic autoantibody (ANCA)–associated GN. Tubular atrophy is also present. This is a pauci-immune form of RPGN, and immunofluorescence will show minimal deposition of immunoglobulins or complement in the glomeruli and renal vessels. MPA typically has an onset in the sixth decade, with fever or weight loss accompanying renal disease with nephrosis in mild cases to nephritis with severe involvement.

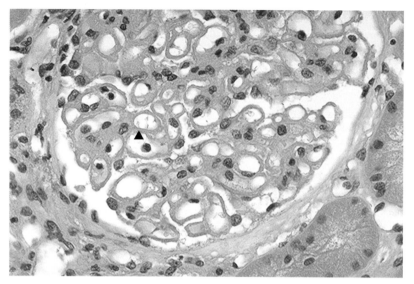

Figure 10-38 Membranous nephropathy microscopic

These capillary loops (▲) are diffusely thickened and prominent, but the overall glomerular cellularity is not increased. Membranous nephropathy is the most common cause of nephrotic syndrome in adults. Nephrotic syndrome is defined as more than 3.5 g of urine protein (mainly albumin) per day per 1.62 m^2 body surface area. With pure nephrotic syndrome, RBCs are typically absent in the urine. About 25% of cases are secondary to an underlying condition, such as a chronic infection (e.g., hepatitis B or C), a carcinoma, drugs (nonsteroidal antiinflammatory drugs [NSAIDs]), or SLE. Most cases are idiopathic. Autoantibodies to M-type phospholipase A$_2$ receptor (PLA$_2$R) are present in about 75% of idiopathic cases but not in those with secondary membranous nephropathy or other renal diseases.

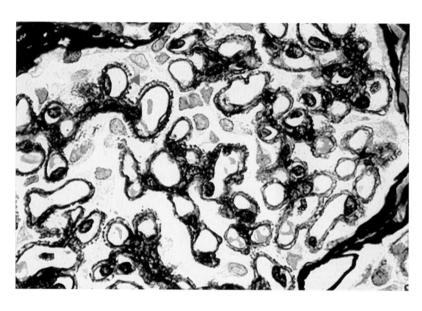

Figure 10-39 Membranous nephropathy, microscopic

A Jones silver stain of this glomerulus highlights the proteinaceous basement membranes of capillary loops in black. There are characteristic "spikes" (◀) involving the capillary loops with membranous nephropathy, shown here with black basement membrane material appearing as small projections distributed within the capillary loops. The immune complexes, not highlighted by the Jones stain, lie between the black spikes. Loss of anticoagulant proteins in nephrosis predisposes to thrombosis, including renal vein thrombosis. Urinalysis with nephrotic syndrome may show lipiduria and proteinuria, whereas blood lipids (cholesterol and triglyceride) are increased.

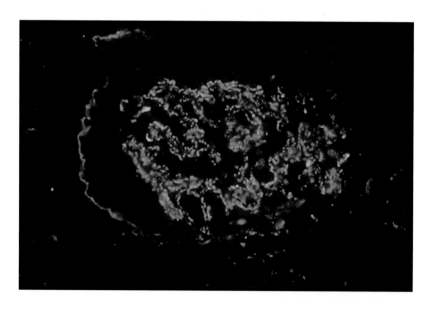

Figure 10-40 Membranous nephropathy, electron microscopy

The immunofluorescence pattern here has a "bumpy" or granular staining pattern as a result of irregular deposition of immune complexes within the basement membranes of the glomerular capillary loops. Various fluorescein-labeled antibodies can be employed, such as those directed against immunoglobulins or complement components, which commonly compose the immune complexes. The onset of membranous nephropathy is often gradual, with nephrotic syndrome a likely presenting finding. Some patients may have hypertension; hematuria is less common. About 10% of patients go on to develop CRF within 10 years.

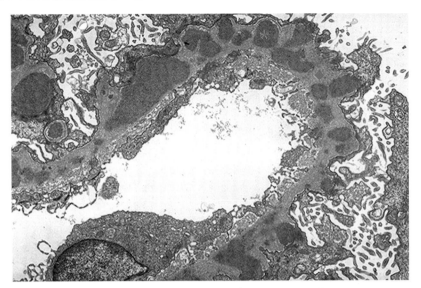

Figure 10-41 Membranous nephropathy, electron microscopy

On electron microscopy, the darker electron-dense immune deposits (✱) appear scattered within the thickened capillary basement membrane. The "spikes" seen with the silver stain are the lighter areas (◆) representing the intervening increased matrix of basement membrane between the darker immune deposits. These deposits invariably contain complement proteins, and the C5b-C9 membrane attack complex damages glomerular capillaries. The loss of basement membrane function leads to proteinuria, which is often "selective" because mostly lower molecular weight proteins such as albumin are lost. Some cases have nonselective proteinuria with hematuria, and up to 40% of cases may eventually progress to chronic renal failure.

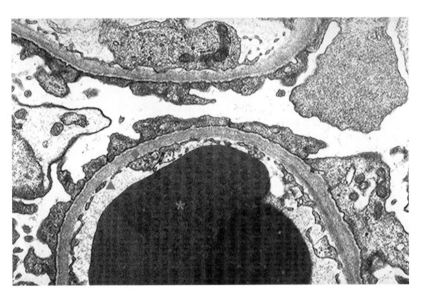

Figure 10-42 Minimal change disease, electron microscopy

On light microscopy the glomerulus is normal with minimal change disease (MCD), the most common cause of nephrotic syndrome in children. In this electron micrograph, the lower capillary loop contains two electron-dense RBCs (✱) in close apposition. Normal fenestrated endothelium (▲) is present, and the basement membranes (◆) are normal in thickness with no immune deposits. Overlying epithelial cell (podocyte) foot processes are effaced (giving the appearance of fusion) and run together (✚), which leads to loss of the normal anionic charge barrier such that albumin selectively leaks out, and proteinuria ensues, often with nephrotic syndrome. Most patients recover completely after a course of corticosteroid therapy.

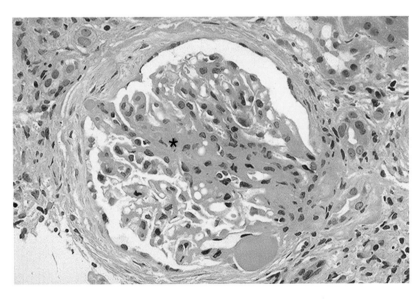

Figure 10-43 Focal segmental glomerulonephritis, microscopic

An area of collagenous sclerosis (✱) traverses the middle segment of this glomerulus. Only 3 of 10 glomeruli in the entire biopsy specimen were involved, a focal process. This podocytopathy is initiated by epithelial cell damage through activation of β_3 integrin signaling by the soluble urokinase-type plasminogen activator receptor (suPAR). Patients with focal segmental glomerulonephritis (FSGS) are more likely than those with MCD to have a poor response to corticosteroid therapy, with nonselective proteinuria, hematuria, and progression to CRF. FSGS may represent the opposite end of the spectrum of MCD because more than half of FSGS patients progress to CRF within 10 years.

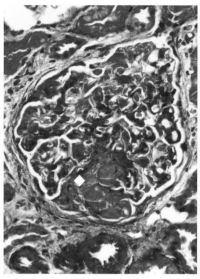
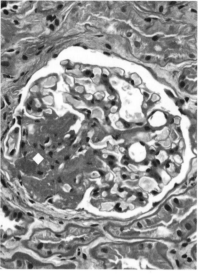

Figure 10-44 Focal segmental glomerulosclerosis, microscopic

The trichrome stain *(blue, left panel)* and PAS stain *(red, right panel)* of a glomerulus in a patient with FSGS shows focal collagen deposition (◆) at the vascular pole. FSGS accounts for about one sixth of cases of nephrotic syndrome in adults and children. This disease is focal, involving some glomeruli, and segmental, involving part of the glomerulus. Patients may have either nephrotic or nephritic syndrome. In some cases, a mutated *NPHS1* gene produces an abnormal nephrin protein, and in others, abnormal podocin is produced by an abnormal *NPHS2* gene. Both proteins are components of the slit diaphragm between podocyte foot processes. Recurrence of FSGS after transplantation is frequent. HIV-associated nephropathy has features of FSGS.

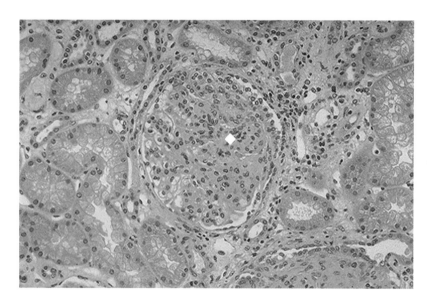

Figure 10-45 Membranoproliferative glomerulonephritis, microscopic

This glomerulus has increased overall cellularity, mainly mesangial (◆). MPGN may be termed *secondary* and follow infections such as hepatitis B or C, malignancies, or immune complex diseases such as SLE. Most cases of MPGN are *primary* (idiopathic), however. On light microscopy there is mesangial proliferation, increased mesangial matrix, mesangial immune complex deposition, accentuation of the lobular architecture, and increased leukocytes. Most cases occur in adolescents and young adults, with both nephrotic and nephritic features. Half of idiopathic cases progress to CRF in 10 years.

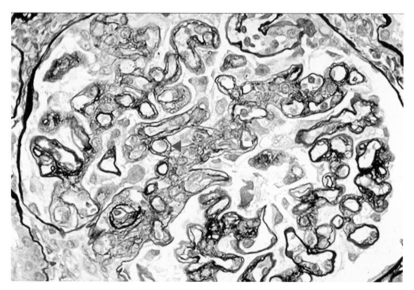

Figure 10-46 Membranoproliferative glomerulonephritis, microscopic

This Jones silver stain shows a double contour (◀) to many basement membranes, or the "tram-tracking" that is characteristic of membranoproliferative glomerulonephritis (MPGN), which results from basement membrane reduplication. (A *tram* is a streetcar on rails.) The disease results from subendothelial immune complex deposition after classic and alternate pathway complement activation, but antigens that trigger this process are often unknown. There is no response to corticosteroid therapy. Some cases progress to RPGN. Recurrence of MPGN after renal transplantation is frequent.

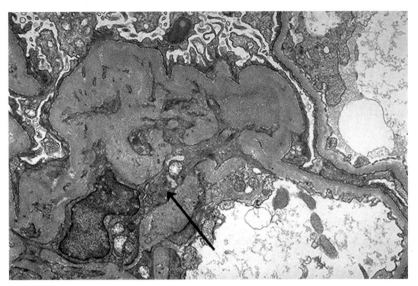

Figure 10-47 Membranoproliferative glomerulonephritis, electron microscopy

A mesangial cell at the lower left is interposing its cytoplasm at the (↑) into the basement membrane, leading to splitting and reduplication of basement membrane that is piled up above the mesangial cytoplasm. These characteristic electron microscopic changes occur when the mesangial cell (which has a macrophage-like function) tries to phagocytose subendothelial immune deposits, but makes a mess of the GBM in the process. Secondary MPGN can complicate SLE, hepatitis B or C infections with cryoglobulinemia, infective endocarditis, HIV infection, non-Hodgkin lymphoma or leukemia, hereditary complement deficiencies, and α_1-antitrypsin deficiency.

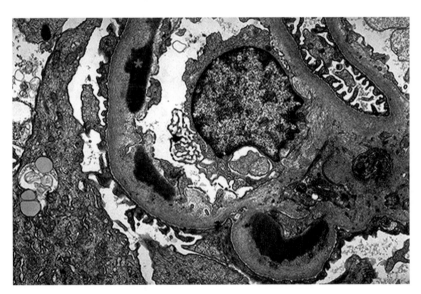

Figure 10-48 Dense deposit disease, electron microscopy

These electron-dense deposits (✱) in the basement membrane are typical of dense deposit disease. The dense deposits within the basement membrane often coalesce to form a ribbon-like mass of deposits. The deposits result from activation of the alternative complement pathway, evidenced by a reduced serum C3 with normal C1 and C4. Patients with dense deposit disease often have circulating C3 nephritogenic factor (C3NeF). The rare condition, called *partial lipodystrophy with C3NeF activity,* may be accompanied by dense deposit disease. The presentation and prognosis are similar to MPGN.

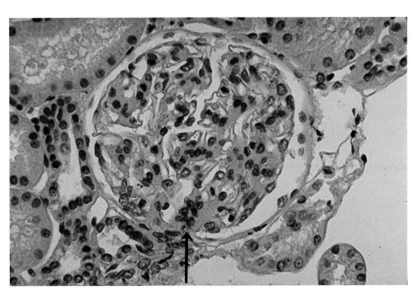

Figure 10-49 IgA nephropathy, microscopic

In IgA nephropathy, there is abnormally glycosylated IgA1. Antiglycan antibodies form and lead to immune complexes deposited within the mesangium of the glomeruli. These complexes attach to fibronectin or type IV collagen in the extracellular matrix and activate mesangial cells to produce extracellular matrix, leading to mesangial hypercellularity (↑), segmental glomerulosclerosis or adhesion, tubular atrophy, and interstitial fibrosis. Some viruses and bacteria express N-acetylgalactosamine on their cell surfaces so that infection may promote antiglycan antibody formation; IgA nephropathy may initially appear in association with an upper respiratory or gastrointestinal infection. IgA nephropathy has now become the most common form of GN.

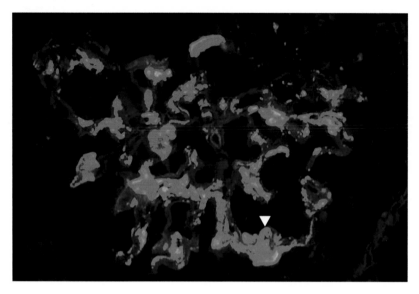

Figure 10-50 IgA nephropathy, immunofluorescence
Note the pattern here of bright green mesangial staining (▼) with antibody to IgA (of the IgA1 subclass); there is often accompanying C3 deposition. This disease most often tends to be mild, but recurrent, and continues with normal renal function for years. One fourth to one half of patients develop CRF within 20 years. Patients with IgA nephropathy who are older tend to have hypertension, or more severe proteinuria, and are more likely to have a worse prognosis, with earlier progression to CRF. Patients rarely present with RPGN. Some cases in children are a manifestation of the systemic illness Henoch-Schönlein purpura. Some cases are associated with celiac disease and some with chronic liver disease from decreased IgA clearance.

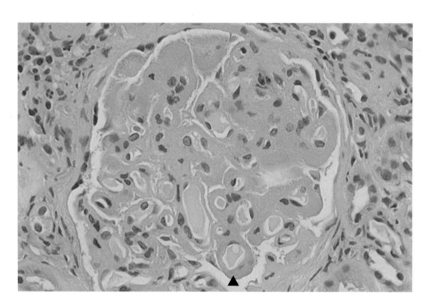

Figure 10-51 Proliferative glomerulonephritis, microscopic
Proliferative GN may involve just a portion of only some glomeruli. This may be idiopathic or the result of an underlying vasculitis, SLE, Goodpasture syndrome, IgA nephropathy, or infection. Glomerular disease with SLE is common, and lupus nephritis can have many morphologic manifestations on renal biopsy. In general, greater immune complex deposition and more cellular proliferation suggest a worse prognosis. In this case there is extensive immune complex deposition in the thickened glomerular capillary loops (▲), giving a wire-loop appearance. A portion of the glomerulus is still intact, however.

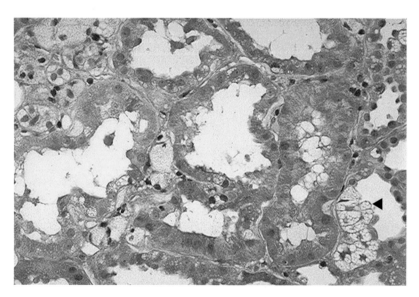

Figure 10-52 Alport syndrome, microscopic
This disease is a form of hereditary nephritis accompanied by nerve deafness and eye problems, such as lens dislocation, cataracts, and corneal dystrophy. Males are more often and more severely affected because of an X-linked dominant inheritance pattern resulting from mutations in the α_2 chain of type IV collagen (COL4A5). Although onset of microscopic hematuria or proteinuria occurs in childhood, renal failure is more likely to occur in adults. The renal tubular cells appear foamy (◄) because of the accumulation of neutral fats and mucopolysaccharides, seen here imparting a pale red appearance with a fat stain. There is thickening and thinning with splitting of the GBM, resulting from defective GBM production in the X-linked form.

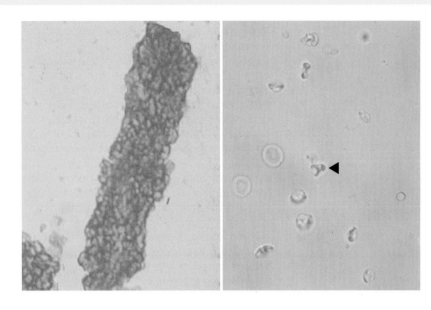

Figure 10-53 Hematuria, urine microscopic

"Nephritic" renal diseases with appearance of RBCs in the urine may have casts on examination of the urine. In contrast, renal diseases that are "nephrotic" are characterized by the presence of protein spilled into the urine. Some renal diseases are both nephritic and nephrotic. The *left panel* shows an RBC cast that formed either in distal convoluted tubules or in collecting ducts. In the *right panel* at high magnification are seen dysmorphic RBCs that are misshapen (◄), suggesting a glomerular disease such as a GN. Dysmorphic RBCs have odd shapes as a result of being distorted by their passage through the abnormal glomerular structure.

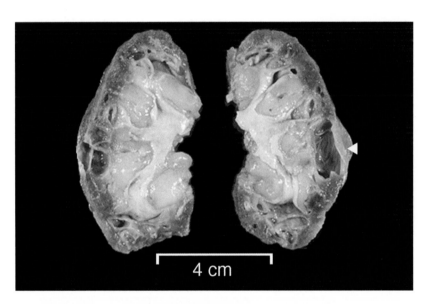

4 cm

Figure 10-54 Chronic glomerulonephritis, gross

Here is the default answer to the question regarding the cause of many cases of CRF: Without a clear history or specific morphologic findings, call it "chronic GN." Seen here are atrophic kidneys with thin cortices from a patient with CRF. About one third to one half of patients with CRF slowly reach end-stage renal disease without significant signs or symptoms along the way, and at the end stage, there are no diagnostic features, so there is no point in performing a renal biopsy. Steadily increasing serum creatinine and urea nitrogen are clues to this progression. Most patients also have hypertension. Some incidental simple cysts (◄) are also seen here.

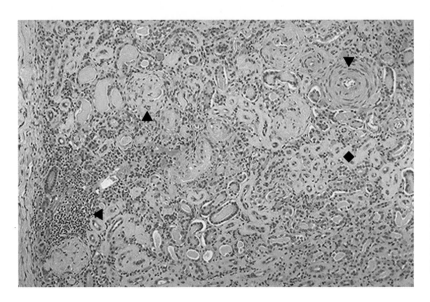

Figure 10-55 End-stage renal disease, microscopic

The microscopic appearance of the end-stage kidney is similar regardless of cause, which is why a biopsy specimen in a patient with CRF may yield little useful information. The cortex is fibrotic (◆), the glomeruli are sclerotic (▲) from hyaline obliteration, there are scattered interstitial chronic inflammatory cell infiltrates (◄), and the arteries (▼) are thickened. Tubules are often dilated and filled with pink casts and give an appearance of "thyroidization." Patients placed on hemodialysis may have extensive deposition of calcium oxalate crystals in tubules and interstitium. Diminished renal clearance of phosphate predisposes to secondary hyperparathyroidism.

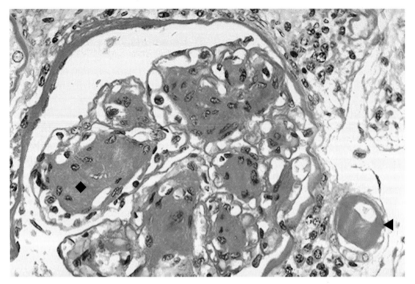

Figure 10-56 Nodular glomerulosclerosis, microscopic

Diabetes mellitus (either type 1 or 2) with nodular glomerulosclerosis (Kimmelstiel-Wilson disease) is characterized by nodules (◆) of pink hyaline material that form in mesangial regions between glomerular capillary loops, made more prominent here with a PAS stain. This glomerulosclerosis is caused by metabolic alterations with hyperglycemia, with a marked increase in mesangial matrix from cellular damage secondary to nonenzymatic glycosylation of proteins. Also note the markedly thickened arteriole (◄) at the lower right, which is typical of hyaline arteriolosclerosis seen in diabetic kidneys. In early stages of this disease, microalbuminuria is present, but it progresses to overt proteinuria that presages renal failure. Hypertension is common.

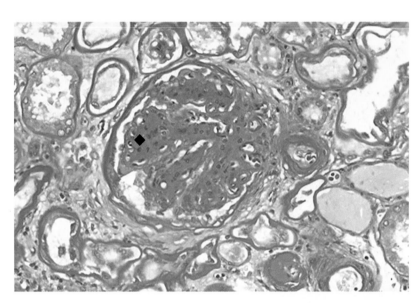

Figure 10-57 Diffuse glomerulosclerosis, microscopic

A PAS stain highlights an increase in mesangial matrix (◆), a slight increase in mesangial cellularity, and capillary basement membrane thickening. Diffuse glomerulosclerosis is associated with long-standing type 1 or 2 diabetes mellitus. These changes gradually advance until the entire glomerulus is sclerotic. Changes of glomerulosclerosis with diabetes mellitus take a decade or longer to develop and gradually worsen. Patients with diabetes mellitus, whether type 1 or 2, are at risk for many renal diseases, including nephrosclerosis, pyelonephritis, and papillary necrosis, in addition to glomerulosclerosis. A major complication of diabetes mellitus is CRF.

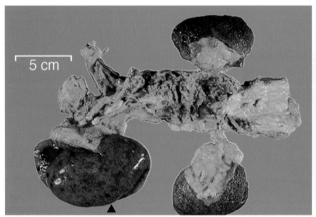
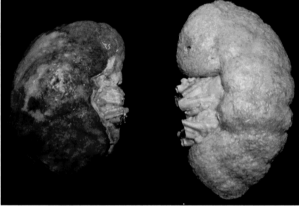

Figure 10-58 Atherosclerosis, gross

Accelerated and advanced atherosclerosis in a patient with diabetes mellitus leads to severe atherosclerosis involving the aorta and its branches, including renal arterial stenosis and nephrosclerosis. The end-stage renal disease seen here with small native kidneys and granular surfaces was treated in the *left panel* with renal transplantation. The transplant kidney is placed in the pelvis because this is technically easier, and there is usually no point in trying to remove the native kidneys, which may still produce erythropoietin. In this case the patient developed chronic rejection, which is why the transplant kidney (▲) is slightly swollen with focal hemorrhages. In the *right panel* the smaller reddish kidney has undergone infarction from renal arterial thrombosis.

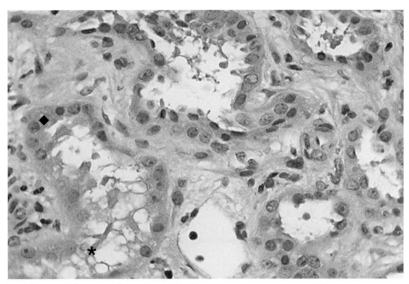

Figure 10-59 Acute tubular injury and necrosis, microscopic
The epithelium of these tubules is ragged (★) from undergoing necrosis with acute tubular necrosis (ATN) from ischemia. In this case, heart failure with hypotension precipitated the ATN. The distribution of necrosis and apoptosis is more segmental with ischemic injuries, as shown here, with some tubules still having intact epithelium (◆), whereas others show considerable damage. Lesser degrees of injury with loss of the brush border and cell swelling are common. This is the most common form of acute tubular injury (ATI), particularly in hospitalized patients, because hypotension from heart failure, sepsis, or disseminated intravascular coagulation is common. ATN is potentially reversible.

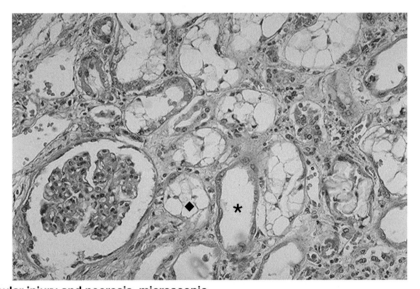

Figure 10-60 Acute tubular injury and necrosis, microscopic
ATN from nephrotoxins is more likely to result in diffuse proximal tubular injury. The tubular vacuolization (◆) and dilation (★) shown here are the result of ethylene glycol poisoning, representative of toxic ATN. The clinical course of ATN is marked by an initiating injury over 1 to 2 days, followed by decreased urine output. The patient can be maintained on dialysis until the recovery phase occurs with polyuria. A nonoliguric form of ATN can be seen in about half of cases of ATN associated with nephrotoxins.

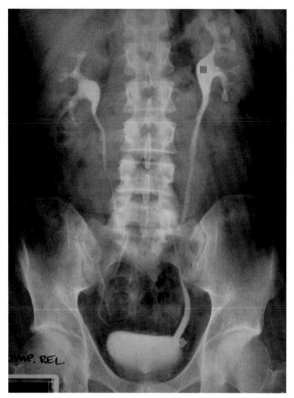

Figure 10-61 Vesicoureteral reflux, radiograph

This intravenous urogram shows dilation of the left ureter, beginning at the left ureteral orifice (♦) and extending to the left renal pelvis (■), which is also dilated along with the calyces. Incompetence of the vesicoureteral valve can predispose to reflux with retrograde flow of urine. In children this is most often caused by congenital shortening of the intravesical portion of the ureter. Decreased bladder contraction from autonomic neuropathy or spinal cord injury can lead to reflux in adults. In either case, there is an increased risk for urinary tract infection, and the inflammation from infection further exacerbates the reflux.

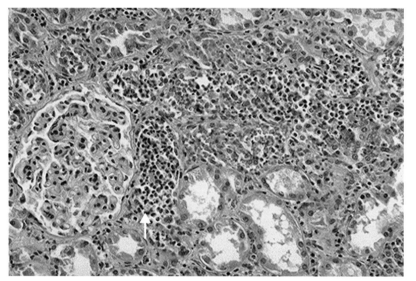

Figure 10-62 Acute pyelonephritis, microscopic

There are various forms of tubulointerstitial nephritis. Shown here are numerous inflammatory cells (↑), mainly neutrophils, filling renal tubules and extending into the interstitium. This case of acute pyelonephritis resulted from an ascending urinary tract infection that started in the bladder. Nearly all such cases are caused by bacterial organisms, including Enterobacteriaceae *(Escherichia, Klebsiella, Proteus, Providencia, Edwardsiella, Enterobacter)* and streptococci and staphylococci. Urinary stasis from congenital anomalies, obstructive uropathy, or decreased bladder emptying may predispose to ascending urinary tract infection.

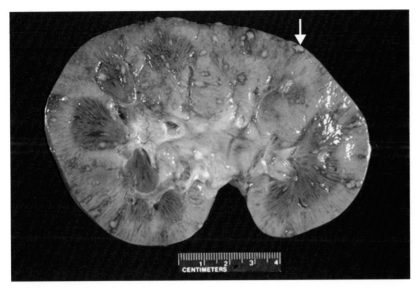

Figure 10-63 Acute pyelonephritis, gross
The cut surface of this swollen kidney reveals many small yellowish microabscesses (↓) involving cortex and medulla. This pattern of acute pyelonephritis is most typical of hematogenous dissemination of infection to the kidney in patients with septicemia. Ascending urinary tract infection leading to acute pyelonephritis is more common than the hematogenous route. Clinical findings of acute pyelonephritis include fever, malaise, and flank pain. Costovertebral angle tenderness may be observed on physical examination. A rare complication not seen here is papillary necrosis, which is more likely to occur in patients with diabetes mellitus or urinary tract obstruction.

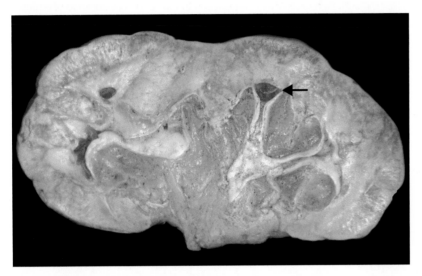

Figure 10-64 Papillary necrosis, gross
These red areas involving some renal papillae (←) are areas of papillary necrosis, a form of focal coagulative necrosis. This is an uncommon but severe complication of acute pyelonephritis, particularly in patients with diabetes mellitus or urinary tract obstruction. Papillary necrosis may also occur with analgesic nephropathy or sickle cell disease. A necrotic, sloughed renal papilla may be recovered from the urine. Acute renal failure may occur.

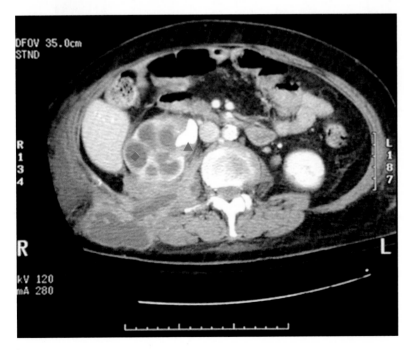

Figure 10-65 Perinephric abscess, CT image
Abdominal CT scan with contrast enhancement shows a staghorn calculus (▲) filling a dilated calyx in this enlarged right kidney, along with marked hydronephrosis (◆) of remaining calyces, as a consequence of chronic urinary tract obstruction. An extensive acute pyelonephritis complicated this process, and the infection became complicated by a perinephric abscess that extended to the right flank region, seen here as irregular areas of decreased attenuation within the skeletal muscle of the posterior flank and back on the right.

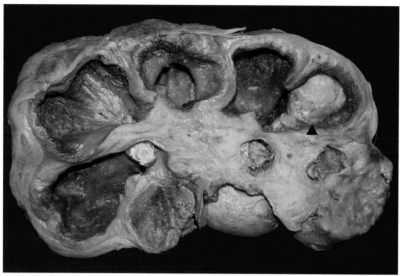

Figure 10-66 Pyonephrosis, gross

Sometimes a very large calculus (▲) nearly fills the calyceal system, with extensions into calyces that give the appearance of a stag's (deer) horns—hence, the name *staghorn calculus*. Appearing here is a hornlike stone extending into a dilated calyx, with nearly unrecognizable pale yellow to tan overlying thinned residual cortex and medulla. This has followed severe inflammation and atrophy from hydronephrosis and pyelonephritis. Nearly complete or total obstruction with extensive inflammation destroys renal parenchyma. Nephrectomy may be done in cases of pyonephrosis because the kidney becomes nonfunctional and serves only as a source of continuing infection.

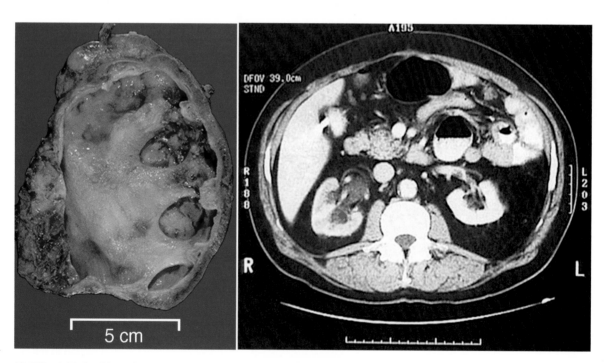

Figures 10-67 and 10-68 Chronic pyelonephritis, gross and CT image

This right kidney has advanced chronic pyelonephritis from reflux and consequent hydronephrosis (◆). There is only a thin rim of remaining renal cortex. If this process is unilateral, the problem originates from a disease involving a location from the ureteral orifice up to the renal pelvis. In this case, an obstructing urinary tract calculus had been present for many years. Vesicoureteral reflux, most often manifesting in childhood, could produce a similar finding. If the obstructive process were bilateral, the underlying disease would originate in the bladder trigone or urethra (or the prostate around the urethra of males) or some process (e.g., a large neoplasm) that could impinge on both ureters or much of the bladder or urethral outlet. Bilateral chronic pyelonephritis is a common cause of end-stage renal disease.

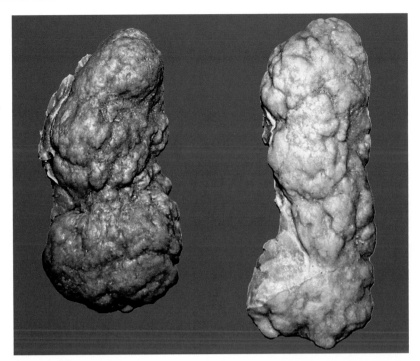

Figure 10-69　Chronic pyelonephritis, gross
The external surfaces of these kidneys show extensive scarring from chronic inflammation with recurrent urinary tract infections. Note the irregular but bilateral involvement. There are coarse, discrete, corticomedullary scars that overlie dilated, blunted, or deformed calyces. The scars vary in number and size. If severe there is loss of concentrating ability with polyuria and urine specific gravity of 1.010.

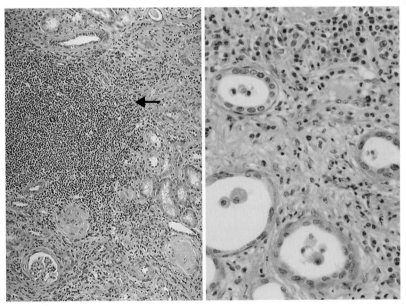

Figure 10-70　Chronic pyelonephritis, microscopic
In the *left panel* at low magnification is a large collection of chronic inflammatory cells (←) in a patient with a long history of multiple recurrent urinary tract infections. Lymphocytes and plasma cells characteristic of chronic pyelonephritis are seen at high magnification *(right panel).* It is common to see interstitial lymphocytes accompany just about any form of chronic renal disease—GN, nephrosclerosis, or pyelonephritis. Plasma cells are most characteristic of chronic pyelonephritis. Over time there is increasing tubular atrophy with prominent proteinaceous casts (so-called thyroidization) and interstitial fibrosis, which eventually affects renal vascular flow, and there is progressive sclerosis of glomeruli leading to CRF.

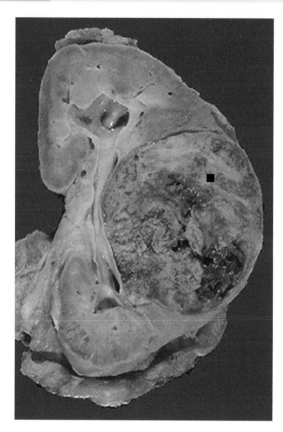

Figure 10-71 Xanthogranulomatous pyelonephritis, gross

Sometimes a long-standing renal infection may be localized and may lead to an uncommon condition termed *xanthogranulomatous pyelonephritis.* Causes include chronic urinary obstruction resulting from a calculus (often a staghorn calculus), stricture, or impinging neoplasm, all conditions that are more frequent in middle-aged adults. The subsequent inflammatory process may form a masslike lesion (■) with circumscribed borders and a gross appearance that is variegated tan to brown to red. It may mimic a renal cell carcinoma grossly and radiographically. Like a malignancy, it may extend into the perinephric fat and adjacent retroperitoneal structures. Fistula formation can occur.

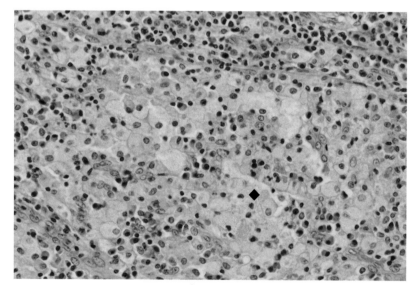

Figure 10-72 Xanthogranulomatous pyelonephritis, microscopic

This inflammatory condition sometimes may be diffuse throughout the kidney, and not localized. In either case, microscopically many pale to foamy macrophages (◆) (xanthoma cells) are present, along with inflammatory round cells from breakdown of renal parenchyma with ongoing inflammation. This inflammatory process can have suppurative and granulomatous features. For obscure reasons, abnormalities in liver function occur in half of affected patients. Urinalysis findings are often absent, although urine culture may yield the typical bacterial organisms found in urinary tract infection.

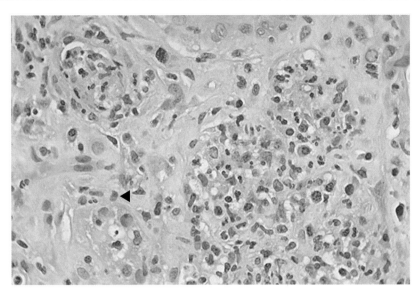

Figure 10-73 Acute interstitial nephritis, microscopic
Cases of tubulointerstitial nephritis may result from drug-induced renal injury. Shown here are scattered eosinophils (◄), along with neutrophils and mononuclear cells in an inflamed interstitium, indicative of acute kidney injury. There may be fever, peripheral blood eosinophilia, a skin rash, oliguria, hematuria, and proteinuria. Half of cases lead to acute renal failure with increasing serum urea nitrogen and creatinine. A type I hypersensitivity reaction is implicated. In more chronic cases, type IV hypersensitivity with granulomas may occur. Antibiotics (methicillin), NSAIDs, and other drugs such as cimetidine acting as a hapten can cause this condition. In one third of cases, the offending agent is unknown.

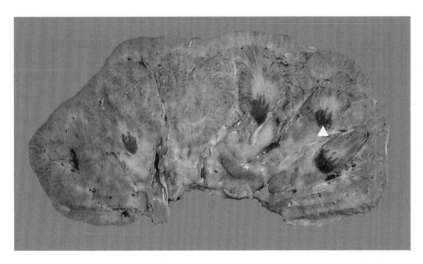

Figure 10-74 Analgesic nephropathy, gross
The excessive use of analgesics containing phenacetin and aspirin over many years can result in papillary necrosis (▲), shown here, followed by tubulointerstitial nephritis. The aspirin inhibits formation of prostaglandin (a vasodilator) to potentiate ischemic injury. Phenacetin is metabolized to acetaminophen, which is nephrotoxic. A urinary tract infection is present in half of cases. Some patients develop transitional cell carcinoma of the renal pelvis. NSAIDs, particularly cyclooxygenase-2 inhibitors, can also produce renal injury from reduced prostaglandin synthesis, leading to acute renal failure or CRF.

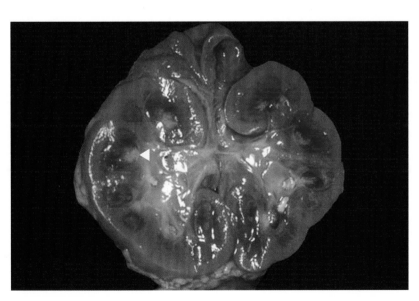

Figure 10-75 Urate nephropathy, gross
Chronic urate deposition has led to pale, yellowish tan tophaceous deposits (◄) in the renal medulla shown. This most often occurs in patients with chronic gout. An acute urate nephropathy can occur with a "lysis" syndrome resulting from massive cellular necrosis of leukemia or lymphoma cells with chemotherapy. The metabolic breakdown of DNA in the many cell nuclei yields large amounts of urate that, when excreted, plugs renal tubules. Precipitation of uric acid is enhanced by an acidic urinary pH. An additional complication of hyperuricemia is nephrolithiasis with uric acid calculi.

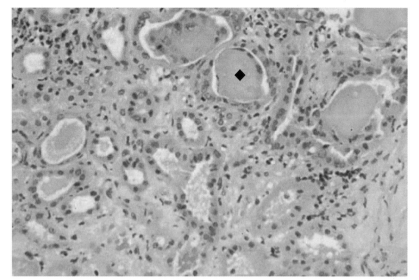

Figure 10-76 Multiple myeloma, microscopic
If there is Bence Jones proteinuria with multiple myeloma, immunoglobulin light chains may precipitate in renal tubules, forming light-chain casts (◆) visible here, which produce cast nephropathy with renal failure. The pale pink casts may act as a foreign body and elicit a multinucleated giant cell reaction around them. Additional renal problems with multiple myeloma include amyloidosis, light-chain glomerulopathy, hypercalcemia with nephrocalcinosis, hyperuricemia with urate nephropathy, and urinary tract infection with pyelonephritis.

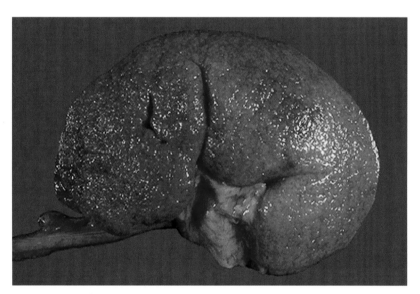

Figure 10-77 Nephrosclerosis, gross
Intrinsic renal vascular disease with sclerosis and progressive luminal narrowing leads to patchy ischemic atrophy with focal loss of parenchyma that gives the kidney surfaces a characteristic granular appearance. The kidneys are usually slightly smaller than normal. The process may be termed benign in most older adults who continue to have normal renal function, as determined by normal serum creatinine and urea nitrogen levels. There may be a mild reduction in the glomerular filtration rate and mild proteinuria. Nephrosclerosis associated with hypertension and diabetes mellitus suggests an increased risk for renal failure.

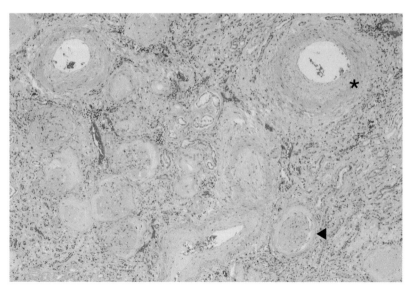

Figure 10-78 Nephrosclerosis, microscopic
The medial thickening of the small arteries (★) leads to progressive luminal narrowing. Nephrosclerosis slowly leads to interstitial fibrosis. Tubular atrophy and cast formation are common. Glomeruli are eventually affected and first undergo collagen deposition within the Bowman space (◄), and periglomerular fibrosis, with eventual total glomerular sclerosis. Nephrosclerosis may lead to mild reduction in glomerular filtration rate and loss of renal reserve capacity. Hyaline arteriolosclerosis with hypertension or diabetes mellitus is also often present.

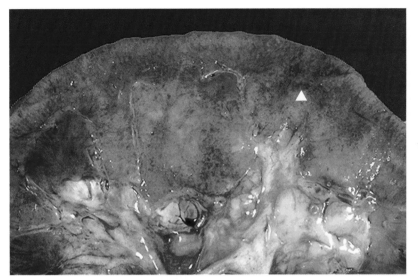

Figure 10-79 Malignant nephrosclerosis, gross

This kidney has many focal small hemorrhages (▲) in cortex and medulla, and the corticomedullary junction is obscured. In this accelerated phase of hypertension blood pressures can become very elevated, with systolic pressures greater than 200 mm Hg and diastolic pressures greater than 120 mm Hg (e.g., 300/150 mm Hg). This condition typically complicates long-standing essential "benign" hypertension, but it may occur de novo. Systemic sclerosis (scleroderma) may be present in some cases. In any case, it is rare. Patients have headache, nausea, vomiting, and visual disturbances. Papilledema may be present. Proteinuria and hematuria are common findings.

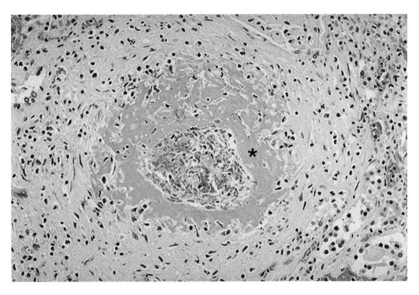

Figure 10-80 Malignant nephrosclerosis, microscopic

Malignant hypertension results from endothelial injury and increased permeability to plasma proteins along with platelet activation, leading to fibrinoid necrosis (★) of small arteries as shown. The damage to this artery is characterized by formation of pink fibrin—hence the term *fibrinoid*. The renin-angiotensin mechanism is stimulated, and very high renin levels develop to produce hypertension. The generation of aldosterone promotes salt retention, which further promotes hypertension. The generation of more renin and angiotensin II leads to further vasoconstriction with ischemic injury.

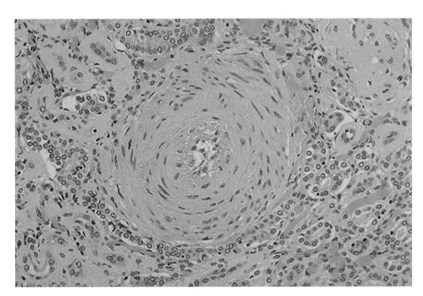

Figure 10-81 Malignant nephrosclerosis, microscopic

Thickening of the arterial wall with malignant hypertension also produces a hyperplastic arteriolitis. The arteriole has an "onion skin" appearance from concentric layering of proliferating smooth muscle along with collagen deposition. This arteriolar lumen is nearly obliterated, promoting ischemic injury. Hematuria and proteinuria are often present. Malignant hypertension is a medical emergency. Patients can develop acute renal failure, heart failure, retinopathy, stroke, and hypertensive encephalopathy. Untreated, half of patients die within 3 months.

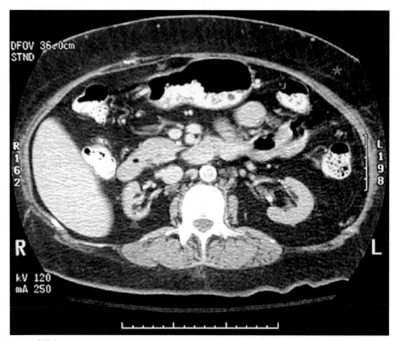

Figure 10-82 Nephrosclerosis, CT image
This patient had a body mass index of 34 (note the large amount of subcutaneous adipose [✱] tissue) accompanied by a long history of poorly controlled diabetes mellitus, with decreasing renal function and increasing blood urea nitrogen and creatinine. This abdominal CT scan with contrast shows decreased size of both kidneys, more pronounced on the right (▲). Nephrosclerosis accounts for most of the changes. Patients with vascular disease, whether from arterial or arteriolar nephrosclerosis, can have a similar fate—continuing loss of renal parenchyma. Most causes of chronic renal disease lead to decreased renal size; exceptions may include polycystic kidney disease, amyloidosis, and glomerulosclerosis.

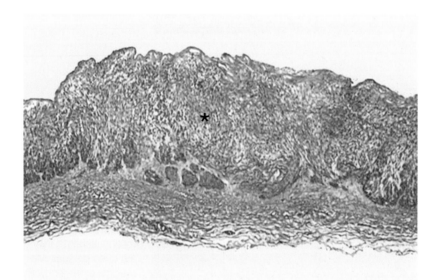

Figure 10-83 Fibromuscular dysplasia, microscopic
An uncommon form of vascular obstruction involving medium-sized muscular arteries is produced by fibromuscular dysplasia. In this condition, there are irregular areas of fibrous thickening (★), mostly involving the media, with an irregular arterial wall and focal, irregular luminal narrowing. This process is seen here with trichrome stain at low magnification in a section through the carotid artery. The renal arteries are most often affected, making this disease one of the surgically correctible causes of hypertension.

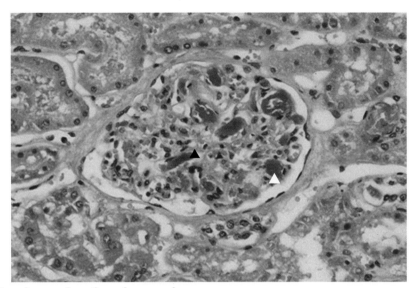

Figure 10-84 Thrombotic microangiopathy, microscopic
Platelet-fibrin thrombi (▲) in glomerular capillaries, shown here with trichrome stain, can occur with thrombotic thrombocytopenic purpura (TTP), which mainly affects the kidneys, heart, and brain with small arteriolar thrombi. Acute renal failure can occur. Difficult to differentiate from TTP is hemolytic-uremic syndrome (HUS), which is a leading cause of acute renal failure in children. Ingestion of certain foods, such as poorly cooked ground beef, introduces a verotoxin-producing *Escherichia coli* infection into the gastrointestinal tract. Such strains are often identified by serotyping, typically type O157:H7. A bloody diarrhea is followed in a few days by renal failure caused by endothelial injury from the toxin, leading to the characteristic fibrin thrombi within glomerular and interstitial capillaries. Most patients recover in a few weeks with supportive dialysis.

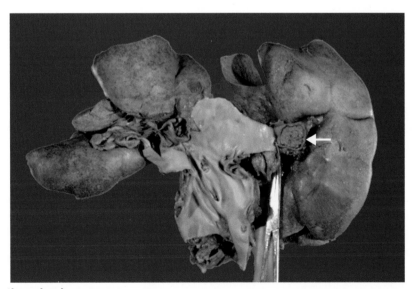

Figure 10-85 Renal vein thrombosis, gross
The (◄) marks the location of a thrombus filling and occluding the left renal vein. The causes of renal vein thrombosis include trauma, coagulopathies, compression by neoplasms, fluid volume loss, renal vein invasion by renal cell carcinoma, and nephrotic syndrome with membranous nephropathy. Renal vein thrombosis is often associated with proteinuria, which may reach the nephrotic range. This condition may occur acutely with flank pain, nausea, vomiting, and hematuria. More commonly, it develops chronically and has few signs or symptoms other than proteinuria leading to edema.

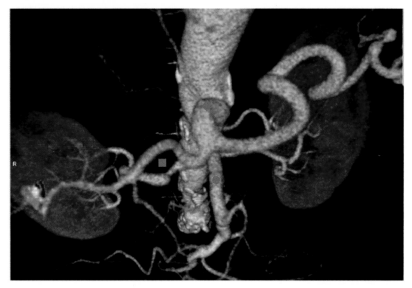

Figure 10-86 Renal artery stenosis, CT angiogram

There is a focal narrowing (■) of the right renal artery consistent with renal artery stenosis. Such focal lesions are typical for more advanced atherosclerosis with occlusive atheroma formation. Atherosclerosis often involves large to medium-sized arteries, particularly the aorta and its major branches. An occlusive lesion reduces renal blood flow to the affected kidney, increasing plasma renin activity to produce hypertension. Long-standing, untreated hypertension damages both kidneys further. Such a focal lesion is a potentially surgically correctable cause of hypertension. The celiac trunk (♦) and the superior mesenteric artery (●) and branches from the aorta are also shown here.

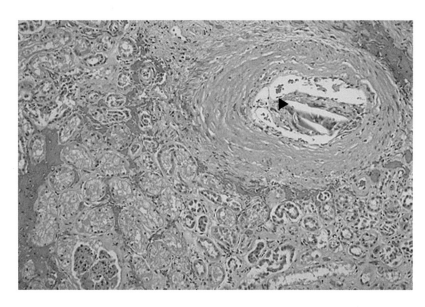

Figure 10-87 Atheroembolic renal disease, microscopic

Despite the frequency of aortic atherosclerosis, complications from cholesterol emboli are rare, or at least many such emboli are small and insignificant most of the time. Shown here in a renal artery branch are cholesterol clefts (▶) characteristic of such an embolus filling the lumen. This patient had severe ulcerative, friable aortic atheromatous plaques and had undergone angiography, which increases the risk for such emboli. Large numbers of these emboli can produce focal ischemia and compromise renal function. Multiple atheroemboli are most likely to be a cause of renal failure in patients with preexisting renal disease.

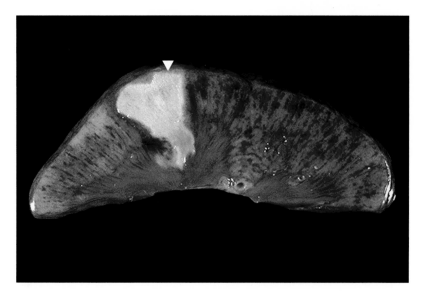

Figure 10-88 Renal infarct, gross

Note the wedge shape of this acute infarct (▼), with the pale zone of coagulative necrosis resulting from loss of blood supply with resultant tissue ischemia that progresses to infarction. The small amount of blood from the capsular arteries supplies the immediate subcortical zone, which is spared. The remaining cortex is congested, as is the medulla. Renal infarcts most often occur with emboli that originate from cardiac diseases, such as endocarditis, rheumatic mitral stenosis with left atrial dilation and mural thrombosis, or ischemic heart disease with ventriculomegaly and mural thrombosis. Patients may be asymptomatic or may have costovertebral angle tenderness and hematuria.

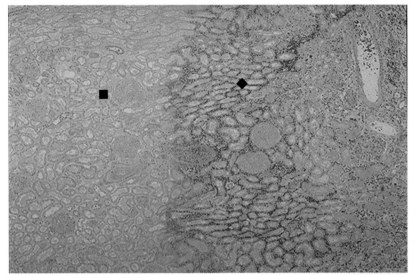

Figure 10-89 Renal infarct, microscopic
On the right is normal kidney; to the left of that, hyperemic parenchyma (◆) is becoming necrotic (■); to the far left is pale pink infarcted kidney, in which tubules and glomeruli have undergone coagulative necrosis, leaving just the cellular outlines of tubules and glomeruli. Renal infarction is most likely a consequence of embolization, although arterial or arteriolar vasculitis may also lead to focal smaller areas of infarction. The renal parenchyma is at increased risk for ischemic injury because there is no collateral blood flow. Infarcts may cause pain and hematuria, but less likely renal failure as a result of their focality.

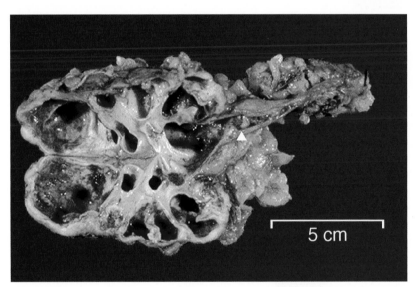

Figure 10-90 Obstructive uropathy, gross
Obstruction to the flow of urine in the urinary tract can occur anywhere from the urethral meatus to the kidney calyces. This kidney has been opened coronally to reveal hydronephrosis, and the cause is a calculus (▲) at the ureteropelvic junction. This kidney shows a marked degree of hydronephrosis with nearly complete loss of cortex. Causes for obstruction may include congenital anomalies such as urethral atresia, neoplasms such as urothelial carcinoma, nodular prostatic hyperplasia, urinary tract calculi, external compression (pregnant uterus), or neurogenic problems such as diabetic neuropathy or spinal cord injury.

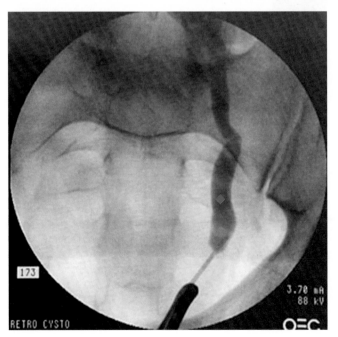

Figure 10-91 Obstructive uropathy, radiograph
Injection of contrast material into the ureter above the bladder reveals marked ureteral dilation (◆) consistent with hydroureter from obstruction at the vesicoureteral junction. Most cases of hydronephrosis are clinically silent, although acute obstruction (as with passage of calculi) may elicit pain poorly localized to the affected portion of the urinary tract. Initially, urine concentrating ability is lost, followed by reduction in glomerular filtration rate and renal failure.

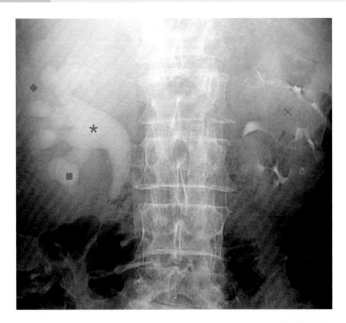

Figure 10-92 Chronic reflux nephropathy, radiograph
The right kidney is decreased in size and shows cortical thinning (◆) with blunted calyces (■) indicative of chronic reflux nephropathy that has led to dilation of the collecting system (✱) and overall atrophy. There is compensatory hyperplasia of the unaffected left kidney (✕) as seen in this intravenous pyelogram. Lesser degrees of hydronephrosis may preserve sufficient cortex to maintain renal function, but there is increased risk for infection.

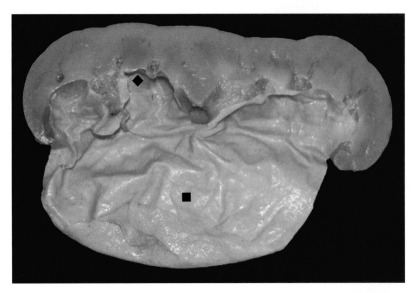

Figure 10-93 Hydronephrosis, gross
This section of kidney shows a marked degree of hydronephrosis. Note the markedly dilated pelvis (■) and calyces (◆). The cortex is present but reduced in thickness. If this process is unilateral (the point of obstruction is at one ureteral orifice or above), then the opposite kidney can compensate and provide sufficient renal function. This adult kidney is most likely hydronephrotic from an acquired condition such as a calculus, neoplasm, or (in men) prostatic hyperplasia.

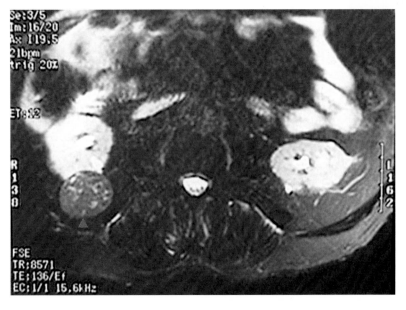

Figure 10-94 Renal angiomyolipoma, MRI
This abdominal MRI image in axial view shows a rounded, discrete angiomyolipoma (▲) eccentrically positioned in the lower pole of the right kidney, which has bright enhancement. The darker areas of the mass represent the "lipoma" component, whereas the brighter areas in this neoplasm correspond to vascular tissue (the "angio" component) similar in attenuation to the adjacent normal renal parenchyma with the contrast enhancement. Angiomyolipomas can be multiple and bilateral (often with tuberous sclerosis) or solitary.

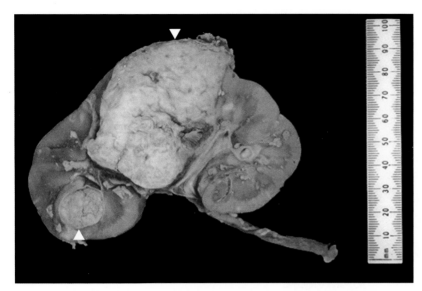

Figure 10-95 Angiomyolipoma, gross
Angiomyolipoma is a rare neoplasm of the kidney. It is solid and has a cut surface (▼) that is tan to yellowish tan. It is also multifocal (a smaller nodule (▲) appears in the upper pole) as shown here. Most of these tumors are incidental findings, but about 25% to 50% of affected persons have a rare condition known as *tuberous sclerosis,* an autosomal dominant condition in which mutations of either the *TSC2* or *TSC1* gene lead to formation of hamartomas in brain and other tissues. Other neoplasms include cutaneous angiofibromas and cardiac rhabdomyomas. Otherwise, angiomyolipoma is an uncommon sporadic renal neoplasm.

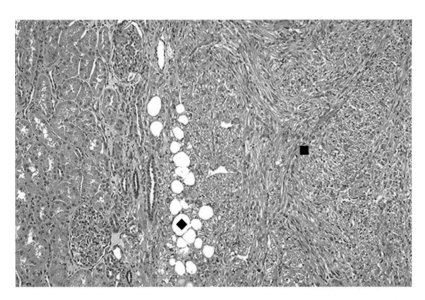

Figure 10-96 Renal angiomyolipoma, microscopic
Normal renal cortical parenchyma with tubules is present at the left. The tumor has a strip of adipocytes (◆), the "lipoma" part, that blends with interlacing bundles of smooth muscle (■), the "myo" component, in which are scattered vascular spaces (the "angio" component). These tumor components closely mimic their non-neoplastic cell counterparts, typical of a well-differentiated benign neoplastic process.

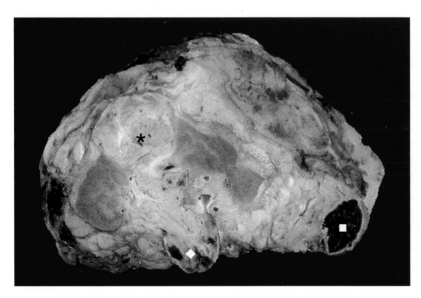

Figure 10-97 Renal cell carcinoma, gross
These carcinomas have a tendency to invade into the renal vein (◆), as shown in the cut surface of a resected kidney surrounded by adipose tissue bounded by Gerota fascia. Tumor may even crawl up the vena cava and into the right side of the heart, but even these invasive lesions can be removed surgically. Here, the tumor (★) extended up the vena cava and occluded the adrenal vein, leading to hemorrhagic adrenal infarction (■). These tumors may also invade through the renal capsule. Renal cell carcinomas are known for unusual behaviors, such as metastases to odd locations, metastases to other neoplasms, regression of the primary site with removal of metastases, and occasional good prognosis after removal of metastases. About one fourth of them first manifest as metastatic lesions.

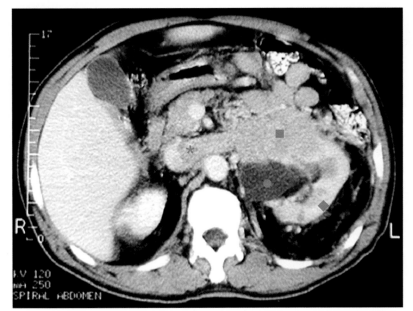

Figure 10-98 Renal vein invasion, CT image

Renal cell carcinomas have a tendency to invade into the renal vein. A renal cell carcinoma (■) arising in the left kidney is shown here. There is remaining renal parenchyma (♦) and hydronephrosis (●). The carcinoma is invading (✳) into the left renal vein, distending the vein, and extending into the inferior vena cava. These lesions may crawl up the vena cava and into the heart, but even then they can often be successfully removed. The most important risk factor is tobacco use. Other risks include obesity, unopposed estrogen therapy, and hypertension. Many cases occur sporadically without an identifiable risk factor. About 4% of cases are familial, occurring with such conditions as von Hippel–Lindau (VHL) disease. Nearly all sporadic renal clear cell carcinomas have a deletion of the *VHL* tumor suppressor gene.

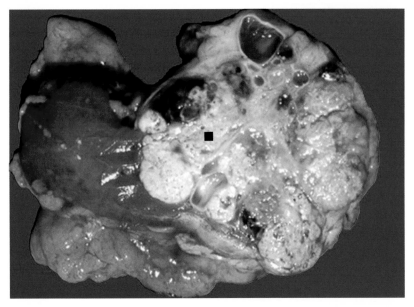

Figure 10-99 Renal cell carcinoma, gross

This malignancy (■) is arising in the lower pole of the kidney. It is large but still fairly circumscribed, typical for the localized growth pattern for years while the neoplasm remains clinically silent. This cut surface has a variegated appearance with white, yellowish, brown, and hemorrhagic red and cystic areas. Early signs and symptoms may not be present because the neoplasm has room to grow in the retroperitoneum, but flank pain, a palpable mass, and hematuria are the most common clinical findings. Some patients have ongoing constitutional symptoms such as fever. Renal cell carcinomas are uncommon in patients younger than 40 years.

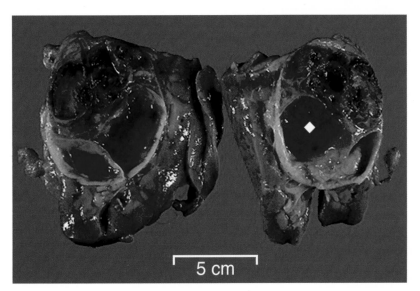

Figure 10-100 Renal cell carcinoma, gross

This renal cell carcinoma on sectioning is mainly cystic with extensive hemorrhage (♦). Large simple renal cysts may develop extensive organizing hemorrhage and mimic this appearance but have a smooth, regular border. Renal cell carcinomas may also develop in acquired cystic disease with hemodialysis. Renal cell carcinomas can often be associated with various paraneoplastic syndromes, including polycythemia from elaboration of erythropoietin; hypercalcemia with tumor production of parathormone-related peptide; and steroid hormone release with Cushing syndrome, feminization, or masculinization.

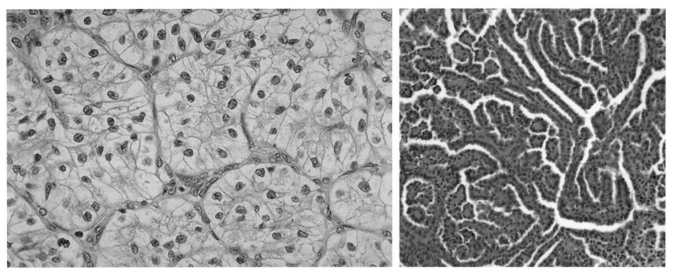

Figures 10-101 and 10-102 Renal cell carcinoma, microscopic

In the *left panel* the neoplastic cells have abundant clear cytoplasm and are arranged in nests with intervening delicate vessels. About three fourths of renal cell carcinomas have this clear cell pattern. Some have a papillary pattern as shown in the *right panel,* with *MET* proto-oncogene mutations and autosomal dominant inheritance. A rare chromophobe variant has cells with abundant pink cytoplasm resembling the benign renal neoplasm known as *oncocytoma.*

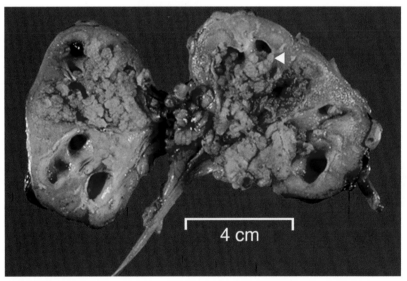

Figure 10-103 Urothelial carcinoma, gross

This sagittally sectioned kidney has a multifocal neoplasm arising in the urothelium of the calyceal system and invading into the renal parenchyma. This neoplasm (◄) of urothelial origin accounts for about 5% to 10% of renal cancers in adults. Other neoplastic foci may be present in other sites with urothelium, such as ureters and bladder. Hematuria is a frequent presenting symptom, and the onset of hematuria occurs earlier in the course of this tumor than with renal cell carcinoma. Most urothelial carcinomas are still discovered at a high stage, however. Similar to renal cell carcinoma, the major risk factor is smoking.

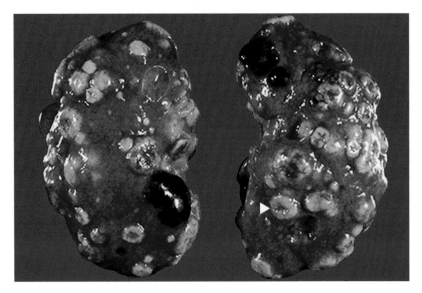

Figure 10-104 Renal metastases, gross

These multiple irregular bilateral masses (▶), many of which show central indentations, or "umbilications" from central necrosis, represent metastases of a carcinoma to the kidneys. Some of these metastases have become dark from hemorrhage. The kidneys are not a usual site for metastases, but they can be involved when there are widespread metastases from a primary neoplasm, typically a carcinoma, such as a lung, gastrointestinal tract, or breast primary. The focal nature of the metastases means that there is sufficient residual renal parenchyma to prevent renal failure. Clinical findings of hematuria and flank pain may occur with larger masses.

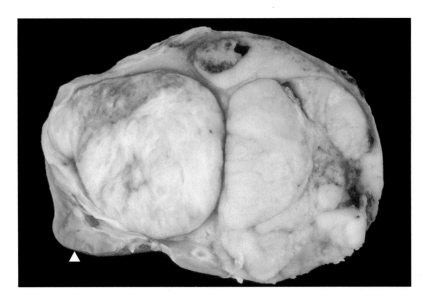

Figure 10-105 Wilms tumor, gross

This large mass with a lobulated cut surface fills and expands the kidney of a child, with a rim of residual cortex (▲) visible at the lower left. The median age at diagnosis is 3 years. The clinical presentation includes abdominal enlargement and pain from mass effect, hematuria, and hypertension secondary to increased renin activity in 25% of cases. Sixty percent of bilateral and 4% of unilateral Wilms tumors are associated with congenital malformations and differing mutations of the *WT1* gene, including WAGR syndrome (*W*ilms tumor, *a*niridia, *g*enital anomalies, *r*etardation), Beckwith-Wiedemann syndrome (macroglossia, organomegaly, hemihypertrophy, neonatal hypoglycemia, embryonal tumors), and Denys-Drash syndrome (intersex disorders, nephropathy).

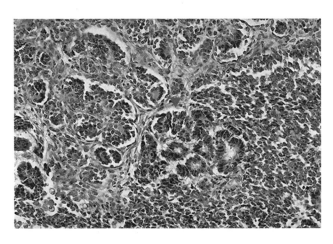

Figure 10-106 Wilms tumor, microscopic

Wilms tumor microscopically resembles the primitive nephrogenic zone of the developing fetal kidney, with primitive glomeruloid structures (▼) and a cellular stroma. Wilms tumor is associated with tumor suppressor genes: *WT1* is located at chromosome 11p13 and encodes a transcription factor crucial to development of normal kidneys and gonads. This neoplasm is treatable with an excellent prognosis and greater than 90% cure rate overall.

The Lower Urinary Tract

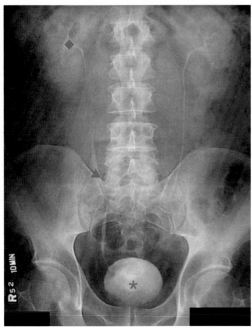

Figure 11-1 Urinary tract, radiograph
This intravenous pyelogram shows a normal urinary tract, with contrast material filling the renal pelves (◆), then the ureters (▲), and finally the bladder (✷).

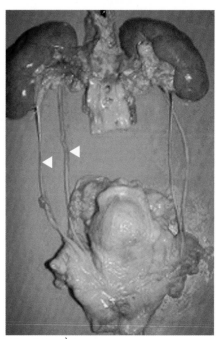

Figure 11-2 Double ureters, gross
Complete ureteral duplication is shown, with two ureters (◄) exiting from each kidney and extending to the bladder, opened anteriorly. A segment of aorta lies between the normal kidneys. A partial or complete duplication of one or both ureters occurs in 1 in 150 people. There is a potential for urinary obstruction because of abnormal flow of urine and the entrance of two ureters into the bladder in close proximity, but most of the time this condition is an incidental finding.

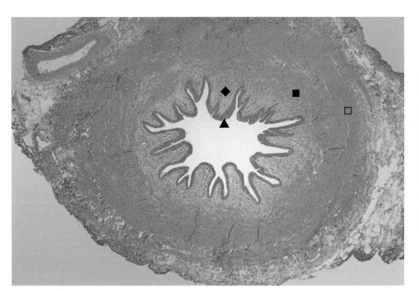

Figure 11-3 Normal ureter, microscopic
This normal ureter in cross-section is shown at low magnification, with an inner longitudinal layer (■) and an outer circular layer (□) of smooth muscle (the opposite of the bowel) to supply peristaltic movement of urine down to the bladder from the renal pelvis. There is a urothelium (▲) and underlying lamina propria (◆). Ordinarily the lumen remains nearly closed because ureters do not store urine. Prolonged stasis of fluids predisposes to infection in the urinary tract.

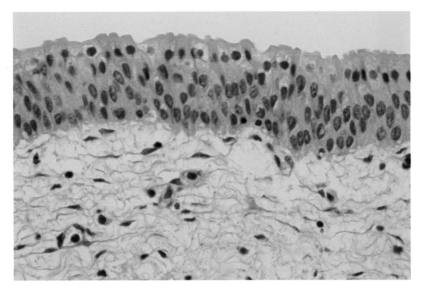

Figure 11-4 Normal urothelium, microscopic
This normal urothelium with an underlying base-ment membrane is stratified and no more than 5 to 7 cell layers thick, and 2 to 3 cells thick in a distended bladder. The topmost superficial layer is composed of plump ("umbrella") cells that have microplicae on the luminal border, have tight junc-tions between them, and can stretch laterally as the urine passes or collects within the lumen. The bladder urothelium produces a mucoid se-cretion with natural antibacterial properties. This feature, along with normal complete emptying of the bladder, helps to prevent urinary tract infec-tions. The underlying lamina propria has connec-tive tissue with scattered small vessels.

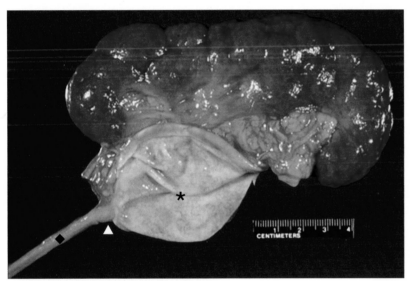

Figure 11-5 Ureteropelvic junction stenosis, gross
There is irregular scarring over the cortical surface of this kidney as a consequence of chronic obstruction and development of acute and chronic pyelonephritis. The renal pelvis (★) is markedly dilated, but the ureter (◆) is not, indicating that the point of obstruction is at the ureteropelvic junction (▲). This condition usually manifests in childhood and most often affects boys. This is the most common cause of hydronephrosis in infants and children.

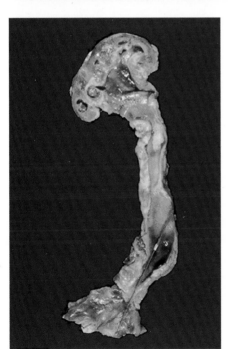

Figure 11-6 Hydroureter, gross
A long-standing obstruction (congenital) at the ureteral orifice through which the metal probe passes led to the marked hydroureter and hydronephrosis shown here. This patient had recurrent urinary tract infections complicated by pyelonephritis.

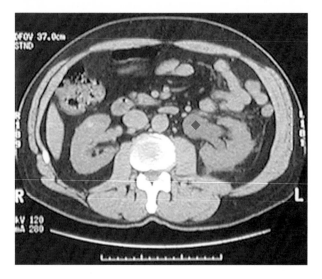

Figure 11-7 Hydroureter, CT image
The left ureter (♦), near the left renal pelvis in this abdominal CT scan, exhibits hydroureter as a consequence of obstruction from the presence of urinary tract calculi.

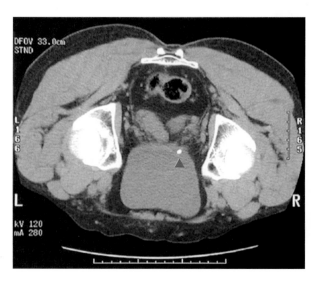

Figure 11-8 Ureteral calculus, CT image
This CT scan was taken with the patient in the prone position (the reverse of the usual CT imaging position with the patient supine) and reveals a bright ureteral calculus (▲) at the vesicoureteral junction. Because most urinary tract calculi contain calcium (calcium oxalate or calcium phosphate), they appear bright with radiographic imaging. Radiolucent stones are likely to be composed of uric acid, and cystine stones are rare. However, even radiolucent material can serve as a nidus for deposition of calcium that imparts brightness with x-rays.

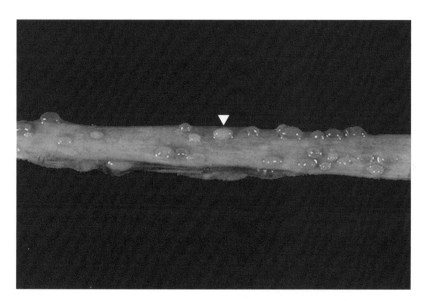

Figure 11-9 Ureteritis cystica, gross
The small, smooth, glistening bumps (▼) shown here over the ureteral mucosa are termed *ureteritis cystica* and represent cystic areas of glandular metaplasia resulting from inflammation, producing cystic nodules 1 to 5 mm in size. They are more commonly seen in the bladder, where they are called *cystitis cystica*.

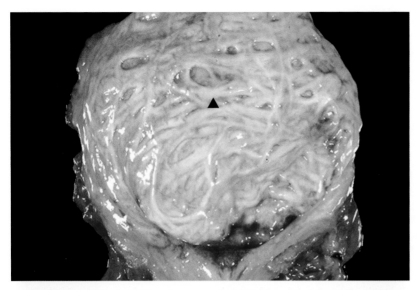

Figure 11-10 Urinary bladder, gross

This urinary bladder is opened anteriorly at autopsy and has a normal shape and size, but there is prominent trabeculation (▲) over the mucosal surface. This is the consequence of bladder muscular hypertrophy from bladder outlet obstruction with nodular prostatic hyperplasia. The outpouchings of mucosa between the muscular trabeculations are pseudodiverticula, which do not have a complete muscular layer. The stasis from obstruction also predisposes to urinary tract infections because there is incomplete emptying of the bladder with residual urine. The urethral obstruction can also lead eventually to bilateral hydroureter and hydronephrosis.

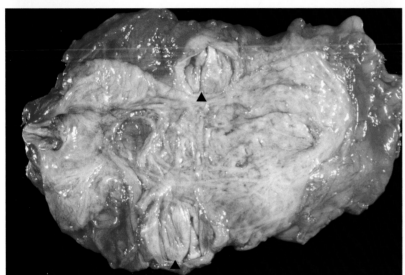

Figure 11-11 Urinary bladder diverticulum, gross

There are two diverticula (▲) in this urinary bladder, opened anteriorly at autopsy. The urethral outlet is on the left, and the dome of the bladder is on the right. A diverticulum is a saccular outpouching. Such a lesion of the bladder may be congenital and a true diverticulum with a complete muscular layer, as shown here, or it may be acquired with obstruction. A diverticulum represents a region prone to stasis and incomplete emptying that increases the risk for urinary tract infections.

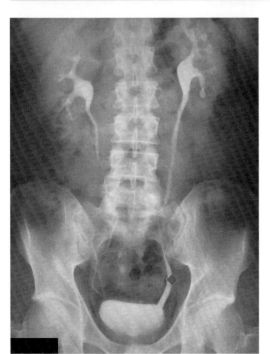

Figure 11-12 Vesicoureteral reflux, radiograph

Incompetence of the vesicoureteral valve allows urine to reflux into the ureter, and this predisposes to urinary tract infection, particularly pyelonephritis, from incomplete voiding with residual urine. This intravenous urogram shows dilation of the right ureter (◆) compared with the normal left ureter in a patient with long-standing vesicoureteral reflux. This condition may be congenital from absence or shortening of the intravesical portion of the ureter, and seen in children, or it may be acquired in adults from loss of bladder innervation after spinal cord injury.

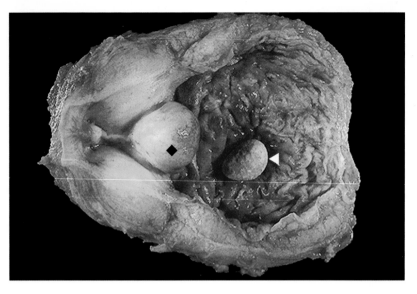

Figure 11-13 Bladder outlet obstruction, gross

The markedly enlarged prostate on the left not only has large lateral lobes, but also has a very large median lobe (◆) that obstructed the prostatic urethra and led to chronic urinary tract obstruction. As a result, the bladder became enlarged and hypertrophied because it had to work against the obstruction with every episode of urination. That is why the surface of the bladder appears trabeculated. Note also the presence of another cause of obstruction—a yellowish brown calculus (◄). Obstruction increases the risk for urinary tract infection. Hydroureter and hydronephrosis may occur as well.

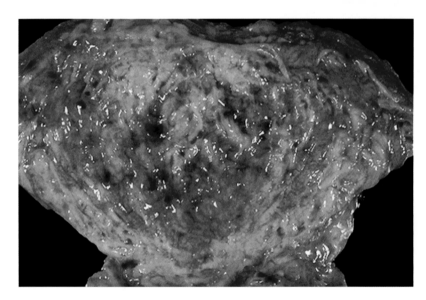

Figure 11-14 Cystitis, gross

This bladder has been opened anteriorly to reveal extensive mucosal hyperemia with an acute cystitis. This is most likely to result from bacterial infection. The most likely organism is *Escherichia coli*, but *Proteus* and *Klebsiella* species, *Staphylococcus saprophyticus*, enterococci, and group B streptococci may also be implicated. With complicated urinary tract infections (infections that are nosocomial or are present with underlying abnormalities, such as obstructions, urinary stones, or indwelling catheters), the range of likely causative agents is wider and includes *Pseudomonas aeruginosa*, *Klebsiella* species (including *Klebsiella pneumoniae*), *Serratia* species, *E. coli*, and other members of the Enterobacteriaceae family.

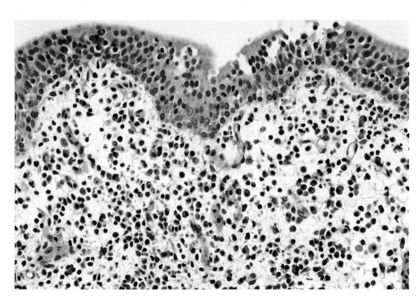

Figure 11-15 Cystitis, microscopic

Increased numbers of inflammatory cells can be seen within the submucosa. Urinary tract infections tend to be recurrent, and so episodes of acute cystitis become chronic cystitis with acute and chronic inflammatory components along with fibrous thickening of the muscularis. The typical clinical findings include increased urinary frequency, suprapubic pain, and dysuria marked by burning or pain on urination. More extensive cases may be marked by fever and malaise. Urinary tract infections are common, particularly in women, in whom the urethra is shorter than in men. Urinary tract obstruction increases the risk for infection.

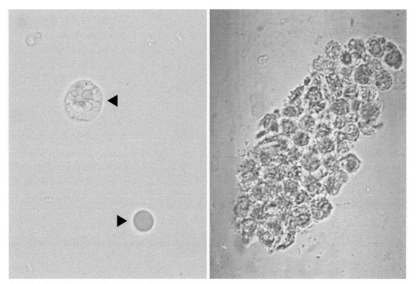

Figure 11-16 White blood cells in urine, microscopic

Inflammation of the urinary tract is often accompanied by the presence of leukocytes, typically neutrophils, and usually from urinary tract infection. Most urinary tract infections are caused by bacterial organisms. In addition to infection, calculi, neoplasms, glomerulonephritis, and trauma may produce inflammation. In the *left panel* is a white blood cell (◄), along with a red blood cell (►) for comparison of size and morphology. A white blood cell cast is shown in the *right panel*. Urinary casts must come from distal tubules or collecting, whereas individual neutrophils may originate with acute inflammation anywhere within the urinary tract. Casts must be caused by renal diseases, such as glomerulonephritis or interstitial nephritis. The "cement" that holds elements of a cast together includes Tamm-Horsfall protein, normally secreted in small quantities from tubular cells. Urine dipstick analysis with positive leukocyte esterase suggests that white blood cells are present even if not intact and recognized on microscopic examination. Urine culture with antibiotic sensitivity testing helps with selection of appropriate antibiotic therapy.

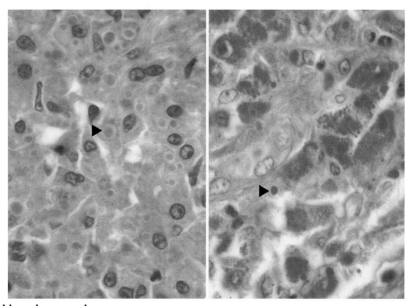

Figure 11-17 Malacoplakia, microscopic

Note the rounded Michaelis-Gutmann bodies (►), which are calcium-containing concretions, within macrophages, shown with H&E stain in the *left panel* and with PAS stain in the *right panel*. Malacoplakia produces grossly visible mucosal plaques on cystoscopy, which must be distinguished from carcinoma on biopsy. Malacoplakia is a peculiar inflammatory response to chronic infection, usually with *Escherichia coli* or *Proteus* species. The increased numbers of macrophages suggest phagocytic defects with accumulation of bacterial products.

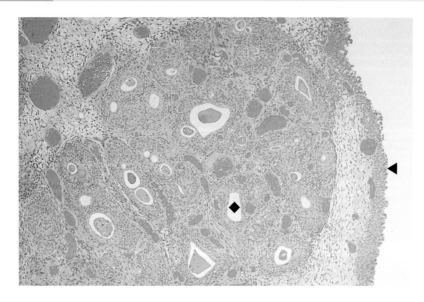

Figure 11-18 Cystitis cystica et glandularis, microscopic

There is a collection of cystically dilated, epithelial-lined glandular spaces (◆) below the surface epithelium (◄) of the bladder at the right. The lesion is formed from Brunn nests of urothelium extending downward into the lamina propria. These nests undergo epithelial transformation into cuboidal or columnar epithelium (*cystitis glandularis*) or cystic spaces lined by flattened urothelium *(cystitis cystica)*. Because the two processes often coexist, the condition is called *cystitis cystica et glandularis.* This is a common incidental finding in adults, and because the cysts can range from 0.1 to 1 cm in size, they form a nodule that is resected for biopsy during cystoscopy when carcinoma is suspected; however, they do not carry a risk for malignancy.

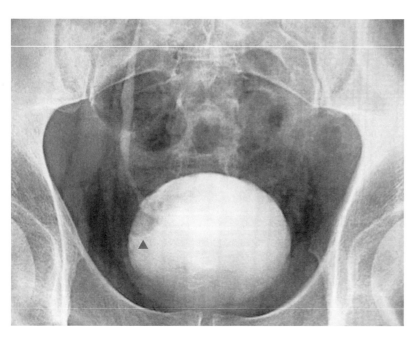

Figure 11-19 Urothelial carcinoma, gross

This opened bladder reveals a large bulky mass (◄). This neoplasm can arise anywhere in the urothelium but is most common in the urinary bladder. Urothelial carcinoma is often multifocal and has a tendency to recur. This bladder was removed surgically from a man with hematuria who had a history of cigarette smoking. In addition to smoking, risk factors include exposure to arylamine compounds (such as 2-naphthylamine), chronic infection with *Schistosoma haematobium,* analgesic abuse, extensive exposure to cyclophosphamide, and prior radiation therapy.

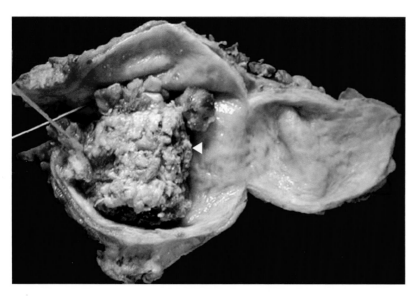

Figure 11-20 Urothelial carcinoma, radiograph

This intravenous pyelogram shows a neoplasm (▲) near the right ureteral orifice that produces a filling defect in the urinary bladder. Urothelial carcinoma occurs when there are genetic alterations of tumor suppressor genes, typically 9p deletions (9p21) involving the tumor suppressor gene *p16/INK4a,* which encodes an inhibitor of a cyclin-dependent kinase, which are seen in papillary tumors. Other mutations involve the *p53* gene, most often with carcinoma in situ (CIS), and *RB* gene, particularly when invasive lesions are present. When a urothelial carcinoma has been treated, the patient must be followed with periodic cytologic examination of urine for atypical cells and subsequent cystoscopic examination because of the risk for subsequent multifocal development of additional urothelial carcinomas.

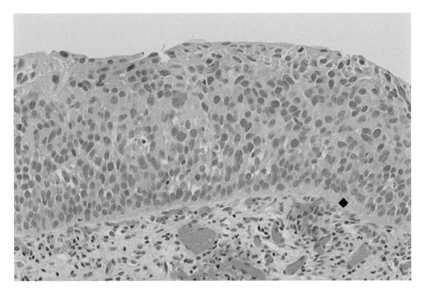

Figure 11-21 Urothelial carcinoma, microscopic

A urothelial CIS is shown. The atypical cells form a disorganized epithelial layer that occupies the full thickness of the urothelium but does not invade through the basement membrane (◆). For the urothelium, *any* malignant cells above the basement membrane qualify as CIS. CIS is often asymptomatic. On cystoscopic examination it may appear only as a flat area of erythema or granularity. It is often multifocal.

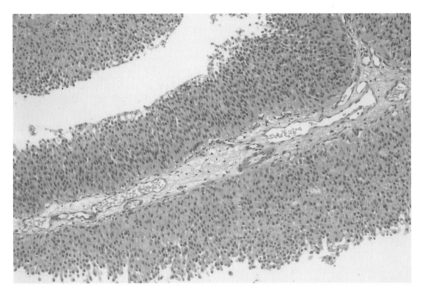

Figure 11-22 Urothelial carcinoma, microscopic

Note the finger-like projection of this papillary frond with a fibrovascular core covered by a very thick, disorganized layer of neoplastic transitional cells having marked atypia. Urothelial carcinomas arising from papillary lesions tend to be exophytic and noninvasive. CIS gives rise to a flat urothelial carcinoma more prone to invasion. The grade and stage determine prognosis. Invasion into the muscularis means that control of the tumor is unlikely to be achieved with local excision alone, and a cystectomy is done.

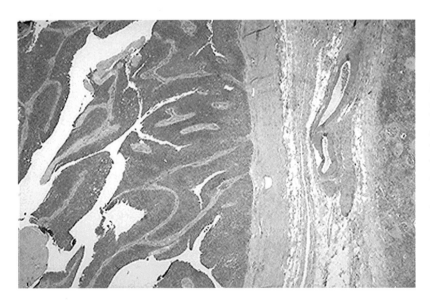

Figure 11-23 Urothelial carcinoma, microscopic

The urothelial carcinoma of the urinary bladder shown here at low magnification reveals the frondlike papillary projections of the tumor above the surface extending to the left. It is differentiated enough to resemble urothelium but is still irregular, with hyperchromatic cells, and is best described as grade 2 (on a scale of 1 to 3). No invasion to the right is seen at this point.

The Male Genital Tract

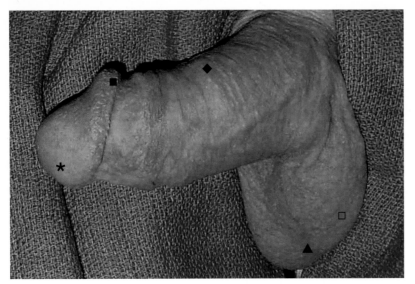

Figure 12-1 Normal external genitalia, gross
The normal appearance of the external male genitalia is shown here. Note the glans (★) and prepuce (■) (mucosal surfaces), but no foreskin in this circumcised penis. The shaft (◆) of the penis is covered by stratified squamous epithelium, as is the scrotum (□), with median (▲) raphe. The erectile tissue beneath the skin is comprised of two corpora cavernosa and one corpus spongiosum, through which the penile urethra passes.

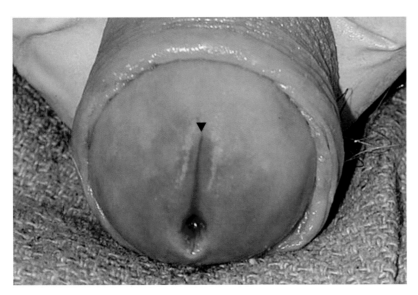

Figure 12-2 Epispadias, gross
This groove (▼) on the dorsal aspect of the penis extending for a short distance upward from the urethral meatus is an abnormality termed *epispadias*. This is an uncommon anomaly of variable severity. The example shown here is not severe. When severe and extensive along the dorsum of the penis, epispadias can lead to problems with urination and ejaculation. The opening may be partially constricted, predisposing to urinary tract infections. The foreskin of this uncircumcised penis is retracted here. This anomaly may be associated with other urinary tract anomalies and may be present along with cryptorchidism.

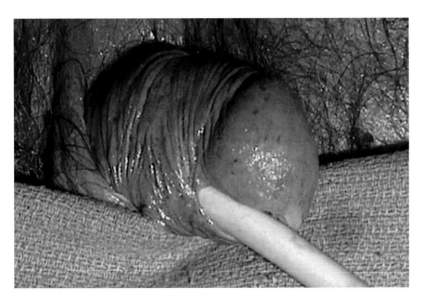

Figure 12-3 Hypospadias, gross
The urinary catheter shown here lies in a groove on the undersurface below the tip of the penis and enters the urethra. This abnormal opening is known as a *hypospadias*. Such an anomaly is present in about 1 in 300 male newborns, but it can lead to problems with urination and ejaculation. Constriction of the opening may be present, increasing the risk for urinary tract infections.

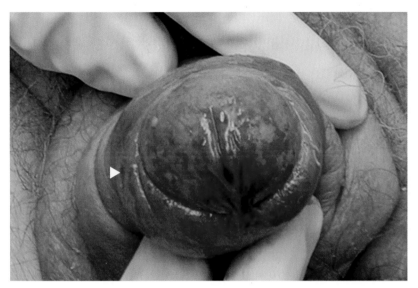

Figure 12-4 Balanoposthitis, gross

This glans penis surrounding the penile urethral meatus shows erythema and focal tan exudate, typical of a balanitis. The retracted foreskin (▶) is also acutely inflamed, a condition called *posthitis.* Together, this inflammatory condition is known as *balanoposthitis.* Infectious agents driving this process include *Candida albicans, Gardnerella* species, and pyogenic bacteria such as *Staphylococcus aureus.* Accumulated smegma (desquamated squamous epithelial cells and debris) beneath the foreskin predisposes to infection. Persistence of this inflammatory process predisposes to phimosis, a condition in which the prepuce cannot be retracted.

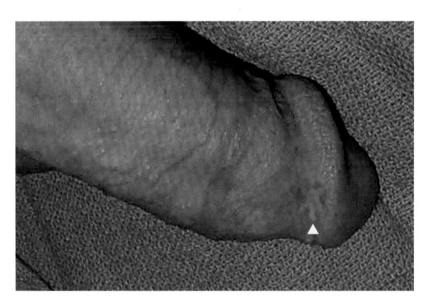

Figure 12-5 Bowen disease, gross

Carcinoma in situ of the external male genitalia is termed *Bowen disease* when there is a plaque-like lesion (▲) as shown. This process is initially painless, but larger lesions may have erythema, ulceration, or crusting. The term *erythroplasia of Queyrat* is reserved for carcinoma in situ of mucosal surfaces (glans or prepuce). Bowenoid papulosis appears in younger patients as multiple, reddish brown papular lesions. Microscopically, all these lesions have dysplastic squamous cells involving the full epithelial thickness without invasion through the basement membrane. Eventually, invasive squamous cell carcinoma occurs in about 10% of cases.

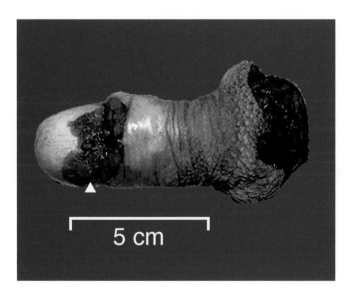

Figure 12-6 Squamous cell carcinoma, gross

This penectomy specimen contains a large invasive carcinoma (▲) that arose in the region of the head of an uncircumcised penis. This neoplasm is reddish tan and nodular, with an ulcerated surface. Such lesions are strongly associated with human papillomavirus infection, particularly types 16 and 18. Other factors, such as a history of smoking and lack of circumcision, are also implicated. Most patients with this disease are older than 40 years. When metastases occur, local inguinal and iliac lymph nodes are most often involved. Denial and fear on the part of the patient may delay treatment.

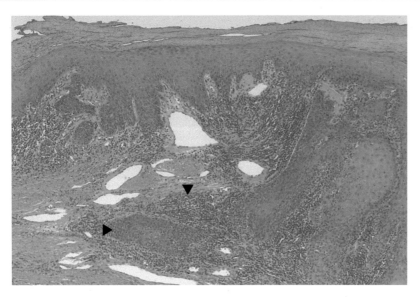

Figure 12-7 Squamous cell carcinoma, microscopic

There are tongues of well-differentiated invasive carcinoma (▼) extending into the penile corpora cavernosum, with inflammatory cell infiltrates (▶). Similar to cervical cancer in women, penile carcinoma is most often correlated with human papillomavirus infection, and the same types (16 and 18) are the most aggressive. Phimosis with increased accumulation of smegma is another risk factor; the incidence of penile cancer is rare in circumcised males. This form of cancer is often slow growing and locally invasive, but metastases can occur if left untreated. Initial metastases occur most often to iliac and inguinal lymph nodes.

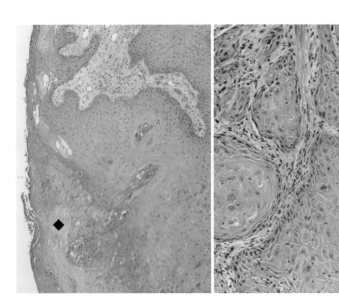

Figure 12-8 Verrucous carcinoma, microscopic

This is a well-differentiated form of squamous cell carcinoma. Note the extensive keratinization (◆) at low magnification in the *left panel* and well-differentiated cells at higher magnification in the *right panel*. Also known as the Buschke-Löwenstein tumor, it is typically a large, exophytic, cauliflower-like lesion of the genital or perianal area, with nonhealing ulceration and sometimes fistulas and sinuses. The surface is warty (verrucous). It arises most often in men and immunocompromised patients, usually on the glans penis of uncircumcised men. A similar verrucous gross and histologic appearance of squamous cell carcinoma may be seen in the oral cavity, larynx, skin of the soles, and anal region.

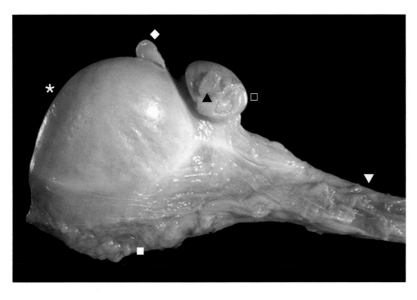

Figure 12-9 Normal testis, gross

Here is a normal testis and adjacent structures, including the body of the testis (★), epididymis (□), and spermatic cord (▼). Note the presence of two vestigial structures, the appendix testis (◆) and the appendix epididymis (▲). The pampiniform plexus of veins (■) lies posterior to the body of the testis. The normal testis descends down into the lower abdomen under the influence of müllerian inhibiting substance. Final descent into the scrotum in the third trimester of fetal development occurs under the influence of increasing androgens. Failure of the testis to descend normally results in cryptorchidism. The Leydig cells of a cryptorchid testis function normally, but the increased body temperature diminishes spermatogenesis.

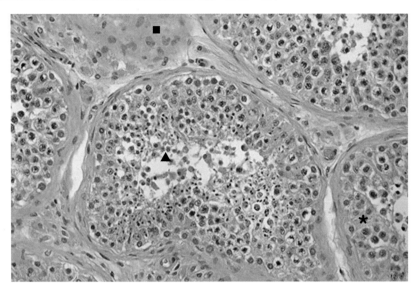

Figure 12-10 Normal testis, microscopic
These seminiferous tubules contain numerous germ cells (★). Sertoli cells (or *nurse cells*) are inconspicuous because their attenuated cytoplasm interdigitates with the germ cells. Small dark oblong spermatozoa (▲) are visible in the center of the tubules because there is active spermatogenesis. The normal sperm count is 80 to 150 million/mL of ejaculate. Small nodular collections of pink Leydig cells (■) are present in the interstitium between the tubules, secreting testosterone under the influence of luteinizing hormone. Note the pale golden-brown pigment in the interstitium, which gives the testicular parenchyma its grossly pale brown color. Sertoli cells secrete inhibin, which feeds back on the adenohypophysis to inhibit release of follicle-stimulating hormone, thus driving spermatogenesis.

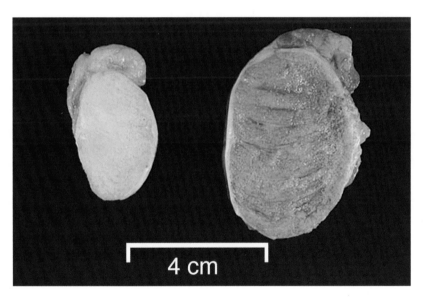

Figure 12-11 Cryptorchidism, gross
The testis shown on the *left* is atrophic, appearing small and pale white, whereas the testis on the *right* appears normal. This left testis did not descend into the scrotum during fetal development, but remained in the abdomen, a condition known as *cryptorchidism,* which is unilateral in 75% of cases. In most cases descent is arrested in the inguinal canal. There may also be an inguinal hernia accompanying 10% to 20% of cases. The abnormal position causes no pain but predisposes to trauma, which does cause pain. About 1% of male newborns have some failure of testicular descent.

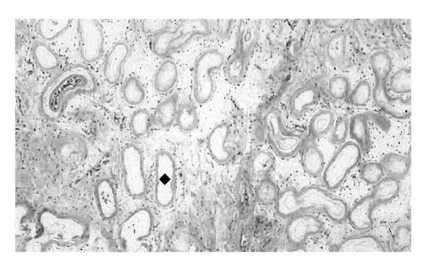

Figure 12-12 Cryptorchidism, microscopic
Note the atrophic, small residual tubules (◆) with no spermatogenesis, and pale surrounding stroma. Leydig cells (not shown here) still retain their function. A cryptorchid testis fails to develop normal spermatogenesis unless placed in the scrotum, because deterioration leading to the appearance shown begins by age 2. If unilateral, spermatogenesis in the remaining normal testis may prevent infertility. Cryptorchidism carries an increased risk for testicular carcinoma in either testis.

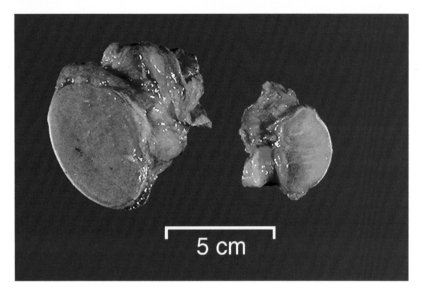

Figure 12-13 Testis, atrophy, gross
On the *left* is a normal testis, and the testis on the *right* has undergone atrophy. Bilateral atrophy may occur with various conditions, including chronic alcoholism, hypopituitarism, atherosclerosis, chemotherapy or radiation therapy, and severe prolonged illness. A cryptorchid testis also becomes atrophic. Inflammation with orchitis may lead to atrophy. Mumps, the most common infectious cause of orchitis, usually has a patchy and bilateral pattern of involvement that decreases the sperm count but does not usually lead to sterility. Bilateral testicular atrophy may accompany Klinefelter syndrome (47,XXY karyotype). Testicular enlargement may occur with fragile X syndrome.

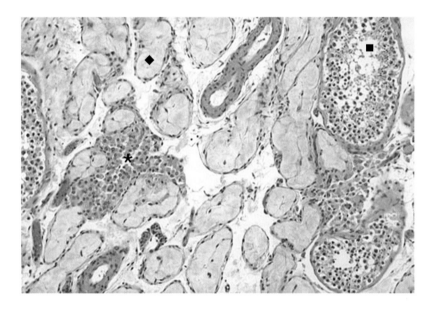

Figure 12-14 Testis, atrophy, microscopic
Here is focal atrophy (◆) of seminiferous tubules along with normal Leydig cells (★) and residual normal tubules (■) with active spermatogenesis. Mumps virus infection may be complicated by orchitis in one fourth to one third of cases. In general, the orchitis is unilateral and patchy, so sterility after infection is uncommon. Other infectious causes of orchitis include echovirus, lymphocytic choriomeningitis virus, influenza virus, coxsackievirus, and arboviruses. In contrast, epididymitis is a more frequent cause of scrotal pain and swelling in men and is most likely to be the result of a sexually transmissible disease, such as *Chlamydia trachomatis* or *Neisseria gonorrhoeae* in younger men or gram-negative bacteria from urinary tract infection in older men.

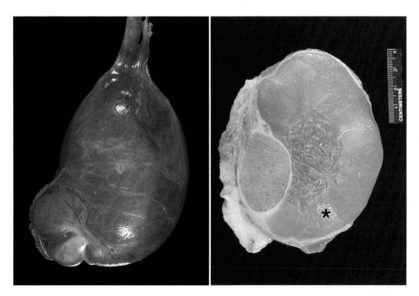

Figure 12-15 Hydrocele, gross
Hydroceles are common accumulations of clear fluid within the sac of tunica vaginalis, which is lined by a serosa. Hydrocele may occur in older men as a result of various inflammatory and neoplastic conditions. The external appearance of a testis with a hydrocele removed from the scrotum at autopsy is shown in the *left panel*. A cross-section through a frozen hydrocele (★) removed at autopsy in the *right panel* shows the relationship of the fluid to the testis. The fluid in a hydrocele is a transudate that accumulates slowly but can produce a mass effect and local discomfort. In many cases, the cause is not determined.

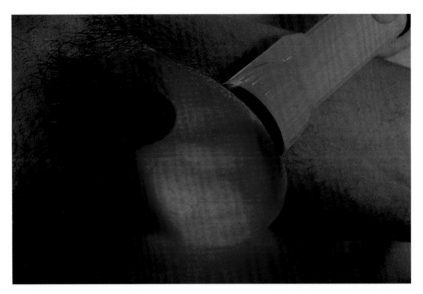

Figure 12-16 Hydrocele, gross
One diagnostic technique to detect a hydrocele is transillumination of the fluid-filled space with a light applied to the scrotum. This effect, shown here, resembles a lunar eclipse. The fluid collection typically occurs slowly and is not painful. A hydrocele must be distinguished from a true testicular mass; transillumination may help in diagnosis because the hydrocele transilluminates, whereas a testicular mass is opaque to the light. Ultrasound examination provides a simple, noninvasive method of diagnosing scrotal masses.

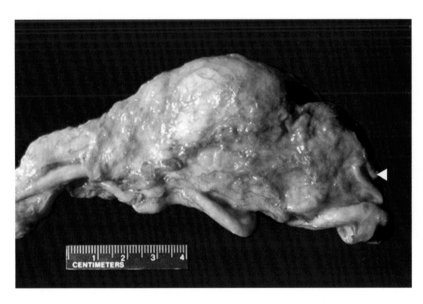

Figure 12-17 Testis, varicocele, gross
A common cause of male infertility is a varicocele, a lesion that consists of prominent dilation of the pampiniform plexus of veins (◄) posterior to the testis, as shown by these prominent blue vessels. Most varicoceles are asymptomatic and detected on palpation with the feel of "a bag of worms." The increased blood flow makes this lesion a radiant heat device that increases the temperature of testicular tubules, inhibiting normal spermatogenesis. It can be present to some degree in up to 20% of men and in 40% of infertile men.

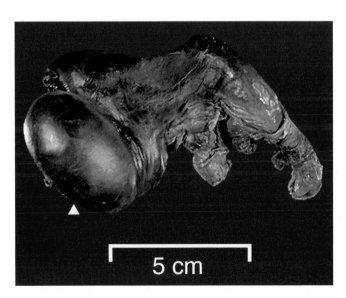

Figure 12-18 Testicular torsion, gross
This testis (▲) appears dark from deoxygenated blood because it has undergone hemorrhagic infarction after torsion, which, although uncommon, is a medical emergency. It occurs when sudden twisting of the spermatic cord cuts off the venous drainage, leading to severe scrotal pain. Torsion in adolescents often occurs when there is greater mobility from abnormal incomplete testicular descent or lack of a scrotal ligament. Perinatal torsion occurs rarely and for no apparent reason. Immediate treatment by surgically untwisting and suturing the cord in place to prevent future torsion prevents infarction and loss of function. Sometimes only the little appendix testis undergoes torsion, producing acute pain.

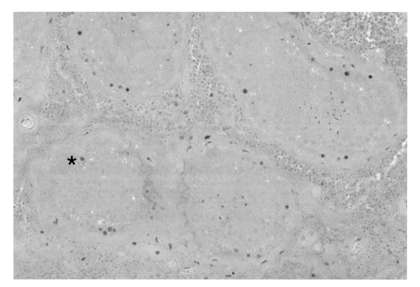

Figure 12-19 Testicular torsion, microscopic
In this case, torsion of the testis has proceeded to hemorrhagic infarction with no viable cells within the seminiferous tubules. Note the pale outlines of the residual tubules (★), but there is loss of nuclear detail, and the interstitium is hemorrhagic. The most common signs and symptoms include a red, swollen scrotum and an acutely painful testicle without evidence of trauma. Nausea and vomiting are common. Doppler ultrasound scan be helpful in showing lack of blood flow, confirming the diagnosis.

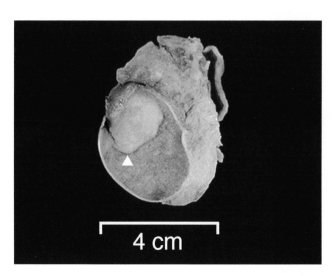

Figure 12-20 Seminoma, gross
The germ cell tumor most likely to be a single histologic type is seminoma, shown here as a uniform solid tan mass (▲) within the body of the testis. Such a small neoplasm may be detectable only with ultrasound. Germ cell neoplasms are the most common forms of testicular neoplasia. The peak incidence is in the 15- to 34-year age range. Such a tumor may be a "mixed germ cell tumor" and have more than one histologic component—seminoma, embryonal carcinoma, yolk sac tumor, teratoma, or choriocarcinoma. Most testicular germ cell tumors arise from a focus of intratubular germ cell neoplasia (ITGCN).

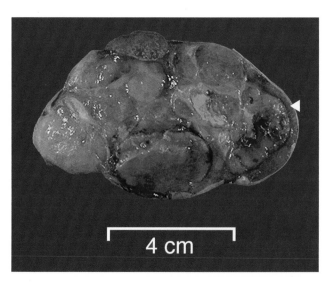

Figure 12-21 Seminoma, gross
A small rim (◀) of remaining normal testis appears at the far right. This tumor is composed of lobulated, soft, tan-to-brown tissue. At least 95% of testicular neoplasms are germ cell tumors. Half of germ cell tumors are seminomas, which have a uniform lobulated tan-to-brown appearance as shown. Many patients exhibit fear and denial, delaying detection and therapy—hence the size this neoplasm attained before treatment. An i(12p) karyotypic abnormality is found in virtually all testicular germ cell (and ovarian germ cell) neoplasms. Female patients with the androgen insensitivity syndrome *(testicular feminization)* are at increased risk for development of seminoma.

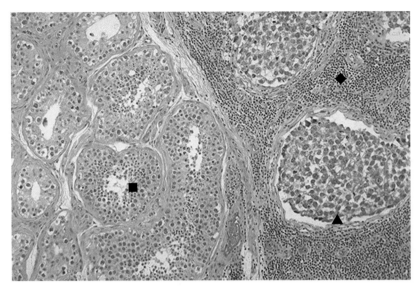

Figure 12-22 Seminoma, microscopic
Normal testis appears on the left, and seminoma is present on the right. Note the difference in size and staining quality of the nests of neoplastic cells compared with normal germ cells (■) in seminiferous tubules. The large seminoma cells (▲) have vesicular nuclei and pale watery cytoplasm. Lobules of neoplastic cells have an intervening stroma with characteristic T-cell lymphoid infiltrates (◆). This classic form of seminoma constitutes 90% of all seminomas, with cells showing positive immunohistochemical staining for human placental lactogen, but not human chorionic gonadotropin (HCG) or α-fetoprotein (AFP). Occasional syncytial cells may be HCG positive. Many of these seminomas are sensitive to radiation and chemotherapy, with a good prognosis.

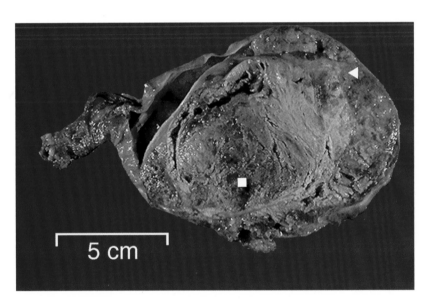

Figure 12-23 Embryonal carcinoma, gross
This large tumor mass is soft and much more variegated than the seminoma, with red, tan, and brown areas, including prominent foci of hemorrhage and necrosis (■). There are a few scattered firmer white areas (◀) that histologically proved to be teratoma. No normal testicular tissue can be seen here. This is mixed embryonal carcinoma plus teratoma (sometimes called *teratocarcinoma*) or mixed germ cell tumor of the testis. Embryonal carcinoma is the second most common testicular tumor and is more aggressive than seminoma. Although most seminomas are stage I at the time of diagnosis, nonseminomatous germ cell tumors (NSGCTs), such as embryonal carcinoma, are more likely to be stage II or III.

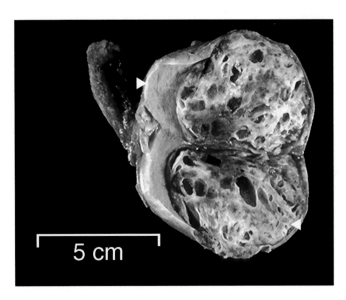

Figure 12-24 Embryonal carcinoma and teratoma, gross
This is an embryonal carcinoma mixed with teratoma in which islands of bluish white cartilage (◀) from the teratoma component are present. A rim of normal pale brown testis (▶) appears at the left of the tumor. From a clinical standpoint, it is most useful to know whether nonseminomatous germ cell elements are present, because this determines a more aggressive course that can be treated with more aggressive chemotherapy. Purely seminomatous neoplasms are more likely to be at a low stage at diagnosis, to remain localized longer, and to be more amenable to chemotherapy and radiation. The *OCT3/4* gene produces a transcription factor in seminomas and embryonal carcinomas. Nonseminomatous germ cell tumors often are accompanied by serum elevations of AFP and HCG.

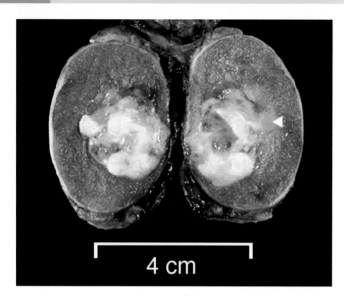

Figure 12-25 Teratoma, gross
This small testicular neoplasm within the body of a normal-sized testis sectioned coronally has a mixture of bluish cartilage (◀) admixed with red and white tumor tissue. Microscopically it contained mainly teratoma, but also areas of embryonal carcinoma. About 60% of all testicular neoplasms are composed of more than one element and are mixed germ cell tumors. Although rare in the pediatric age group (second in frequency to yolk sac tumor), testicular teratomas in children are likely to act in a benign fashion. Germ cell tumors of the testis tend to metastasize first to para-aortic lymph nodes, but hematogenous spread to lungs and other sites occurs. Metastases may have different microscopic germ cell tumor components than the primary.

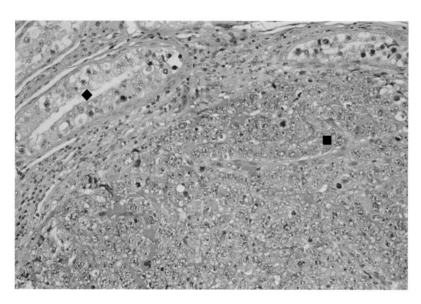

Figure 12-26 Embryonal carcinoma, microscopic
The neoplastic cells (■), compared with the residual seminiferous tubule (◆) at the upper left, appear more primitive than seminoma. Sheets of large pale blue cells with indistinct borders are trying to form primitive tubules. Occasional syncytial cells may stain positively for HCG, and some cells with yolk sac differentiation are positive for AFP. HCG and AFP may be elevated in the serum of patients with testicular germ cell tumors.

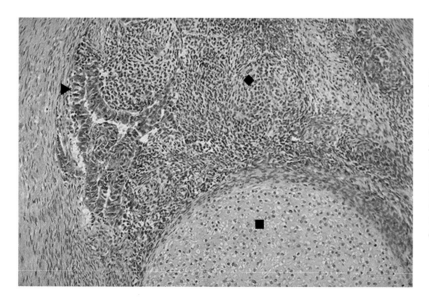

Figure 12-27 Mixed testicular germ cell tumor, microscopic
At the bottom is a focus of primitive but benign-appearing cartilage (■), representing a teratoma component of a mixed germ cell neoplasm. Above this is a primitive mesenchymal stroma (◆), and to the left is a focus of primitive cells (▶) most characteristic of embryonal carcinoma. This is embryonal carcinoma mixed with teratoma (teratocarcinoma). Over half of testicular malignancies have more than one histologic component.

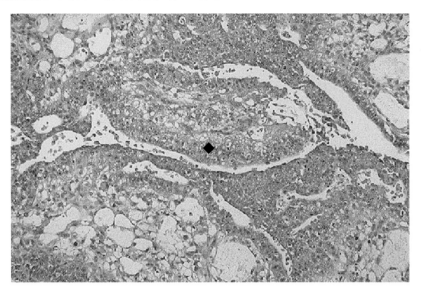

Figure 12-28 Yolk sac tumor, microscopic
This endodermal sinus tumor (yolk sac tumor, or infantile embryonal carcinoma) of the testis is composed of primitive germ cells that form glomeruloid (◆), or embryonal-like structures (Schiller-Duval bodies). These tumors are most frequent in children younger than 3 years, but overall they are a rare type of germ cell neoplasm. The prognosis for most patients is good. The cells of this tumor produce AFP, which can be detected in the serum as a tumor marker. An element of yolk sac differentiation is often present in embryonal carcinomas, so AFP is often detected in patients with embryonal carcinoma.

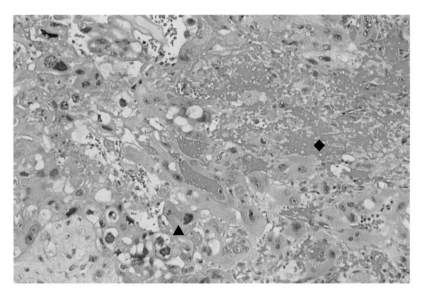

Figure 12-29 Choriocarcinoma, microscopic
Pure testicular choriocarcinomas are rare. The primary is often small at the time of detection because these tumors are aggressive and metastasize early. Some cases may exhibit the phenomenon of the "disappearing primary" tumor, in which the rapidly growing tumor outgrows its blood supply and infarcts with hemorrhage (◆) and necrosis, eventually leaving only a small scar, although the metastases continue to grow. Shown here are large syncytiotrophoblastic cells (▲) with abundant pink cytoplasm (positive for HCG) and a highly pleomorphic nuclei. Smaller cytotrophoblastic cells with clear cytoplasm are present.

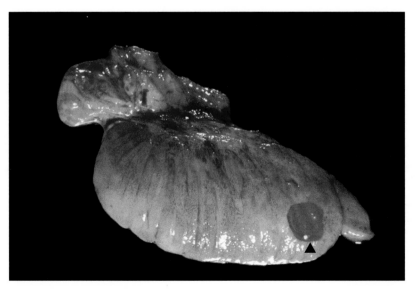

Figure 12-30 Leydig cell tumor, gross
The cut surface of this normal-sized adult testis reveals a small discrete brown mass (▲). Most of these interstitial (Leydig) cell tumors arise in men 20 to 60 years old. They may elaborate androgens, estrogens, or other steroid hormones such as glucocorticoids. Although often less than 1 cm in diameter, some may reach several centimeters in size, enough to produce palpable testicular enlargement. Significant hormone production may lead to gynecomastia in adults. In prepubertal children, such a neoplasm could be a cause of sexual precocity.

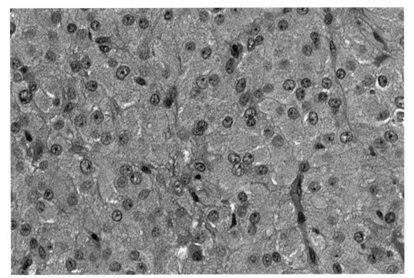

Figure 12-31 Leydig cell tumor, microscopic
The small round cells of this tumor are found in nests or clusters, and there are many intervening capillaries, typical of endocrine tissue. A distinctive electron microscopic feature is the cytoplasmic rod-shaped crystalloid of Reinke. About 10% of these neoplasms act in an aggressive fashion, with local invasion or metastases. Most, similar to the one shown here, are benign.

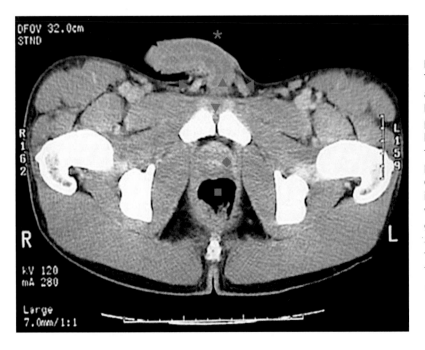

Figure 12-32 Normal prostate, CT image
This pelvic CT scan shows the normal penis (✱) and penile urethra (▲), right spermatic cord (▶), left spermatic cord (◀), pubic symphysis (▼), prostate (◆), and rectum (■). The prostate lies below the bladder, and the prostatic portion of the urethra traverses the prostate gland. The prostate is derived embryologically from epithelial evaginations along the urethra. There is little increase in size of the prostate until puberty when, under the influence of testosterone, growth and differentiation occur. The enzyme 5α-reductase in nuclei of prostatic cells converts testosterone produced by Leydig cells of the testes to dihydrotestosterone (DHT), which promotes prostatic growth.

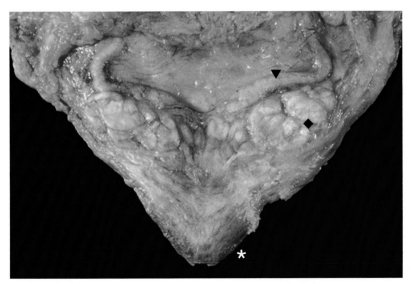

Figure 12-33 Normal prostate, gross
The normal prostate (✱) is shown here from a posterior view. Anterior to the rectum and posterior and superior to the prostate are the paired seminal vesicles (◆), which produce about 70% of the secretions constituting seminal fluid. The vas deferens (▼) from each testis is shown to extend to the prostate as well. The seminal vesicles are rarely a site at which pathologic lesions arise. They can occasionally be infiltrated by carcinomas from surrounding organs such as the prostate.

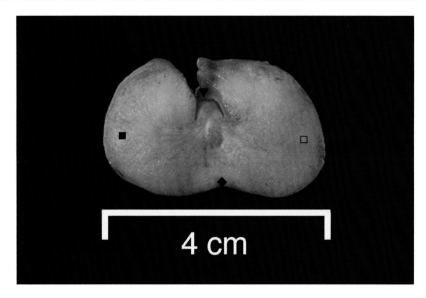

Figure 12-34 Normal prostate, gross
This is a transverse (axial) section through a normal prostate. There is a central urethra (▼) at the depth of the cut made to open this prostate anteriorly at autopsy, with the left lateral lobe (■), the right lateral lobe (□), and the posterior lobe (◆). The consistency is uniform, without nodularity. The normal prostate is 3 to 4 cm in diameter and weighs 20 to 30 g. About 75% of the prostate is composed of the peripheral zone, or what is traditionally described as the lateral and posterior lobes. The small anterior zone contains mostly fibromuscular stroma. The central zone lies between the ejaculatory ducts. A transitional zone lies anterior to the central zone around the internal urethral sphincter.

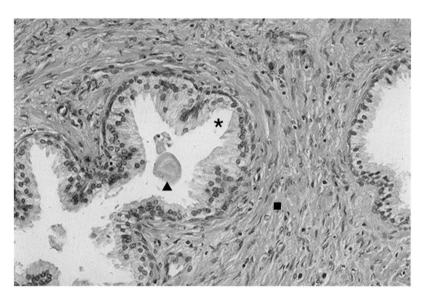

Figure 12-35 Normal prostate, microscopic
The normal histologic appearance of prostate glands (★) and surrounding fibromuscular stroma (■) is shown here at high magnification. A small pink concretion (▲) (typical of the corpora amylacea seen in benign prostatic glands of older men) appears in the gland just to the left of center. Note the well-differentiated glands with a double layer of inner tall columnar epithelial lining cells and basal low cuboidal cells. These cells normally do not have prominent nucleoli. The peripheral, central, and transitional zones typically have this appearance. By immunohistochemical staining, prostate-specific antigen (PSA) can be identified within the glandular epithelial cell cytoplasm, and small amounts of PSA can normally be detected in the serum.

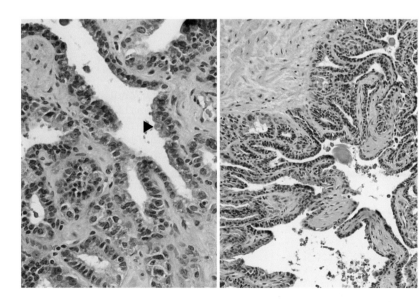

Figure 12-36 Normal seminal vesicle, microscopic
The normal mucosa is extensively folded with a mazelike appearance that is multichanneled on cross-section. Columnar to cuboidal mucosal cells on lamina propria are surrounded by inner circular and outer longitudinal smooth muscle layers. The epithelial cells contain light brownish yellow cytoplasmic pigment (▶) that imparts a slightly yellowish color to secretions. The seminal vesicle contributes over half the volume of ejaculate and imparts a high fructose content to nourish spermatozoa.

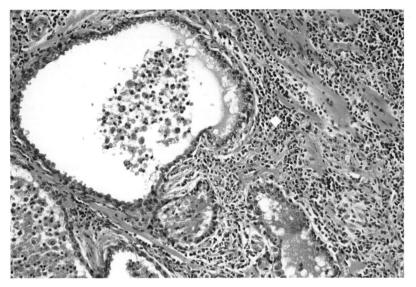

Figure 12-37 Prostatitis, microscopic
Numerous small, round, dark-blue lymphocytes (♦) are visible in the stroma between the glands. There may be a bacterial agent accompanying this inflammation, and urinary tract infection with cystitis or urethritis may be present. More commonly in men older than 50 years, chronic prostatitis is abacterial, with no history of urinary tract infection, with negative cultures but with at least 10 leukocytes per high-power field in prostatic secretions. Patients with prostatitis often have perineal or back pain with dysuria, although some are asymptomatic. The serum PSA may be slightly elevated, typically up to twice the upper limit of the normal range. Acute prostatitis is caused by bacteria similar to those with urinary tract infections.

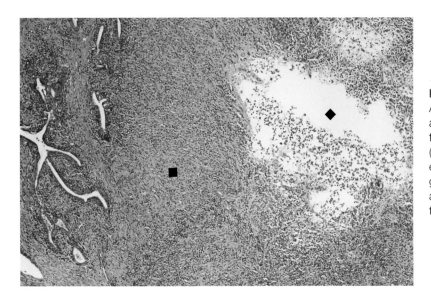

Figure 12-38 Prostatic abscess, microscopic
An acute prostatitis is typically caused by bacterial organisms similar to those involved with urinary tract infections. Note the liquefied, clear center (♦) of the abscess at the right, surrounded by extensive inflammatory infiltrate (■), and prostatic glands at the left. Patients have dysuria with fever and chills. The prostate is tense and extremely tender on digital rectal examination.

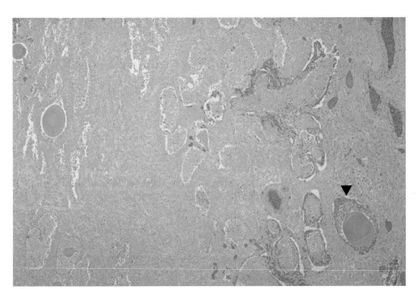

Figure 12-39 Prostatic infarction, microscopic
Shown on the left is an area of pale pink prostatic infarction. Such infarcts do not occur often; they are typically small but may cause discomfort and may increase the serum PSA, similar to prostatitis or prostatic adenocarcinoma. The glands surrounding a prostatic infarct can have squamous metaplasia (▼). Note also the rounded pink corpora amylacea within glands.

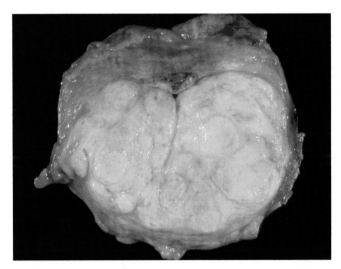

Figure 12-40 Prostatic hyperplasia, gross
This 5-cm diameter prostate is enlarged and nodular as a result of prostatic hyperplasia. This condition is termed either *benign prostatic hyperplasia* (BPH) or *nodular prostatic hyperplasia*. The hyperplasia is most pronounced in the lateral lobes. This is a process that occurs gradually over many years, typically after age 50; by age 80, more than 90% of men have some degree of BPH, although only a few are symptomatic. An enlarged prostate can obstruct urinary outflow from the bladder and lead to an obstructive uropathy. BPH is detected as diffuse prostatic enlargement on digital rectal examination. Symptoms relate to inability to void completely, with residual urine causing increasing urinary frequency, along with difficulty starting and stopping the urinary stream. The larger the prostate, the more likely urinary tract symptoms will be present. On average older men have a 2% increase in prostate size and a 2% decrease in peak urine flow rate per year.

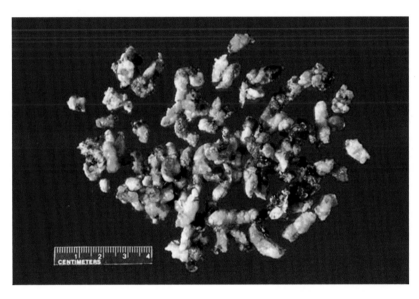

Figure 12-41 Prostatic hyperplasia, gross
A frequently performed operation for symptomatic nodular prostatic hyperplasia is a transurethral resection, which yields the small "chips" of rubbery prostatic tissue shown here. Prostatic hyperplasia is the result of increased sensitivity of the prostatic glands and stroma to DHT because there are increased numbers of androgen receptors induced by increasing estradiol levels with aging. The enzyme 5α-reductase type 2, found mainly in prostatic stromal cells, converts circulating testosterone to DHT. Pharmacotherapy for BPH is aimed at blocking either this enzyme or α_{1a}-adrenoreceptors to relax the smooth muscle of the bladder neck and improve urine flow, affording a greater, earlier effect on symptoms but not reducing prostate size.

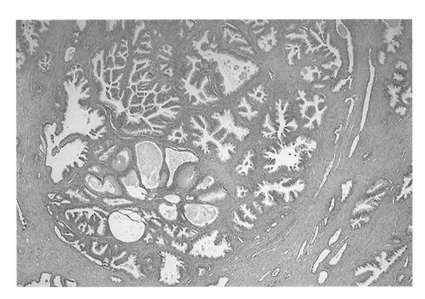

Figure 12-42 Prostatic hyperplasia, microscopic
Both glands and stroma may be involved, although hyperplasia of the former is usually more prominent. A large hyperplastic nodule with numerous crowded glands is present here. There is still stroma between the glands. The glands are larger than normal, with more complex infoldings, but are still lined by a double layer of uniform columnar cells and basal cuboidal cells that show no atypia. The periurethral zone often enables an initial increase in these hyperplastic nodules, although the bulk of prostatic enlargement often comes later from pronounced nodular growth in the peripheral zone.

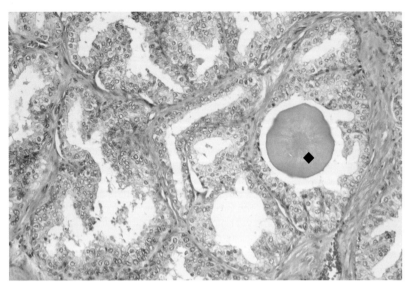

Figure 12-43 Prostatic hyperplasia, microscopic

A nodule with crowded glands is shown. A rounded pink concretion (◆), typical for corpora amylacea found in benign prostatic glands, is present. These columnar cells lining the glands are normal, as well as the indistinct surrounding layer of basal cells. About 70% of men will have some microscopic hyperplasia by age 60, but only half of them have prostatic enlargement, and just a subset of those are symptomatic from urinary obstruction. With aging, DHT induces growth factors to increase the proliferation of stromal cells and decrease the death of epithelial cells.

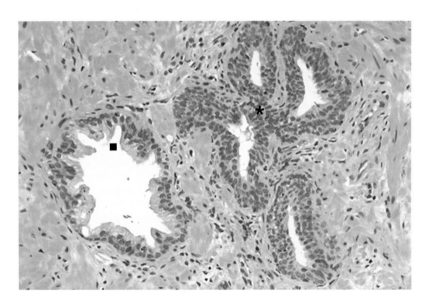

Figure 12-44 Prostatic intraepithelial neoplasia, microscopic

Prostatic intraepithelial neoplasia (PIN) is a potentially precancerous cellular proliferation found in a single acinus or more commonly in a small group of prostatic acini. A normal prostatic gland (■) is shown on the left for comparison, with the acini showing PIN (★) on the right. The PIN can be low grade or high grade (as shown here). Androgen receptor gene mutations that shorten CAG repeat sequences increase androgen sensitivity, which plays a role in driving prostatic neoplasia. Germline mutations may also be present.

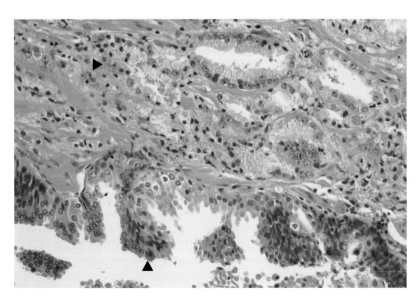

Figure 12-45 Prostatic intraepithelial neoplasia and adenocarcinoma, microscopic

The finding of PIN suggests that prostatic adenocarcinoma may also be present, and an adenocarcinoma accompanies high-grade PIN over half the time. Shown here are irregular glands (▶) of adenocarcinoma at the top, and foci of PIN (▲) at the bottom. A molecular alteration common to both is chromosomal rearrangements putting the *ETS* family transcription factor gene adjacent to the androgen-regulated *TMPRSS2* promoter gene. Men with germline mutations of the tumor suppressor *BRCA2* have a 20-fold increased risk of prostate cancer.

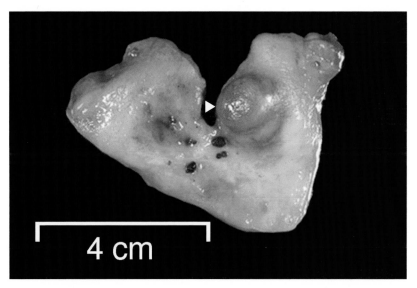

Figure 12-46 Adenocarcinoma, gross
This axial section reveals a single prominent nodule (▶) of adenocarcinoma. Such a nodule may be palpable on digital rectal examination or may be detected on ultrasound. Some small dark glandular concretions are also shown here in the adjacent normal prostate. This prostate is not significantly enlarged, and no nodularity is present. Although the incidence of BPH and adenocarcinoma increases with age, BPH is not a risk factor for carcinoma. Prostate cancer is the most common nonskin malignancy in elderly men. It is rare before age 50, but autopsy studies have found prostatic adenocarcinoma in more than half of men older than 70 years.

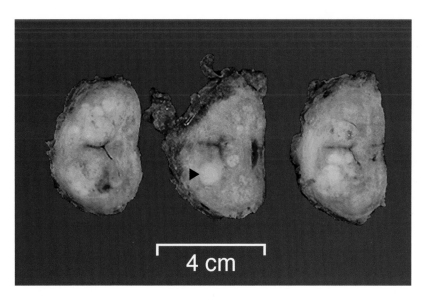

Figure 12-47 Adenocarcinoma, gross
These sections through a prostate removed by radical prostatectomy reveal irregular yellowish nodules (▶) of adenocarcinoma, mostly in the posterior region. Prostate glands containing adenocarcinoma are not always enlarged. Adenocarcinoma may coexist with BPH. Staging of prostatic adenocarcinoma is based on how extensive the tumor is. Many of these carcinomas are small and clinically insignificant. Some, such as the one shown here, are more extensive. Prostatic adenocarcinoma is second only to lung carcinoma as a cause of tumor-related deaths among men. More than 90% of prostatic carcinomas show hypermethylation of the glutathione S-transferase $(GSTP1)$ gene promoter.

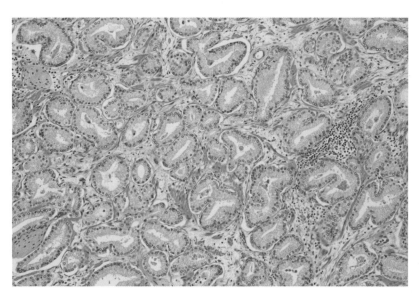

Figure 12-48 Adenocarcinoma, microscopic
Note how the glands of the carcinoma are small, irregular, and crowded, with no intervening stroma. Prostatic adenocarcinomas are given a histologic grade. The Gleason grading system is used most often and includes a score of 1 to 5 (increasing as the carcinoma becomes less differentiated) for the most prominent component, added to a score of 1 to 5 for the next most common pattern. This adenocarcinoma could be given a Gleason grade of 3/3. The grade gives an indication of prognosis and how aggressive therapy should be. In general, a combined score of less than 6 suggests that the neoplasm will be indolent. Advanced cancers tend to have scores of 8 or higher.

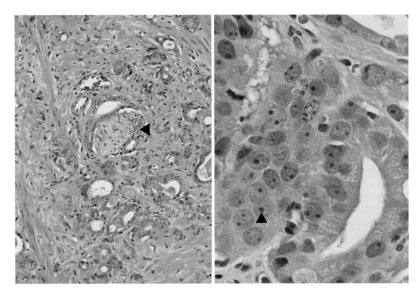

Figure 12-49 Adenocarcinoma, microscopic
Prominent nucleoli (▲) are a characteristic histologic feature of prostatic adenocarcinoma *(right panel)* as well as perineural (◄) invasion *(left panel)*. Prostate cancers may be detected by screening with a blood test for PSA. PSA is a glycoprotein produced almost exclusively in the epithelium of the prostate glands. The PSA level tends to increase gradually with age. A mildly increased PSA (4 to 10 ng/mL) in a patient with a very large prostate can be a result of nodular hyperplasia or of prostatitis, rather than carcinoma. An increasing PSA suggests carcinoma, even if the PSA is in the normal range. A small focus of cancer confined to the prostate may not be accompanied by an increase in PSA. Transrectal needle biopsy is useful to confirm the diagnosis of adenocarcinoma.

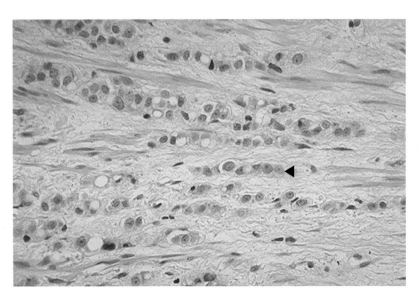

Figure 12-50 Adenocarcinoma, microscopic
This adenocarcinoma is so poorly differentiated (Gleason grade 5) that no glandular structure is recognizable, only individual cells infiltrating (◄) in rows. Advanced prostatic adenocarcinomas typically cause urinary obstruction and metastasize to regional (pelvic) lymph nodes and to the bones, causing osteoblastic (bone-forming) metastases in many cases. The most typical site of bone metastases is the vertebral column, with accompanying chronic back pain. Metastases to the lungs and liver occur in a few cases.

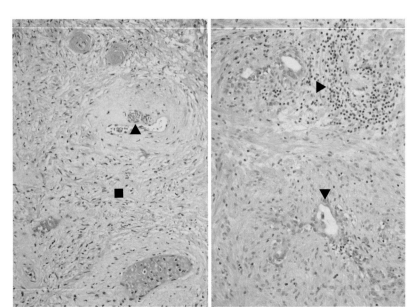

Figure 12-51 Prostate, postradiation changes, microscopic
Radiation therapy may be given for advanced-stage prostatic adenocarcinoma. Shown here are typical tissue changes following therapeutic radiation. In the *left panel* there is extensive stromal fibrosis (■) and thickened blood vessels and narrowed lumens (▲). In the *right panel* there are a few remaining atrophic glands (▼) with stroma containing chronic inflammation (▶). Tissue hypoxia and inflammation reduce functionality.

The Female Genital Tract

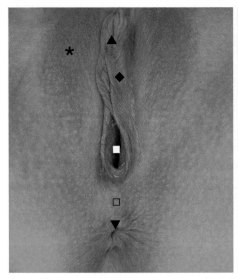
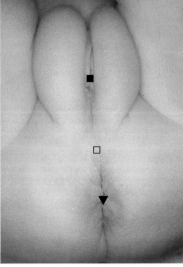

Figure 13-1 Normal external genitalia, gross

In the *left panel,* adult external genitalia include the labia majora (★), labia minora (◆), clitoris (▲), vaginal orifice (■), and perineum (□) extending to the anus (▼). In the *right panel,* the appearance of the genitalia at birth illustrates the relationship of the vaginal orifice (■), perineum (□), and anus (▼). The external genitalia are covered by keratinizing stratified squamous epithelium.

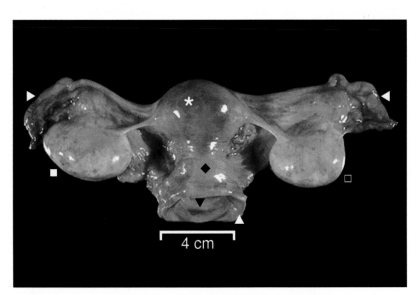

Figure 13-2 Normal internal genitalia, gross

The gross appearance of a normal uterus from a young woman includes the fundus (★), lower uterine segment (◆), cervix (▼), vaginal cuff (▲), right fallopian tube (▶), left fallopian tube (◀), right ovary (■), and left ovary (□). In the developing embryo, primordial germ cells from the yolk sac wall migrate to the urogenital ridge to become ovarian germ cells within the epithelium and stroma derived from urogenital ridge mesoderm. The unfused portions of the müllerian (paramesonephric) ducts form the fallopian tubes, and the fused portions become the uterus and vagina, whereas the distal fused ducts contact the urogenital sinus to become the vestibule of the external genitalia.

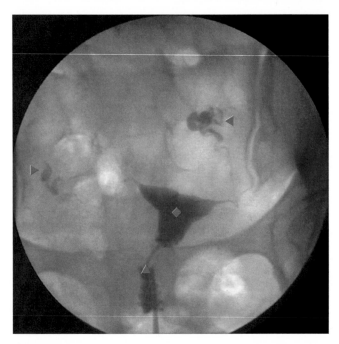

Figure 13-3 Normal internal genitalia, radiograph

This is a hysterosalpingogram, in which a catheter is introduced through the cervix (▲) to fill the endometrial cavity (◆) with contrast material. Contrast material extends into the right fallopian tube and left fallopian tube, eventually spilling out through the fimbriated ends of the fallopian tubes (oviducts) in the right adnexal (▶) and left adnexal (◀) regions, indicating normal tubal patency. Some contrast material here has also backfilled into the vagina. This radiographic study may be undertaken as part of an infertility workup.

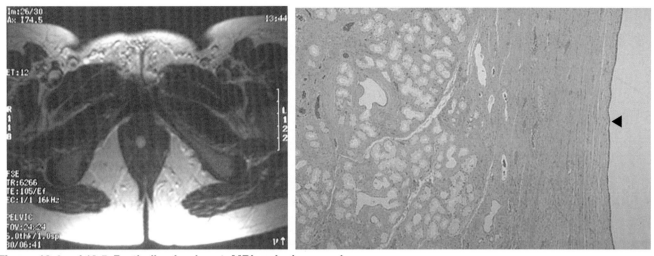

Figures 13-4 and 13-5 Bartholin gland cyst, MRI and microscopic

A small, bright, cyst (▶) of the Bartholin gland is shown in the *left panel.* These paired glands produce mucinous secretions and have ducts that empty into the vaginal orifice. The duct to a gland can become obstructed, leading to cystic glandular enlargement with inflammation and infection, producing pain and discomfort. A Bartholin cyst can reach 3 to 5 cm in size. In the *right panel,* the cyst with flattened transitional or squamous lining (◀) is at the far right, with remaining adjacent normal glands at the left.

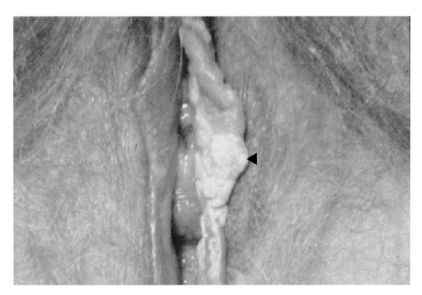

Figure 13-6 Lichen sclerosus, gross

The pale white patches (◀) of leukoplakia appearing here on the vulva with atrophy and fibrosis can narrow the introitus and produce discomfort. This process can develop slowly and involve progressively more labial skin surface in women, particularly after menopause. Lichen sclerosus increases the risk for secondary infection.

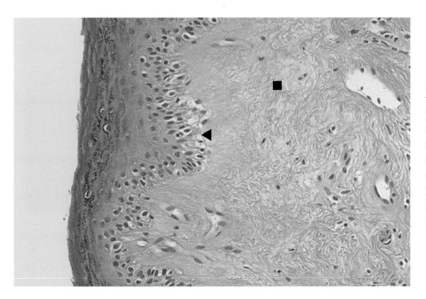

Figure 13-7 Lichen sclerosus, microscopic

There is atrophy of the vulvar squamous epithelium with thinning, loss of rete pegs, hydropic degeneration of basal keratinocytes (◀), dermal dense band collagenous fibrous thickening (■), and sometimes a bandlike infiltrate of lymphocytes. These findings suggest an autoimmune process. Although lichen sclerosus is not premalignant, vulvar squamous cell cancer eventually develops in less than 4% of these women.

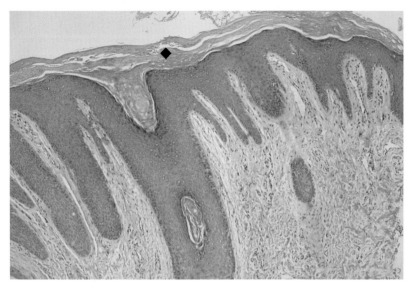

Figure 13-8 Squamous cell hyperplasia, microscopic

Note the thickened (acanthotic) epidermis and overlying keratin (◆) layer (hyperkeratosis), giving a grossly white appearance (leukoplakia). There is no atypia of the keratinocytes. Formerly known as *lichen simplex chronicus,* this lesion arises from mechanical irritation with rubbing or scratching pruritic skin to relieve pruritus. Squamous cell hyperplasia is not considered premalignant.

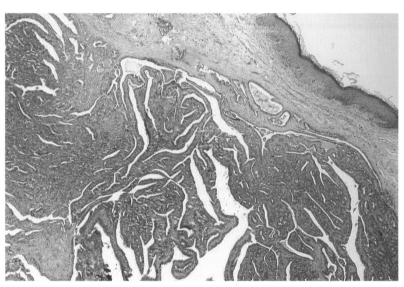

Figure 13-9 Papillary hidradenoma, microscopic

The vulva has modified apocrine sweat glands from which a papillary hidradenoma may arise. It forms a sharply circumscribed nodule, most commonly in the labia majora or interlabial folds. A vulvar carcinoma may be suspected because the hidradenoma tends to ulcerate. It has a histologically similar appearance to an intraductal papilloma of the breast. As shown here, there is a regular papillary growth pattern with tubular ducts lined by a single or double layer of nonciliated columnar cells, with a layer of flattened "myoepithelial cells." This lesion underlies the epithelium at the upper right. Myoepithelial elements are characteristic of sweat glands and sweat gland tumors.

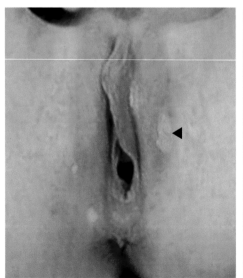

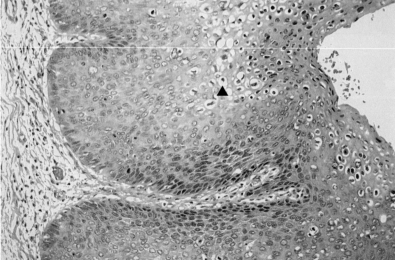

Figures 13-10 and 13-11 Condyloma acuminata, gross and microscopic

Note the pale pink lesions (◀) on the vulva shown in the *left panel.* These warty (verrucous) excrescences can involve the perineum, vulva, and perianal region, typical of sexually transmitted human papillomavirus (HPV) infection, often HPV subtypes 6 and 11. The lesions can be solitary or multiple. The squamous epithelium becomes thickened, and there is perinuclear vacuolization to produce the characteristic cytologic "koilocytotic atypia" (▲) shown in the *right panel.* Condylomata are benign and do not progress to malignancy. They may remain the same size, regress spontaneously, or enlarge slowly.

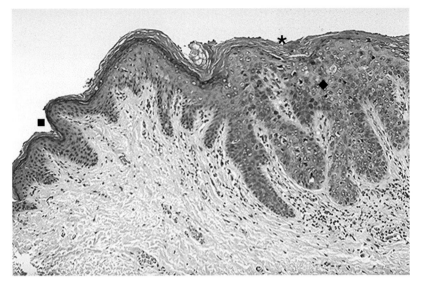

Figure 13-12 Vulvar dysplasia, microscopic
Dysplasia (◆) may involve the vulvar epithelium as a consequence of HPV infection. Note the overlying hyperkeratosis (★) (which produces a grossly visible area of leukoplakia), with more normal (but atrophic) keratinizing squamous epithelium (■) on the left. Most cases of vulvar intraepithelial neoplasia (VIN) do not progress to invasive cancer, but the risk is greater with HPV subtypes 16 and 18. Many lesions are multicentric, and some occur in association with cervical or vaginal squamous carcinoma. In older women, vulvar carcinomas may be preceded by lichen sclerosus, not HPV infection.

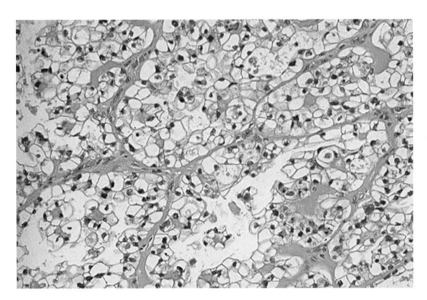

Figure 13-13 Clear cell carcinoma, microscopic
Neoplasms of the vagina are rare. Note the vacuolated cells forming irregular clusters with ill-defined glandular lumens. Red, granular foci that appear on the vaginal mucosa are called *adenosis* and may precede clear cell carcinoma, a lesion most likely to occur in a young woman whose mother was given diethylstilbestrol (DES) during pregnancy. These cancers are rare, even in women with this history. DES exposure increases the risk for clear cell carcinoma arising in the upper vagina and cervix of adolescents and young adults. Clear cell carcinoma often becomes invasive before detection and is difficult to cure.

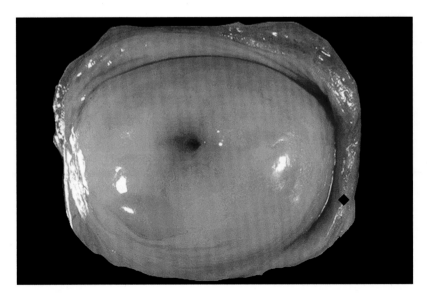

Figure 13-14 Normal cervix, gross
The normal cervix has a smooth, glistening mucosal surface. There is a small rim of vaginal cuff (◆) in this hysterectomy specimen. The cervical os is small and round, typical of a nulliparous woman. The os attains a fish-mouth shape after one or more pregnancies.

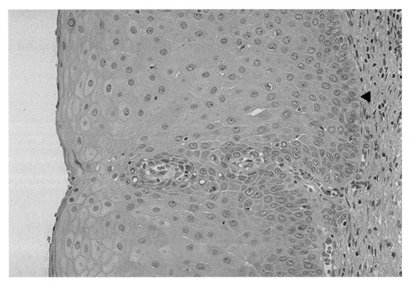

Figure 13-15 Normal cervix, microscopic
This is normal cervical nonkeratinizing squamous epithelium. The squamous cells show maturation from the basal layer (◄) to the overlying surface. A Pap smear is obtained by scraping or brushing the surface of the cervix (and sometimes the vagina) to obtain cells that are placed in a fixative solution and stained. The maturation pattern of these cells gives an indication of a woman's hormonal status and changes during the normal menstrual cycle. Inflammatory cells and infectious agents can be seen on a Pap smear. Dysplastic changes can also be detected.

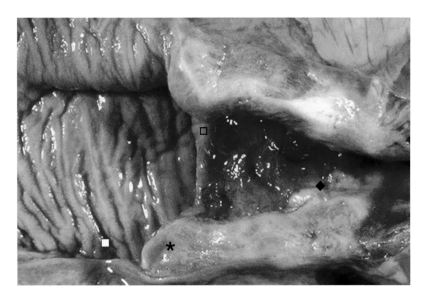

Figure 13-16 Normal cervix and vagina, gross
The normal adult vaginal mucosa (■) in reproductive-age women has a wrinkled appearance. The cervix (★) has been opened anteriorly at autopsy to reveal an endocervical canal leading to the lower uterine segment (◆) on the right that has an erythematous appearance extending to the cervical os (□), consistent with chronic inflammation. The cervix has an underlying dense fibromuscular stroma that appears white on cut section.

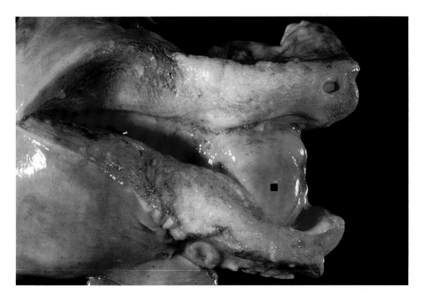

Figure 13-17 Nabothian cyst, gross
A large translucent nabothian cyst (■) extends from the stroma around the outer endocervical canal in an exophytic manner into the canal. Inflammation with cervicitis may produce submucosal gland obstruction so that glandular cystic dilation occurs. These cysts are filled with a clear, mucoid fluid. These are common lesions, generally ranging from a few millimeters to 1 cm in size. They are benign.

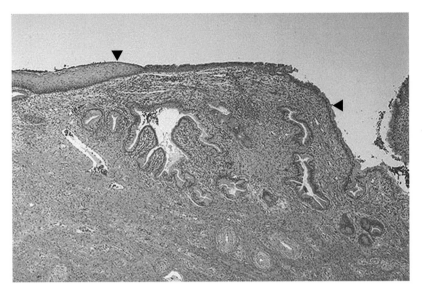

Figure 13-18 Normal cervical transformation zone, microscopic
Normal cervix with stratified nonkeratinizing squamous epithelium (▼) merges at the transformation zone (squamocolumnar junction) into endocervix lined by tall mucinous columnar cells (◀), as shown here at low magnification. The endocervix has underlying endocervical glands in the stroma that are also lined by tall mucinous columnar cells.

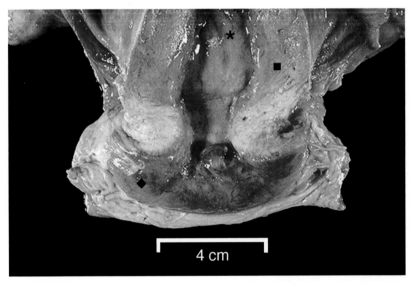

Figure 13-19 Chronic cervicitis, gross
Chronic cervicitis typically begins at the squamocolumnar junction of the cervix and can extend to involve the ectocervical squamous epithelium. The uterus has been opened anteriorly here to reveal the endocervical canal (★) and lower uterine segment (■). Note the erythematous appearance (◆) of this inflamed cervical epithelium. During reproductive years, estrogen levels promote maturation with glycogen uptake of cervical and vaginal squamous epithelium, and this glycogen provides a substrate for the normal vaginal bacterial flora that keeps the pH low to inhibit proliferation of pathogenic organisms.

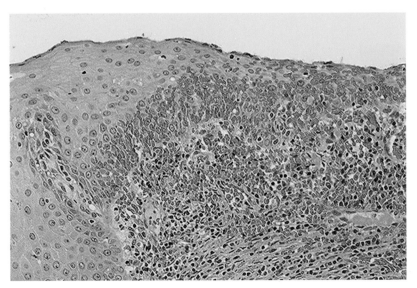

Figure 13-20 Chronic cervicitis, microscopic
Chronic cervicitis, shown here at the squamocolumnar junction of the cervix, has small, round, dark-blue lymphocytes in the submucosa; there is also hemorrhage. Chronic cervicitis is quite common. Common bacterial organisms, including streptococci, staphylococci, enterococci, and coliforms, and the fungus *Candida* and the protozoan *Trichomonas vaginalis* may contribute to cervicitis and vaginitis, which typically have a clinical course marked by episodes of acute inflammation that blend into chronic inflammation. The repair reaction to the inflamed and eroded epithelium may produce mildly atypical–appearing cells ("inflammatory" atypia) on a Pap smear.

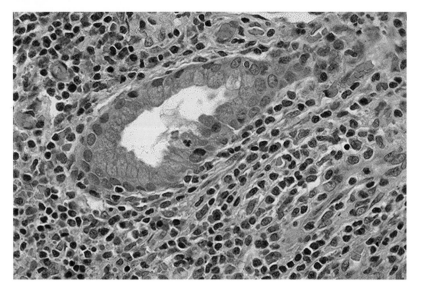

Figure 13-21 Chronic cervicitis, microscopic
A predominantly lymphocytic infiltrate extends around this endocervical gland in the stroma of the cervix beneath the epithelium. Epithelial erosion, ulceration, and repair may accompany this inflammation. There is some degree of cervicitis in nearly all women, but the amount of inflammation is minimal, and usually no significant health problems are related to it.

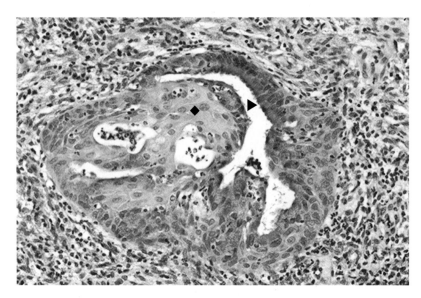

Figure 13-22 Cervical squamous metaplasia, microscopic
In this endocervical gland, the normal columnar epithelium (▶) is transforming to a squamous-appearing epithelium (♦) as a consequence of the ongoing inflammatory process. Metaplasia is a potentially reversible process in which one type of epithelium is exchanged for the normal epithelium. Metaplasia may be the first step in epithelial cellular alteration leading to dysplasia.

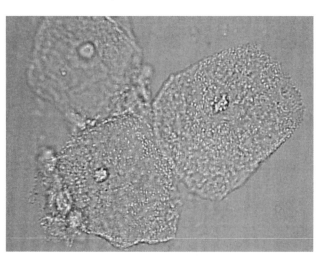

Figure 13-23 Bacterial vaginosis, wet mount, microscopic
The squamous epithelial cells shown have refractile bacteria plastered over their surfaces, a morphologic appearance called *clue cells* (their appearance is a clue to the diagnosis) and indicative of bacterial vaginosis. Normal vaginal flora includes large gram-positive rods of lactobacilli. Bacterial vaginosis includes gram-negative cocci of *Gardnerella* species and small curved rods of *Mobiluncus* species. Inflammatory cells and infectious agents such as *Candida albicans,* trichomonads, and clue cells of bacterial vaginosis (e.g., *Gardnerella vaginalis*) can be seen on a Pap smear.

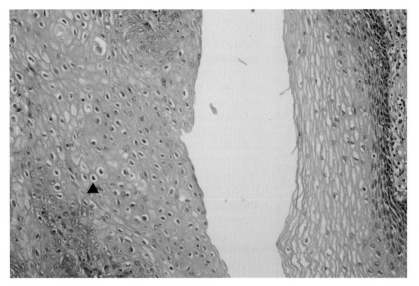

Figure 13-24 Human papillomavirus effect, microscopic

This cervical biopsy specimen shows a thickened squamous epithelium at the left with a vacuolated appearance (▲), called *koilocytotic change* (compare with normal cervical epithelium at the right). Condyloma acuminatum of external genitalia has a similar appearance. These changes typically result from HPV infection. Most healthy women clear an HPV infection after several years. HPV can be subtyped into high-risk and low-risk varieties. High-risk varieties include HPV subtypes 16 and 18. The E6 and E7 oncoproteins in these HPV subtypes bind to p53 and promote its degradation, whereas E7 binds to RB and upregulates DNA synthesis.

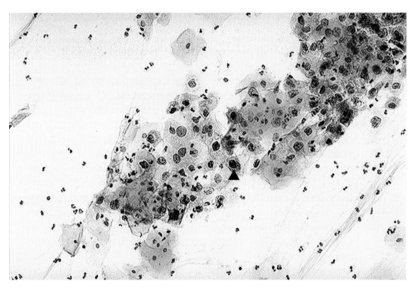

Figure 13-25 Cervical squamous dysplasia, Pap smear

Pap smear screening has reduced the incidence of and death rate from cervical carcinoma because dysplasias and early carcinomas can be detected and treated to prevent invasive carcinomas. The cytologic features of normal squamous epithelial cells can be seen at the center top and bottom, with orange to pale blue, platelike squamous cells that have small pyknotic nuclei. The dysplastic cells in the center extending to the upper right are smaller overall with darker, more irregular nuclei (▲). Dysplastic lesions are classified as grades I, II, or III cervical intraepithelial neoplasia (CIN). CNI I may be termed low-grade squamous intraepithelial lesion (LSIL), while CIN II and III are consistent with a high-grade squamous intraepithelial lesion (HSIL).

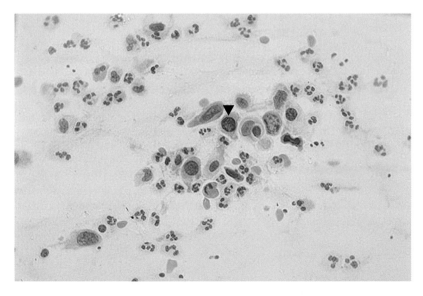

Figure 13-26 Cervical squamous carcinoma, Pap smear

This Pap smear shows more pleomorphic, darker, and larger cells (▼) indicative of a carcinoma. The inflammation and hemorrhage in the background are characteristic of a more aggressive, ulcerative, and invasive lesion. It is essential to follow up an abnormal Pap smear showing CIN or carcinoma with a biopsy and treatment. Risk factors for cervical neoplasia include early age at first intercourse, multiple sexual partners, increased parity, male sexual partners with multiple previous sexual partners, and exposure to high-risk HPV subtypes 16 and 18.

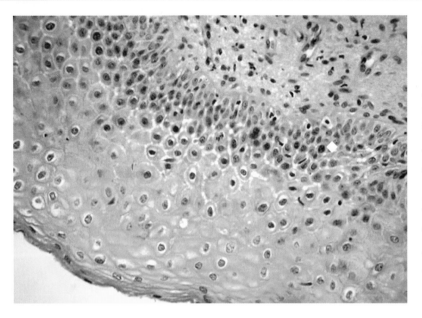

Figure 13-27 Cervical intraepithelial neoplasia grade I, microscopic
In this biopsy sample, the dysplastic, disordered cells (◆) occupy less than one third of the squamous epithelial thickness above the basal lamina, so this is CIN I. Note the koilocytotic change in some cells, consistent with HPV effect. The term *atypical squamous cells of undetermined significance* (ASCUS) may be applied in some Pap smear reports when there are abnormal cells but a CIN classification is impossible, and further follow-up is warranted. The term *squamous intraepithelial lesion* (SIL) may also be used in Pap smear reports, and CIN I typically correlates with a low-grade squamous intraepithelial lesion (LSIL).

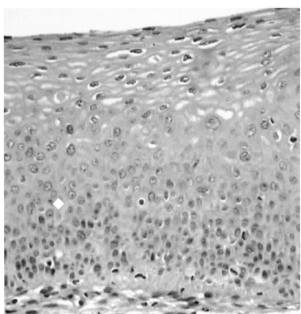

Figure 13-28 Cervical intraepithelial neoplasia grade II, microscopic
In this cervical biopsy sample, the dysplastic, disordered cells (◆) occupy about one third to one half the thickness of the epithelium, and the basal lamina is still intact, so this is CIN II. Moderate to severe dysplasias (CIN II and III) tend to correlate with a high-grade squamous intraepithelial lesion (HSIL) and infection with more aggressive forms of HPV. There is continued expression of *E6/E7* oncogenes with destabilizing influences on the cell cycle. There is upregulation of *p16/INK4* with increased expression of *p16*, a cyclin-dependent kinase inhibitor. Nevertheless, dysplasias tend to progress over many years, giving plenty of opportunity to find early lesions with periodic Pap smear screening and to treat with excision of the dysplastic areas. Colposcopy may aid in detection of the abnormal areas for removal.

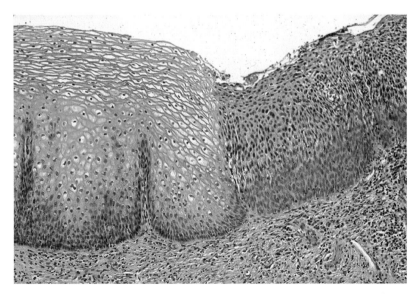

Figure 13-29 HSIL (CIN III), microscopic
In this biopsy specimen, there is severe cervical squamous dysplasia extending from the center to the right, compared with nondysplastic epithelium at the left. Note how the dysplastic cell nuclei are larger and darker, and the dysplastic cells have a disorderly arrangement within the epithelium. This dysplastic process involves the full thickness of the epithelium, but the basal lamina is intact, so this is an HSIL, also designated as severe dysplasia/carcinoma in situ (CIS) under the CIN III heading. HSIL has significant risk for progression to invasive carcinoma.

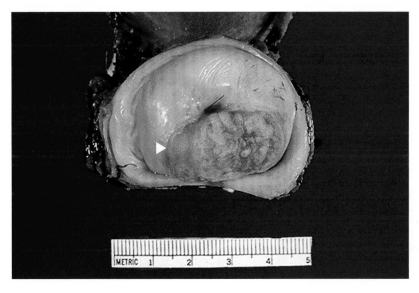

Figure 13-30 Squamous cell carcinoma, gross

This hysterectomy specimen shows the gross appearance of a cervical squamous cell carcinoma (▶) that is still limited to the cervix (stage I). The 5-year survival rate for CIN is essentially 100%, and it is more than 95% for microinvasive carcinomas (stage Ia). Five-year survival rates of 80% to 90% occur when the neoplasm is more invasive but still confined to the cervix (stage Ib). The tumor appearing here from the 3 o'clock to 7 o'clock positions around the cervical os is a red to tan to yellow mass that is exophytic (growing outward and extending above the surrounding normal smooth tan epithelium). There is a natural history of progression of dysplasia to carcinoma. Cervical carcinomas may begin appearing in the second decade, but the peak incidence is in the fifth decade.

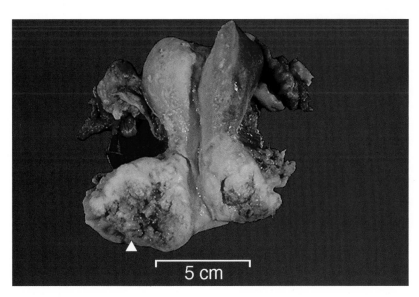

Figure 13-31 Squamous cell carcinoma, gross

This total abdominal hysterectomy with bilateral salpingo-oophorectomy (TAH-BSO) on sectioning in half shows an advanced cervical squamous cell carcinoma (▲) that has spread to the vagina. This stage II cervical carcinoma has extended beyond the cervix, but not to the pelvic side wall. The 5-year survival rate is 75%. In stage III, the carcinoma has spread to the pelvic side wall, and the 5-year survival is less than 50%.

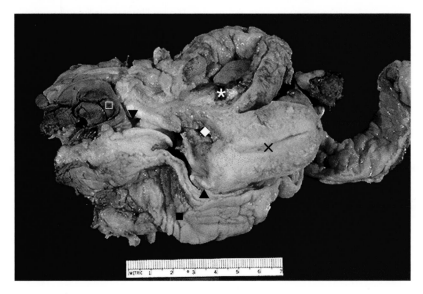

Figure 13-32 Squamous cell carcinoma, gross

This is a pelvic exenteration done for stage IV cervical carcinoma, which involves the bladder or rectum or extends beyond the true pelvis. On the left, dark vulvar skin (□) leads to the vagina (▼) and to the cervix (▲) in the center, where an irregular tan tumor mass (◆) is infiltrating upward into the bladder (✱). A slitlike endometrial cavity (✕) is surrounded by myometrium at the mid right. The rectum (■) and sigmoid colon are at the bottom extending to the right. The 5-year survival rate approaches 5%, but that is still 1 in 20, and the quality of life with a reconstructed ileal bladder and colostomy (or Koch pouch) after exenteration is adequate for an active lifestyle. Advanced cancers require a realistic, but not futile, approach.

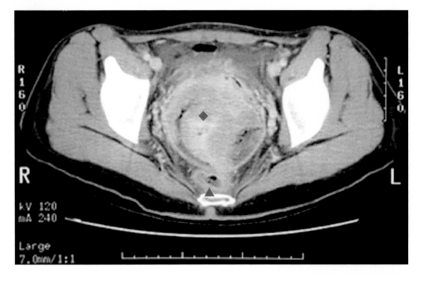

Figure 13-33 Squamous cell carcinoma, CT scan

CT scan of the pelvis shows a large mass (◆) with heterogeneous attenuation from necrosis and air-filled spaces arising in the cervix and extending anteriorly to the bladder (▼) and posteriorly to the rectum (▲). This squamous cell carcinoma of the cervix has invaded the rectum and bladder and is stage IV.

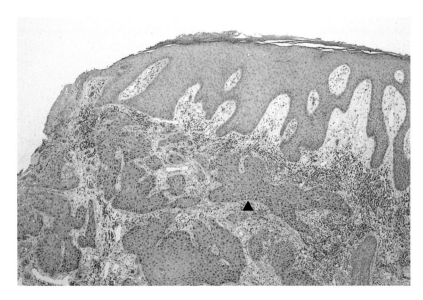

Figure 13-34 Squamous cell carcinoma, microscopic

Nests (▲) of squamous cell carcinoma are invading downward and undermining the mucosa. There is loss of the epithelial surface from ulceration at the left. Nests of neoplastic squamous cells are invading through a chronically inflamed stroma. Most cervical carcinomas are composed of large pink keratinizing or nonkeratinizing squamous cells. Less than 5% are composed of small undifferentiated cells or neuroendocrine cells. Adenocarcinomas arising in the cervix are uncommon.

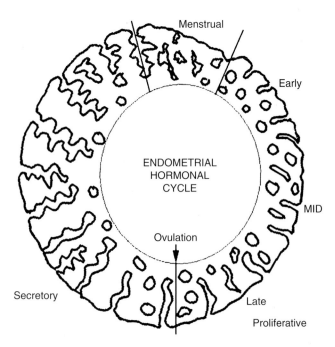

Figure 13-35 Endometrial hormonal cycle, diagram

The normal endometrial hormonal cycle is diagrammed here. The average cycle is 28 days. The proliferative (follicular) portion of the cycle varies among women but tends to remain the same for any one woman. The time from ovulation to menstruation in the secretory (luteal) portion of the cycle is a constant 14-day period. The menstrual portion of the cycle averages 3 to 7 days. The menstrual cycle is controlled by follicle-stimulating hormone (FSH) and luteinizing hormone (LH) secretion from the adenohypophysis, which is under negative feedback control by ovarian steroids, mainly estradiol, and by inhibin (which selectively suppresses FSH). FSH secretion is inhibited as estrogen levels increase about 8 to 10 days before ovulation. In the latter half of the follicular phase, LH begins to increase, reaching a peak, along with estradiol secretion, that is driven by positive feedback from increasing progesterone levels, to trigger ovulation. The luteal phase is marked by decreasing FSH and LH with increasing progesterone and estrogen levels. If fertilization does not occur, estrogen and progesterone levels decrease to trigger menses with sloughing of the stratum functionale layer of endometrium.

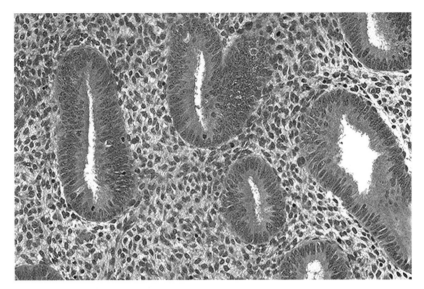

Figure 13-36 Endometrium, proliferative, microscopic

The proliferative (follicular) phase is the variable part of the menstrual cycle but averages about 14 days. In this phase, tubular endometrial glands lined by tall columnar cells and surrounded by a dense stroma are proliferating to build up the amount of functional endometrium after the previous cycle with shedding from menstruation. Mitoses within these proliferating glands can be seen.

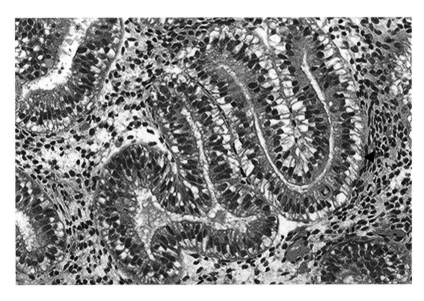

Figure 13-37 Endometrium, early secretory, microscopic

This appearance with prominent subnuclear vacuoles (◄) in the tall columnar cells lining these larger endometrial glands is consistent with postovulatory day 2 of the luteal phase of the menstrual cycle. The histologic changes after ovulation are constant over the next 14 days to menstruation and can be used to date the endometrium with biopsy for diagnostic purposes.

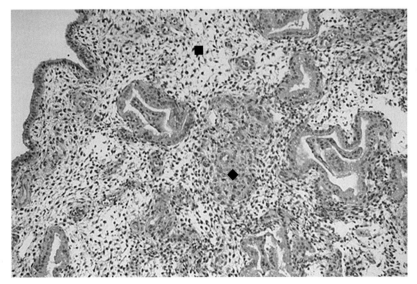

Figure 13-38 Endometrium, mid-secretory, microscopic

The mid-secretory endometrium of the normal menstrual cycle shows prominent stromal edema (■). The endometrial glands are becoming larger and more tortuous as well. Some of the stromal cells have pink cytoplasm, representing the decidualizing effect (◆) of the increasing estrogen and progesterone levels in the luteal phase of the cycle after the LH surge with ovulation.

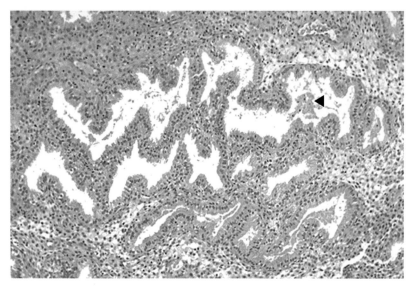

Figure 13-39 Endometrium, late secretory, microscopic
The tortuosity of the endometrial glands is apparent in this late secretory endometrium of the luteal phase of the normal menstrual cycle, and there are intraluminal secretions (◄) within the glands. There is more pronounced pink decidualization of the surrounding stroma. Such an endometrium is now able to support implantation of a fertilized ovum.

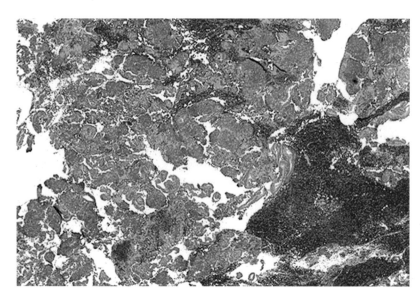

Figure 13-40 Endometrium, menstrual, microscopic
The menstrual phase endometrium is marked by breakdown of the glands and stroma from apoptosis triggered by declining estrogen and progesterone levels. There is hemorrhage and leukocyte infiltration. The upper two thirds of the endometrium, the functionale layer, is shed. From the lower third, the basale layer, which does not respond in similar manner to the ovarian hormones, will arise a new endometrial lining in the next cycle.

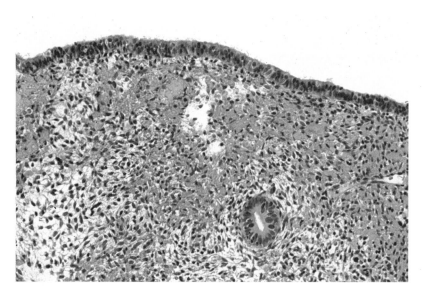

Figure 13-41 Endometrium, anovulatory cycle, microscopic
Dysfunctional uterine bleeding is most often caused by anovulatory cycles, which are most apt to occur during the reproductive years just after menarche and just before menopause. Endocrine abnormalities of the pituitary or ovary may also be implicated, as may obesity or any chronic disease state. The failure of ovulation leads to an inadequate luteal phase with prolonged estrogenic stimulation without the progestational phase. This produces a persistent proliferative endometrial pattern and eventual stromal breakdown with bleeding. The biopsy sample shown here, on what should be postovulatory day 8, shows minimal glandular development and stromal hemorrhage.

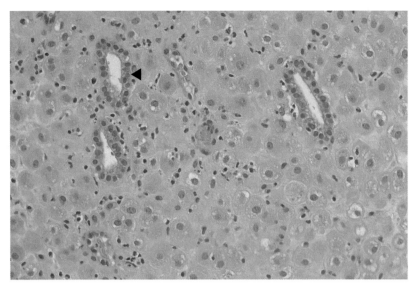

Figure 13-42 Endometrium, oral contraceptive effect, microscopic
The endometrial stroma here is markedly decidualized, with large cells having abundant pink cytoplasm, whereas the few endometrial glands (◄) are small and inactive. These changes prevent successful implantation of the blastocyst, but the primary effect of contraceptive agents is prevention of ovulation. The effect on the endometrium is not permanent, and the endometrium returns to normal cyclic changes when the oral contraceptives are discontinued.

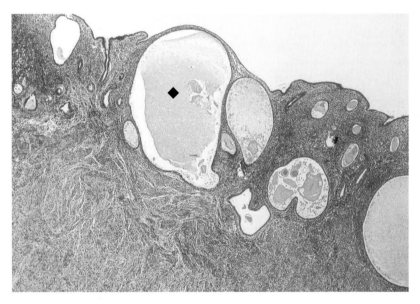

Figure 13-43 Endometrium, postmenopausal, microscopic
Note the thin endometrial layer with dense stroma containing small tubular endometrial glands scattered amid other cystically dilated glands (◆) that are lined by flat, atrophic-appearing epithelial cells. After menopause, which typically occurs in the late 40s to early 50s, there is reduced ovarian function with subsequent loss of regular hormonal cycles and decreased ovarian output of the estrogen and progesterone necessary to drive endometrial growth and cycling. Levels of FSH and LH from the pituitary increase as a result of the loss of the feedback loop through the ovaries.

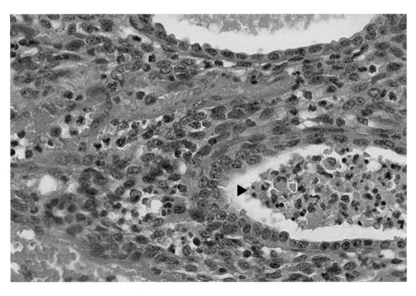

Figure 13-44 Acute endometritis, microscopic
There are scattered neutrophils (►) within these endometrial glands and stroma, indicative of acute endometritis, a condition that is most often a complication of childbirth (puerperal sepsis or postpartum fever); causative organisms include group B *Streptococcus* and *Staphylococcus aureus*. Retained products of conception after delivery increase the risk for endometritis. With good obstetric care, this condition is uncommon, but throughout human history it has accounted for significant maternal morbidity and mortality. Chlamydial infections also may produce an acute or chronic endometritis.

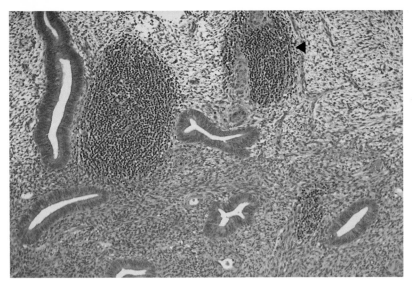

Figure 13-45 Chronic endometritis, microscopic

Collections of lymphocytes (◄) within the endometrial stroma are shown. At higher magnification, plasma cells would be identified. Chronic endometritis is present to a milder degree when an intrauterine device is present (the low-grade inflammation induced by some of these devices, designed to create a spermicidal environment, secondarily prevents implantation). The more marked inflammation shown here can occur postpartum, typically with retained products of conception, after abortion, or with chronic pelvic inflammatory disease (PID). In one sixth of patients, there is no definable cause. Affected women can have pelvic pain, fever, vaginal discharge, and infertility.

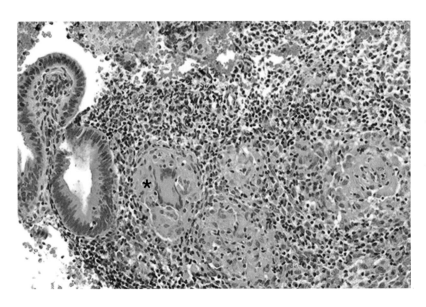

Figure 13-46 Granulomatous endometritis, microscopic

The endometrial stroma contains ill-defined granulomas (★) with epithelioid cells having abundant pink cytoplasm. Note the Langhans giant cell. The granulomatous form of chronic endometritis shown is caused by drainage of tuberculous salpingitis into the endometrial cavity. This can occur in a patient with disseminated tuberculosis.

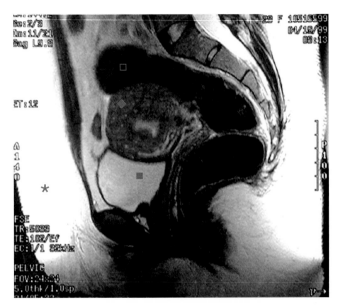

Figure 13-47 Adenomyosis, MRI

In this T2-weighted MRI image of the pelvis in sagittal view, the uterus shows abnormally low T2 signal intensity with obliteration of the junctional zone, consistent with adenomyosis (◆). The uterus is enlarged by this process. The bladder anteriorly (■) is filled with bright contrast material, whereas the sigmoid (□) and rectum posteriorly appear dark. Note the normal appearance of the sacrum (✚). This obese patient has abundant subcutaneous adipose tissue (✱).

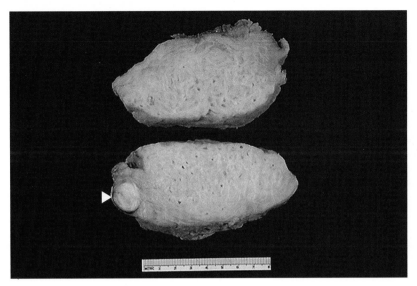

Figure 13-48 Adenomyosis, gross
The thickened and spongy-appearing myometrial wall of this sectioned uterus is typical of adenomyosis, a condition in which endometrial glands with (or without) stroma are located within the myometrium. Twenty percent of uteri examined after hysterectomy have some degree of adenomyosis, usually not as florid as in this case. The uterus may be enlarged, usually symmetrically, and there may be menometrorrhagia, dysmenorrhea, dyspareunia, or pelvic pain. (An incidental small round white leiomyoma [▶] also is shown.)

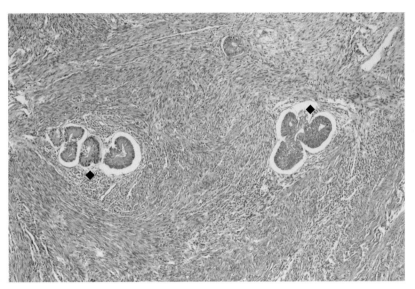

Figure 13-49 Adenomyosis, microscopic
Down-growth of the endometrium more than 2 mm from the stratum basale into the myometrium may account for adenomyosis. In this section through the myometrium, a cluster of endometrial tissue can be seen with glands (◆) and surrounding stroma, typical of adenomyosis. Because these foci are derived from the endometrial stratum basale, there is usually no significant bleeding within the foci themselves. This condition can lead to uterine enlargement and menorrhagia, dysmenorrhea, and pelvic pain.

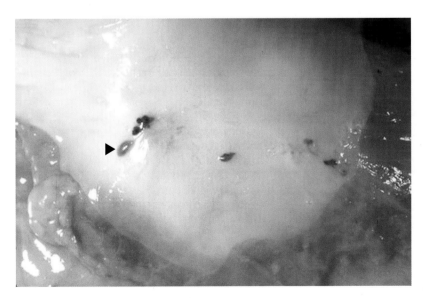

Figure 13-50 Endometriosis, gross
About 10% of women have endometrial glands and stroma found outside the uterus, a very disabling and painful condition, even when just a few of these small foci are present. Clinical features include dysmenorrhea, dyspareunia, pelvic pain, and infertility. There is bleeding into these foci of endometriosis, and the blood is dark (from deoxygenation and from breakdown to hemosiderin), giving them the gross appearance of powder burns. The small nodular foci here (▶) are just beneath the serosa of the posterior uterus in the pouch of Douglas. Such endometriotic lesions can be identified and obliterated by cauterization during laparoscopy.

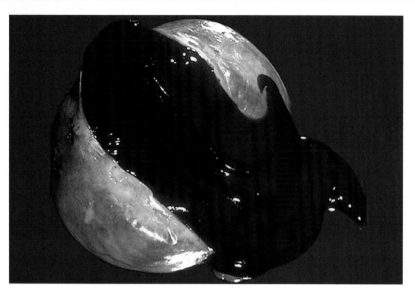

Figure 13-51 Endometriosis, gross
Typical locations for endometriosis include ovaries, uterine ligaments, rectovaginal septum, pelvic peritoneum, and laparotomy scars. Endometriosis may be found at more distant locations, such as the appendix and vagina. This is a section through an enlarged 12-cm ovary to show a cystic cavity filled with old blood typical of endometriosis with formation of an endometriotic or chocolate cyst. The chocolate cyst is so named because the old blood in the cystic space formed by the hemorrhage is broken down to produce hemosiderin, which has a brown-to-black color.

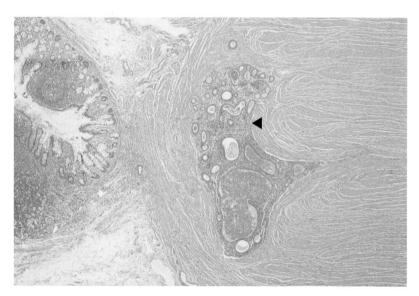

Figure 13-52 Endometriosis, microscopic
A focus of endometriosis (◄) with a small cluster of endometrial glands and stroma with hemorrhage appears in the center, adjacent to appendix at the left. Theories for the origin of endometriosis include metaplastic change in coelomic epithelium, regurgitation of menstrual tissue out the fallopian tube with implantation onto the peritoneum, or vascular dissemination of endometrial tissues through veins or lymphatics. Endometriotic stromal cells express high levels of aromatase that increase estrogen production, and proinflammatory cytokines such as prostaglandin are released. There is an increased risk for development of endometrioid and clear cell carcinomas in foci of endometriosis.

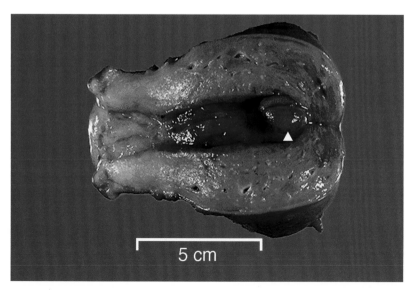

5 cm

Figure 13-53 Endometrial polyp, gross
This uterus has been opened anteriorly through the cervix and into the endometrial cavity. High in the fundus and projecting into the endometrial cavity is a small endometrial polyp (▲). Such benign polyps may ulcerate, undergo necrosis, and cause uterine bleeding. They are typically 0.5 to 3 cm in size. Some polyps may be composed of functioning endometrium, but most are associated with endometrial hyperplasia. Rarely, an endometrial carcinoma may arise within a polyp. There is an increased incidence of endometrial polyps in women treated with tamoxifen for estrogen receptor–positive breast cancer.

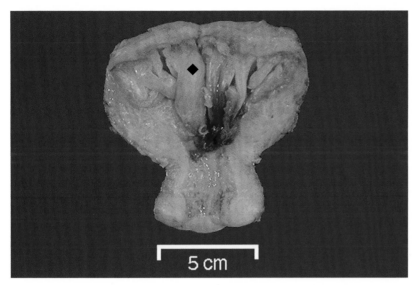

Figure 13-54 Endometrial hyperplasia, gross
This normal-sized uterus is opened to reveal an endometrial cavity filled with lush fronds (◆) of hyperplastic endometrium. Atypical hyperplasia, also known as *endometrial intraepithelial neoplasia,* usually develops under conditions of prolonged estrogen excess in conjunction with relative or absolute decreased progesterone. Hyperplasia can lead to metrorrhagia (uterine bleeding at irregular intervals), menorrhagia (excessive bleeding with menstrual periods), or menometrorrhagia. Predisposing factors include menopause, prolonged administration of estrogenic agents, estrogen-producing ovarian neoplasms, and polycystic ovary syndrome.

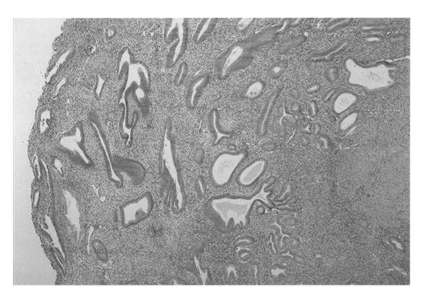

Figure 13-55 Endometrial (non-atypical) hyperplasia, microscopic
In endometrial hyperplasia, the amount of endometrium is abnormally increased and not cycling as it should. The glands are enlarged and irregular, with columnar cells that have some atypia. Some glands are cystic. This is the pattern of simple, non-atypical hyperplasia. Simple hyperplasias can cause bleeding, but these are not thought to be premalignant. Atypical (adenomatous) hyperplasia is premalignant. Excess, unopposed estrogen can lead to hyperplasia. Inactivation or deletion of the *PTEN* tumor suppressor gene makes endometrial cells more sensitive to estrogenic stimulation, driving this proliferative process.

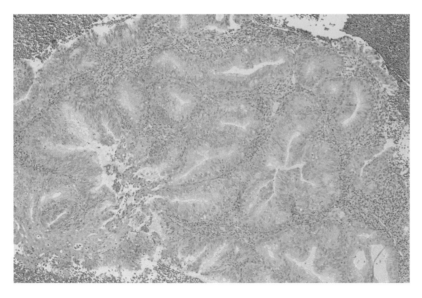

Figure 13-56 Endometrial atypical hyperplasia, microscopic
This biopsy specimen shows endometrial intraepithelial neoplasia with a complex proliferation of back-to-back glands with complex outlines and branching structures. These glands are lined by columnar cells with crowded hyperchromatic nuclei, indicating that the hyperplasia of the endometrium has atypical features. The presence of these changes increases the risk for subsequent development of endometrial carcinoma. Complex hyperplasia and endometrial carcinomas often have inactivation of the *PTEN* tumor suppressor gene. This condition can be treated by hysterectomy.

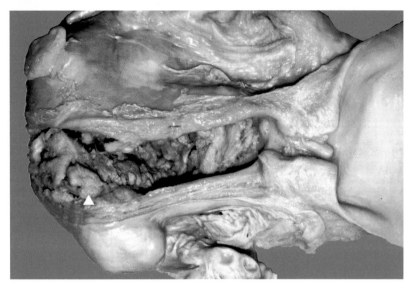

Figure 13-57 Endometrial carcinoma, gross
This uterus is not enlarged, as is often the case with many endometrial carcinomas when signs such as vaginal bleeding first appear. The irregular masses (▲) in the upper fundus can be detected by endometrial biopsy. These carcinomas are more likely to occur in postmenopausal women, with a peak incidence from 55 to 65 years. They are rare before age 40. Any postmenopausal bleeding should raise concern about the possibility of endometrial carcinoma. Any condition that increases the exposure to estrogen is associated with an increased risk. Although the overall risk for cancer increases with obesity, the strongest association of obesity and cancer occurs with endometrial carcinoma.

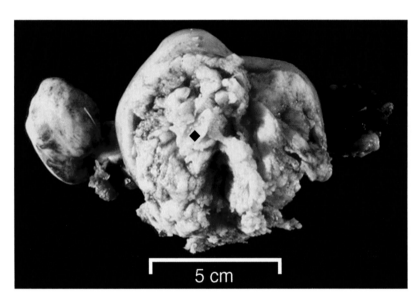

Figure 13-58 Endometrial carcinoma, gross
This total abdominal hysterectomy specimen with uterus opened anteriorly shows an advanced adenocarcinoma of the endometrium that enlarges the entire uterus. This enlargement is palpable on physical examination. Irregular masses (◆) of white tumor are filling and expanding the endometrial cavity and extending into the uterine wall. Such a neoplasm often manifests with abnormal bleeding. Endometrial carcinomas termed type I often develop in the setting of prior complex atypical endometrial hyperplasia, driven by relative estrogen excess, and increased signaling through the PI3K/AKT pathway. A less common type II subset of endometrial carcinomas arises from the surface epithelium, has *p53* mutations, and resembles serous peritoneal carcinoma.

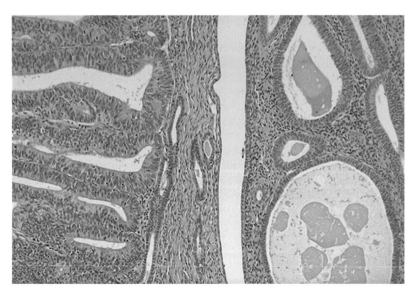

Figure 13-59 Endometrial carcinoma, type I, microscopic
The adenocarcinoma on the left is moderately differentiated because a glandular structure can still be discerned. Note the architectural atypia, cellular crowding with hyperchromatism, and pleomorphism of the cells compared with the underlying endometrium with cystic hyperplasia on the right. More than 80% of endometrial carcinomas have this endometrioid adenocarcinoma pattern, and most of these have *PTEN* mutations. The diagnosis is most often made with endometrial biopsy because exfoliated cells are unlikely to be present or diagnostic on a Pap smear. Most are detected while confined to the uterus (stage I), and the 5-year survival is about 90%.

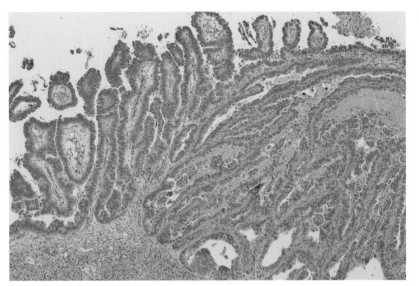

Figure 13-60 Endometrial carcinoma, type II, microscopic

The papillations with cuboidal epithelium are characteristic for the serous type of endometrial carcinoma. It occurs about 10 years later than type I and follows endometrial atrophy. It accounts for a sixth of endometrial carcinomas. *TP53* mutations are present in most of them. Like the endometrioid type I carcinomas, type II carcinoma is preceded by endometrial intraepithelial carcinoma, but it tends to invade and metastasize early. Postmenopausal bleeding may be the first sign.

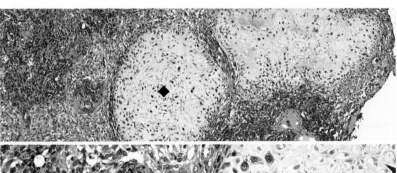

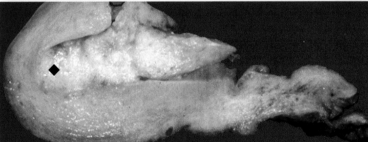

Figure 13-61 Carcinosarcoma (malignant mixed müllerian tumor), gross

This irregular, infiltrative neoplasm (◆) involves the endometrium and myometrium. These neoplasms form bulky, polypoid masses that have a fleshy cut surface. They may be so large as to protrude through the cervical os. The typical clinical presentation is similar to that of endometrial carcinoma, with postmenopausal bleeding. Some patients have had prior radiation therapy to the pelvis.

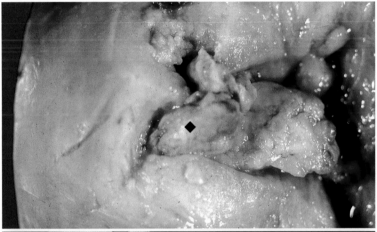

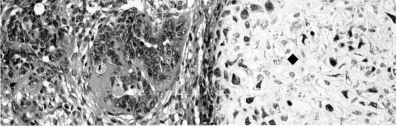

Figure 13-62 Carcinosarcoma (malignant mixed müllerian tumor), microscopic

There are carcinomatous elements along with "heterologous" sarcomatous (◆) elements (here resembling chondrosarcoma). Mutations in *PTEN, TP53,* and *PIK3CA* are typical for endometrial carcinomas. The malignant sarcomatous mesodermal components can have muscle, bone, adipose tissue, and cartilage differentiation. Most of these neoplasms act in an aggressive fashion. Metastases are most likely to have the microscopic appearance of adenocarcinoma.

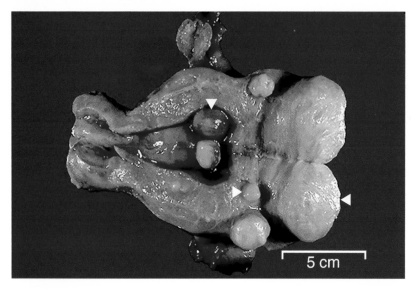

Figure 13-63 Leiomyomata, gross
Benign smooth muscle tumors of the uterus are common and often multiple—75% of women may have one. These neoplasms are sharply circumscribed, firm, and white on cut section. They are uncommon in the genital tract outside of the myometrium. Submucosal (▼), intramural (▶), and subserosal (◀) leiomyomata are shown here. Such benign tumors of the myometrium may cause irregular bleeding or infertility, if present in a submucosal location. Larger leiomyomas may also produce bleeding or pelvic discomfort, and they may cause spontaneous abortion in pregnancies. Most are asymptomatic, however.

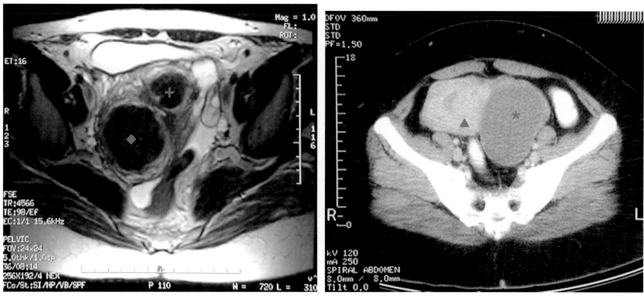

Figures 13-64 and 13-65 Leiomyomata, MRI and CT image
The pelvic axial T1-weighted MRI image in the *left panel* shows a large, nodular uterus containing a larger (◆) and smaller (✚) leiomyoma of the uterus. The CT scan in the *right panel* shows another patient with an enlarged uterus in which there is a submucosal leiomyoma (▲); the fluid-filled structure (✳) displacing the uterus to the left is an endometrioma of the left ovary.

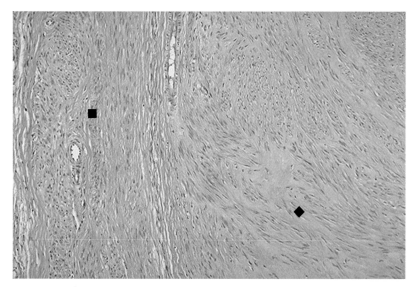

Figure 13-66 Leiomyoma, microscopic
Interlacing bundles of uniform spindle cells resembling smooth muscle compose this benign leiomyoma (◆). Mitoses do not appear here (and are rare in leiomyomas). Normal myometrium is on the left, and the neoplasm is so well differentiated that the leiomyoma hardly appears different from the normal myometrium (■). Leiomyomas may undergo enlargement during the reproductive years, then regress after menopause. Larger leiomyomas may have central softening with hemorrhage (red degeneration). Although cytogenetic abnormalities such as chromosome 12q14 and 6p rearrangements can be identified within these tumors, as well as *MED12* gene mutations, malignant transformation is quite rare, which is fortunate, given their prevalence.

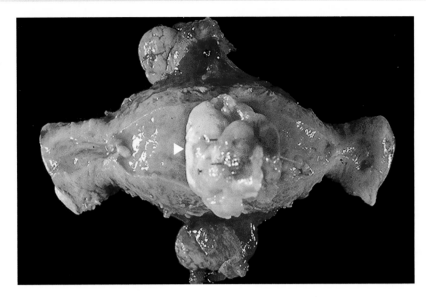

Figure 13-67 Leiomyosarcoma, gross
This total abdominal hysterectomy specimen reveals a large, bulky, polypoid, exophytic mass (▶) protruding from the myometrium into the endometrial cavity. (An endophytic growth pattern would produce extensive myometrial invasion.) This uterus has been opened coronally so that the halves of the cervix appear at right and left. Fallopian tubes and ovaries project from top and bottom. The irregular nature of this mass suggests that it is not just an ordinary leiomyoma. Leiomyosarcomas are much less common than leiomyomas, and they do not tend to arise from leiomyomas, though both often have *MED12* mutations. Their biologic behavior is unpredictable, but the larger and less differentiated tumors tend to recur or metastasize.

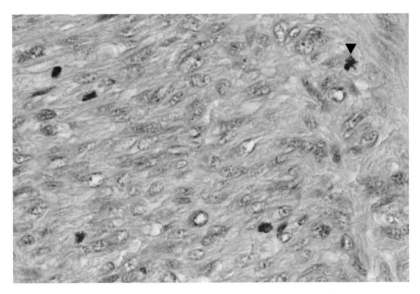

Figure 13-68 Leiomyosarcoma, microscopic
This malignant smooth muscle neoplasm is much more cellular than a leiomyoma, and the cells shown here display pleomorphism and hyperchromatism. Multiple mitoses (▼) are present—five in just one field. The degree of cellular atypia, the number of mitoses (five per 10 high-power microscopic fields), and the presence of zonal necrosis aid in making this diagnosis. These neoplasms arise most commonly in the fifth to seventh decades. They have a tendency to recur and metastasize.

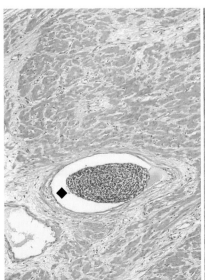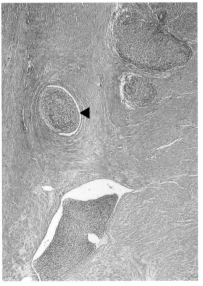

Figure 13-69 Endometrial stromal sarcoma, microscopic
In the *left panel* is a dilated myometrial lymphatic space (◆) containing stromal cells, a low-grade stromal sarcoma. In the *right panel* there is more extensive stromal proliferation (◀) within lymphatic spaces, with invasion into surrounding myometrium, typical of high-grade endometrial stromal sarcoma. Half of stromal sarcomas recur after resection.

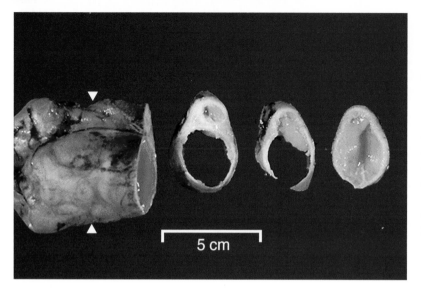

Figure 13-70 Tubo-ovarian abscess, gross
This condition followed *Neisseria gonorrhoeae* infection, although other organisms, including *Chlamydia trachomatis,* can cause this disease. Gonorrhea leads to multiple complications in the female genital tract, including acute inflammation with abscess formation and chronic inflammation with tubal scarring (and a greater likelihood of ectopic pregnancy) and PID. There is no clear boundary here between tube (▼) and ovary (▲), and this dilated ovary on sectioning is filled with purulent material.

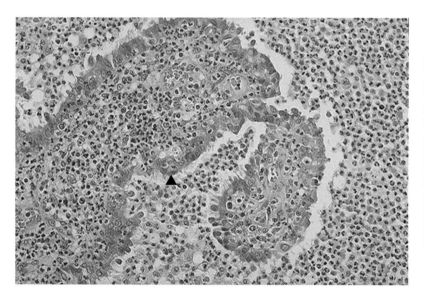

Figure 13-71 Acute salpingitis, microscopic
A remnant of tubal epithelium (▲) is surrounded and infiltrated by numerous neutrophils. *N. gonorrhoeae* was cultured. The next most likely causative organism for this acute suppurative process is *C. trachomatis.* Multiple pyogenic bacterial species may be present with acute salpingitis that evolves to PID, including enteric bacteria, staphylococci, streptococci, and clostridia. Clinical findings include pelvic pain and fever. Infertility may result from this process. Laboratory findings include leukocytosis with a left shift.

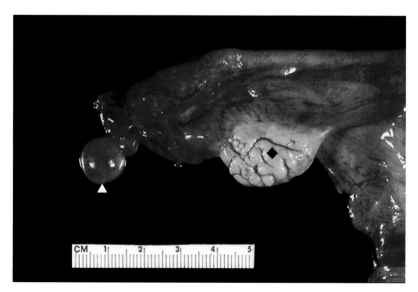

Figure 13-72 Paratubal cyst, gross
This small fluid-filled cyst (▲) is a common incidental finding. It is an embryologic remnant of the müllerian duct. Sometimes such simple cysts are found adjacent to the ovary (◆) and are called *parovarian cysts*. They are filled with clear serous fluid and lined by flattened cuboidal epithelium. They can range from barely visible to about 2 cm in size. This cyst at the fimbriated end of the tube (or in broad ligament) may also be designated as a *hydatid of Morgagni.*

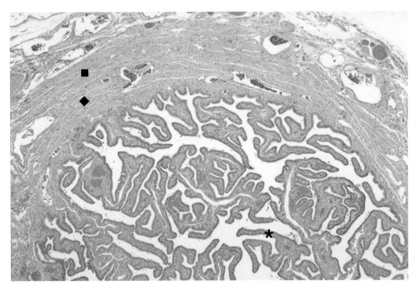

Figure 13-73 Normal fallopian tube, microscopic
Note the smooth muscular coat composed of ill-defined inner circular (◆) and outer longitudinal (■) layers, and an inner complex branching pattern of finger-like projections (★) of connective tissue lined by a tall columnar epithelium. Some epithelial cells have cilia. Some of the cilia beat upward to help sperm ascend, whereas others beat downward to conduct ova toward the uterus. Some epithelial cells with a secretory function are called *peg cells.* The secretion products of peg cells function in capacitation of spermatozoa, which causes them to mature and become capable of fertilizing any ovum lurking in the tube. (Few sperm get this far, because, being male, they don't ask for directions.)

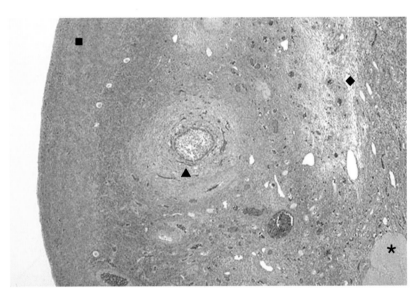

Figure 13-74 Normal adult ovary, microscopic
The adult ovary consists of a cortex (■) and a medulla (◆). A mesothelium, also known as the *germinal epithelium,* surrounds the ovary. The outer cortex consists mainly of a stroma, or interstitium, composed of small fusiform cells that can transform under hormonal influence to support the developing ova. The normal adult cortex contains only scattered ova and consists mainly of stroma. A primordial follicle (▲) consists of just the oocyte surrounded by a flattened layer of stromal cells. Shown here at low magnification is ovarian cortex with abundant dense stroma and few follicles. A developing primary follicle with prominent granulosa cells appears near the center. At the lower right is a pink cloudlike corpus albicans (★).

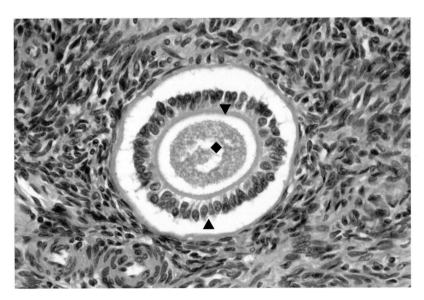

Figure 13-75 Normal ovary, microscopic
Shown here is a primary ovarian follicle with the central ovum (◆) and surrounding thin zona pellucida (▼) through which sperm must pass to fertilize the ovum. A layer of granulosa cells (▲) is present. Surrounding the follicle are theca cells. The number of follicles begins to decrease even before birth. Beginning in late gestation and throughout childhood, ova disappear, until at the time of reproductive maturity at menarche, less than a few hundred ova remain in each ovary, which can be released during each menstrual cycle throughout the next 30 to 40 reproductive years.

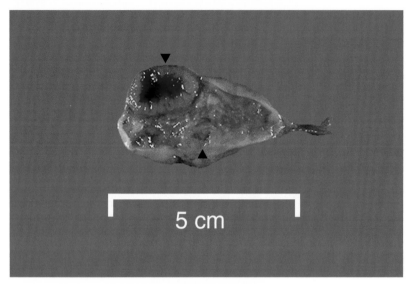

Figure 13-76 Corpus luteum, gross
An adult ovary with two prominent yellow corpora lutea is shown. The larger one (▼) at the top bulging from the surface is a hemorrhagic corpus luteum of menstruation, and the smaller one (▲) at the bottom is involuting after a previous menstrual period. If implantation of a fertilized ovum occurs, the corpus luteum persists because of human chorionic gonadotropin (HCG) elaborated from the developing placenta. Of 400,000 ovarian follicles present at birth, only about 400 mature to the point of ovulation during childbearing years.

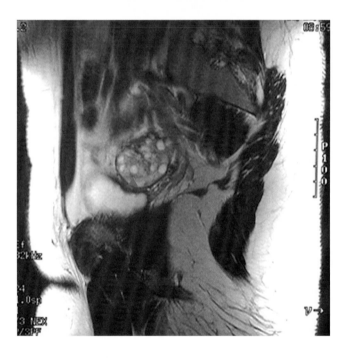

Figure 13-77 Polycystic ovary, MRI
This T1-weighted sagittal MRI image of the pelvis shows multiple small, peripheral, fluid-filled cysts (▲) of an enlarged ovary consistent with polycystic ovarian syndrome (PCOS). The cysts average 0.5 to 1 cm in size. Clinical findings include anovulatory cycles with oligomenorrhea or amenorrhea, acne, and hirsutism. PCOS may be related to insulin resistance, and half of patients are obese, often with type 2 diabetes mellitus. An increased LH pulse frequency results in increased LH secretion and decreased FSH (altered LH/FSH ratio), driving androgen production by follicles with elevated serum testosterone. The decreased FSH is not enough to convert testosterone to estradiol adequately and does not sustain follicular maturation, but because FSH is not totally depressed, new follicular growth occurs, although not to the point of full maturation and ovulation. Multiple cysts result. There is an increased risk for hyperlipidemia and heart disease, endometrial cancer, and pregnancy loss.

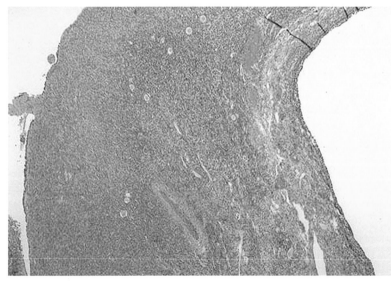

Figure 13-78 Polycystic ovarian syndrome, microscopic
Polycystic ovarian syndrome (PCOS) is characterized by ovarian enlargement with thickening of the outer cortex (at left) and many follicle cysts (a large one is at the right). A variation of this syndrome is known as *stromal thecosis,* or *cortical stromal hyperplasia*. There are no cysts, but only a cortex up to 7 cm thick containing many luteinized stromal cells. A physiologic response to elevated gonadotropins in pregnancy can lead to theca lutein hyperplasia of pregnancy.

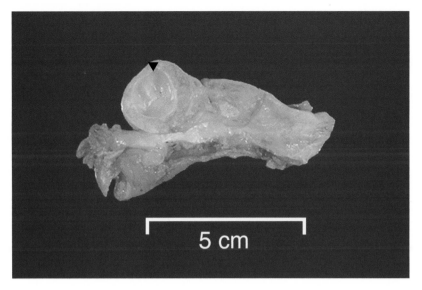

Figure 13-79 Follicle cyst, gross
A benign follicular cyst (▼) is shown, which is larger than a normal developing cystic follicle. Such cysts can be multiple. They contain clear fluid. Occasionally such cysts may reach several centimeters in size and if they rupture can cause abdominal pain. They represent unruptured graafian follicles or follicles that ruptured in ovulation and immediately sealed.

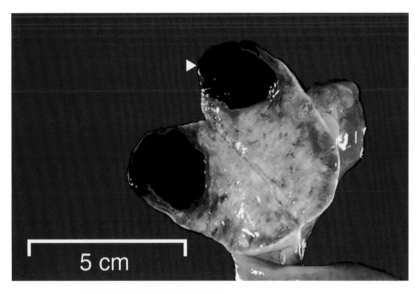

Figure 13-80 Hemorrhagic corpus luteum, gross
This normal adult ovary has been sectioned to reveal a hemorrhagic corpus luteum (▶). Note the dark red-black hemorrhagic region surrounded by a thin rim of yellow corpus luteum. This appearance may be present after ovulation. The hemorrhage may produce lower abdominal or pelvic pain. Larger luteal cysts that persist may resemble the chocolate cysts of endometriosis.

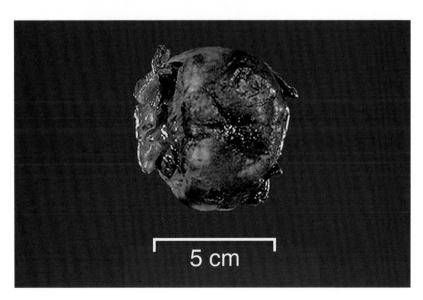

Figure 13-81 Ovarian torsion, gross
This ovary is dark and enlarged from hemorrhage after torsion on its ligament. Torsion of the ovary is uncommon but may occur in adults in conjunction with benign ovarian cysts or neoplasms, and in children or infants spontaneously. Some cases occur during pregnancy. It leads to a presentation similar to that of acute appendicitis, but this adnexal mass may be palpable on examination. The disruption of the blood supply results in hemorrhagic infarction and loss of ovarian function.

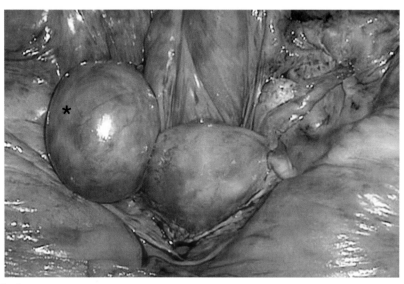

Figure 13-82 Serous cystadenoma, gross

Shown here in the pelvis adjacent to the uterus in the midline is a smooth-surfaced tumor (✷) arising from ovarian müllerian surface epithelium—a serous cystadenoma—of the right ovary. Such tumors can reach a large size because they grow slowly and do not impinge on surrounding structures until they are quite large. They may cause some local discomfort. They are typically unilocular cysts filled with serous fluid. Benign and borderline serous tumors most often occur between the ages of 20 and 45. The left ovary here is atrophic, consistent with a normal postmenopausal state. The uterus is also normal in size.

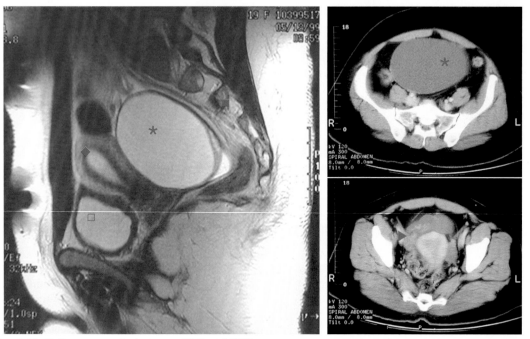

Figures 13-83 and 13-84 Serous cystadenoma, MRI and CT image

In the *left panel,* a sagittal T1-weighted pelvic MRI image shows a large fluid-filled mass (✷). The uterus (◆), bladder (□), and sacrum (■) are visualized as well. In the *upper right panel,* a large, unilocular, cystic, fluid-filled mass (✷) fills much of the pelvis in the CT scan. The inferior margin of the mass can be seen in the *lower right panel* to attach (▶) to the right ovary next to the bladder, where the wall is thickened and irregular.

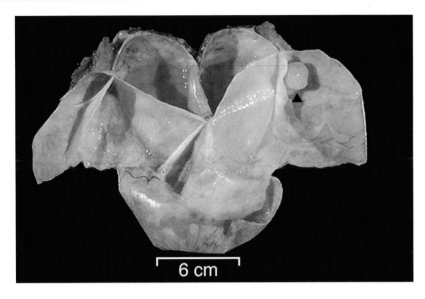

Figure 13-85 Multiloculated ovarian tumor, gross

This ovary has been sectioned to reveal multiple fluid-filled cavities, which are smooth-surfaced with a rare nodular excrescence (▲). This is a mucinous cystadenoma, and 80% of all mucinous tumors are benign. Serous and mucinous tumors of the ovary are derived from müllerian epithelium. Although slightly less common overall than serous tumors, mucinous tumors of the ovary are more likely to be multiloculated and to reach a larger size. Together, serous and mucinous tumors constitute more than half of all ovarian neoplasms (40% are serous, and 25% are mucinous).

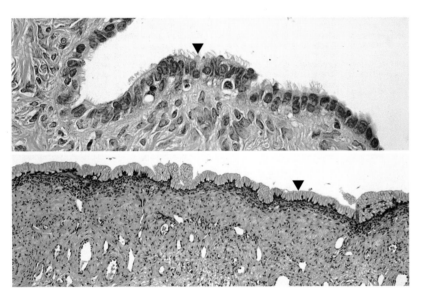

Figure 13-86 Cystadenoma, serous, mucinous, microscopic

In the *top panel* is a thin epithelial lining of tall, ciliated cuboidal cells (▼) with minimal infolding and complexity overlying a fibromuscular wall that is not invaded by these epithelial cells. Such a serous ovarian neoplasm is benign and tends to form a unilocular cyst. In the *bottom panel* the epithelium lining (▼) is mucinous, resembling endocervical mucosa, and is termed a *mucinous cystadenoma*. It would likely have a grossly multilocular appearance. Mucinous tumors have *KRAS* mutations.

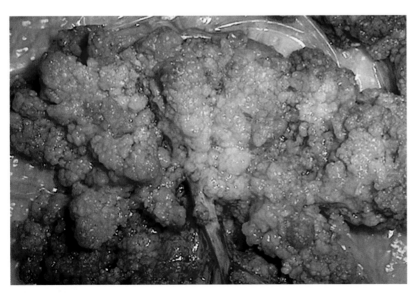

Figure 13-87 Borderline tumor, gross

This ovarian mass had a smooth surface, but on opening revealed the papillary appearance shown here. Borderline tumors have increased numbers of papillary excrescences, larger masses of solid tumor, and greater irregularity or nodularity, and microscopically have a multilayered epithelial lining with cells having some nuclear atypia. Invasion is absent. Such borderline tumors are not clearly malignant, and conservatively just the ovary can be resected. Some borderline tumors may be accompanied by implants on peritoneal surfaces, but such implants still do not invade, although they may enlarge slowly.

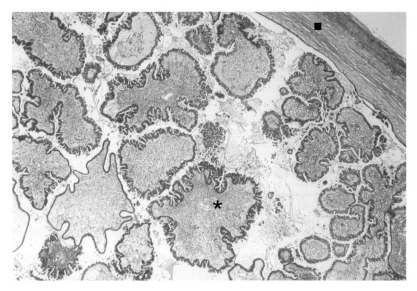

Figure 13-88 Borderline serous tumor, microscopic

Here are increased numbers of papillations (★) with complex borders, but with one or two cell layers and minimal atypia. A thick collagenous capsule (■) has not been invaded. A borderline tumor must be removed completely but is unlikely to metastasize or to recur. *KRAS, BRAF,* or *HER2* mutations are often present. *BRCA* mutations, present in about 10% of sporadic ovarian cancers, are unlikely to be present in borderline tumors.

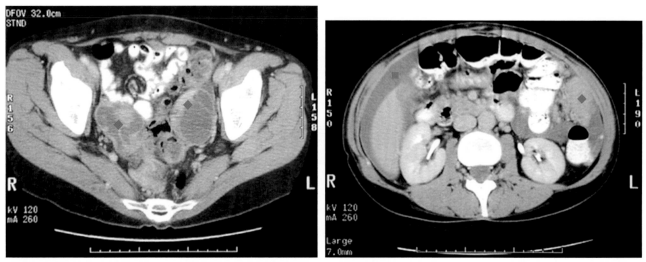

Figures 13-89 and 13-90 Cystadenocarcinoma and peritoneal metastases, CT images

The bilateral pelvic masses (◆)in the *left panel* have cystic and solid components, and they arise in the region of the ovaries. These masses proved to be bilateral ovarian serous cystadenocarcinomas. In the *right panel,* the CT scan shows a mass lesion (◆) on the left lateral abdominal wall from seeding of an ovarian serous cystadenocarcinoma. Often, the first sign is abdominal enlargement with ascites. Note the ascitic fluid (■) around the liver and elsewhere in the peritoneal cavity.

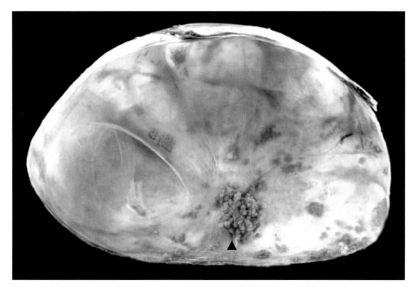

Figure 13-91 Cystadenocarcinoma, gross

Papillations (▲) are visible on the surface of the wall of this neoplasm. These invade through the wall. By the time they are detected, cystadenocarcinomas have often spread by seeding the peritoneal surfaces, giving them a more advanced stage and poorer prognosis. The ovary can expand considerably in size before symptoms or signs, such as abdominal enlargement with ascites, occur. A serum tumor marker for ovarian serous and endometrioid tumors is CA-125. Some of them are associated with *BRCA1* and *BRCA2* mutations. *TP53* mutations are usually present.

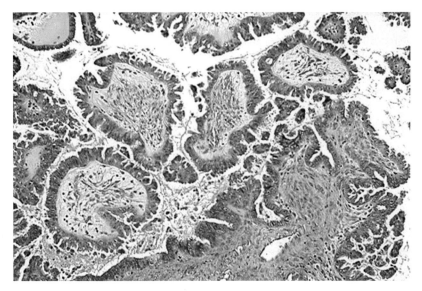

Figure 13-92 Cystadenocarcinoma, microscopic

Note the pronounced papillary growth pattern, more complex infolding, more layers of cells, and cells with more mitoses, hyperchromatism, and pleomorphism than a borderline tumor. Invasion is also likely to be present into the underlying stroma or through the capsule of the ovary with this cystadenocarcinoma.

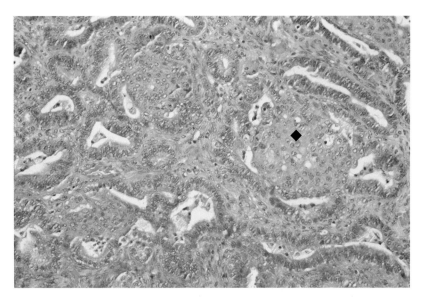

Figure 13-93 Endometrioid tumor, microscopic

This neoplasm, although arising in the ovary, resembles an endometrial carcinoma with a glandular pattern. Foci of squamous metaplasia (◆) may be present. Endometrioid tumors constitute up to 15% of all ovarian cancers. In about 15% to 30% of cases, there is synchronous occurrence of an endometrial carcinoma. About 15% of cases are associated with preexisting endometriosis. Grossly, they tend to have solid and cystic components. *PTEN* mutations are often present, and *TP53* mutations in high-grade lesions.

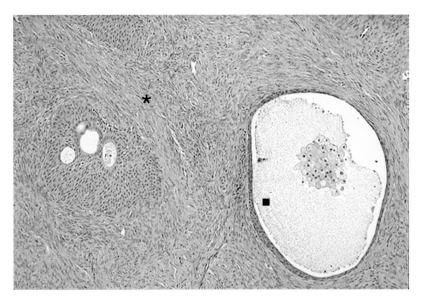

Figure 13-94 Brenner tumor, microscopic

This uncommon benign ovarian tumor, a variant of an adenofibroma, has nests of cells resembling transitional epithelium (urothelium) of the urinary bladder. These epithelial nests (■) lie within a fibrous stroma (★) resembling the stroma of a normal ovary. Grossly, they can be solid or cystic. Most are unilateral, and they range from 1 to 20 cm in size. There may be a Brenner component within a malignant cystadenocarcinoma.

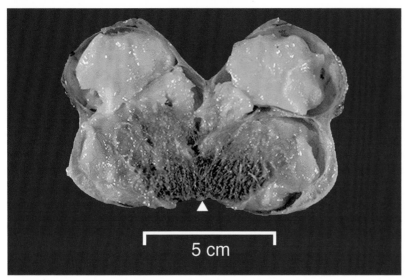

Figure 13-95 Mature cystic teratoma, gross
This cystic mass has been opened to reveal mostly ectodermal elements; the most frequently found tissue element in these cysts is skin, so large amounts of hair (▲) and sebum are produced, as shown. A variety of mature, well-differentiated tissue elements may be found from all three embryologic germ layers (ectoderm, mesoderm, and endoderm). They are often called *dermoid cysts* because they are mostly cystic ectodermal derivatives. If these tumors are mostly solid, they are often "immature" teratomas with less differentiated tissue and may behave more aggressively. Rarely, there are frankly carcinomatous areas. They are bilateral in a sixth of cases.

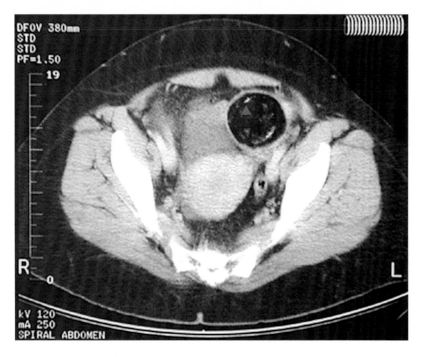

Figure 13-96 Mature cystic teratoma, CT image
There is a large but sharply circumscribed, rounded mass involving the left adnexal region of the pelvis adjacent to the uterus and next to the urinary bladder. This mass has variegated contents, including soft-tissue densities with low (dark) attenuation and bright calcification (▲). Most of the contents of this left ovarian mass have the same attenuation as the abdominal fat, indicative of the fact that most teratomas contain only mature (benign) tissue elements, mostly oily fluid elaborated by sebaceous glands. Immature teratomas have malignant elements, occur in adolescence, grow rapidly, and can metastasize. About 1% of the time, a mature teratoma can undergo malignant degeneration, typically with development of squamous cell carcinoma.

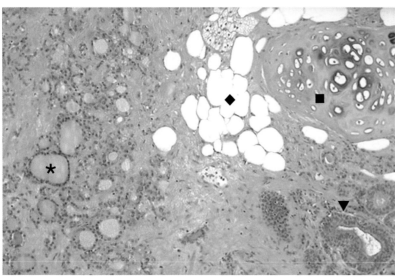

Figure 13-97 Mature cystic teratoma, microscopic
Histologically, teratomas contain tissues with differentiation that resembles all three embryonic germ layers (mesoderm, endoderm, and ectoderm). In most benign teratomas, the ectodermal elements predominate. The benign teratoma shown here contains cartilage (■), adipose tissue (♦), and intestinal glands (▼) on the right; on the left, there are numerous thyroid follicles (✶). This is a specialized form of teratoma termed *struma ovarii*. Rarely, struma ovarii can be a cause of hyperthyroidism.

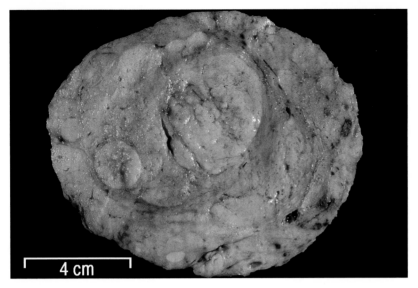

Figure 13-98 Dysgerminoma, gross

This mass is another form of ovarian germ cell tumor, which is the female counterpart of the male testicular seminoma. This cut surface reveals a lobulated tan appearance. Such tumors are usually solid. Only 10% to 20% are bilateral. They occur most often in young women in their second and third decades. They may express *OCT-3, OCT-4,* and *NANOG.* Some have *KIT* gene mutations. Dysgerminomas account for only about 2% of all ovarian cancers; 90% are unilateral.

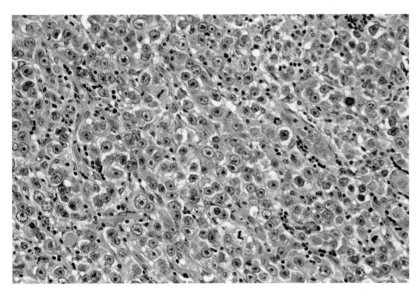

Figure 13-99 Dysgerminoma, microscopic

This neoplasm is composed of sheets and cords of large polyhedral cells with large nuclei and pale pink to watery vesicular cytoplasm. There is a scant lymphoid infiltrate and virtually no fibrous stroma. Although not shown here, there may be syncytiotrophoblastic cells producing HCG. Although classified as malignant, only one third behave in an aggressive manner. They are radiosensitive. Those confined to the ovary have an excellent prognosis.

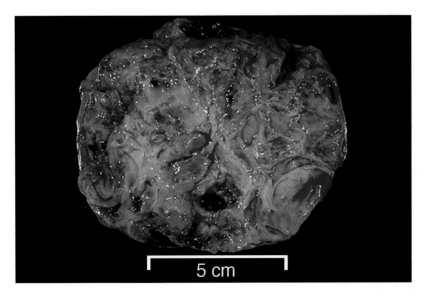

Figure 13-100 Granulosa–theca cell tumor, gross

This tumor has a variegated cut surface with solid and cystic areas. These sex cord–stromal tumors are derived from ovarian stroma and have varying amounts of granulosa cell differentiation and a component of thecoma. They are often hormonally active, with grossly yellowish areas from increased lipids, and can produce large amounts of estrogen such that the patient may initially have bleeding from endometrial hyperplasia or endometrial carcinoma. Occasionally, androgens are produced in excess, leading to virilization. Their biologic behavior is impossible to predict from histologic characteristics, and some may have an aggressive granulosa component.

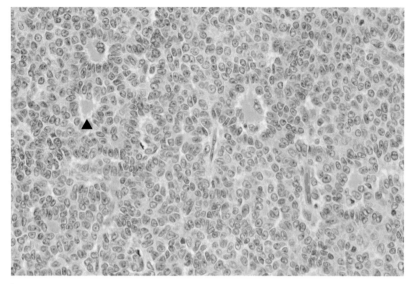

Figure 13-101 Granulosa cell tumor, microscopic
Microscopically, the granulosa cell tumor attempts to form structures that resemble primitive follicles. This tumor has nests of cells that are forming primitive follicles filled with an acidophilic material, termed *Call-Exner bodies* (▲). Most of these tumors are histologically benign, but all are potentially malignant, and some invade and recur. There is often an elevated serum inhibin and positive immunohistochemical staining of the tumor cells with antibody to inhibin. *FOXL2* gene mutations are found in nearly all of them.

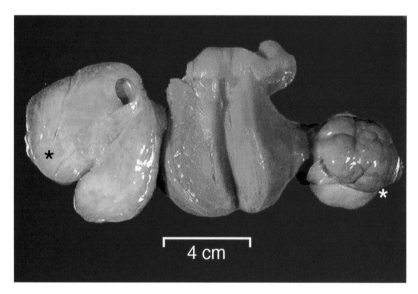

Figure 13-102 Thecoma-fibroma, gross
Here are bilateral, solid, sharply circumscribed, benign ovarian tumors (✶). The thecoma component of the neoplasm gives the tumor a yellowish cast (shown on cut surface of the neoplasm on the left) because of the lipid content. They can also produce abundant estrogen, which leads to endometrial hyperplasia and to endometrial carcinoma. These are tumors that arise from the ovarian stroma. They are bilateral in only about 10% of cases. Most are biologically benign. Ascites accompanies about 40% of cases. The additional finding of a right-sided hydrothorax in association with this tumor is known as *Meigs syndrome.* They can also be associated with basal cell nevus syndrome.

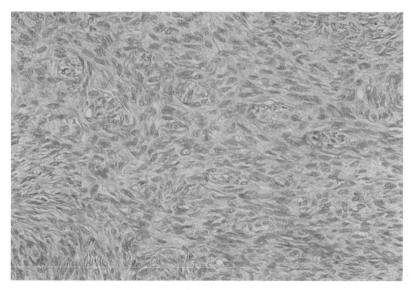

Figure 13-103 Thecoma-fibroma, microscopic
The elongated fibroblastic-appearing cells of the fibroma component are fairly uniform. In contrast, the thecoma component is composed of clusters or sheets of plumper cuboidal to polygonal cells. The pale to clear cytoplasmic appearance of the thecoma cells is a consequence of the amount of lipid present, and there can be elaboration of estrogens. Fibromas are hormonally inactive. There is some collagenous stroma present, more fibroma-like. In either case, this neoplasm acts in a benign fashion. Clinical findings include pelvic pain, palpable adnexal mass, and ascites.

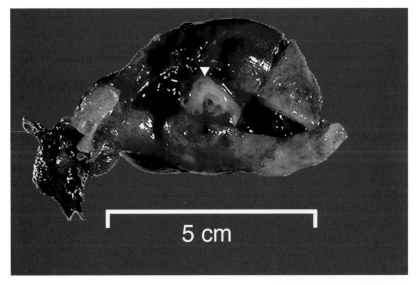

Figure 13-104 Ectopic pregnancy, gross
Note the small embryo (▼) within the blood clot emanating from the point of rupture in this resected fallopian tube. This is a medical emergency because of the sudden rupture with hemoperitoneum. Ectopic pregnancy should be considered in the differential diagnosis of severe acute abdominal pain in a woman of childbearing age. About half of ectopic pregnancies occur because of an identifiable lesion, such as chronic salpingitis from PID or from adhesions after appendicitis, endometriosis, or previous laparotomy.

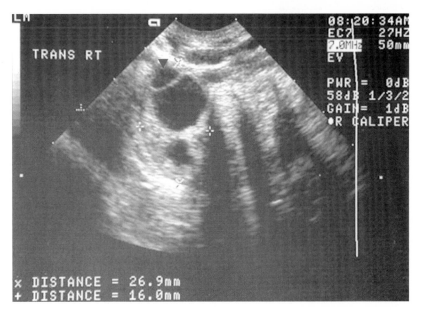

Figure 13-105 Ectopic pregnancy, ultrasound
On transvaginal ultrasound, a ringlike structure (▼) is present in the right adnexal region, highly characteristic of an ectopic pregnancy because no gestational sac was present in the uterine cavity, only a thickened endometrium. HCG was also elevated, indicating that a pregnancy had occurred. A culdocentesis may yield blood in cases of ruptured ectopic pregnancy. Isthmic tubal pregnancies tend to rupture at 6 to 8 weeks' gestation, ampullary pregnancies usually rupture at 8 to 12 weeks' gestation, and interstitial pregnancies rupture at 12 to 16 weeks' gestation.

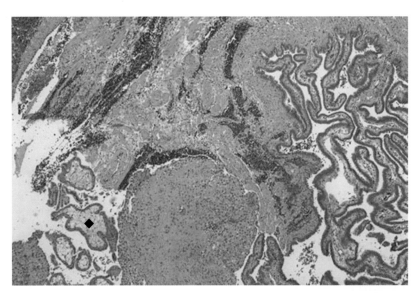

Figure 13-106 Ectopic pregnancy, microscopic
A positive pregnancy test (from presence of HCG), ultrasound examination, and culdocentesis with presence of blood are helpful in making the diagnosis of ectopic pregnancy. Shown here is normal tubal epithelium on the right, with rupture site and chorionic villi (◆) on the lower left. These chorionic villi are characteristic of an early pregnancy. If an endometrial biopsy were performed, it would show decidualized endometrium, but no implantation site, fetal parts, or chorionic villi.

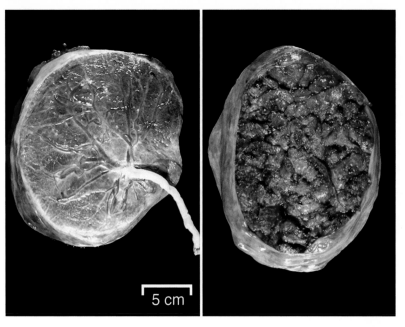

5 cm

Figure 13-107 Normal placenta, gross
The umbilical cord inserts into the fetal surface of the placenta, as in the *left panel.* Note the vessels radiating out from the cord over the fetal surface in this normal term placenta. The insertion point is typically just a bit off center (paracentral). Any insertion onto the disc, including the margin, is of no consequence. The maternal surface of this normal term placenta is shown in the *right panel.* The cotyledons that form the placenta are reddish brown and indistinct.

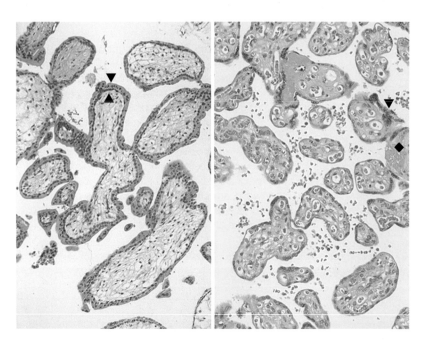

Figure 13-108 Normal placenta, microscopic
In the first trimester, as in the *left panel,* the chorionic villi are large and covered by two layers of cells—cytotrophoblast (▲) and syncytiotrophoblast (▼)—and the blood vessels in the villi are not prominent. As the placenta matures in the second trimester, the villi become smaller and more vascular. The syncytiotrophoblast cell layer draws up into "syncytial knots" (▼), which are small clusters of cells, leaving a single cytotrophoblast layer. Clumps of pink fibrin (♦) begin to appear between the villi. A mature placenta in the third trimester, as in the *right panel,* has small and highly vascularized chorionic villi to support the blood gas and nutrient exchange of maternal-fetal circulation required by the growing fetus approaching term gestation. Syncytial knots and intervillous fibrin are prominent.

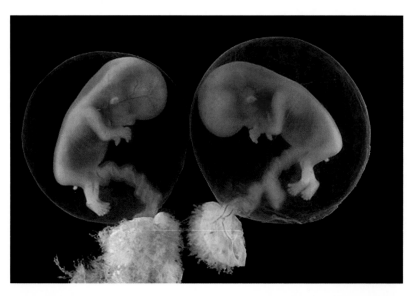

Figure 13-109 Twinning, gross
The process of twinning may be monozygous (identical twins derived from one fertilized ovum) or dizygous (separate fertilizations). The former may have one or two amniotic cavities, whereas the latter always has two. A histologic section through the dividing membranes is useful to help determine these possibilities. A dividing membrane that is monochorionic implies monozygous twinning. A dichorionic twin placenta could result from either dizygous or monozygous twinning (the former is more likely). The dizygous twin boys shown here are at 9 weeks' gestational age, and each has his own amnionic cavity. These amnions eventually fuse to form a diamnionic dividing membrane.

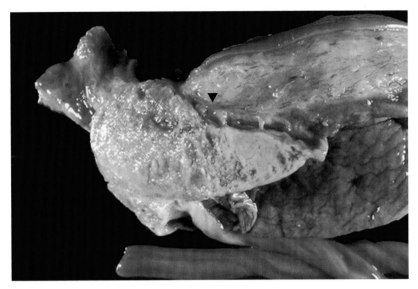

Figure 13-110 Placenta accreta, gross
The portion of placenta shown here has invaded (▼) into the myometrial wall in the region of the endocervical canal. There is lack of normal separation at delivery, leading to marked hemorrhage. This is also a low-lying placenta previa, which is present in 60% of such cases. The classification of these disorders is as follows: placenta accreta—superficially into myometrium; placenta increta—deep into myometrium; placenta percreta—through the myometrium.

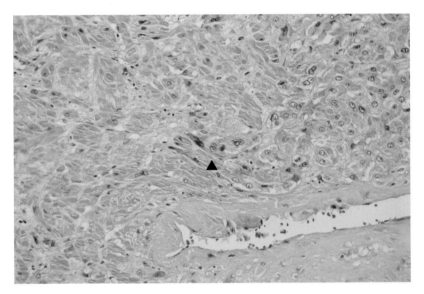

Figure 13-111 Placenta accreta, microscopic
These placental trophoblastic cells (▲) are extending into and interdigitating directly with uterine myometrium, without an intervening decidual plate. Bleeding can be profuse and life-threatening from the many large vascular spaces. Hysterectomy can be life-saving, along with blood product transfusion. Risk factors include prior caesarean delivery and placenta previa.

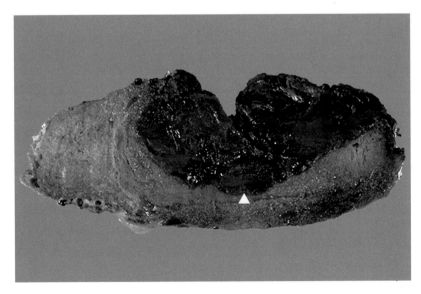

Figure 13-112 Abruptio placenta, gross
Placental abruption occurs from premature separation of the placenta in late pregnancy, with formation of a retroplacental blood clot. A blood clot (▲) is shown here in cross-section of the placenta. Larger abruptions are more likely to compromise the vascular supply to the fetus and produce distress. This abnormal hemorrhage before delivery can lead to sudden onset of severe lower abdominal pain in the mother. Ultrasound is useful to demonstrate separation. Emergent delivery is required.

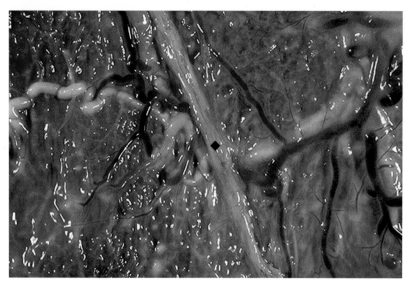

Figure 13-113 Twin-twin transfusion syndrome, gross
A twin-twin transfusion syndrome occurs from a vascular anastomosis in a monochorionic placenta between the two fetal circulations that leads to diminished blood flow to one twin (the donor) and increased blood flow to the other twin (the recipient). The donor may die from lack of blood, or the recipient may die from congestive heart failure. The placental blood vessels shown here have been injected with a white fluid to reveal the anastomosis across the dividing membranes (◆) on the placental fetal surface. In general, this syndrome can be suspected when one twin is at least 25% larger than the other. With survival the size differential eventually disappears.

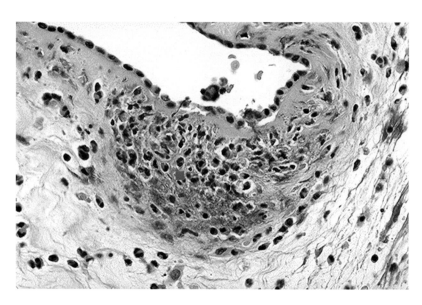

Figure 13-114 Chorioamnionitis, microscopic
Note the neutrophilic infiltrates (■) beneath the amnion in these fetal membranes. Premature or prolonged rupture of fetal membranes increases the risk for an ascending infection because bacteria in the vaginal canal can pass into the normally sealed amniotic cavity. Transplacental spread hematogenously is also possible but much less common. This leads to acute inflammation and premature labor with premature birth. The fetus may become infected in utero, and intrauterine fetal demise may result.

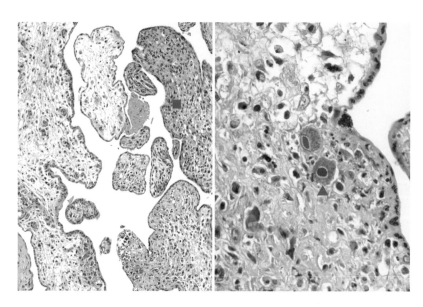

Figure 13-115 Villitis, microscopic
There are acute and chronic inflammatory cells (■) infiltrating villi *(left panel)* and large cells (▲) with large intranuclear inclusions typical of cytomegalovirus (CMV) infection *(right panel)*. Villitis may occur with congenital infections reaching the placenta from maternal circulation, including CMV, listeriosis, syphilis, parvovirus, and toxoplasmosis. Severe infections may interfere with placental function and lead to fetal loss. Some degree of noninfectious chronic villitis may occur in up to 5% of third trimester placentas.

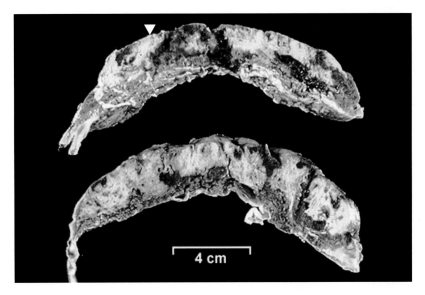

Figure 13-116 Placental infarction, gross
A placenta is cut in cross-sections to reveal pale yellow areas (▼) of infarction involving more than half of the parenchyma. This was so extensive that fetal demise resulted from these infarctions. Small infarcts are common and are of no consequence to the fetus, but if more than one third or one half of the placental parenchyma is infarcted or damaged in some fashion, blood supply to the fetus becomes severely compromised.

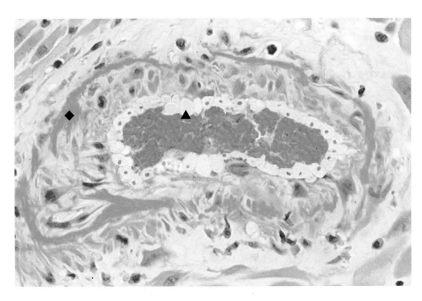

Figure 13-117 Placental atherosis, microscopic
This decidual arteriole shows atherosis consisting of prominent intimal macrophage (▲) proliferation along with fibrinoid necrosis (the irregular pink strands [◆] in the arteriolar wall) and edema. This decidual arteriopathy can be seen with pregnancy-induced hypertension and with maternal antiphospholipid antibody. Altered placental perfusion can underlie cases of toxemia of pregnancy, manifested in up to 5% of pregnancies by hypertension, proteinuria, and edema, called *preeclampsia;* presence of convulsions in addition to these defines *eclampsia.*

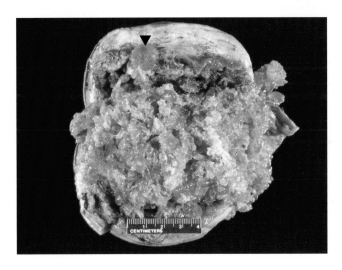

Figure 13-118 Hydatidiform mole, gross
The enlarged uterus opened here has numerous grapelike villi (▼), but no fetus, typical for complete hydatidiform mole, the most common form of gestational trophoblastic disease. HCG levels are markedly elevated. Patients with this "complete" mole are often large for dates and have hyperemesis gravidarum more frequently. Patients may have bleeding and may pass some of the grapelike villi. Molar pregnancies occur when there is fertilization of an ovum by a sperm but subsequent loss of maternal chromosomes (or, less commonly, fertilization of an empty ovum by two sperm), most often leaving a 46,XX karyotype with only paternal chromosomes, enough to form placental tissue but not a fetus.

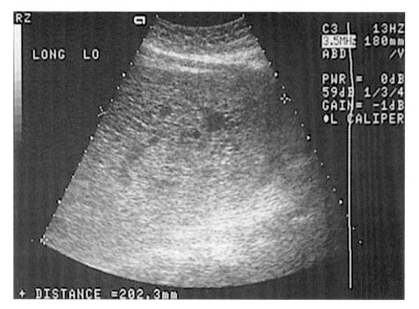

Figure 13-119 Hydatidiform mole, ultrasound
Ultrasound of the pelvis shows a large cystic mass in the uterine cavity, giving a snowstorm (◆) appearance without a fetus present, which is consistent with a complete hydatidiform mole. The uterus is typically large for gestational age. Ultrasound confirms the diagnosis before curettage is done to evacuate this tissue. After evacuation, the patient is followed with serial HCG levels to determine whether an invasive mole or choriocarcinoma has occurred as a complication. Up to 15% of complete moles develop into invasive moles; choriocarcinoma follows only 2.5% of complete moles.

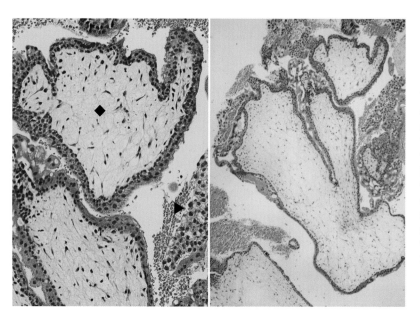

Figure 13-120 Hydatidiform mole, microscopic
The complete hydatidiform mole has large avascular chorionic villi (◆) and areas of cytotrophoblastic proliferation (▶). This must be distinguished from spontaneous abortion with passage of the fetus and retained products of conception with hydropic degeneration of villi. Normal placental villi have immunohistochemical staining for *p57*, a cell cycle inhibitor that is paternally imprinted. Villi of a complete mole, with only paternal X chromosomes, would be *p57* negative; 90% are 46,XX with only paternal genetic material, and 10% result from dispermy.

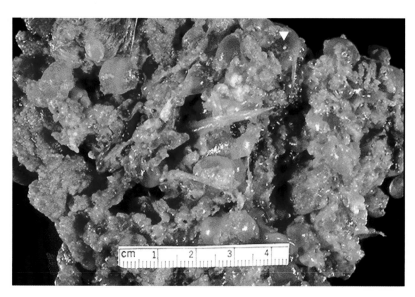

Figure 13-121 Partial hydatidiform mole, gross
A partial mole occurs and is diandric when two sperm fertilize a single ovum (or is digynic when the polar body of the last meiotic division is not lost). The result is triploidy (69 chromosomes). Only some of the villi are grapelike (▼), and a growth-retarded fetus with anomalies is typically present but rarely survives past 15 weeks. Scattered grapelike masses are shown here, but not as large as those of complete mole, with intervening normal-appearing spongy pale red placental tissue. When triploidy is digynic, the placenta is unlikely to have partial mole features, but the fetus still exhibits anomalies, and fetal loss occurs.

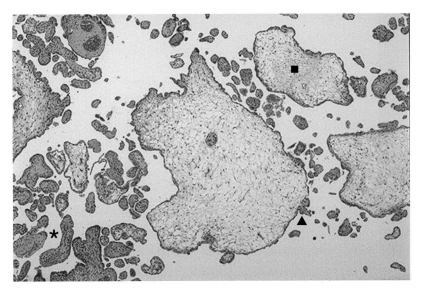

Figure 13-122 Partial hydatidiform mole, microscopic

In partial moles, some villi (as shown here at the lower left) appear normal (★), whereas others are swollen and grapelike (■). There is minimal trophoblastic proliferation (▲). The likelihood of subsequent development of invasive mole or choriocarcinoma is much lower for a partial mole than for a complete mole. A characteristic fetal anomaly with triploidy is 3-4 syndactyly of the digits of the hands. The karyotype is likely 69,XXY.

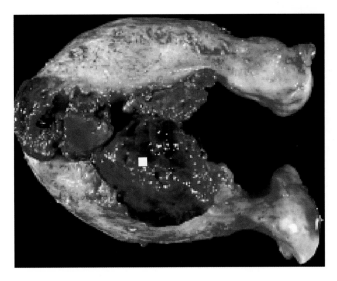

Figure 13-123 Choriocarcinoma, gross

The uterus has been opened to reveal a hemorrhagic mass (■) in the upper fundus. A choriocarcinoma is the most aggressive of the molar pregnancies. The serum HCG level can be markedly elevated. The patient may not have much uterine enlargement, and vaginal bleeding may be the first clue to its presence. These neoplasms have a propensity to spread locally to the vagina. Distant metastases are most commonly seen in the lungs. Brain, liver, and kidneys are also potential sites of metastases.

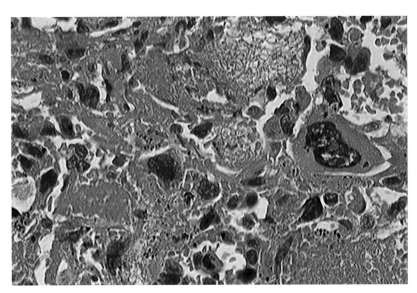

Figure 13-124 Choriocarcinoma, microscopic

Chorionic villi are not present within a choriocarcinoma, the most serious form of gestational trophoblastic disease (GTD), but only a proliferation of bizarre trophoblastic cells (◄) with loose cohesion and interstitial hemorrhage. This gives the lesion a grossly soft and hemorrhagic appearance. These tumors are very aggressive and are associated with very marked HCG levels. Half of them arise in preceding hydatidiform moles. Metastases are common, particularly to the lungs distantly and vagina locally, and chemotherapy results in a near-100% cure rate. Metastases to liver or brain, a very high HCG, and persistent disease indicate high-risk disease with a cure rate of about 75%.

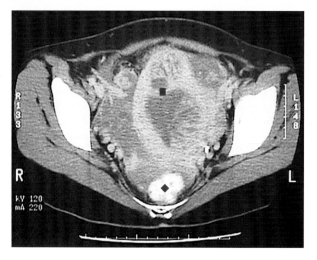

Figure 13-125 Choriocarcinoma, CT image
CT scan of the pelvis shows an irregular solid and cystic mass (■) in the region of the uterus extending into the pelvis. There is bright contrast material in the rectum (◆). Clinical findings that may suggest GTD in pregnancy include preeclampsia, prolonged hyperemesis gravidarum, and hyperthyroidism (resulting from production of thyrotropin by the molar tissue, or similarities between HCG and thyroid-stimulating hormone, both glycoprotein hormones).

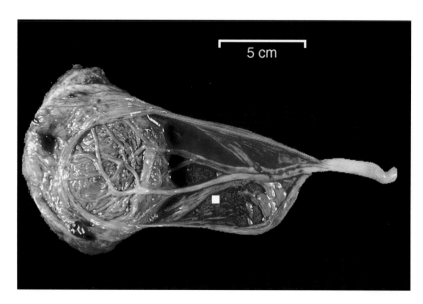

Figure 13-126 Placenta, velamentous insertion, gross
A velamentous insertion (■) of the umbilical cord occurs when the three major umbilical vessels separate within the fetal membranes before reaching the placental disc. Such a condition is usually of no major consequence in utero, but it could lead to a greater chance for cord trauma with tearing of one of the vessels and bleeding during the delivery process.

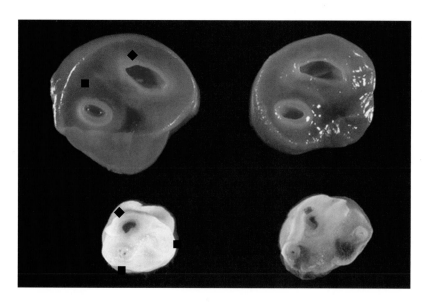

Figure 13-127 Umbilical cord vessels, gross
Cross-sections from an abnormal two-vessel umbilical cord with a single artery (■) and vein (◆) above are compared with the normal three-vessel cord with an artery (■), a second artery (■), and a vein (◆). By itself, the lack of one umbilical artery, which may occur from agenesis or atrophy, has minimal impact on the developing fetus. Less than 1% of singleton and about 5% of twin live births are accompanied by a two-vessel cord. The significance of this umbilical cord anomaly is its association with other fetal anomalies. Observation of a two-vessel cord on inspection of the placenta at the time of delivery should prompt one to look carefully for additional anomalies in a newborn.

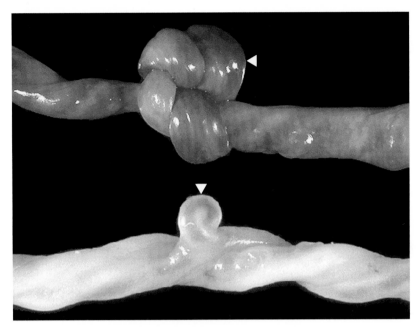

Figure 13-128 Umbilical cord, true versus false knot, gross
A true knot (◀) of the umbilical cord *(upper panel)* is more likely to occur with an abnormally long umbilical cord that may develop in association with increased fetal movement. A true knot is uncommon but could potentially constrict the blood vessels and lead to fetal demise. The consistency of the cord is like a rubber band, difficult to completely tighten. An umbilical cord pseudoknot *(lower panel)* is quite common and is an incidental finding. It is an exaggerated loop of one umbilical artery (▼), because it is longer than the vein. The abnormal vessel shown here has the shape of a clothoid loop, which should be recognizable to aficionados of roller coaster rides, because this loop maintains lower, constant gravitational force in transit around the loop.

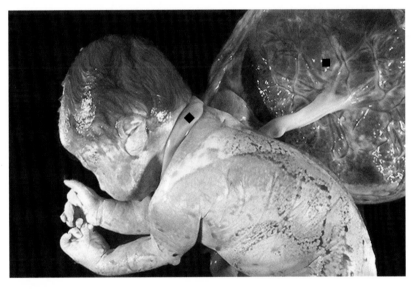

Figure 13-129 Nuchal cord, gross
The amniotic cavity has been opened here to reveal the normal fetal surface of the placenta (■). The umbilical cord inserts centrally into the placental disc. The abnormal finding here is a "nuchal cord," in which one or more loops of umbilical cord are wrapped around the fetus's neck (◆). A single loop may be present in 20% and multiple loops in 5% of deliveries. This is usually an incidental finding, but a nuchal cord could interfere with descent through the birth canal during delivery and increases the risk for umbilical cord trauma or constriction of the blood flowing through the cord.

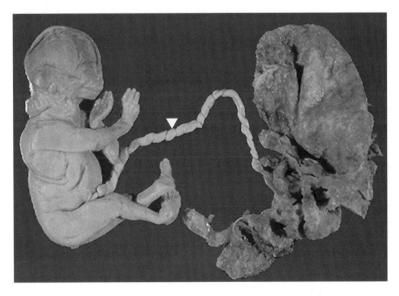

Figure 13-130 Umbilical cord torsion and fetal demise, gross
The fetus and the placenta shown here are macerated from prolonged demise in utero. The cause of the demise in this case is the marked twisting (▼), or torsion, of the umbilical cord. Torsion compromises blood flow through the cord. Torsion may result from increased fetal movement, which abnormally lengthens the cord, allowing the fetus to rotate more freely.

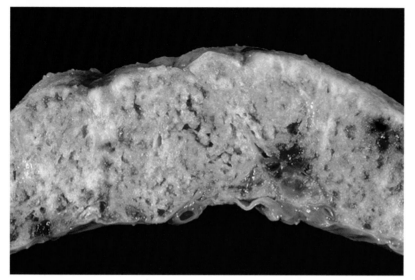

Figure 13-131 Maternal floor infarction, gross
The cross-section of the placenta shown here is quite abnormal, with a pale tan appearance rather than the normal spongy pink appearance. This represents the consequence of extensive, diffuse fibrin deposition, associated with a condition known as *maternal floor infarction,* and sometimes called a "gitterinfarkt." A related condition known as *massive perivillous fibrin deposition* has a similar appearance, although the fibrin deposition is most pronounced at the maternal base with maternal floor infarction.

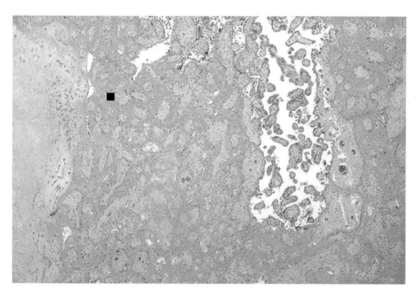

Figure 13-132 Maternal floor infarction, microscopic
The placental villi have extensive deposits of fibrin (■) between them, and the villi are becoming infarcted because of the perivillous fibrin deposition. The amount of fibrin in this condition is far greater than the scattered, small deposits of intervillous fibrin regularly observed within a term placenta. It is as though cement were poured into the placenta. This condition can cause uteroplacental insufficiency and fetal demise. This condition is uncommon, but it has a tendency to recur in subsequent pregnancies. Some cases may be associated with maternal coagulopathies, such as antiphospholipid syndrome.

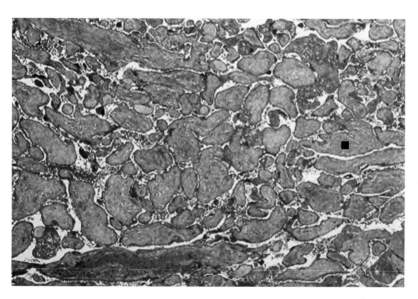

Figure 13-133 Placenta with fetal demise, microscopic
A trichrome stain shows extensive blue-staining collagen representing fibrosis within the placental villi (■) in this case of prolonged fetal demise. The villi are also quite small, even though this is a second-trimester placenta. Such placental dysmaturity is a finding with prolonged demise. Syncytial knots may increase in number in the placenta during the first week after demise.

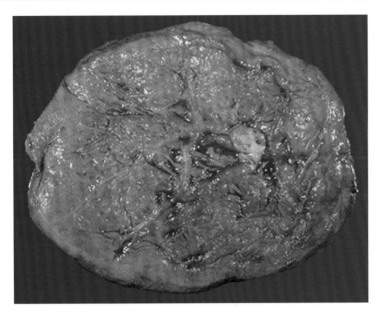

Figure 13-134 Meconium staining, gross
Meconium is a thick solution forming within fetal intestine after 34 weeks' gestation that contains intestinal secretions, mucosal cells, and solid elements of swallowed amniotic fluid, and it appears dark green because of bile staining. Meconium spillage is a complication occurring at or near term, typically when there is fetal distress with loss of anal sphincter tone and passage of meconium into amniotic fluid. A clue to this occurrence is greenish staining of fetal skin or fetal surface of the placenta as shown here. Evidence of fetal distress, followed by observation of greenish staining to the fetal or placental surfaces, should raise suspicion for meconium spillage.

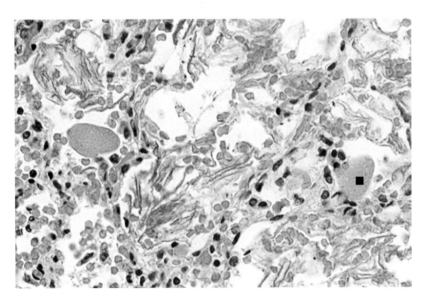

Figure 13-135 Meconium aspiration, microscopic
The worst consequence of meconium spillage is meconium aspiration into the lungs, when fetal distress leads to reflex gasping efforts by the fetus. Orange-brown balls (■) of meconium (shaped like a rugby ball) and numerous flattened squames or desquamated fetal skin cells that are found in the amnionic fluid are shown here within alveoli. Meconium is an irritant that leads to respiratory distress and chemical pneumonitis. It can diminish surfactant function. Large amounts of meconium may cause airway obstruction and atelectasis. At birth, tracheal suction and lung lavage may be useful to help remove the meconium.

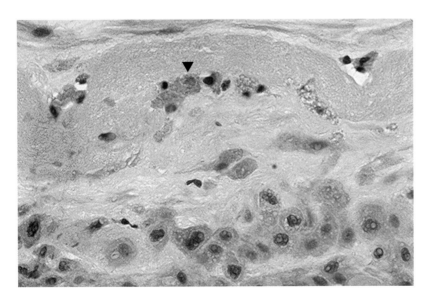

Figure 13-136 Meconium in fetal membranes, microscopic
If the fetus lives in utero after the meconium spillage, the microscopic yellow-brown pigment (▼) can be taken up into macrophages in the membranes, as shown here, which can give an indication that meconium was present in the amnionic cavity.

The Breast

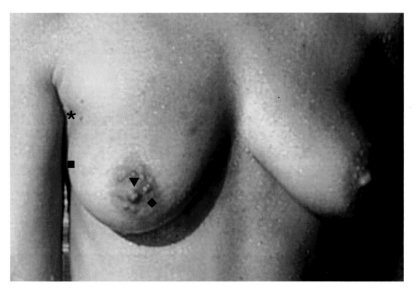

Figure 14-1 Normal breast, gross
The normal appearance of female breasts is shown here. The nipple (▼) is surrounded by a darker areola (◆). Some breast tissue extends into the axillary tail of Spence (■). Breast size is primarily determined by the amount of adipose tissue. There may be some asymmetry in development. Macromastia may occur unilaterally or bilaterally with increased sensitivity to hormonal stimulation and may be called *juvenile hypertrophy* when it occurs at the time of puberty. Rarely, a supernumerary breast may produce a subcutaneous mass anywhere from the axilla (★) to the perineum.

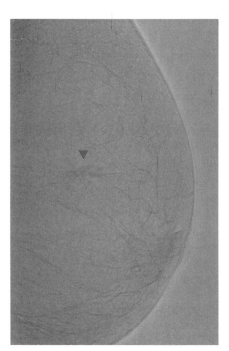

Figure 14-2 Breast, mammogram
A mammogram uses a small amount of x-radiation to visualize the breast parenchyma. This mammogram shows the normal pattern of lactiferous sinuses and ducts. There is one suspicious density (▼), however, which could be a carcinoma or just an area of pronounced sclerosis with fibrocystic changes. A mammogram is a useful screening tool to find such lesions and to determine the need for further workup. A mammogram may detect lesions that are not palpable. Women in their 30s begin to have some involution of lobules and adjacent stroma, and the breast tissue becomes more radiolucent from an increased composition of adipose tissue replacing fibrous stroma and lobules.

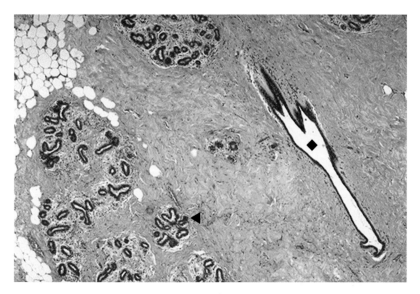

Figure 14-3 Normal breast, microscopic
The normal microscopic appearance of female breast tissue is shown. There is a larger duct (◆) to the right and lobular units (◀) to the left. A collagenous stroma extends between the structures. A variable amount of adipose tissue can be admixed with these elements. During the normal menstrual cycle, after ovulation under the influence of estrogen and increasing progesterone levels, lobular acini increase, epithelial cells become vacuolated, and the interlobular stromal edema increases, leading to increased breast fullness. With menstruation and a decrease in hormone levels, apoptosis of epithelial cells and a reduction in stromal edema occur.

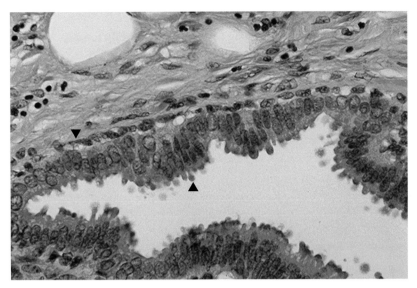

Figure 14-4 Normal breast, microscopic
The appearance of a normal breast acinus is shown at high magnification. The epithelial cells lining the lumen show apocrine secretion with snouting, or cytoplasmic extrusions (▲), into the lumen. A layer of myoepithelial cells (▼), some of which are slightly vacuolated, is seen just around the outside of the acinus.

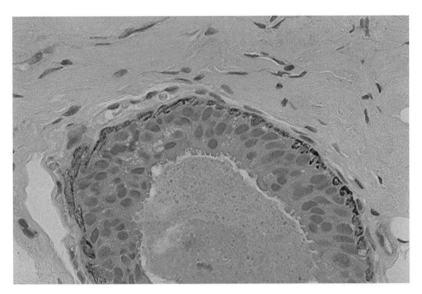

Figure 14-5 Normal breast, microscopic
Immunostaining with antibody to actin shows the red-brown myoepithelial cell layer around the breast acinus. The myoepithelial cells are contractile and are very sensitive to oxytocin. After pregnancy and delivery of the infant, suckling by the infant results in release of oxytocin from where it is stored in the posterior pituitary gland. The oxytocin induces myoepithelial cell contraction with expression of milk. Breast secretory activity is driven by prolactin from the anterior pituitary. The initial peripartum secretions are known as *colostrum;* they are low in lipid but high in protein, including maternal immunoglobulins.

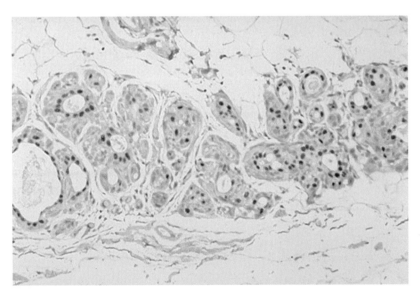

Figure 14-6 Normal breast, microscopic
The normal microscopic appearance of female breast tissue is shown here with a terminal duct lobular unit. Note the cluster of lobules lined by epithelial cells that show focal dark-brown positivity for estrogen receptor (ER) with immunohistochemistry. This steroid hormone receptor is located in the cell nucleus. Normal breast tissue is responsive to estrogen and progesterone. Assessment of estrogen and progesterone receptors is done on tissues removed by biopsy or surgery to evaluate the biologic characteristics of breast carcinomas. Carcinomas that are hormone sensitive may respond to therapy with agents such as letrozole or tamoxifen.

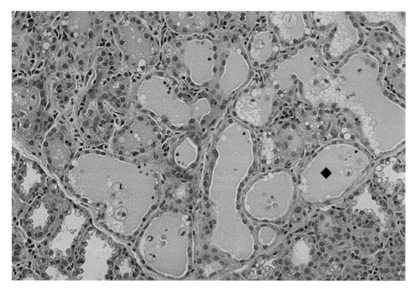

Figure 14-7 Normal lactating breast, microscopic

The female breast during pregnancy undergoes hyperplasia and hypertrophy, so that after birth, lactation can occur. Under the influence of estrogen, terminal ducts and ductal epithelium proliferate, and progesterone promotes development of increased acini in the lobular units. Lobules filled with pink-appearing secretions (◆) are seen here. The breast, a modified sweat gland, secretes by budding off of portions of cell cytoplasm (apocrine secretion) to form breast milk with high lipid content. After delivery, estrogen and progesterone levels decrease, increasing the lactogenic effect of prolactin. The acinar epithelial cells become vacuolated with increased secretions.

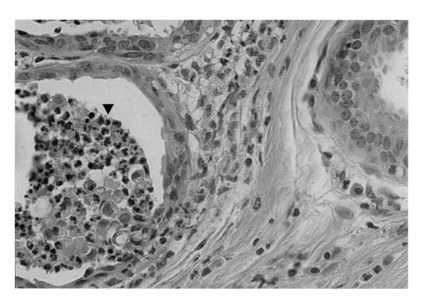

Figure 14-8 Acute mastitis, microscopic

During breastfeeding of an infant, usually in the first month, the skin of the breast may become irritated and inflamed. This skin may fissure, predisposing to infection with entry of microorganisms into underlying breast tissue. Acute mastitis typically involves just one breast and is most often caused by bacterial organisms such as *Staphylococcus aureus,* although streptococci can produce this condition, with neutrophilic infiltrates (▼) seen here microscopically. If untreated by antibiotic therapy, spread of infection and abscess formation can occur.

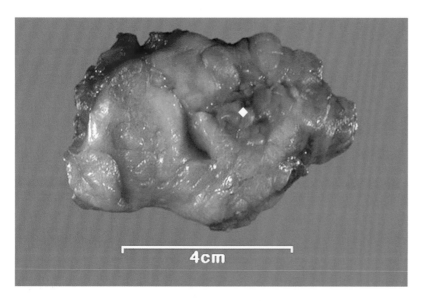

Figure 14-9 Breast abscess, gross

During lactation, or at other times with dermatologic conditions that allow cracks and fissures to form in the skin of the nipple, infectious organisms can invade into breast and result in acute inflammation, and this may progress to breast abscess (◆) formation. The most common organism is *Staphylococcus aureus*. Streptococcal organisms are more likely to produce a diffuse cellulitis. Organization with fibrous scar formation around the abscess can form a firm mass that can mimic a carcinoma on physical examination, on mammography, and grossly in the resected tissue specimen.

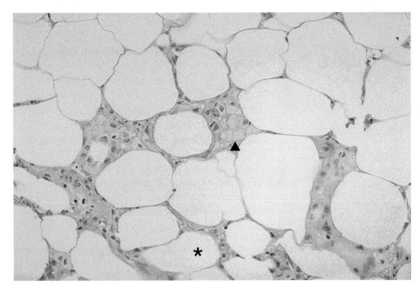

Figure 14-10 Fat necrosis, microscopic
The most common cause of fat necrosis of breast is trauma. The resulting lesion can be a localized, firm area with scarring that can mimic a breast carcinoma. Microscopically, fat necrosis consists of irregular steatocytes with loss of their peripheral nuclei and intercellular pink amorphous necrotic material and inflammatory cells, including macrophages and foreign body giant cells responding to formation of the necrotic debris. In this view of fat necrosis at high magnification, some lipid-laden macrophages (▲) are seen among the necrotic adipocytes (★).

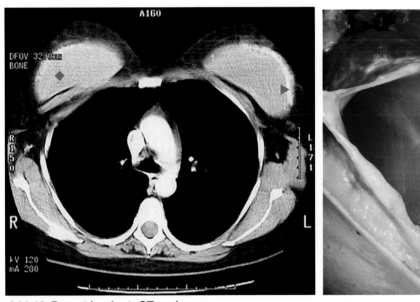

Figures 14-11 and 14-12 Breast implant, CT and gross
The chest CT scan in the *left panel* reveals bilateral silicone breast implants (◆). These implants have resulted in the formation of a fibrous capsule that has partially calcified (▶). The thin connective tissue capsule (▶) around a silicone breast implant is shown grossly in the *right panel.* Note the overlying skin and adipose tissue at the upper left with the chest wall below the implant and to the right. This is a typical capsule that is pliable and nondeforming, without scarring.

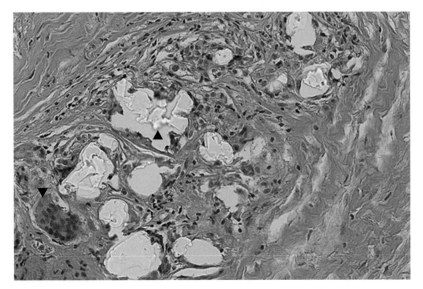

Figure 14-13 Breast implant capsule, microscopic
Microscopic examination of the fibrous capsule from a silicone breast implant often reveals the refractile silicone material (▲) as shown here because this material gradually leaks out from the implant into surrounding connective tissues. This process induces a foreign-body granulomatous response (▼). This is a localized reaction not associated with systemic disease, such as autoimmune disease. The fibrosis with scar formation around a breast implant may produce deformity and pain in some women. Rupture of an implant is uncommon.

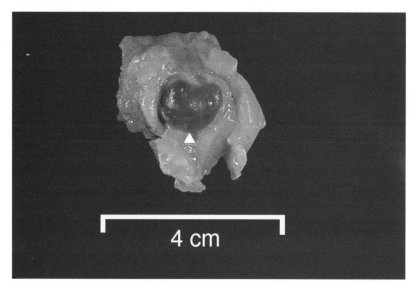

Figure 14-14 Fibrocystic changes, gross
A 1.5-cm parenchymal breast cyst (▲) is shown. Its presence led to palpation of an ill-defined but focal lump in the breast to be distinguished from other lesions, including carcinoma. Sometimes, fibrocystic changes in the breast, particularly in women of childbearing age, produce a more diffusely lumpy breast. One or more mammographic densities, with or without calcifications, are present. Fine-needle aspiration (FNA) of fluid from a cyst found in conjunction with fibrocystic changes typically yields benign-appearing cells visible on cytologic preparations, and the cyst may disappear after aspiration.

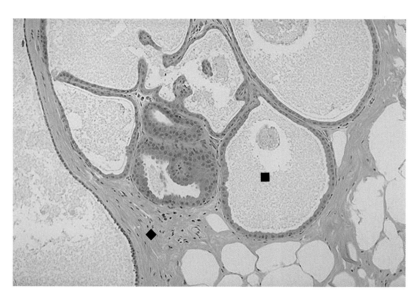

Figure 14-15 Fibrocystic changes, microscopic
The appearance of fibrocystic changes in breast includes irregular, cystically dilated ducts (■) and intervening stromal fibrosis (◆). The cysts are lined by uniform benign cuboidal to columnar epithelial cells. This is a "nonproliferative" breast change. Fibrocystic changes account for most breast lumps that are found in women of reproductive years, particularly between the age of 30 and menopause.

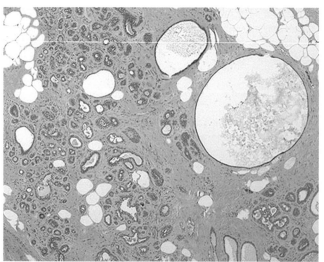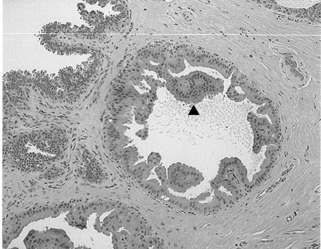

Figures 14-16 and 14-17 Fibrocystic changes, microscopic
Additional fibrocystic changes are shown, including the irregular duct and lobule size in the *left panel*. There is prominent apocrine change with abundant pink-staining cytoplasm (▲) of tall columnar epithelial cells lining the cysts in the *right panel*. These appearances are benign.

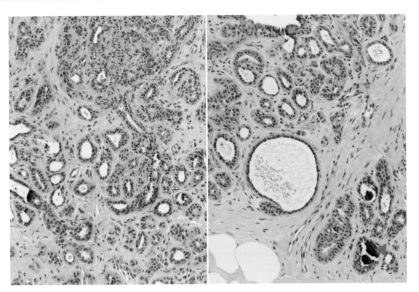

Figure 14-18 Sclerosing adenosis, microscopic

Prominent sclerosing adenosis, one of the proliferative breast diseases and a feature that is often seen in association with fibrocystic changes, is shown by the appearance of a proliferation of small ducts in a fibrous stroma as well as cystically dilated ducts. Microcalcifications (◄) can be present. The number of acini per terminal duct is more than double the normal number found in normal lobules. This lesion may produce a palpably firm and irregular mass. Although benign, the gross and mammographic appearance may mimic carcinoma, and it can be difficult to distinguish from carcinoma on frozen section of a biopsy specimen.

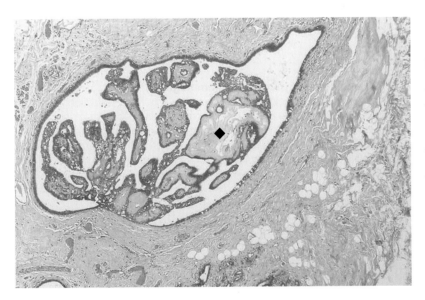

Figure 14-19 Intraductal papilloma, microscopic

This small papilloma appears in a breast duct, typically in one of the large main lactiferous ducts beneath the areola, where it can be palpated as a lump. The epithelial cells show no atypia, and there is a fine pink collagenous stroma (◆) within branching fibrovascular cores of this papilloma. There can be associated proliferative and nonproliferative breast changes. An intraductal papilloma may be associated with a serous or bloody nipple discharge, or it may cause some nipple retraction.

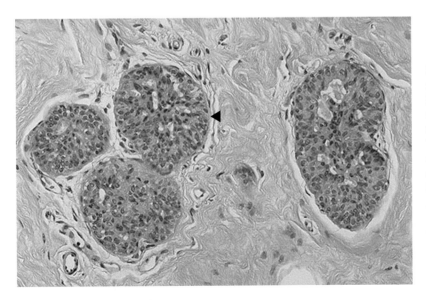

Figure 14-20 Epithelial hyperplasia, microscopic

Proliferative breast disease includes the florid ductal epithelial hyperplasia (◄) shown here. This can occur within areas of fibrocystic changes. The epithelial cells are multilayered, filling and expanding the ducts or acini; myoepithelial cells are increased. There is no epithelial cell atypia, however. There is a slightly increased risk (1.5 to 2 times normal) for development of breast carcinoma when such changes (more than four layers of epithelial cells) are present.

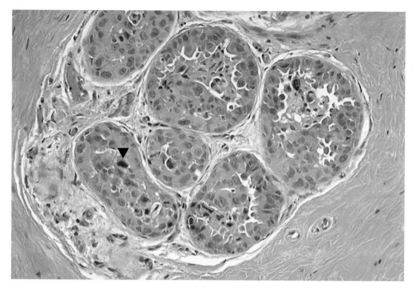

Figure 14-21 Atypical ductal hyperplasia, microscopic

Proliferative breast disease with atypia is shown by this cluster of ductular structures, which has irregular proliferation of epithelial cells that show variation in size and shape. Some of the epithelial cell nuclei are enlarged and slightly hyperchromatic (▼). These atypical changes indicate an increased risk for subsequent malignancy, although atypical hyperplasia itself is not yet malignant, remaining confined to the ducts, and closely resembles ductal carcinoma in situ (DCIS) or lobular carcinoma in situ (LCIS). Atypical ductal hyperplasia does not fill the entire ductal space, however, and lacks the monomorphism seen in the in situ carcinomas.

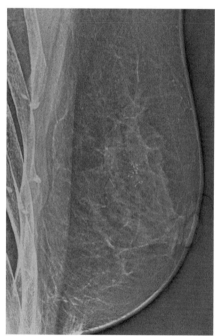

Figure 14-22 Atypical ductal hyperplasia, mammogram

This mammogram shows a suspicious dense area (▲) with microcalcifications that could be a carcinoma, proliferative breast disease, or an area of fibrocystic changes. On biopsy, this lesion had areas of fibrocystic changes along with atypical epithelial hyperplasia. Microcalcifications can be seen in either benign or malignant breast lesions. There are no pathognomonic criteria on radiologic imaging for either benign or malignant breast lesions, but imaging serves to confirm the presence and extent of palpable lesions, to find nonpalpable lesions as part of screening for breast disease, and to provide an index of suspicion for the nature of the lesions to determine further workup.

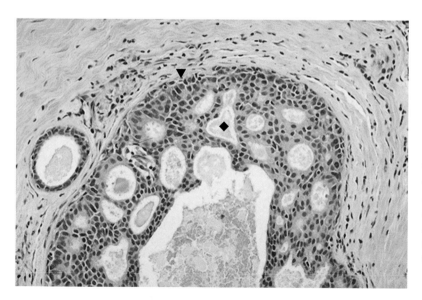

Figure 14-23 Ductal carcinoma in situ, microscopic

The classic cribriform pattern of noncomedo DCIS is shown. The neoplastic epithelial cells within the duct are monomorphous, with minimal hyperchromatism and pleomorphism, but they surround irregular spaces with sharp margins (◆), as though punched out by a cookie cutter. This neoplasm is limited to the duct, confined by the basement membrane (▼). DCIS may produce an ill-defined lump on palpation, but most of these non-invasive carcinomas are detected as an irregular density on mammogram; DCIS may be found incidentally on biopsy. Excision is curative in more than 95% of cases.

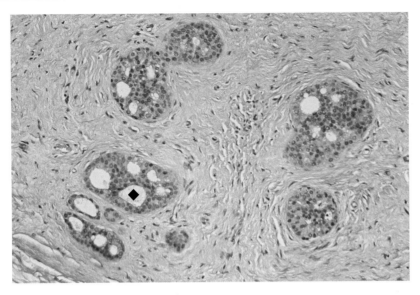

Figure 14-24 Ductal carcinoma in situ, microscopic

The expanded ducts shown here have neoplastic cells with a few cookie-cutter (◆) spaces. This is the noncomedo type of DCIS. The basement membrane remains intact. DCIS produces a subtle lesion grossly and mammographically, making it difficult to detect. It is bilateral in 10% to 20% of cases. DCIS constitutes about 15% to 30% of all cancers in women receiving screening for breast cancer. If DCIS is not treated, the risk for development of invasive carcinoma is 1% per year.

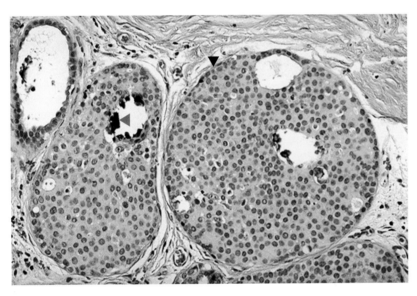

Figure 14-25 Ductal carcinoma in situ, microscopic

The intraductal carcinoma seen here has a solid pattern with neoplastic cells that fill and expand the duct lumina, but are still within the ducts and have not broken through the basement membrane (▼) into the adjacent stroma. The two large ducts in the center contain microcalcifications (◀), a form of dystrophic calcification in response to focal necrosis in the neoplasm. Such microcalcifications can appear on mammography. Prominent central necrosis would indicate the comedo pattern of DCIS. Microcalcifications may also appear in benign breast lesions, including fibrocystic changes and proliferative breast diseases.

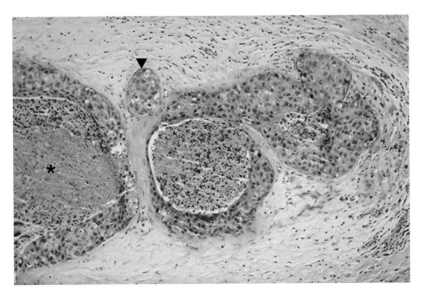

Figure 14-26 Ductal carcinoma in situ, microscopic

The comedo pattern of DCIS is characterized by the presence of rapidly proliferating, high-grade malignant cells. Note the prominent central necrosis (★) in these ducts. There is prominent periductal fibrosis with minimal chronic inflammation. This central necrosis leads to the gross characteristic of extrusion of cheesy material from the ducts with pressure (similar to a comedone). This pattern is uncommon, but the overall prognosis for patients with comedocarcinoma is generally good. Even with microinvasion (<1 mm) shown here (▼), the prognosis is still similar to that of DCIS overall.

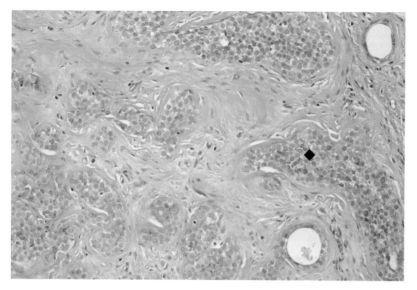

Figure 14-27 Lobular carcinoma in situ, microscopic

Note the neoplastic cells (◆) expanding the lobules, but not invading the stroma. LCIS is unlikely to form a palpable mass or radiologic density, but it can be multicentric and is bilateral in 20% to 40% of cases. LCIS does not usually form microcalcifications. LCIS consists of a proliferation of small, round, monomorphic epithelial cells within the terminal breast ducts and acini. E-cadherin gene (CDH1) mutations are frequent. Although low grade, there is an increased risk for development of invasive carcinoma in the same or the opposite breast (greater for the ipsilateral breast).

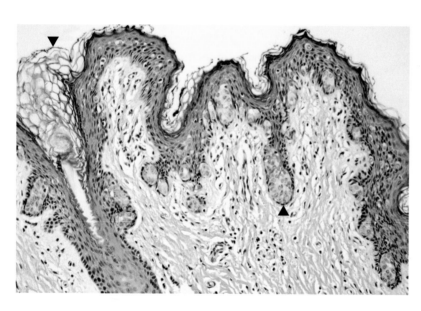

Figure 14-28 Paget disease of breast, microscopic

Note the overlying hyperkeratosis (▼) of the skin seen here, which contributes to the pruritus with rough, red, scaling eczematous appearance seen grossly; there is often skin ulceration. The large cells (▲) infiltrating into the epidermis represent intraepithelial extension of an underlying DCIS or invasive ductal carcinoma. The large Paget cells of Paget disease of the breast have abundant clear cytoplasm and appear within the epidermis either singly or in clusters. The nuclei of the Paget cells are atypical and, although not seen here, often have prominent nucleoli. They are often ER negative and HER2 positive. Over half of cases have a palpable underlying mass.

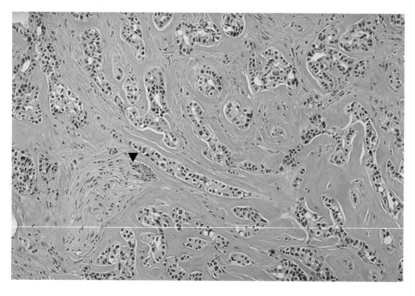

Figure 14-29 Invasive ductal carcinoma, microscopic

Note small nests and infiltrating strands of neoplastic cells with prominent bands of collagen between them. Ductal carcinoma here infiltrates outward into the surrounding stroma. As it does so, the marked increase in the dense fibrous tissue stroma produces the characteristic hard, scirrhous appearance of the typical infiltrating ductal carcinoma. Note the nerve surrounded by the neoplasm (▼) at the lower left. Perineural invasion is a frequent feature of invasive carcinoma and can account for the dull but constant character of neoplastic pain. Multiple immunopatterns of ER and HER2 are found in ductal cancers and aid in treatment selection.

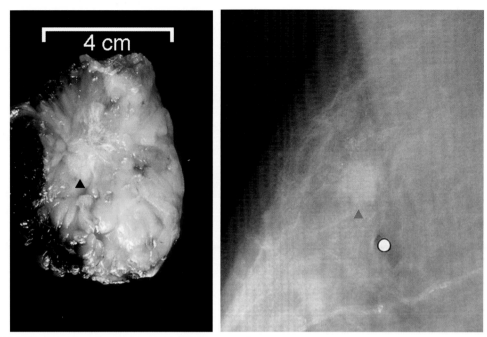

Figures 14-30 and 14-31 Invasive ductal carcinoma, gross and mammogram

Note the grossly irregular margins and varied cut surface of this breast carcinoma (▲) in the *left panel*. This lesion felt firm on physical examination with palpation and was not freely movable. The cut surface of this excised lesion felt gritty because of desmoplasia and microcalcifications. The margins of the specimen were inked with green dye after removal to assist in determining whether cancer extended to the margins after histologic sections were made. The mammogram in the *right panel* shows tiny peripheral calcifications within a lesion (▲) consistent with a neoplasm in the upper portion above and just to the left of the (●) marking the point at which the patient felt some pain on palpation.

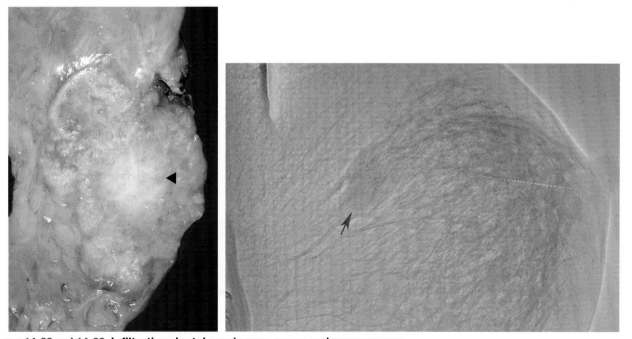

Figures 14-32 and 14-33 Infiltrating ductal carcinoma, gross and mammogram

The grossly irregular mass lesion (◄) seen in the *left panel* is an infiltrating ductal carcinoma of the breast. The center is very firm (scirrhous) and white because of the desmoplasia. There are areas of yellowish necrosis in the portions of neoplasm infiltrating into the surrounding breast and adipose tissue. Such tumors are very firm and immobile on physical examination. The mammogram in the *right panel* shows a large, irregular mass lesion (↑).

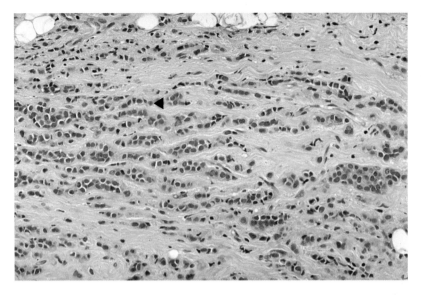

Figure 14-34 Infiltrating lobular carcinoma, microscopic

This neoplasm arises in the terminal ductules of the breast. The characteristic "Indian file" strands (◀) of infiltrating lobular carcinoma cells are seen here within the fibrous stroma. Pleomorphism of these neoplastic cells is not marked. About 10% to 15% of breast cancers are of this type. There is about a 20% chance that the opposite breast will also be involved, and many of these neoplasms arise multicentrically in the same breast. The may metastasize to meninges, peritoneum, and/or retroperitoneum. Most are ER positive and HER2 negative.

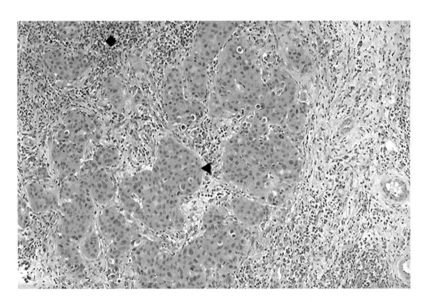

Figure 14-35 Medullary carcinoma, microscopic

Medullary carcinomas account for about 2% of breast cancers. They can sometimes be large, fleshy masses that measure 5 cm. They are composed of cells with pleomorphic nuclei that have prominent nucleoli. Although not seen here, foci of necrosis and hemorrhage can be found. Shown here at low power, sheets and nests (◀) of cells are surrounded by a lymphoid stroma (◆) with little desmoplasia. Some of these tumors occur in association with *BRCA1* gene mutations. *HER2/neu* overexpression is not observed. The prognosis with medullary carcinoma is better than for infiltrating ductal or lobular carcinoma, despite ER and HER2 negativity.

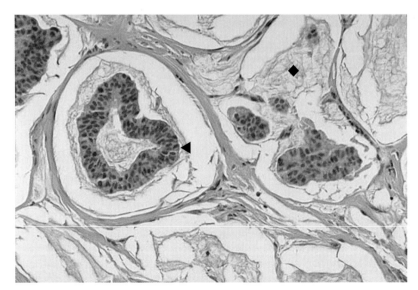

Figure 14-36 Colloid carcinoma, microscopic

This variant of breast cancer is known as *colloid,* or *mucinous,* carcinoma because of the abundant bluish mucin (◆) shown. The carcinoma cells (◀) appear to be floating in the mucin. This mucinous matrix gives the tumor a grossly soft, blue-to-gray appearance. Some of these tumors occur in association with *BRCA1* gene mutations. This variant tends to occur in older women as a small, circumscribed mass. It is slow growing, and when it is the predominant histologic pattern present in a breast cancer, the prognosis is better than for nonmucinous, invasive carcinomas. They are ER positive and HER2 negative.

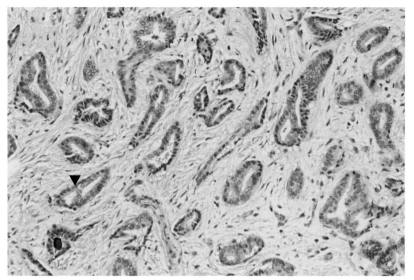

Figure 14-37 Tubular carcinoma, microscopic
This variant of breast cancer accounts for about 2% of all cases. These cancers tend to be small and often are detected only mammographically. These well-differentiated neoplastic cells form a single cuboidal layer in small, round to teardrop-shaped ductules (▼) widely spaced in a fibrous stroma. The prognosis tends to be better than for an intraductal carcinoma, despite the multifocal nature and bilaterality that are more common with this variant, because of the well-differentiated nature of the cells and the younger average age at onset (40s). Most are ER positive and HER2 negative.

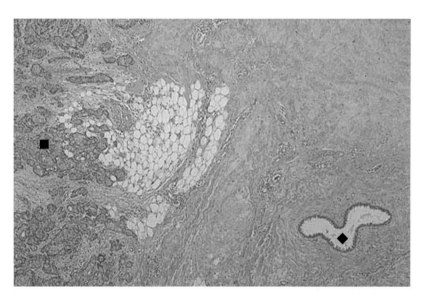

Figure 14-38 Male breast carcinoma, microscopic
Male breast cancers are much less common than female breast cancers, perhaps by a ratio of 100:1. Most occur as a subareolar mass with nipple discharge in elderly men and have spread to contiguous structures, giving them a high stage at diagnosis. Some are related to the *BRCA1* and *BRCA2* gene mutations; some are associated with Klinefelter syndrome. The same diagnostic techniques, such as mammography, can be used for screening and diagnosis.
At low power on the right can be seen a duct (◆) in a fibrous stroma, with absence of lobules, typical of male breast. On the left is an infiltrating carcinoma (■). Most male breast cancers are of the infiltrating ductal carcinoma variety. More than 80% are ER positive.

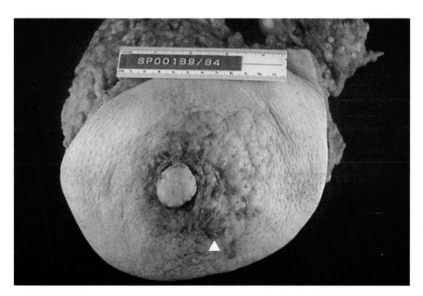

Figure 14-39 Inflammatory carcinoma, gross
This mastectomy specimen shows the gross findings of an inflammatory carcinoma of the breast. This is not a specific histologic type of breast cancer; rather, it implies dermal lymphatic invasion by some type of underlying breast carcinoma (usually invasive ductal carcinoma). Such involvement of dermal lymphatics gives the grossly thickened, erythematous, and rough skin surface (▲) with the appearance of an orange peel *(peau d'orange)*. There may not be an obvious underlying mass lesion.

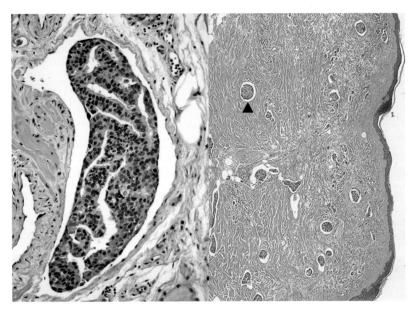

Figure 14-40 Inflammatory carcinoma, microscopic
The skin overlying this breast shows prominent dilated dermal lymphatic spaces (▲) filled with small clusters of metastatic cells from an underlying breast carcinoma. Carcinomas typically metastasize first to lymphatics. Breast cancers most often metastasize to the axillary lymph nodes, and these nodes can be sampled or removed at the time of surgery. Rarely, a metastasis is detected first because the primary site is occult and not detectable by physical examination or radiographic imaging techniques. Conversely, the nodes may contain micrometastases seen only with microscopy.

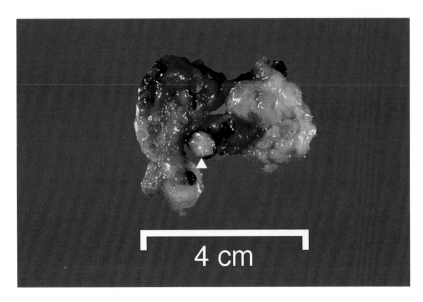

Figure 14-41 Fibroadenoma, gross
A small mass (▲) surgically excised from the breast is shown. This mass is well circumscribed. On physical examination, it felt firm and rubbery and was movable. The blue dye around this fibroadenoma was used to mark the lesion during needle localization in radiology so that the surgeon could find this small mass within the breast tissue. Fibroadenomas are common causes of breast lumps and the most common benign breast tumor in women. During reproductive years they may gradually increase in size, then they regress after menopause. During menstrual cycles they may cause some pain with transient enlargement in response to increasing estrogen levels.

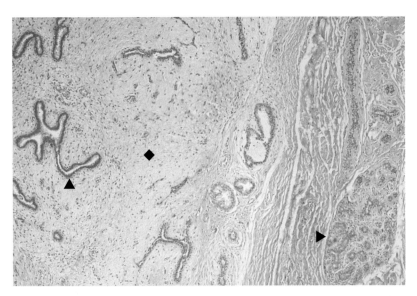

Figure 14-42 Fibroadenoma, microscopic
Compared with normal breast (▶) at the right, this solid mass is composed of a proliferating fibroblastic stroma (◆) containing elongated compressed ducts (▲) lined by benign-appearing cuboidal epithelium. These lesions are most likely to be found as a breast lump on examination in young women. They are palpably discrete, firm, rubbery masses that are freely movable. After menopause, they become more dense and may calcify. Some fibroadenomas are true neoplasms, whereas others represent polyclonal proliferations.

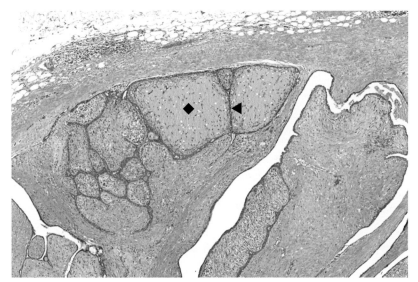

Figure 14-43 Phyllodes tumor, microscopic
A phyllodes tumor of the breast arises from the interlobular stroma, but in contrast to fibroadenomas, it is uncommon and is often much larger in size. Phyllodes tumors are low-grade neoplasms that rarely metastasize but can recur locally after excision. Microscopically, they are more cellular than fibroadenomas. Projections of stroma (◆) between the ducts (◀) create the leaflike pattern for which these tumors are named (from the Greek word *phyllodes,* meaning "leaflike").

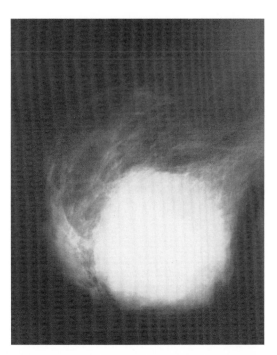

Figure 14-44 Phyllodes tumor, mammogram
This mammogram shows a bright, solid 10-cm rounded mass lesion consistent with a phyllodes tumor. It still has discrete margins, similar to a fibroadenoma, but is much larger. The biologic behavior of a phyllodes tumor is difficult to predict, and it may recur locally, but rarely are there high-grade lesions that can metastasize. These neoplasms tend to occur at an older age than do fibroadenomas, most commonly in the sixth decade.

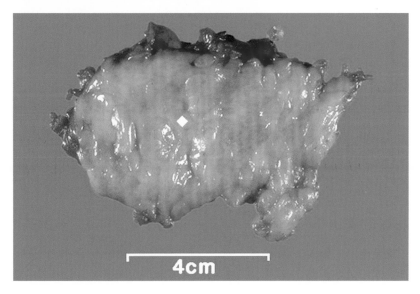

Figure 14-45 Gynecomastia, gross
An increased amount of breast tissue (◆) in a male is known as *gynecomastia.* This condition is uncommon. In pubertal boys, it may be idiopathic and resolve spontaneously or may persist and require surgical removal, as in this case. In older men, it results from hyperestrinism and may be a result of cirrhosis of the liver (from decreased hepatic clearance of estrogenic substances), pharmacologic agents, Klinefelter syndrome (47,XXY), or neoplasms such as a Leydig cell tumor of the testis.

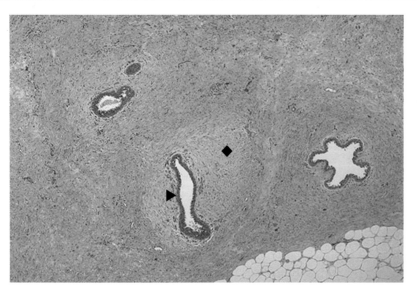

Figure 14-46 Gynecomastia, microscopic
The normally small amount of male breast tissue consists of just a few ducts, without lobules, in a fibrous stroma. With gynecomastia, this stromal and ductular (▶) tissue is increased, and there can be ductal epithelial hyperplasia, or prominent periductular edema (◆) as here. Lobule formation does not occur. Gynecomastia can be unilateral or bilateral.

The Endocrine System

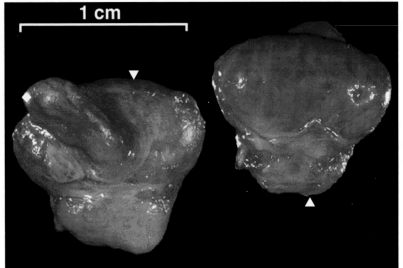

Figure 15-1 Normal pituitary gland, gross
The normal adult pituitary, situated in the sella turcica, weighs about 1 g. Embryologically, the anterior pituitary (▼) (adenohypophysis) is derived from an upward evagination of the oral cavity, called *Rathke pouch*. The posterior pituitary (▲) (neurohypophysis) is derived from the diencephalon and consists of modified glial cells (pituicytes) and their axons extending down the pituitary stalk (◆) (seen here superiorly) from supraoptic and paraventricular hypothalamic nuclei. The adenohypophysis has a dual blood supply, with a hypophyseal portal system and small perforating arteries. Seen inferiorly at the right, the neurohypophysis appears at the bottom.

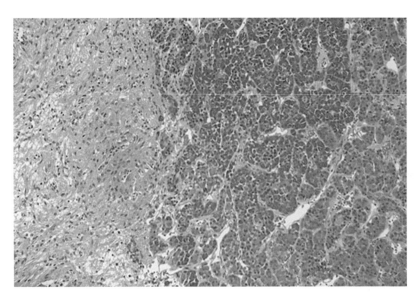

Figure 15-2 Normal pituitary, microscopic
The neurohypophysis, which resembles neural tissue because it is composed of modified glial cells along with the axons of hypothalamic nerve cell bodies, is on the left. The highly vascularized adenohypophysis is on the right. The neurohypophyseal hormones oxytocin and vasopressin (antidiuretic hormone) are synthesized in the hypothalamus and transported along axons to the neurohypophysis, from which they are released into the bloodstream and carried systemically to act on cells in target organs.

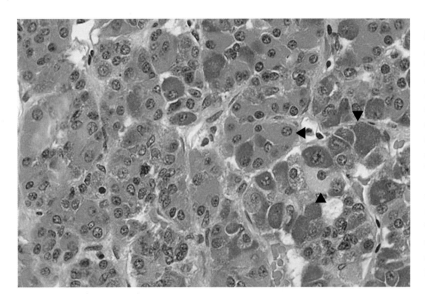

Figure 15-3 Normal pituitary, microscopic
At higher magnification in the adenohypophysis, the pink acidophils (◄) that produce prolactin (lactotrophs) and growth hormone (somatotrophs) can be seen. The dark-purple basophils (▼) can produce luteinizing hormone and follicle-stimulating hormone (gonadotrophs), thyroid-stimulating hormone (TSH) (thyrotrophs), and adrenocorticotropic hormone (ACTH) (corticotrophs). The paler cells are the chromophobes (▲). As in all endocrine glands, there is prominent vascularity with many capillaries into which the hormones are secreted for distribution throughout the body. The secretions of these cells are under control of hypothalamic-releasing factors, which are all positive acting except for dopamine, which inhibits lactotrophs.

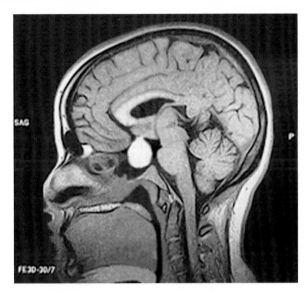

Figure 15-4 Pituitary macroadenoma, MRI
This T1-weighted sagittal MRI image shows a large bright pituitary mass (▶) larger than 1 cm. Pituitary adenomas arise in the adenohypophysis. They may be null-cell adenomas producing a mass effect, but without detectable hormonal secretion, or composed of either acidophils or basophils secreting an excess of one hormone (or, less commonly, several hormones). Overall, the most common types of pituitary adenomas (and their clinical outcomes) include prolactinoma (amenorrhea-galactorrhea in women, decreased libido in men), followed by null-cell adenoma, corticotroph adenoma (Cushing disease), gonadotroph adenoma (paradoxical hypogonadism), and somatotroph adenoma (acromegaly in adults and gigantism in children). About 3% of pituitary adenomas are associated with multiple endocrine neoplasia type 1 (MEN 1).

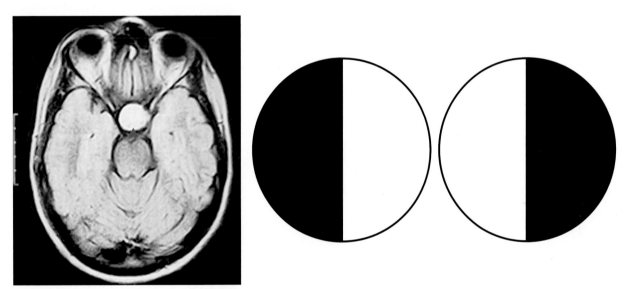

Figure 15-5 Pituitary macroadenoma, MRI and diagram
This T1-weighted MRI image in axial view shows a bright pituitary macroadenoma (▲). Macroadenomas by their size can erode the sella turcica to produce headaches and impinge on the optic chiasm to produce visual field defects, most commonly bitemporal hemianopsia, as shown by the diagram.

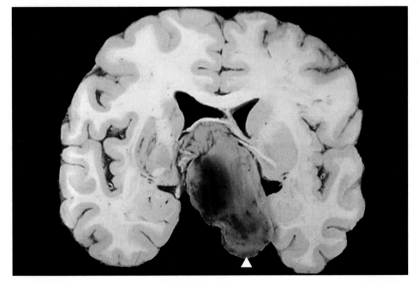

Figure 15-6 Pituitary macroadenoma, gross
This large pituitary adenoma (▲), a macroadenoma, impinges on the ventricular system, as shown here, with subsequent elevation in intracranial pressure producing symptoms of headache, nausea, and vomiting. Occasionally there can be acute hemorrhage into the adenoma to increase the mass effect. Some pituitary adenomas have mutations in *GNAS* that result in activation of the α subunit of a G-stimulatory protein, increasing cyclic adenosine monophosphate (cAMP) production, which drives cellular proliferation. About 5% of these adenomas arise with familial syndromes such as MEN1.

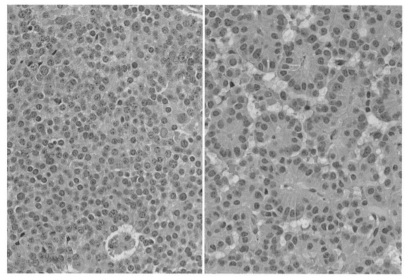

Figure 15-7 Pituitary adenoma, microscopic

Note solid *(left panel)* and fetal *(right panel)* patterns of monotonous pattern of fairly uniform rounded cells and capillary channels. The H&E staining pattern is variable. The most common pituitary adenoma (30% of cases) in adults secretes prolactin, whereas 20% are null-cell adenomas that do not secrete a hormone but can exert a mass effect, diminish pituitary function (hypopituitarism), or have a "stalk section" effect to disrupt prolactin-inhibiting factor release into the anterior pituitary, leading to hyperprolactinemia. Growth hormone–secreting adenomas are most common in children but are uncommon in adults.

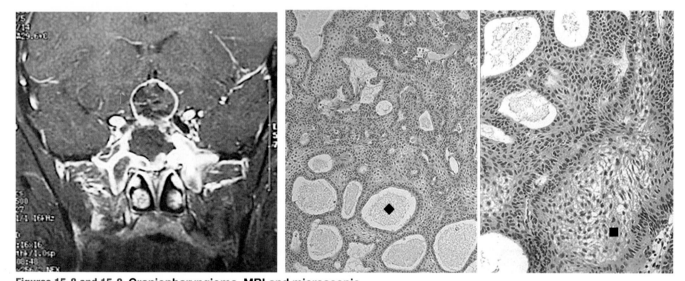

Figures 15-8 and 15-9 Craniopharyngioma, MRI and microscopic

This coronal MRI image shows an expansile suprasellar mass (▶) derived from Rathke pouch remnants eroding surrounding structures. Microscopically, there are cystic spaces (♦), and nests of squamoid cells (■) are surrounded by columnar cells. Dystrophic calcifications may be present. Although histologically benign, these neoplasms are difficult to eradicate because of their location and their extension to adjacent structures such as brain and bone. Some arise in children, and some in older adults. They can produce headache, visual field defects, and hypopituitarism. Those less than 5 cm in diameter are less likely to recur after resection.

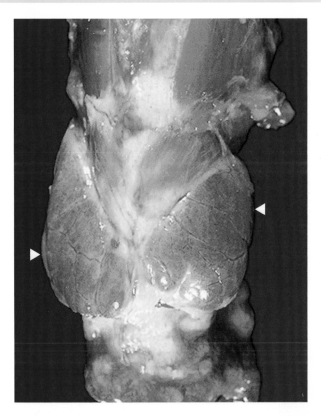

Figure 15-10 Normal thyroid in situ, gross

The thyroid gland is present over the anterior trachea. It normally has a reddish brown, firm appearance and is difficult to palpate on physical examination. The normal adult thyroid gland weighs 10 to 30 g. There is a right lobe (◀), a left lobe (▶), and a connecting isthmus (from which a small pyramidal lobe may project superiorly along the track of the embryologic thyroglossal duct). The thyroid in embryogenesis is derived from an evagination from the foramen cecum of the tongue that migrates downward along the thyroglossal duct to a position over the thyroid cartilage in the anterior neck. The C cells are derived from the fifth branchial pouches. The thyroid produces the thyroid hormones triiodothyronine (T_3) and tetraiodothyronine (T_4). A small amount of dietary iodine is required for thyroid hormone synthesis. In the past, many cases of adult goiter with myxedema were caused by a diet lacking in iodine, whereas in infants and children this manifested as cretinism. Mostly T_4 is released, but peripherally T_4 is deiodinated within cells to the more biologically active T_3. T_3 and T_4 increase the basal metabolic rate, including anabolic and catabolic processes.

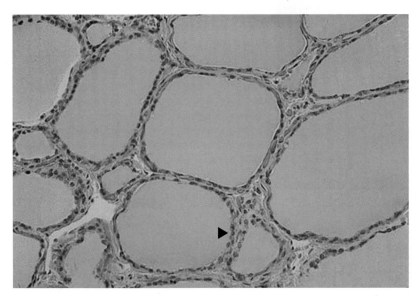

Figure 15-11 Normal thyroid, microscopic

The normal thyroid gland is composed of round follicles lined by cuboidal epithelial cells (▶) and filled with colloid, a storage product containing thyroglobulin that is metabolized to release thyroid hormones (T_4 and T_3) under the influence of TSH released from the anterior pituitary thyrotrophs, which sense levels of circulating thyroid hormone. Thyroid hormone acts on nuclear thyroid hormone receptor in target cells to upregulate transcription of proteins that drive carbohydrate and lipid metabolism, while stimulating protein synthesis.

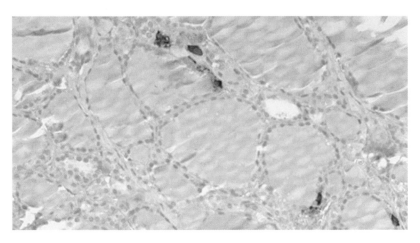

Figure 15-12 Normal C cells, microscopic

This immunohistochemical stain of normal thyroid with antibody to calcitonin identifies the C cells by the brown reaction product. The C cells (parafollicular cells) of the thyroid interstitium are located between the follicles, adjacent to the epithelium of follicles. The C cells secrete calcitonin, which can inhibit resorption of bone by osteoclasts and reduce the serum calcium, but which has a much smaller role to play in calcium hemostasis than parathyroid hormone (PTH).

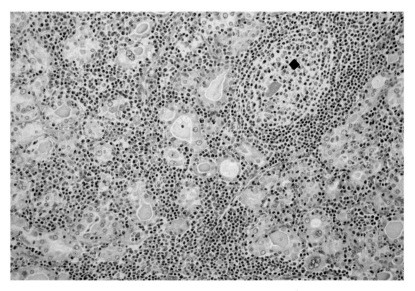

Figure 15-13 Hashimoto thyroiditis, microscopic

This autoimmune disease can be associated with HLA-DR3 and HLA-DR5 alleles. It results in chronic inflammation characterized by infiltrates of CD8+ and CD4+ T lymphocytes forming much of the lymphoid infiltrates, including a lymphoid follicle (◆) seen here. The remaining thyroid follicles become atrophic, and the epithelial cells undergo Hürthle cell change, with abundant pink cytoplasm. Initially there can be painless enlargement of the thyroid. Laboratory findings include antithyroglobulin and antimicrosomal (thyroid peroxidase) antibodies detected in serum. Polymorphisms in both *CTLA4* and *PTPN22* are present in many cases, along with other autoimmune manifestations.

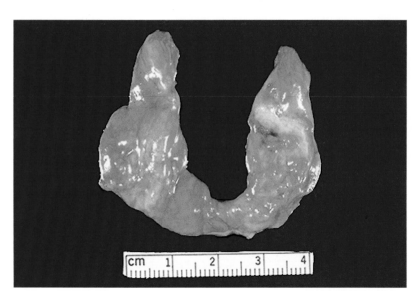

Figure 15-14 Hashimoto thyroiditis, gross

There is relentless destruction of thyroid follicles over the years, with eventual atrophy, so that the thyroid is often not palpable when a patient presents with myxedema from hypothyroidism, and the serum TSH is elevated. Early in the course of this disease, there may be transient hyperthyroidism from excessive release of thyroid hormones from damaged follicles. Women are affected far more often than men. Other autoimmune diseases, such as Addison disease or pernicious anemia, may also occur in patients with Hashimoto thyroiditis. There is an increased risk for subsequent development of B-cell non-Hodgkin lymphoma.

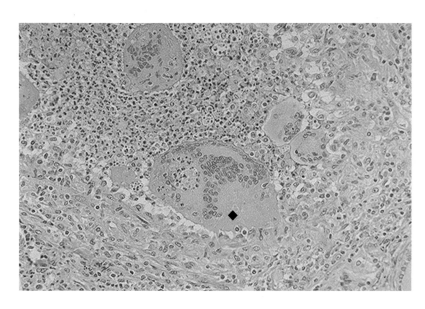

Figure 15-15 Granulomatous thyroiditis, microscopic

Also known as *de Quervain disease,* this uncommon form of thyroiditis begins with diffuse painful thyroid enlargement. It most often occurs in the fourth to the sixth decades and is more common in women, similar to other thyroid diseases. Note the marked acute inflammation along with lymphocytes, macrophages, and prominent giant cells (◆). There is destruction of thyroid follicles. This condition typically follows a viral infection that activates cytotoxic T lymphocytes. It usually follows a course of 1 to 3 months during which transient hyperthyroidism or hypothyroidism along with fever can occur. Most patients recover completely within months and remain euthyroid.

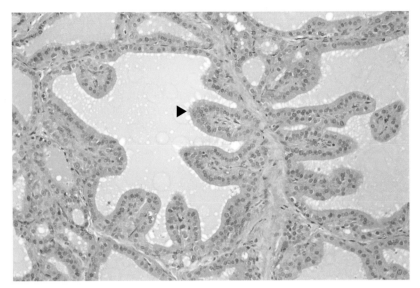

Figure 15-16 Graves disease, microscopic
At low magnification, this thyroid hyperplasia is characterized by many papillary infoldings (▶) within follicles. This is an autoimmune disease in which autoantibodies to TSH receptors stimulate growth of follicular epithelial cells and stimulate adenylate cyclase to increase thyroid hormone output. There is an association with the HLA-DR3 allele. The entire thyroid gland becomes diffusely enlarged to double or triple normal size. Patients can have β-adrenergic excess with fever, diarrhea, heat intolerance, tachycardia, weight loss, tremor, and nervousness. Exophthalmos and infiltrative dermopathy (pretibial myxedema) are clinical features characteristic of Graves disease.

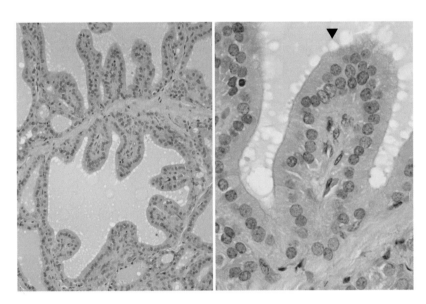

Figure 15-17 Graves disease, microscopic
At higher magnification, the tall columnar appearance of the hyperplastic follicular epithelial cells is evident. Small, clear vacuoles (▼) appear next to each cell, indicating increased processing of colloid to produce increased output of thyroid hormone leading to hyperthyroidism. The feedback on the adenohypophyseal thyrotrophs decreases the serum TSH, whereas the serum T4 is high. Antithyroid antibodies may be present. An uncommon but serious complication is thyroid storm with malignant hyperthermia. Graves disease can be treated with a β-blocker to diminish β-adrenergic effects, with antithyroid drugs such as propylthiouracil, and with subtotal thyroidectomy.

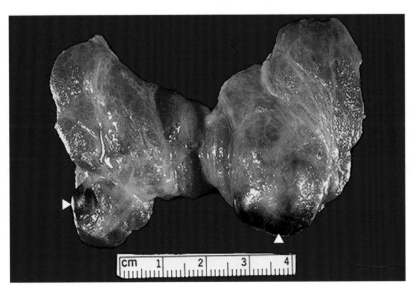

Figure 15-18 Thyroid with colloid cysts, gross
One of the most common lesions to produce a palpable nodule of the thyroid gland is a colloid cyst. The cyst is filled with colloid and surrounded by flattened cuboidal epithelium. It is just an exaggerated follicle in an otherwise normal thyroid. Patients are euthyroid. Seen here is a larger colloid cyst (▲) anteriorly and inferiorly in the left lower lobe and a smaller cyst (▶) laterally in the right lower lobe. Such nodules can mimic a neoplasm on physical examination or imaging studies. They can mimic a nodular goiter, although the overall size of the thyroid is not enlarged here. On radionuclide imaging, this would be a "cold" nodule, as are most neoplastic and non-neoplastic thyroid nodules.

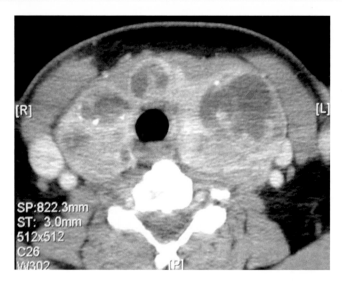

Figure 15-19 Thyroid, multinodular goiter, CT scan
This large thyroid surrounds the trachea and contains several nodular areas (♦) with diminished attenuation (brightness). This is a multinodular goiter in a patient who is euthyroid, the most typical clinical picture accompanying goiter. The painless enlargement produces discomfort and cosmetic deformity to the neck. Multinodular goiters usually arise from simple goiters after many years. Simple goiters may be endemic in populations with decreased dietary iodine intake. Sporadic goiters can be caused by goitrogens in foods such as Brussels sprouts, cauliflower, cassava, and turnips (favorites of mine, but perhaps not yours) that interfere with thyroid hormone synthesis and promote development of goiter. Most patients with goiters remain euthyroid. Inborn errors of metabolism that interfere with thyroid hormone production are rare but can lead to goiter with cretinism in children.

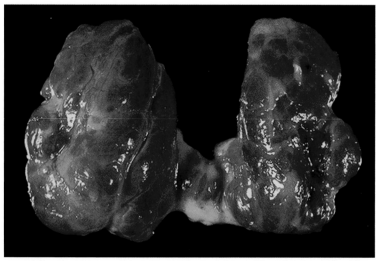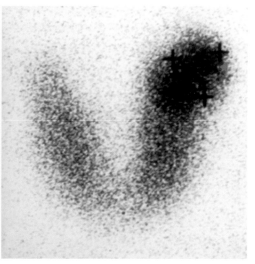

Figure 15-20 Thyroid, multinodular goiter, gross and scintigraphic scan
Multinodular goiters are often asymmetric, although both lobes become enlarged. Most patients remain euthyroid, bothered only by the mass effect. Larger masses may be removed because of fixed airway obstruction, dysphagia, or superior vena cava syndrome. In about 10% of patients, a hyperfunctioning "toxic" nodule (Plummer syndrome) may develop, producing T_4 and causing hyperthyroidism. Such a "hot" nodule (◀) with increased activity on radionuclide scintigraphic scanning is shown in the *right panel*.

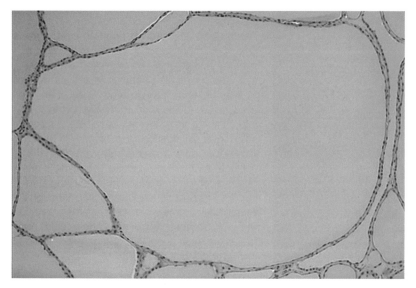

Figure 15-21 Thyroid, goiter, microscopic
Shown here from a goiter are enlarged thyroid follicles lined with inactive, flattened epithelial cells and filled with abundant stored colloid. The process starts as a simple, diffuse, nontoxic goiter. Over time, there can be irregular nodular enlargement with fibrosis, hemorrhage, and calcification in areas of cystic change. The irregular growth and enlargement may mimic thyroid carcinoma. Mutations in TSH-receptor signaling pathway (*TSHR* or *GNAS*) may lead to autonomous growth and function of a nodule within a goiter.

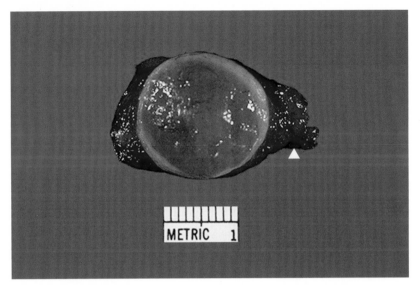

Figure 15-22 Thyroid, follicular neoplasm, gross

This cross-section through a resected lobe of thyroid gland reveals an encapsulated round neoplasm with a uniform brown appearance, surrounded by a rim of normal thyroid (▲). This is a follicular adenoma, which typically manifests as a painless mass. This lesion is often diagnosed on microscopic examination as a follicular neoplasm because in 10% of cases, although it is benign histologically, such a lesion proves to act in a malignant fashion. A follicular neoplasm forms a palpably firm nodule and is more common in middle-aged women. Most are hypofunctioning cold nodules on radionuclide scanning.

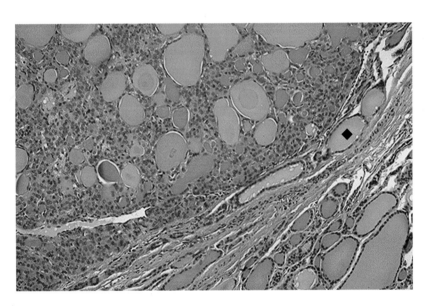

Figure 15-23 Thyroid, follicular neoplasm, microscopic

This well-differentiated follicular neoplasm is composed of recognizable follicles that are small and packed closely, whereas the adjacent normal thyroid (◆) has compressed and flattened follicles at the lower right. There is no invasion visible here, so this neoplasm is more likely to act in a benign fashion. Most follicular neoplasms do not function, but a rare hyperfunctioning adenoma, or toxic adenoma, can be a cause of hyperthyroidism. Some toxic adenomas have a G protein–coupled receptor mutation encoding the stimulatory α subunit *(GNAS1)* that upregulates adenyl cyclase and cAMP to drive thyroid hormone output.

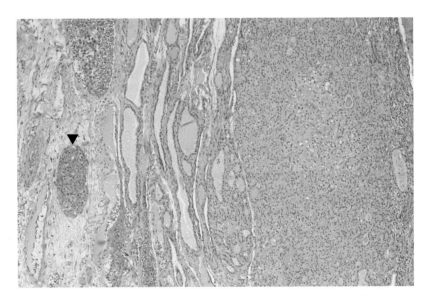

Figure 15-24 Thyroid, follicular carcinoma, microscopic

This follicular neoplasm is composed of small, closely packed but recognizable follicles. There is invasion (▼) seen here into venous spaces at the left (lymphatic invasion is uncommon), so this neoplasm is likely to act in a malignant fashion. These carcinomas account for 5% to 15% of thyroid cancers, and more in persons with iodine deficiency. Most are cold nodules on scintigraphic scans and enlarge slowly. Even minimally invasive follicular carcinomas have a good prognosis.

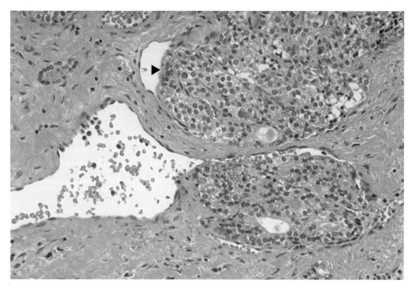

Figure 15-25 Thyroid, follicular carcinoma, microscopic
Vascular invasion (▶) is evidence of malignancy in a neoplasm that is vaguely follicular, with absence of microscopic features of papillary carcinoma. Follicular carcinomas often have mutations in the PI-3K/AKT signaling pathway, including gain-of-function point mutations of *RAS* and *PIK3CA*, amplification of *PIK3CA*, and loss-of-function mutations of *PTEN*. Half of them have chromosome 2,3 translocations with *PAX8-PPARG* fusion gene. Follicular carcinoma is the second most common thyroid malignancy. It tends to be indolent and metastasizes hematogenously to locations such as lung or liver.

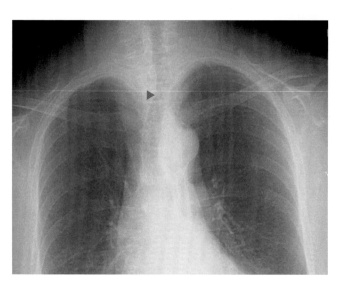

Figure 15-26 Thyroid, neoplasm, chest radiograph
The subtle evidence of a mass involving the thyroid is seen here as tracheal deviation (▶) to the right as a consequence of displacement by the mass effect. Thyroid neoplasms may be palpable on physical examination, although less so in corpulent individuals. Radiologic procedures such as CT can help document the size, extent, and consistency of the thyroid; scintigraphic scans can determine the amount and distribution of isotopic uptake into the thyroid parenchyma. Fine-needle aspiration with cytologic examination of the aspirated cells is a useful tool to determine the histologic nature of thyroid lesions. Removal of part (subtotal) or all (total) of the thyroid (thyroidectomy) may be undertaken for diagnostic and therapeutic purposes.

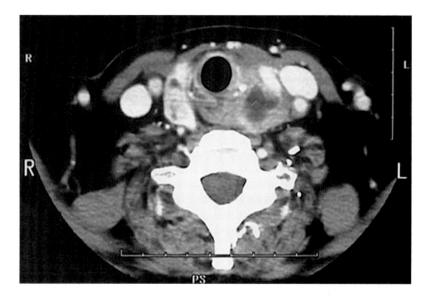

Figure 15-27 Thyroid, papillary carcinoma, CT image
CT scan of the neck reveals a left thyroid lobe mass with an irregular cystic area (◆) of decreased attenuation within the mass. This neoplasm often manifests as a painless palpable thyroid nodule. In some cases, the carcinoma is not palpable, but metastasis results in a nearby enlarged cervical lymph node (called a *Delphian node,* after the ancient Greek oracle of Delphi, who predicted future events). Underlying molecular mechanisms for development of this neoplasm include chromosomal rearrangement of the tyrosine kinase receptors *RET* (with formation of the *RET/PTC* fusion gene) or *NTRK1*, *BRAF* oncogene–activating mutations, and *RAS* mutations.

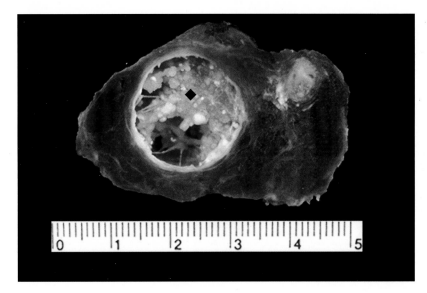

Figure 15-28 Thyroid, papillary carcinoma, gross
These neoplasms may be multifocal, as seen here, because of the propensity to invade lymphatics within thyroid, and metastases to adjacent lymph nodes not only are common, but also may be the presenting feature. The larger mass (◆) shown here in this cross-section through an excised thyroid gland is cystic and contains papillary excrescences. Papillary carcinoma, which constitutes up to 85% of all thyroid carcinomas, invariably produces a cold nodule by radionuclide scanning.

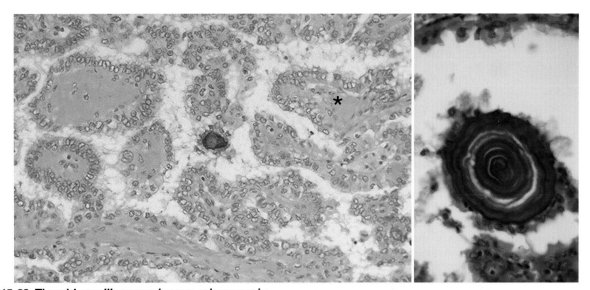

Figure 15-29 Thyroid, papillary carcinoma, microscopic
This carcinoma in the *left panel* has fronds of tissue with thin fibrovascular cores (★) that form a papillary pattern with papillations lined by cells with nuclei that appear clear (empty) on H&E staining after formalin fixation. Another microscopic feature, seen at high magnification in the *right panel,* is the round laminated concretion, a psammoma body. Papillary carcinomas are indolent tumors that have a long survival, even with metastases.

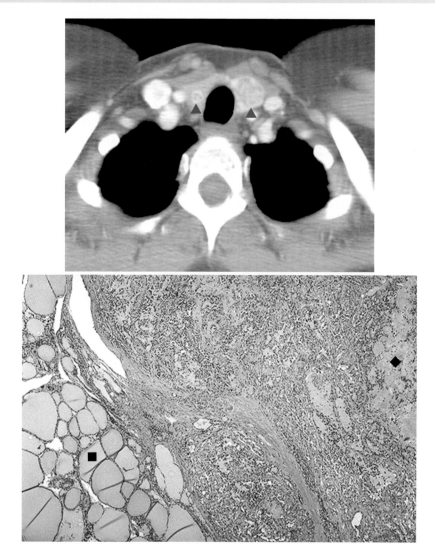

Figures 15-30 Thyroid, medullary carcinoma, CT image and microscopic

There is a mass lesion (▲) in each thyroid lobe *(upper panel)* representing the multifocal origin that is most likely to occur with familial disease. The carcinoma cells are at the top and right *(lower panel),* with adjacent normal thyroid (■) follicular tissue visible at the lower left. At the far right is pink hyaline material (◆) with the appearance of amyloid (it stains positively with Congo red). These neoplasms, derived from thyroid C cells, have neuroendocrine features, such as secretion of calcitonin (but without hypocalcemia). C-cell hyperplasia may be present in surrounding thyroid. Medullary carcinomas can be sporadic or familial. The familial form has a better prognosis and can be multifocal and associated with MEN syndromes. *RET* gene mutations are present in most familial and half of sporadic medullary carcinomas.

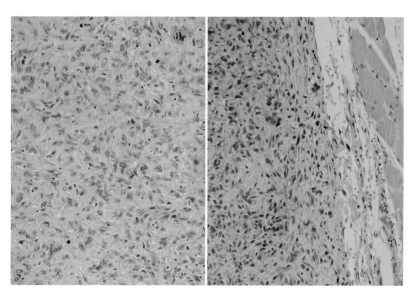

Figure 15-31 Thyroid, anaplastic carcinoma, microscopic

The least common thyroid malignancy, but the most aggressive, is rapidly growing and invasive to involve adjacent esophagus with dysphagia or trachea with dyspnea. Shown here *(right panel)* are highly pleomorphic spindle cells infiltrating into adjacent skeletal muscle on the right. Both epithelioid and spindle cells with desmoplasia are seen in the *left panel.* Some cases arise in a multinodular goiter. Multicentricity and foci of papillary or follicular carcinoma can be present in 20% to 30% of cases, suggesting origin from a prior differentiated carcinoma. They occur in elderly individuals. A mutated *p53* gene is often present.

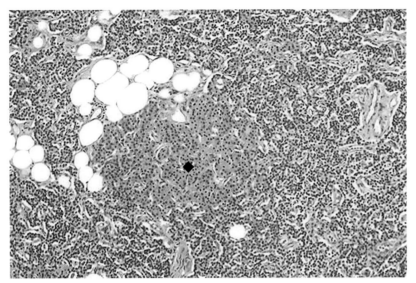

Figure 15-32 Parathyroid gland, normal
In the normal parathyroid gland, there are variable numbers of adipocytes, seen here mostly on the left, which are mixed with the small nests of chief cells that secrete PTH. There are typically small nodules of pink oxyphil cells (◆) whose function is obscure. The parathyroid gland has a rich vascular supply, as in all endocrine tissues secreting hormonal products directly into the bloodstream. Embryologically, parathyroids are derived from the third and fourth pharyngeal pouches and are present on the posterior aspect of the thyroid gland as superior and inferior pairs. Occasionally an ectopic parathyroid is located substernally in thymus. PTH is released inversely to ionized calcium and magnesium levels in the blood.

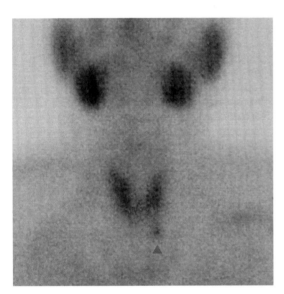

Figure 15-33 Parathyroid, adenoma, scintigraphic scan
This parathyroid scan after intravenous administration of technetium-99m shows, in addition to radiotracer uptake in both thyroid lobes and salivary glands, a small area of increased activity inferior to the left lobe of the thyroid, consistent with a left lower parathyroid adenoma (▲). Clinical findings with hyperparathyroidism include bone pain, nephrolithiasis, constipation, peptic ulcer disease, pancreatitis, cholelithiasis, depression, weakness, and seizures. Metastatic calcification of tissues such as lung, kidney, and gastric mucosa is rare. Surgical exploration to find the adenoma can be difficult, and a second adenoma may be present, or there may be parathyroid hyperplasia with asymmetric enlargement of the parathyroids. Parathyroid surgery is the most common cause of hypoparathyroidism, so serum calcium levels are checked postoperatively. Clinical findings with hypoparathyroidism include neuromuscular irritability, behavioral changes, including either anxiety or depression, papilledema, cataract formation, and cardiac dysrhythmias with prolonged Q–Tc interval.

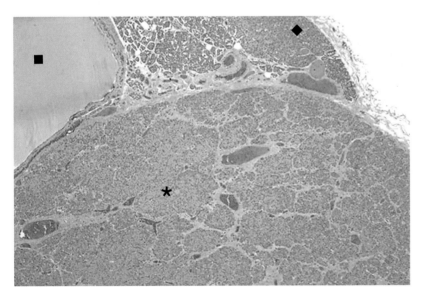

Figure 15-34 Parathyroid adenoma, microscopic
Adjacent to this parathyroid adenoma (★) is a rim of normal parathyroid, with a pink oxyphil cell nodule (◆) at the *upper right*, and a small benign parathyroid cyst (■), an incidental finding filled with pink proteinaceous fluid at *the upper left*. Adenoma accounts for nearly 85% to 95% of all cases of primary hyperparathyroidism. In addition to elevated serum ionized calcium with hypophosphatemia, a PTH assay reveals a high-normal to elevated level of PTH. Overexpression of the cyclin D1 gene is present in 40% of cases. In 20% to 30% of these adenomas there are *MEN1* gene mutations.

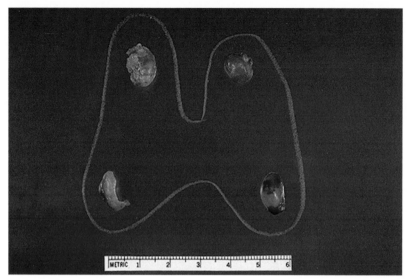

Figure 15-35 Parathyroid hyperplasia, gross
Three and one half hyperplastic parathyroid glands have been removed (only half the gland at the lower left is present) from this patient. Although all these glands are enlarged, they may be asymmetrically enlarged. Microscopically, chief cell hyperplasia is most common, but other parathyroid cell types may proliferate, too. Parathyroid hyperplasia is the second most common form of primary hyperparathyroidism, accounting for 10% to 15% of cases. Parathyroid hyperplasia is less commonly seen in association with MEN 1 or MEN 2A syndromes. Renal failure with reduced phosphate excretion may lead to secondary hyperparathyroidism.

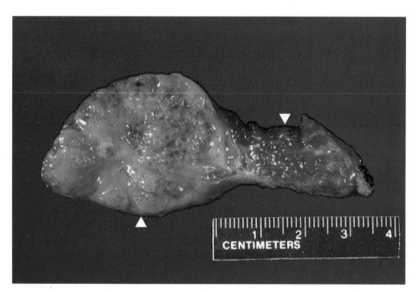

Figure 15-36 Parathyroid carcinoma, gross
An irregular tan mass (▲) invading into adjacent red-brown thyroid tissue (▼) is shown. Parathyroid carcinoma is the least common form of primary hyperparathyroidism, accounting for less than 1% of cases. These carcinomas tend to invade into surrounding tissues in the neck, complicating their removal. The serum calcium level is often quite high. Markedly elevated serum calcium levels also can be seen in association with nonparathyroid malignancies elsewhere, particularly those that produce a paraneoplastic syndrome from elaboration of PTH-related peptide.

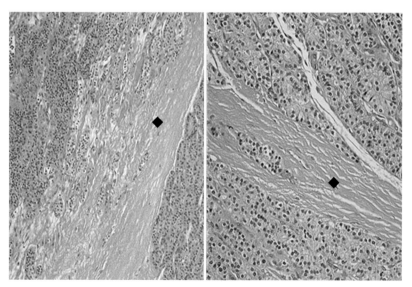

Figure 15-37 Parathyroid carcinoma, microscopic
This parathyroid carcinoma, seen at medium power in the *left panel* and higher power in the *right panel,* shows distinctive bands of fibrous tissue (◆) between the nests of carcinoma cells. The nests of neoplastic cells are not very pleomorphic, so invasion and metastases are the only reliable indicators of malignancy. The high serum PTH levels with parathyroid carcinomas, adenomas, and hyperplasia can increase bone osteoclast activity and bone remodeling to produce osteitis fibrosa cystica and brown tumor of bone.

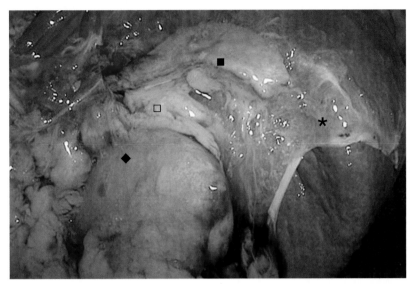

Figure 15-38 Normal adrenal gland, gross
This normal right adrenal gland (■) is positioned between the liver (★) and the kidney (◆) in the retroperitoneum. There is surrounding retroperitoneal adipose tissue (□). Each normal gland weighs 4 to 6 g. Embryologically, the adrenals develop from induction of coelomic epithelial cell proliferation by the ureteric bud, forming fetal adrenal cortex, which eventually becomes the zona reticularis. This is invaded by neural crest–forming neuroblasts to become adrenal medulla. Another proliferation of coelomic epithelium surrounds the fetal cortex to become the adult cortical zona glomerulosa and zona fasciculata.

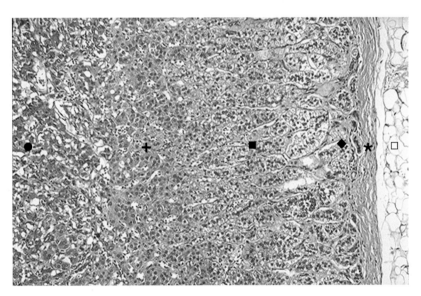

Figure 15-39 Normal adrenal gland, microscopic
The normal layers of the adrenal gland are not that distinctive. At the far right is the surrounding adipose tissue (□). Moving left in the image, next is the fibrous tissue capsule (★). Adjacent to the capsule is the zona glomerulosa (◆), whose cells produce mineralocorticoids such as aldosterone. Then comes the zona fasciculata (■) in the center of this image, whose cells produce glucocorticoids, mainly cortisol. Next is the zona reticularis (✛), composed of darker and slightly smaller pink cells producing sex steroid hormones. At the far left is the medulla (●), which produces catecholamines, mainly norepinephrine and some epinephrine and dopamine.

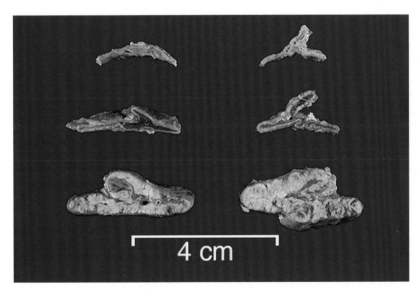

Figure 15-40 Comparison of atrophic, normal, and hyperplastic adrenal glands
The topmost pair of adrenal glands are atrophic, characteristic of either idiopathic Addison disease or long-term use of corticosteroids. The normal adrenals at the center have a well-defined rim of golden cortex and a center of reddish medulla. The hyperplastic pair of adrenals at the bottom are typical of increased ACTH secretion with ectopic production either from a neoplasm, such as a small cell lung carcinoma, which results in Cushing syndrome, or from a pituitary adenoma, resulting in Cushing disease. The adrenals may become hyperplastic from enzymatic defects in steroidogenesis or, rarely, without the stimulus of ACTH, as a primary idiopathic process.

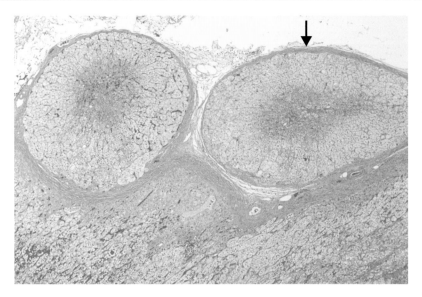

Figure 15-41 Adrenal nodular hyperplasia, microscopic
Sporadic primary cortical macronodular hyperplasia is independent of ACTH, with nodules larger than 3 mm. Note that the nodules (↓) here have both lipid-rich (clear, like fasciculata) and lipid-poor (pink, like reticularis) cells. Receptors for gastric inhibitory polypeptide, luteinizing hormone (LH), antidiuretic hormone (ADH), and serotonin are overexpressed in the hyperplastic nodules. Some cases of macronodular hyperplasia occur with McCune-Albright syndrome. Diffuse hyperplasia with few or small nodules is ACTH dependent.

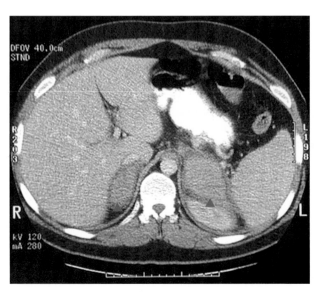

Figure 15-42 Waterhouse-Friderichsen syndrome, CT
Abdominal CT scan shows the typical locations of the adrenal glands (▲), but these glands are enlarged because of bilateral adrenal gland hemorrhage from Waterhouse-Friderichsen syndrome with *Neisseria meningitidis* (meningococcal) infection. Less commonly, infection with other organisms, such as *Pseudomonas aeruginosa*, *Streptococcus pneumoniae*, or *Haemophilus influenzae*, may lead to this condition. This condition causes acute adrenal insufficiency along with endotoxin-induced vasculitis and disseminated intravascular coagulopathy (DIC).

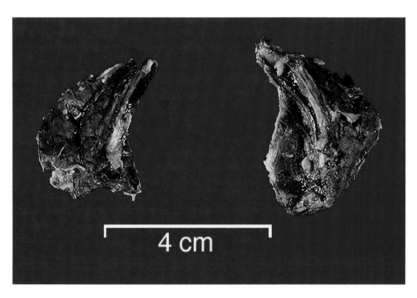

Figure 15-43 Waterhouse-Friderichsen syndrome, gross
These adrenals have a dark-red to black color from extensive hemorrhage with disseminated intravascular coagulopathy as a consequence of endotoxin release from *Neisseria meningitidis* organisms causing septicemia. This condition is known as *Waterhouse-Friderichsen syndrome* and is more likely to complicate infections in children. Infection with *N. meningitidis* can start initially as a mild pharyngitis but become a florid septicemia with hypotension and shock within hours. Destruction of more than 90% of the adrenal cortex leads to adrenal cortical insufficiency.

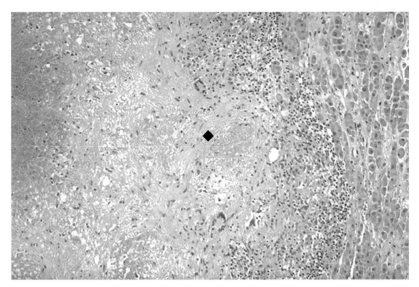

Figure 15-44 Tuberculous adrenalitis, microscopic

Although most cases of Addison disease are now idiopathic (presumably autoimmune in cause), there are still cases resulting from disseminated *Mycobacterium tuberculosis* infection. Shown here is a granuloma (◆) with central pink areas of caseous necrosis and surrounding inflammation with lymphocytes, epithelioid cells, and Langhans giant cells. Residual adrenal is present on the right. This infection proceeds over months to years, and adrenocortical destruction leads to chronic adrenal insufficiency. The decreased plasma cortisol leads to increased ACTH and precursors that can stimulate melanocytes, leading to skin hyperpigmentation.

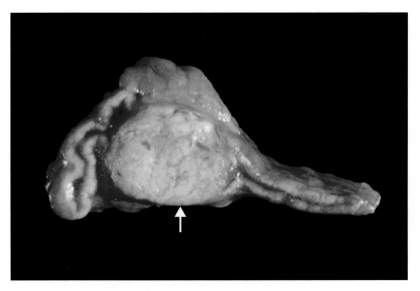

Figure 15-45 Adrenal adenoma, gross

This circumscribed, uniformly yellow-tan mass (↑) is an adenoma found in a patient with hypertension and hypokalemia. Further workup revealed high serum aldosterone and low plasma renin activity, findings consistent with an aldosterone-secreting adenoma (Conn syndrome). Adenomas account for about a third of primary hyperaldosteronism cases, and idiopathic nodular hyperplasia for most of the rest. Such adenomas are typically smaller than 2 cm and have a yellow hue on cut surface. If the adenoma were secreting cortisol, the patient would have Cushing syndrome.

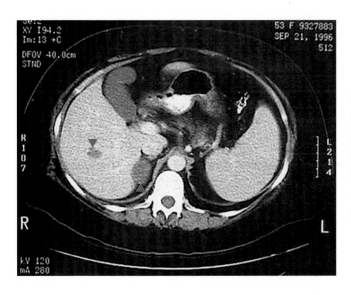

Figure 15-46 Adrenal adenoma, CT

Abdominal CT scan shows a small adrenal adenoma (▲) with decreased attenuation adjacent to the liver on the right. There is also an incidental simple cyst (▼) of the liver. Some adrenal adenomas are incidental findings ("incidentaloma") on an abdominal CT scan performed for other indications, and adenomas smaller than 2 cm without signs or symptoms of adrenal hyperfunction may be left alone (as in fishing—"catch and release"). The hepatic cyst is the other incidentaloma.

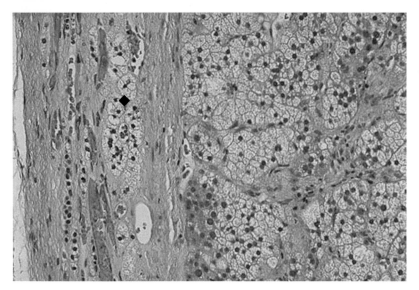

Figure 15-47 Adrenal adenoma, microscopic
The adrenocortical adenoma on the *right* is well differentiated and resembles normal adrenal fasciculata. It appears histologically nearly the same as the compressed normal adrenal (◆) on the *left,* just outside the capsule of the adenoma. There may be minimal cellular pleomorphism within these adenomas. If such an adenoma does not function, it may not be detected except by imaging studies done for other reasons. Adenomas secreting cortisol may lead to Cushing syndrome with central fat redistribution, hypertension, secondary diabetes, purpura, and osteoporosis.

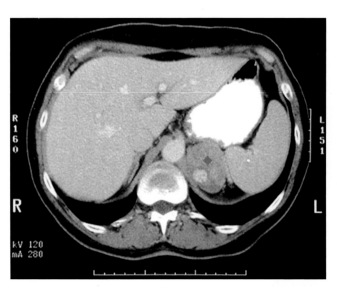

Figure 15-48 Adrenocortical carcinoma, CT image
A large mass is arising in this left adrenal gland (◆). These carcinomas tend to be larger than adrenal adenomas and more variegated in their radiographic and gross pathologic appearance, typically from areas of hemorrhage and necrosis. Most weigh more than 100 g. They can occur over a wide age range. After administration of intravenous contrast material, there is a focus of brighter attenuation seen here in the posterior aspect of the mass that corresponds to an area of hemorrhage. The major differential diagnosis for this mass, in the absence of clinical or laboratory evidence of endocrine function, is a metastasis, most often from a lung primary. Metastases to both adrenals may lead to adrenocortical insufficiency, whereas many cortical carcinomas function hormonally.

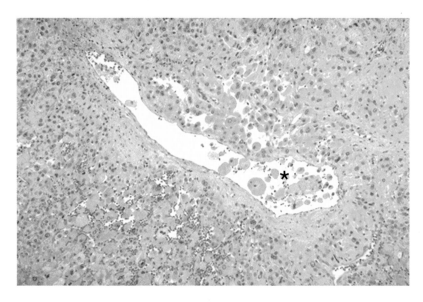

Figure 15-49 Adrenocortical carcinoma, microscopic
This adrenocortical carcinoma has a microscopic appearance that closely resembles normal adrenal cortex. It is difficult to determine malignancy in endocrine neoplasms based on cytologic features alone. Invasion (as seen here in a vein [★]) and metastases are the most reliable indicators of malignancy. Adrenocortical carcinomas often are hormonally functional and can lead to Cushing syndrome from glucocorticoid secretion, or there can be sex steroid hormone secretion with clinical features of masculinization in a woman or feminization in a man. These carcinomas rarely produce mineralocorticoids in excess.

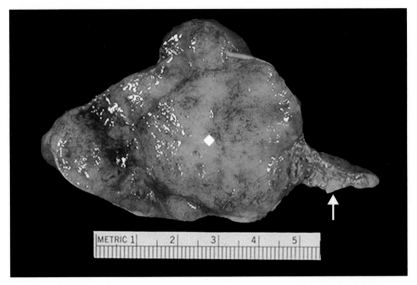

Figure 15-50 Pheochromocytoma, gross
Note the gray-tan color of this neoplasm (◆) arising from the adrenal medulla, and compare it with the yellow color of the residual cortex (↑) of normal adrenal stretched around it, and a small remnant of remaining adrenal gland at the lower right. This patient had episodic hypertension from secretion of catecholamines (norepinephrine and epinephrine) acting on α-adrenergic and β-adrenergic receptors in various cells. Although most pheochromocytomas occur sporadically, they may be associated with MEN 2A or 2B syndromes, neurofibromatosis 1, Sturge-Weber disease, and von Hippel–Lindau disease. Pheochromocytomas follow the 10% rule—10% are bilateral, malignant, pediatric, nonhypertensive, or extraadrenal in location.

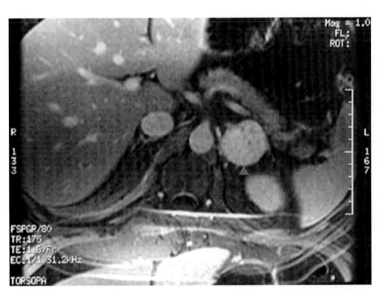

Figure 15-51 Adrenal pheochromocytoma, MRI
Axial postgadolinium T1-weighted MRI image of the abdomen with fat saturation shows diffuse contrast enhancement (because of this neoplasm's vascularity) in a mass (▲) that is replacing the left adrenal gland. This patient had hypertension, tachycardia, palpitations, headache, tremor, and diaphoresis, along with an elevated catecholamine level. The hypertension is most often sustained and less often of the more suggestive episodic variety. The patient also had increased free urinary catecholamines, vanillylmandelic acid, and metanephrines. Cardiac dysrhythmias may lead to sudden death. The anesthesiologist can report elevation of the blood pressure when the surgeon manipulates this tumor during removal.

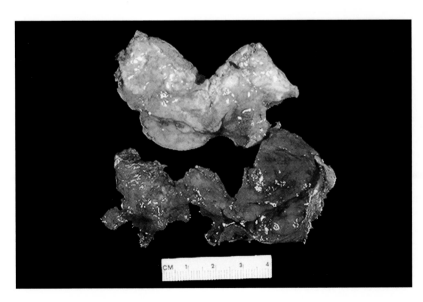

Figure 15-52 Adrenal pheochromocytoma, chromaffin reaction, gross
It is a traditional pathology "magic trick" to display the chromaffin reaction, in which the tissues of a pheochromocytoma turn from tan to brown when placed in a freshly made solution of potassium dichromate. This reaction occurs because large amounts of biogenic amines (catecholamines) in the cytoplasm of the neoplastic cells are oxidized by this solution. In addition to catecholamines, these neoplasms may secrete ACTH (leading to Cushing syndrome) or somatostatin. Up to 25% of cases may be familial and have a genetic basis, including *RET, NF1,* and *VHL* gene mutations.

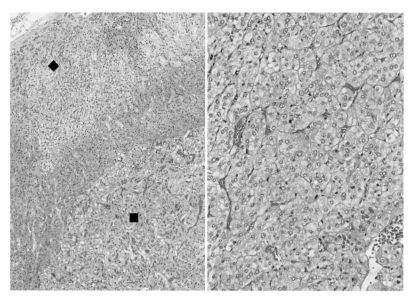

Figure 15-53 Pheochromocytoma, microscopic

Note the normal (◆) adrenal cortex *(left panel)*, with the medullary neoplasm (■) composed of large polygonal to spindle chromaffin (chief) cells that have pink to mauve cytoplasm. The cells are arranged in nests *(Zellballen)* with adjacent smaller sustentacular cells, surrounded by abundant intervening capillaries *(right panel)*. Immunohistochemical staining for chromogranin and synaptophysin is usually positive. The microscopic appearance gives no reliable clue to biologic behavior, so determination of malignancy is based on presence of invasion or metastases. The symptoms can be treated with adrenergic-blocking agents before surgical removal.

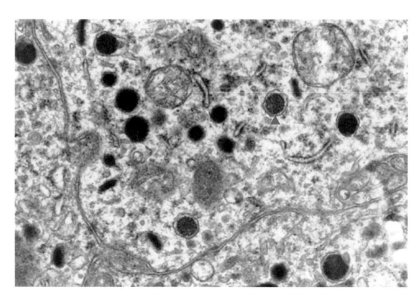

Figure 15-54 Adrenal pheochromocytoma, electron microscopy

By electron microscopy, these chromaffin (chief) cells of a pheochromocytoma, similar to the chief cells of other neoplasms with neuroendocrine differentiation, contain dark round membrane-bound neurosecretory granules (▲) in their cell cytoplasm. These granules contain the catecholamines in a pheochromocytoma. Immunohistochemical staining for chromogranin and synaptophysin is present in chief cells, whereas the sustentacular cells are positive for S100, a calcium-binding protein. Persistently elevated catecholamine levels can produce a catecholamine cardiomyopathy complicated by congestive heart failure and arrhythmias.

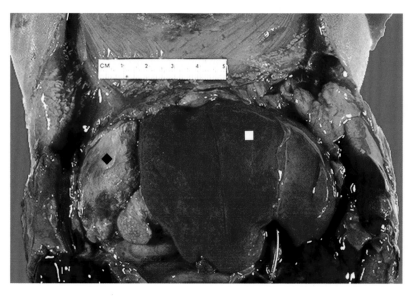

Figure 15-55 Adrenal neuroblastoma, gross

Abdominal enlargement palpated in this neonate resulted from a congenital neuroblastoma arising within the right adrenal gland. This irregular tan mass (◆) with focal hemorrhage is a neuroblastoma large enough to displace the liver (■) to the left. Most of these neoplasms arise during the first 3 years of life, and despite the higher stage seen here, neuroblastomas arising in infancy have a better overall prognosis. *MYCN* gene amplification is often present and affects prognosis. Similar to adult pheochromocytomas, they may also arise in extra-adrenal paraganglia. Familial cases may have anaplastic lymphoma kinase *(ALK)* germline mutations.

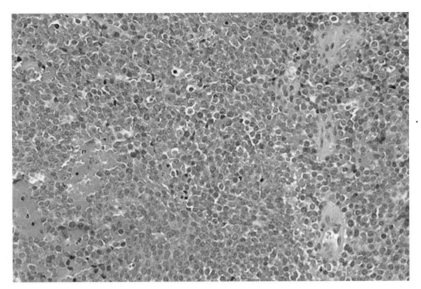

Figure 15-56 Adrenal neuroblastoma, microscopic

This is one of the "small round blue cell" tumors most typically seen in children. Note the population of round blue cells resembling embryonic neuroblasts. These neoplasms can reach a large size in the retroperitoneum before they are detected. They often contain focal areas of necrosis and calcification. Hypertension may be present in some cases. They may be detected because they secrete homovanillic acid, a precursor in catecholamine synthesis, and vanillylmandelic acid, dopamine, and norepinephrine, although not in as large quantities as pheochromocytomas. Age younger than 18 months or lower stage predicts better prognosis.

The Skin

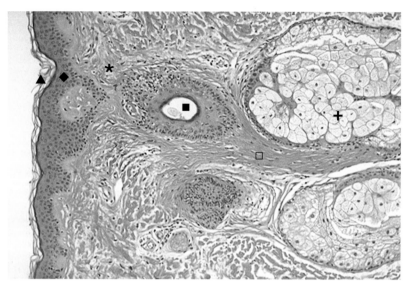

Figure 16-1 Normal skin, microscopic
The normal histologic appearance of the skin is shown. At the left is the epidermis. A thin layer of keratin (▲) overlies this epidermis. This keratinized layer is thicker on the palms and soles and over areas of the body surface where the skin is persistently rubbed or irritated. Beneath the epidermis (◆) is the dermis (✱), containing connective tissue with collagen and elastic fibers. A hair follicle (■) can be seen at the center with surrounding sebaceous glands (✚). Associated with the hair follicle is a small bundle of smooth muscle (□) known as the *arrector pili,* which can cause the hair to "stand on end" and dimple the skin to form "goose bumps" when exposed to a cold environment.

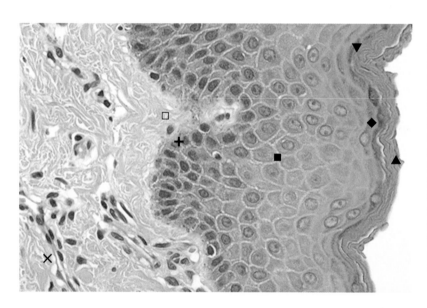

Figure 16-2 Normal skin, microscopic
At high magnification, the skin has an overlying acellular keratin layer called the *stratum corneum* (▲) that continually desquamates. Beneath this is the nearly indistinguishable thin, darker red stratum lucidum (▼). The outer layer of epidermal cells has prominent purplish cytoplasmic granules and is called the *stratum granulosum* (◆). Below this is the thickest layer, the *stratum spinosum* (■), with polyhedral cells that have prominent intercellular bridges. A basal layer (✚) of cells rests on a basement membrane. In this case, there is also prominent brown melanin pigmentation in the basal region. The upper papillary dermis (□) has small capillary blood vessels (✖) that play a role in temperature regulation.

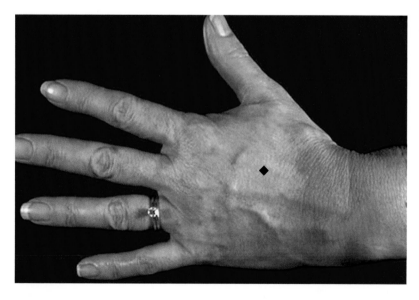

Figure 16-3 Vitiligo, gross
Irregular areas of hypopigmentation (◆) of the skin are shown here on the hand. This is a localized form of hypopigmentation (as contrasted with the diffuse form known as *oculocutaneous albinism*). Many localized cases are idiopathic, although sometimes a systemic disease may be present. Microscopically, melanocytes are absent in the areas of vitiligo. The degree of skin pigmentation is related to melanocyte activity through the enzyme tyrosinase, with formation of pigmented melanin granules, which are passed off to adjacent keratinocytes by long melanocyte cytoplasmic processes.

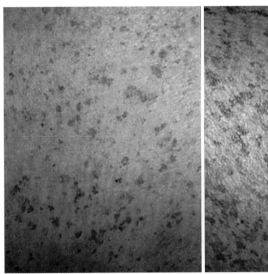

Figure 16-4 Freckles, gross

Ephelis is a fancy word for a freckle. Freckles represent hyperpigmentation that can occur in some fair-skinned individuals, particularly those with red hair. The onset occurs in childhood, and the extent is related to the amount of sun exposure. Microscopically, the number of melanocytes in the skin is normal, but there is focally increased melanin production from each melanocyte. There is no increased risk for malignancy from an ephelis. The cosmetic industry benefits from them.

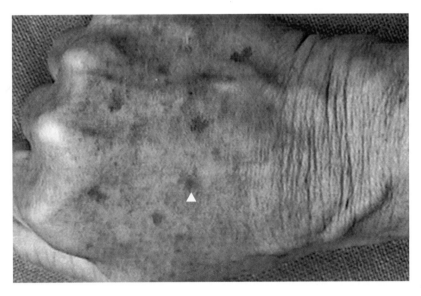

Figure 16-5 Age spots, gross

Appearing on the hand are age spots or liver spots, termed *senile lentigines* (▲), which are common on areas of sun-exposed skin of older individuals. Perhaps 90% of whites older than 70 years have one or more age spots. They are flat lesions with irregular borders, can be pinpoint to 1 cm in size, and are often multiple. They have no significance except for their cosmetic appearance. They do not change in response to sun exposure.

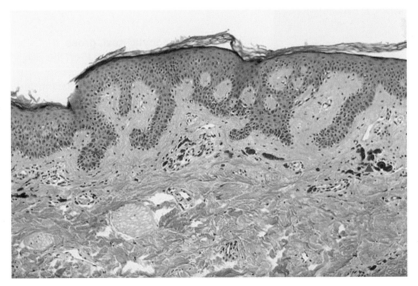

Figure 16-6 Lentigo senilis, microscopic

The microscopic appearance of lentigo senilis, commonly known as an age or liver spot, is shown. The rete ridges (✱) of the epidermis are elongated and appear club shaped or tortuous. Melanocytes are increased in number along the basal layer of the epidermis, and melanophages (▲) filled with brown melanin granules appear in the paler pink lower papillary dermis, just above the darker pink reticular dermis. This process is localized and benign.

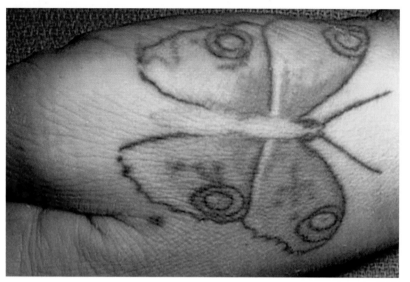

Figure 16-7 Tattoo, gross
Tattooing is a practice that is thousands of years old. In many human cultural groups, tattoos have great significance. Rituals can have usefulness for social groups, as long as no one gets hurt. The pigment in tattoos is transferred into the dermis with a needle, so there can be a risk for infection from the tattooing procedure. The tattoo itself over time tends to lose sharpness and intensity of color. Removal of a tattoo can be difficult; a laser light can be used to vaporize the pigment granules beneath the epidermis, but this is a laborious, time-consuming process. Removal at a later date is more likely to be undertaken when the blood ethanol level was high at the time of the tattooing procedure, or social relationships have changed.

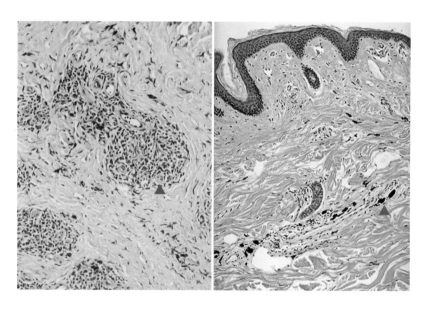

Figure 16-8 Tattoo, microscopic
The tattoo pigment shown here as black granules (▲) is introduced into the dermis with a needle. This pigment is deep within the dermis *(right panel)*, so removing or changing a tattoo is difficult. Over time, the pigment can be taken up into dermal macrophages, which can concentrate it or redistribute it, blurring the pattern, particularly on intricate designs. Granulomatous inflammation or hypertrophic scarring may occur. Different tattoo pigments account for different colors. Some pigments, such as those creating a green color, can impart photosensitivity with inflammation (▲) *(left panel)*. Red, green, yellow, or blue pigments may cause an allergic reaction.

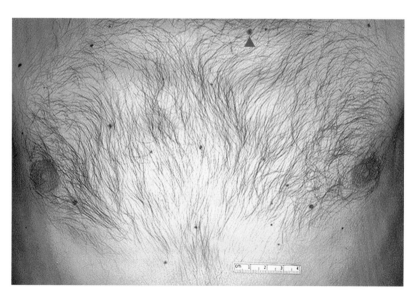

Figure 16-9 Melanocytic nevi, gross
Note the discrete brown lesions (▲) on the skin of the anterior chest. A melanocytic nevus (pigmented nevus) is a small, brown, flat (macular) to slightly raised (papular) lesion with sharp borders that is quite common in light-skinned individuals. Such lesions are commonly called *moles.* These nevi are usually less than 0.6 cm in diameter, and they tend to grow very slowly and retain the same uniform degree of pigmentation and same sharp outlines, so that they seem hardly to change over time. These nevi are benign, with no risk for subsequent malignancy, but they must be distinguished from more aggressive lesions.

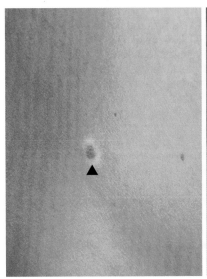
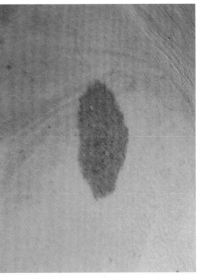

Figure 16-10 Melanocytic nevi, gross

The *left panel* shows a halo nevus, so called because the central pigmented area is surrounded by a lighter zone (▲), caused by an immune response to nevus cells. Nevi can show considerable variation in appearance: flat to raised and pale to darkly pigmented. Most are small, well-circumscribed lesions that hardly seem to change at all or change very slowly over time. The *right panel* shows a larger, flat, pigmented nevus on the upper back that sometimes is termed a *café au lait spot.*

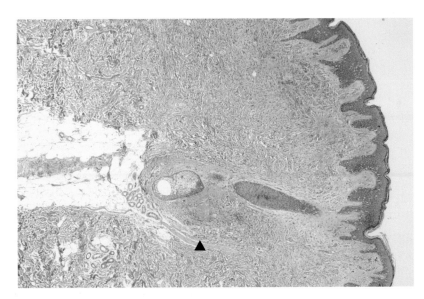

Figure 16-11 Congenital nevus, gross

Larger nevi are congenital if present from birth; they remain relatively unchanged, and microscopically extend into the deep dermis. Congenital nevi can be found in approximately 1% to 2% of newborns. This lesion is usually raised, dark to medium brown, with a sharp border (as shown) and a smooth or papillomatous surface. Very large congenital nevi have an increased risk for malignant melanoma.

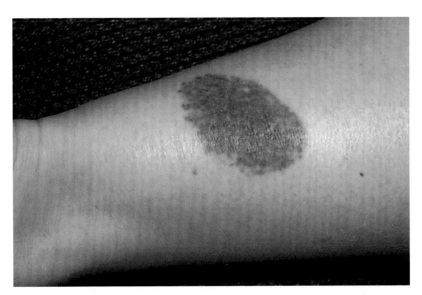

Figure 16-12 Congenital nevus, microscopic

The microscopic features shown here include nevus cells (▲) extending to deep dermal appendages and neurovascular structures and subcutaneous fat, infiltration of nevus cells among collagen bundles, and a subepidermal region with few nevus cells. Although extending downward without a distinct border, the cells are quite uniform, and the lesion is benign. Acquired nevi appearing later in life usually do not involve deeper structures. Abnormalities in the melanocortin-1 receptor (MC1R) may be present.

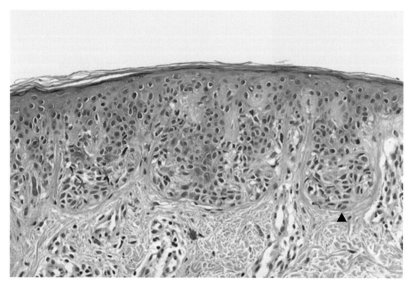

Figure 16-13 Junctional nevus, microscopic
This is the early stage of a junctional, or nevocellular, nevus. It is termed a *junctional nevus* because there are nevus cells in nests (✱) in the lower epidermis. As nests of cells continue to drop off (▲) into the upper dermis, the lesion could then be termed a *compound nevus*. In contrast to a melanoma, there is no significant atypia of these nevus cells and no adjacent dermal inflammation. In addition, there is a maturation effect so that the nevus cells in the lower epidermis tend to be larger, with pigment, whereas the cells that extend deeper into the dermis are smaller, with little or no pigment. This microscopic maturation with differentiation to smaller cells helps distinguish this lesion from a malignant melanoma.

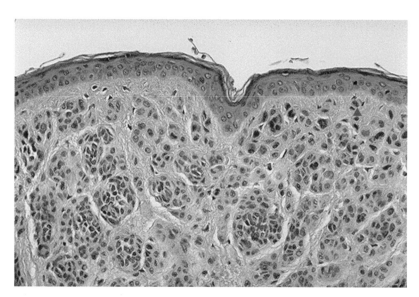

Figure 16-14 Intradermal nevus, microscopic
This lesion is termed an *intradermal nevus* because the nevus cells (melanocytes that are transformed to rounded cells that proliferate as aggregates or nests [✱]) are found solely within the dermis, although close to (▲) the overlying epidermis. This is considered to be a later stage of a junctional (nevocellular) nevus in which the connection of the nevus cells to the epidermis has been lost. The benign nature of the nevus cells is confirmed by their small, uniform appearance. The cells form small aggregates in nests and cords, which are not encapsulated and may interdigitate with adnexal structures. The nevus cells (derived from melanocytes) have clear cytoplasm and small round blue nuclei without prominent nucleoli or mitoses.

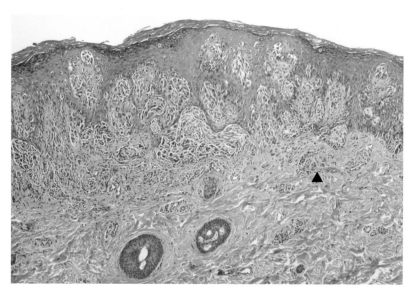

Figure 16-15 Spitz nevus, microscopic
Spitz nevi are more common in children, appear red like a hemangioma, and are generally larger than other forms of nevi. They are composed of spindled or epithelioid melanocytes or both, as shown here. The melanocytes display uniform features; cytoplasm is abundant and varies from eosinophilic to slightly basophilic. The visible skin lesion has a symmetrical profile and circumscribed margins (▲). Nested melanocytes have fairly uniform cytologic features. There is a gradual transition from larger nests of melanocytes in the superficial dermis to smaller melanocytes in smaller nests, to dispersed aggregates and single units within the deep dermal component, often appearing adjacent to adnexa.

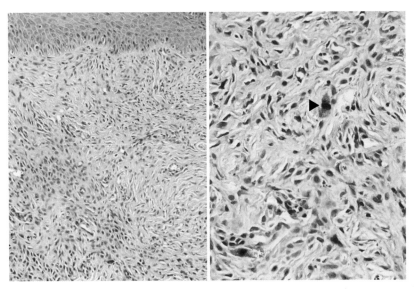

Figure 16-16 Blue nevus, microscopic

The nevus shown has uniform highly dendritic spindle cells with abundant melanin (▶), giving them their grossly blue-black appearance. This color suggests melanoma, but the blue nevus has regular borders and more uniform pigmentation and tends to grow slowly. The cells extend into the dermis, but not as nests. They are most common in Asian populations, arising in teenage years and affecting 3% to 5% of adults and twice as many women as men.

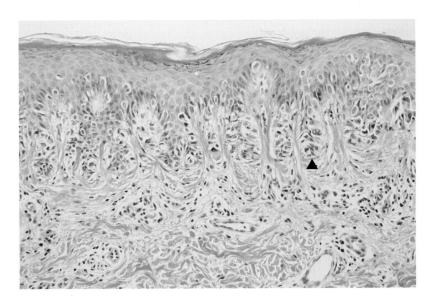

Figure 16-17 Dysplastic nevus, microscopic

This atypical melanocytic hyperplasia is "in between" a clearly benign melanocytic nevus and a malignant melanoma. There are an increased number of melanocytes, some with atypical features, such as enlarged, irregular nuclei, at the dermal-epidermal junction (▲). They are generally larger than 0.5 cm and have an irregular pigment distribution. Patients with autosomal dominant dysplastic nevus syndrome (or familial melanoma syndrome) have many such lesions, and there is an increased risk for eventual development of malignant melanoma, although most lesions act benignly. A *CDNK2* gene mutation leads to production of an abnormal *p16/INK4A* cyclin-dependent kinase inhibitor. Activating mutations in the *NRAS* and *BRAF* genes are often present.

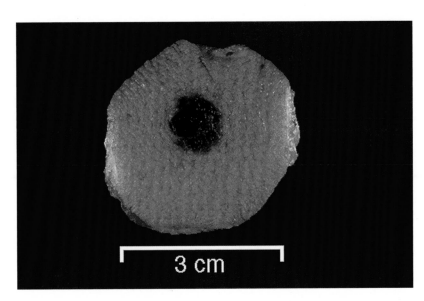

3 cm

Figure 16-18 Malignant melanoma, gross

This pigmented lesion has been excised with a wide margin. Although this lesion is only about 1 cm in size, it shows asymmetry, irregular borders, variable pigmentation, and an irregular surface—all worrisome signs. Increasing diameter and evolution in the appearance are also suspicious for malignancy. Melanomas begin with a radial growth phase, but then over time start a vertical growth phase, invading down into the dermis and developing the potential for metastases to lymph nodes and distant sites. Larger lesions are more likely to have invaded more deeply. Sun exposure (ultraviolet [UV] radiation) in light-skinned individuals leads to an increased risk for malignant melanoma.

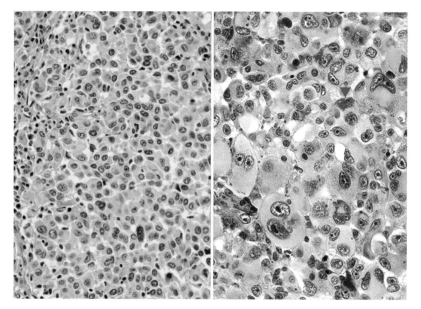

Figure 16-19 Malignant melanoma, microscopic

This neoplasm is composed of large polygonal cells (or spindle cells in some other cases) that have very pleomorphic nuclei that contain prominent nucleoli. The neoplasm in the *right panel* is making abundant brown melanin pigment (▼). Melanoma cells can make variable amounts of melanin pigment, even within the same lesion (leading to the characteristic variability in pigmentation, which helps distinguish it from a benign nevus). Some melanomas may make so little pigment that grossly they appear amelanotic *(left panel)* but microscopically still have atypical cellular features with the hyperchromatism and pleomorphism shown here.

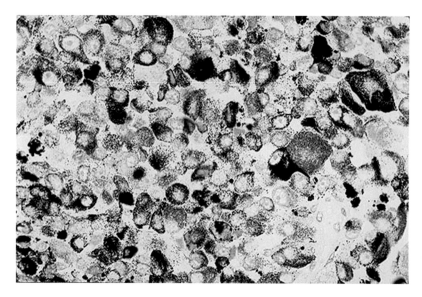

Figure 16-20 Malignant melanoma, microscopic

This Fontana-Masson silver stain (melanin stain) shows a fine black dusting of melanin pigment within the cytoplasm of the neoplastic cells of this malignant melanoma. Familial and sporadic malignant melanomas can have the *CDKN2A (p16/INK4A)* gene mutation, a cyclin-dependent kinase inhibitor. Mutations in the *BRAF* and *NRAS* genes also occur. *TERT* gene mutations that activate telomerase can be found in up to 70% of melanomas. A sixth of melanomas may have a genetic basis with autosomal dominant inheritance and variable penetrance.

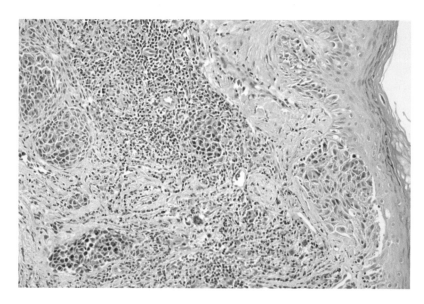

Figure 16-21 Malignant melanoma, microscopic

Nests of neoplastic cells have infiltrated downward as part of the ominous vertical growth phase. There was likely development of a nodule in the lesion. The nests here contain abundant brown melanin pigment. Note the marked inflammatory reaction of lymphocytes around the tumor nests. This immunologic response is rarely effective on its own in controlling the growth. The depth of invasion determines the prognosis. T1 stage with invasion of less than 1 mm has a better prognosis. Suspicious pigmented lesions should be completely excised.

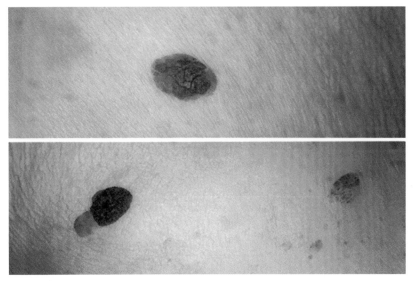

Figure 16-22 Seborrheic keratosis, gross
Shown here are examples of a very common lesion of older individuals—seborrheic keratoses. These warty lesions are usually distributed over the skin of the face, neck, and upper trunk. They develop into rough-surfaced, coinlike plaques that vary from a few millimeters in size to several centimeters. They slowly enlarge over time. They are usually brown, but the amount of pigmentation can vary from one lesion to the next. On close inspection of a lesion, keratin appears to erupt out of small pores on the surfaces.

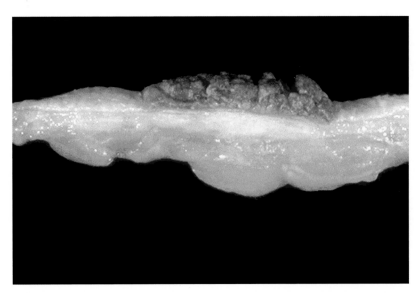

Figure 16-23 Seborrheic keratosis, gross
This seborrheic keratosis looks as though it has just been pasted or "stuck" on the skin, as shown here in cross-section of an excised lesion. The brownish, nodular, rough-surfaced lesion extends above the level of the surrounding epidermis. In some cases, seborrheic keratoses can have a downward growth phase, in which case they are termed *inverted follicular keratoses.* Seborrheic keratoses enlarge slowly over time. Their unsightliness is their only real consequence. They are never malignant.

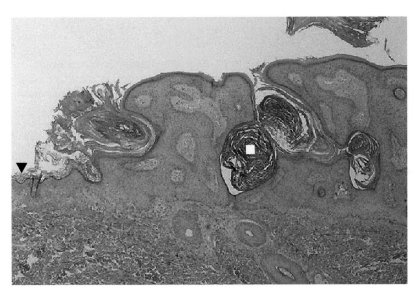

Figure 16-24 Seborrheic keratosis, microscopic
This seborrheic keratosis is formed of benign-appearing, well-differentiated squamous epithelium, and the lesion extends above the level of the surrounding epidermis (▼) shown on the left, giving it the raised appearance as though it were "stuck onto" the skin surface. Broad bands of normal-appearing epidermal cells have large keratin-filled "horn cysts" (■) within them. When irritated by scratching or rubbing, they can enlarge from inflammation with swelling. Activating mutations in the fibroblast growth factor receptor 3 *(FGFR3)* gene may drive their growth.

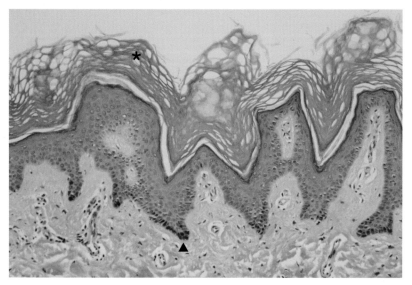

Figure 16-25 Acanthosis nigricans, microscopic

These hyperpigmented lesions occur most commonly in areas of flexure, such as at the elbow, axilla, neck, or groin. Their hyperpigmentation is caused by increased melanin granules in the epidermal basal layer. There are activating mutations in the receptor tyrosine kinase FGFR3, leading to increased growth factor receptor signaling in the skin. Shown here is epidermal papillomatosis with hyperkeratosis (★) and patchy hyperpigmentation (▲) of the basal cell layer. Most cases occur in childhood and are the result of either an autosomal dominant condition or a manifestation of obesity or an endocrinopathy. The appearance of acanthosis nigricans in adults may presage signs and symptoms of an underlying malignancy such as gastric adenocarcinoma.

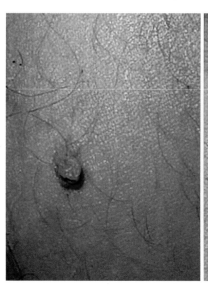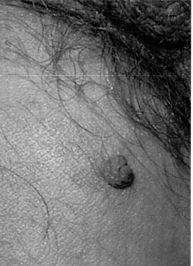

Figure 16-26 Fibroepithelial polyp, gross

Two examples of *skin tags,* each about 0.6 cm long, are shown. These are also termed *soft fibromas* or *acrochorda*. They appear as papules or baglike pedunculated growths connected by a narrow pedicle to the skin of the neck, trunk, or extremities. They are covered by epidermis and composed centrally of a loose overgrowth of connective tissue from the reticular dermis. They can be a nuisance when they appear at the belt line or axillary line, where rubbing and irritation can occur. Similar to hemangiomas and nevi, they may become more numerous during pregnancy.

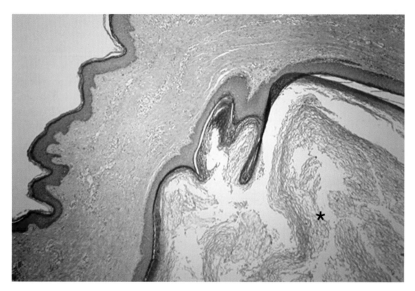

Figure 16-27 Epithelial cyst, microscopic

An epithelial cyst (also known as a *wen,* or *sebaceous cyst*) is palpably fluctuant and freely movable. It becomes filled with soft keratinaceous debris. A wen forms when there is down-growth of the overlying epidermis or epithelium of a hair follicle into the underlying dermis. There is continued desquamation of keratin into the center of the expanding cyst (★). These lesions are common. Larger cysts may become traumatized and rupture, inducing a surrounding inflammatory reaction that can include acute, chronic, and granulomatous elements.

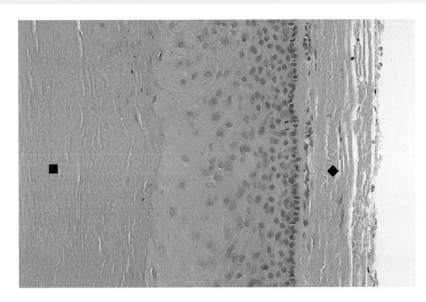

Figure 16-28 Epithelial cyst, microscopic
This epithelial cyst was excised from beneath the skin surface, with a rim of dermal connective tissue (◆) on the right. These cysts occur most frequently on the face, scalp, neck, and trunk. They are about 1 to 5 cm in size. They have a wall of epidermis that desquamates keratin, visible here as the laminated pink material (■) on the left, which forms the soft cyst contents that give the cyst characteristics that lead to the clinical description *sebaceous cyst.* The cyst can rupture and lead to marked foreign-body inflammation. The lack of a granular cell layer in this example is most characteristic of the variant known as a *pilar cyst* beneath the scalp.

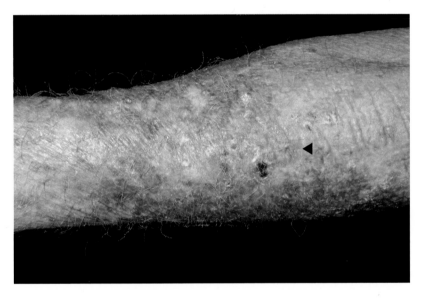

Figure 16-29 Actinic keratosis, gross
The irregular, tan to red, plaquelike lesion (◀) with a rough surface here in a sun-exposed area (the forearm) may enlarge over time. These lesions are usually smaller than 1 cm. This is a potentially premalignant lesion that can give rise to squamous cell carcinoma (SCC) in situ, which can evolve into an invasive squamous carcinoma. It is common for patients to have more than one such lesion in sun-exposed areas of skin. If such a lesion appears on the lips, it is termed *actinic cheilitis.* Because SCCs often arise in areas of actinic keratosis, removal of these lesions, or topical chemotherapy (imiquimod that activates Toll-like receptors, or 5-fluorouracil), is recommended.

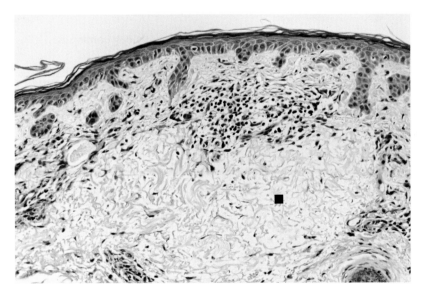

Figure 16-30 Actinic change, microscopic
With extensive, prolonged exposure to sunlight with UV radiation, particularly in light-skinned persons, there is homogenization of the dermal collagen and elastic fibers. Note the pale blue connective tissue (■) shown here in the dermis. The overlying epidermis is atrophic, consistent with aging. The loss of elastic fibers increases visible skin features such as wrinkles. More sun exposure leads to more wrinkling.

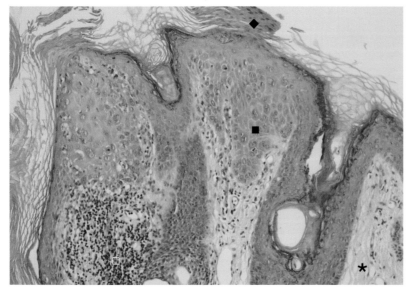

Figure 16-31 Actinic change, microscopic
Actinic damage from increased skin exposure to UV light (exposure to sunlight) is shown here. There is parakeratosis (◆) along with keratinocyte atypia (■) limited to the lower epidermal layers. The damaged collagen and elastic fibers appear as homogeneous pale blue areas (★) in the dermis, termed *solar elastosis.* With more extensive solar damage, there can be dermal inflammation (□), as here. Fair-skinned individuals are at greater risk for development of this condition. This actinic damage is cumulative and nonreversible. The loss of dermal elastic fibers contributes to skin aging with wrinkling.

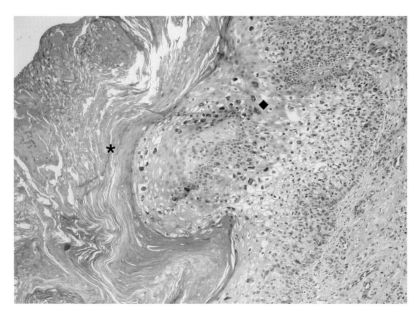

Figure 16-32 Squamous carcinoma in situ, microscopic
This actinic keratosis has marked overlying hyperkeratosis with a dense layer of keratin (★) on the left. Sometimes the hyperkeratosis is so pronounced that there is formation of a "cutaneous horn" of projecting keratin. Actinic keratoses are predisposed to progress to SCCs. Note the epithelial atypia (◆) here involving the full thickness of the epidermis, which qualifies this lesion as an SCC in situ. *TP53* mutations are often present as the first step toward loss of growth control.

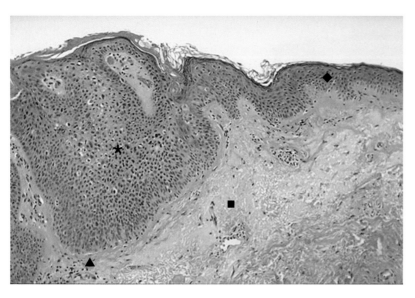

Figure 16-33 Squamous cell carcinoma, microscopic
Because this neoplasm does not extend below the basement membrane (▲), this lesion is termed a *squamous cell carcinoma in situ.* This condition is sometimes called *Bowen disease.* Note the normal skin (◆) on the right adjacent to the thicker carcinoma (★) on the left with more cellular pleomorphism and hyperchromatism. There is also extensive solar elastosis (■), marked by the pale-blue homogeneous appearance of the underlying dermal collagen, a result of chronic sun damage. Loss of normal p53 tumor suppressor gene function in such lesions is common; *RAS* mutations may also be present. The cells of these neoplasms are often aneuploid.

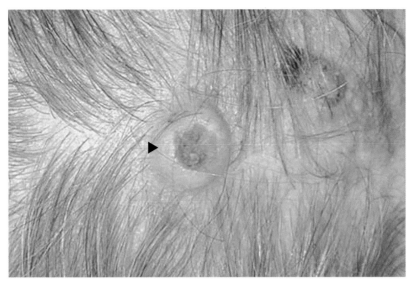

Figure 16-34 Squamous cell carcinoma, gross

This small nodule (▶) on the scalp is an SCC, although a basal cell carcinoma could have a similar appearance. Such small tumors are often noticed by the patient before reaching a larger size, and smaller, more localized lesions are less likely to have invaded far or metastasized. This explains the high "cure" rate for nonmelanoma skin cancers. SCCs of the skin are related to the amount of past sun exposure; ultraviolet B (UVB) rays are the most damaging. The surrounding skin may show actinic keratoses (premalignant actinic change from sun damage). Human papillomavirus (HPV) infection may play a role in development of some of these cancers, particularly with immunosuppression (chemotherapy or transplantation).

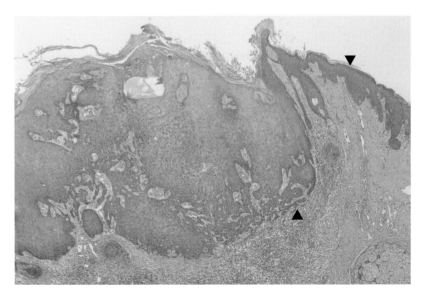

Figure 16-35 Squamous cell carcinoma, gross

This is an ulcerated SCC (▽) that arose on the dorsum of the hand. In addition to sun exposure, risk factors for SCC of skin include carcinogens such as tars, chronic ulcers, burn scars, arsenic poisoning, and radiation exposure. In this case, there was a history of sun exposure and exposure to carcinogens. Patients with the rare autosomal recessive disorder xeroderma pigmentosum have defects in nucleotide excision and repair *(NER)* genes so that pyrimidine dimers formed in cellular DNA from UV light exposure lead to a 2000-fold increased risk for SCCs, which can arise even in childhood.

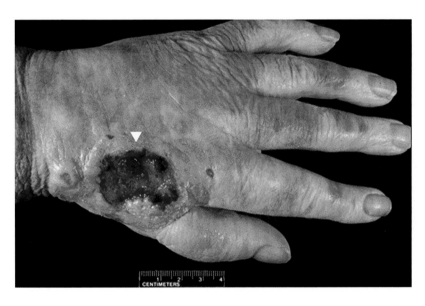

Figure 16-36 Squamous cell carcinoma, microscopic

This well-differentiated lesion has large polygonal cells with extensive pink keratinization. However, it is nodular and infiltrates as tongues and nests of cells (▲) into the underlying dermis. Compare with noncancerous squamous epithelium (▽) at the upper right. In spite of the size of these lesions, they typically remain localized and rarely metastasize. HPV subtypes 5 and 8 may play a role in development of some SCC cases, including the rare autosomal recessive condition known as epidermodysplasia verruciformis.

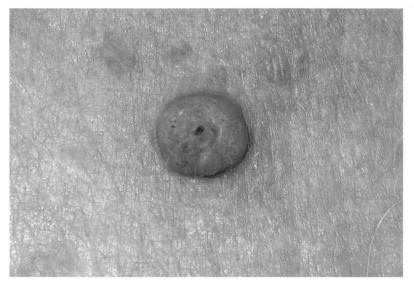

Figure 16-37 Keratoacanthoma, gross
This lesion arises in pilosebaceous glands and can grow rapidly over weeks to months, reaching a size of 1 cm to several centimeters, suggesting a more aggressive behavior. A period of rapid growth in weeks to months is followed by stabilization, then regression in a year, leaving a residual scar. Keratoacanthomas (KAs) most often occur on sun-exposed skin in men older than 50 years. Grossly, the lesion shown here appears as a symmetrical dome-shaped nodule with a central keratin-filled crater.

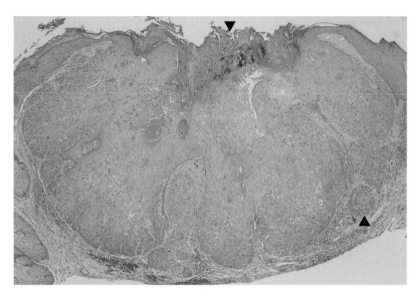

Figure 16-38 Keratoacanthoma, microscopic
This endophytic crater-like lesion has a proliferation of well-differentiated squamous epithelium extending downward in tongues and nests (▲) into the dermis, without invasion. The large cells have prominent glassy pink cytoplasm and minimal atypia. Abundant keratin production results in the central collection of keratinaceous material (▼) that erupts outward. KA resembles a well-differentiated SCC but the course and biology are different. *HRAS* mutations, as well as cyclin D1 overexpression coupled with functional p16, are more frequent in KA than in SCC.

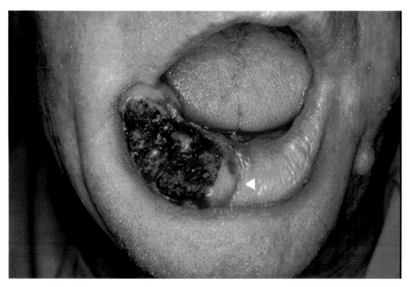

Figure 16-39 Basal cell carcinoma, gross
This large basal cell carcinoma of the lower lip has a pearly pink papular border (◄) and an ulcerated center. These lesions rarely metastasize, but they are slowly growing and progressively infiltrative over time (a "rodent ulcer" that keeps eating away at normal tissues). Leaving them to get larger just makes the plastic surgeon's job that much harder, with more disability to the patient, so early detection and excision are a must. Most basal cell carcinomas occur in the head and neck area of adults. There is an increased risk for development of basal cell carcinoma with prolonged sun exposure, specifically damaging UVB rays.

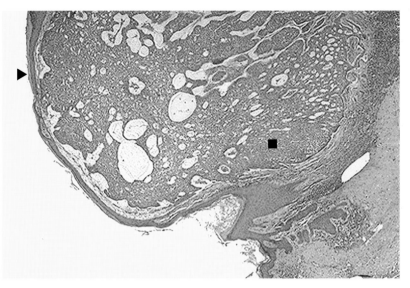

Figure 16-40 Basal cell carcinoma, microscopic

Basal cell carcinoma and SCC are the most common skin malignancies. Note here the densely packed dark-blue cells (■) expanding in a nodular growth pattern beneath the thin overlying epidermis (▶). This tumor can grow quite large and invade surrounding tissues, but it virtually never metastasizes. Basal cell carcinomas around the eye present a challenge to the surgeon to remove and retain functionality of the eyelid. It is best to detect these carcinomas early and excise them when they are small. Most have mutations in *PTCH,* a tumor suppressor gene producing a protein receptor for the sonic hedgehog (SHH) signaling pathway, as does the rare basal cell nevus syndrome.

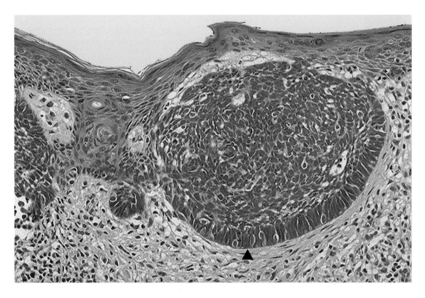

Figure 16-41 Basal cell carcinoma, microscopic

The cells of a basal cell carcinoma are dark blue and oblong with scant cytoplasm, resembling the cells along the basal layer of normal epidermis. These cells are arranged into nests or trabeculae that infiltrate downward into the dermis. A nest of tumor often has a palisaded arrangement of cells (▲) around its periphery. These tumor cell nests have an intervening fibrous stroma with variable inflammatory cell component. Nests of basaloid cells dropping off into the upper dermis are shown here. These neoplasms can often be multifocal in areas of chronic sun exposure. They also occur frequently in patients with xeroderma pigmentosum and in patients with immunosuppression.

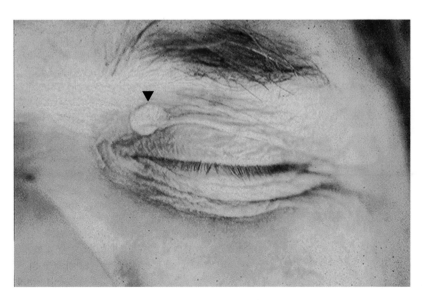

Figure 16-42 Xanthoma, gross

Xanthomas are collections of lipid-laden (foamy) histiocytes (macrophages) within the dermis, producing a grossly visible yellowish nodule or plaque (▼). This little yellow plaque on the upper eyelid here from a patient who did not have any abnormality of blood lipids is called a *xanthelasma.* In contrast, eruptive xanthomas may appear in patients who have familial or acquired forms of hyperlipidemia. Xanthomas tend to increase or decrease in size in proportion to blood lipid levels.

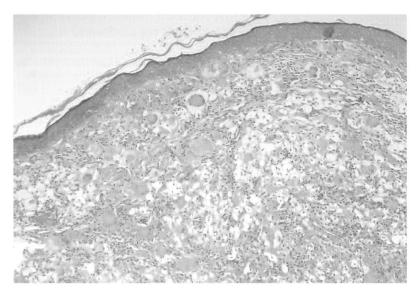

Figure 16-43 Xanthoma, microscopic
Numerous foamy macrophages (histiocytes) with a pale appearance to their cytoplasm are shown here within the dermis. This foamy appearance of the cells results from extensive lipid deposition, including cholesterol, phospholipids, and triglycerides, contained within the macrophage cytoplasm.

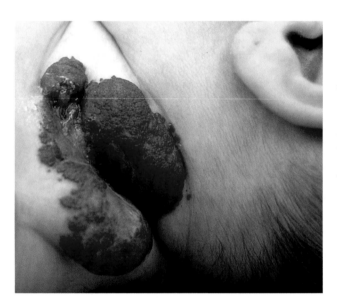

Figure 16-44 Hemangioma, gross
The red nodular lesion shown is benign, with sharp borders. It is composed of proliferations of small blood vessels. Some of these lesions may be present from birth, such as this one, suggesting that they are hamartomas rather than true neoplasms. In any case, they are so slow growing that they seemingly never change. They can range in color from blue to reddish blue to purple to bright red. They generally average a few millimeters to several centimeters in size, although some congenital lesions (typically cavernous hemangiomas) can be more extensive (port-wine stain). Some juvenile hemangiomas may grow rapidly in the first few months of infancy but then regress by age 5 years.

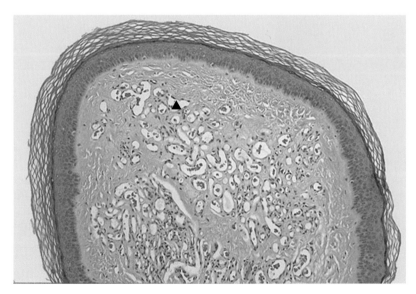

Figure 16-45 Hemangioma, microscopic
A reddish "mole" that is small, round, and raised may represent a hemangioma, here composed of vascular spaces in the upper dermis. These small vascular channels, which may vary in size and shape, are lined by flattened endothelial cells (▲). These lesions appear to change slowly, if at all, over time and seem to have been present as long as the patient can remember. In a capillary hemangioma, the vascular spaces are small or collapsed, as shown here, and the intervening loose connective tissue stroma may contain larger arterioles or venules. In contrast, a cavernous hemangioma has large, dilated vascular spaces that may extend into the underlying adipose tissue.

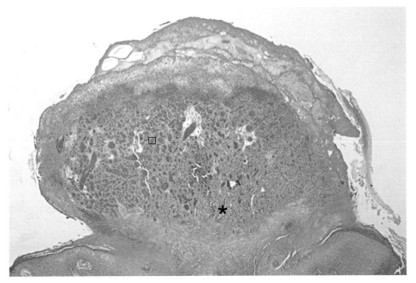

Figure 16-46 Pyogenic granuloma, microscopic

Also known as a *lobular capillary hemangioma,* a pyogenic granuloma is a lesion that can grossly resemble a hemangioma, but it is characteristically rapidly growing, arising and then receding within weeks to months, rather than persisting for years unchanging, as a typical hemangioma would. They may develop during pregnancy and disappear after delivery. Local inflammation or irritation may result in formation of a nodule of granulation tissue (★) with prominent capillaries (☐), as shown here. Around the capillaries are inflammatory cell infiltrates. The lesion often ulcerates. Similar lesions can appear on the gingiva.

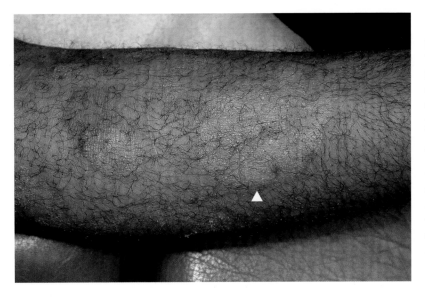

Figure 16-47 Mycosis fungoides, gross

This cutaneous T-cell lymphoma can remain localized to skin for years but may evolve into a generalized lymphoma in a few cases. Well-demarcated, erythematous, slightly scaly plaques (▲) are shown here on the skin of the dorsal arm. They may resemble psoriatic or eczematous lesions. Over time, the lesions may become more numerous on many skin surfaces; they may become nodular and ulcerate. In some patients the malignant T cells seed into the bloodstream *(Sézary syndrome)* and are distributed diffusely to large areas of the body, leading to erythroderma, characterized by extensive erythema and scaling of skin.

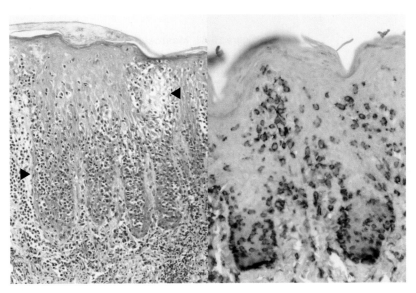

Figure 16-48 Mycosis fungoides, microscopic

Shown here is psoriasiform hyperplasia of the epidermis with infiltration by atypical T cells (▶), shown with H&E staining in the *left panel* and immunohistochemical staining for CD5 in the *right panel,* which highlights epidermotropism, where the intraepidermal lymphocytes are aligned along the basal cell layer in short linear arrays. These cells are also CD4+, and they have folded cerebriform nuclei. They are known as *Sézary-Lutzner cells,* and they can form small epidermal clusters known as *Pautrier microabscesses* (◀).

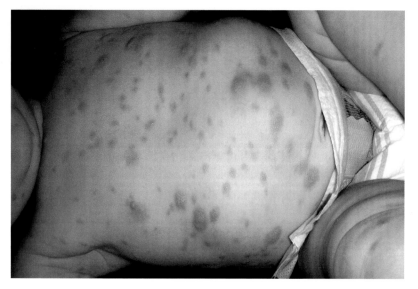

Figure 16-49 Mastocytosis, gross
This red-brown maculopapular eruption called *urticaria pigmentosa* results from focal dermal infiltration by mast cells. It is a localized form of mastocytosis, accounting for half of all cases of mastocytosis, occurring most often in children. These lesions often arise in groups, or they may be solitary, and appear as a brown pruritic papule. Rubbing a lesion leads to development of surrounding edema and erythema from the release of mediators such as histamine from mast cells, called *Darier sign*.

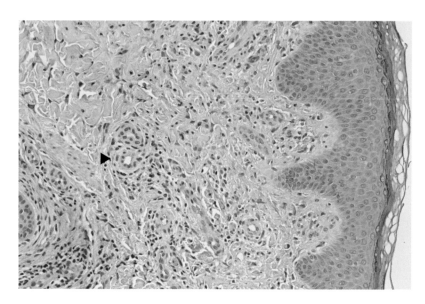

Figure 16-50 Mastocytosis, microscopic
The dermis here is heavily infiltrated in a perivascular distribution (▶) by cells with uniform, round nuclei and abundant pink cytoplasm, typical of mast cells. A mutation in the KIT receptor tyrosine kinase can activate a receptor tyrosine kinase that leads to this mast cell proliferation. The release of preformed cytokines and biogenic amines such as histamine leads to urticaria, vasodilation, and swelling. Plasma tryptase levels can be increased with systemic disease.

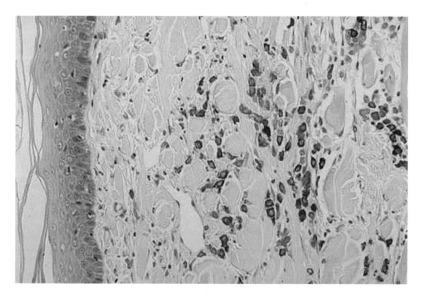

Figure 16-51 Mastocytosis, microscopic
A Giemsa stain highlights numerous purple cytoplasmic granules of mast cells within the dermis in this case of urticaria pigmentosa. The mast cells contain numerous metachromatic cytoplasmic granules; the granules contain many substances, including vasoactive amines such as histamine, which are released on activation and degranulation of the mast cells to cause symptoms such as itching and wheal formation. In systemic mastocytosis, which usually occurs in adults, tissues of the mononuclear phagocyte system, including spleen, liver, lymph nodes, and bone marrow, are often infiltrated by mast cells. Release of tryptase and heparin may drive bone remodeling with osteoporosis or osteosclerosis.

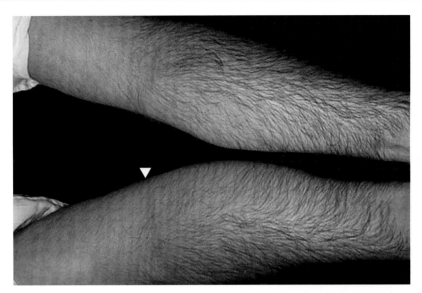

Figure 16-52 Urticaria, gross
The skin (▼) of the right arm is swollen (edematous) from angioedema and reddened (erythematous) from vasodilation compared with the left arm. Cardinal signs of inflammation are rubor (redness), calor (heat), tumor (swelling), dolor (pain), and loss of function. This urticarial response resulted from an insect sting leading to a systemic allergic reaction with type I hypersensitivity. These manifestations resulted from IgE-mediated mast cell degranulation with release of vasoactive substances such as histamine. More localized anaphylaxis, typically occurring with food allergy, may also result in urticaria (hives). These lesions usually appear and disappear within hours.

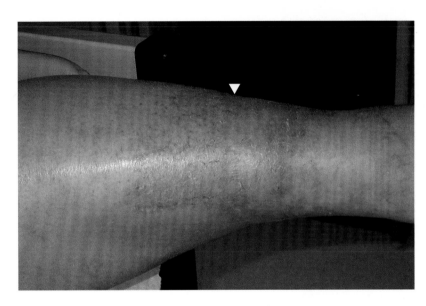

Figure 16-53 Acute eczematous dermatitis, gross
Eczema is a generic clinical term for any red, papulovesicular area of skin eruption (▼) that can develop oozing of fluid with crusting and scaling. Forms of eczematous dermatitis include reactions to insect bites, contact dermatitis, atopic dermatitis, drug-induced dermatitis, and photodermatitis. Many irritants (those with fine print on the warning label of the container reading "avoid contact with skin") produce this pattern of skin disease. Eczema can be caused by something that was ingested. Type IV hypersensitivity plays a role in many cases.

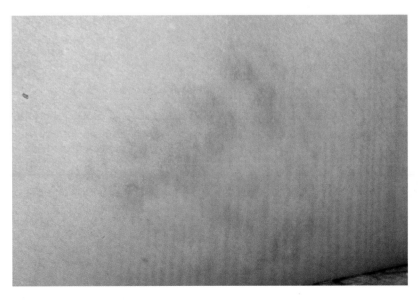

Figure 16-54 Contact dermatitis, gross
Focal, slightly raised areas of erythema are shown here on skin exposed to poison oak, a plant containing resin with the compound urushiol. The lesions may produce a burning or itching sensation. Cases of contact dermatitis, a form of eczematous dermatitis, are typically self-limited from focal exposure to an antigen, subsiding in days to a couple of weeks. The irritant antigen is processed by Langerhans cells and presented to CD4 cells, which migrate to the site of exposure, releasing cytokines that recruit additional inflammatory cells. More severe forms may progress to papulovesicular lesions with oozing and crusting that can persist as scaling plaques.

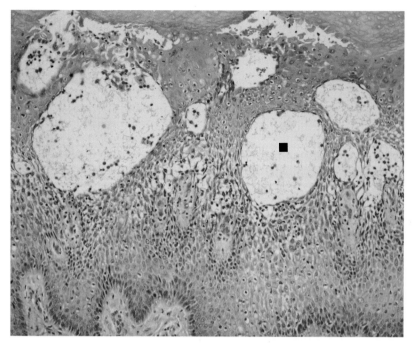

Figure 16-55 Acute eczematous dermatitis, microscopic

A key microscopic feature with any form of eczema is spongiosis, consisting of edema fluid that collects within the epidermis, forming vesicles (■). Many cases of eczema are related to type IV hypersensitivity with initial antigen exposure resulting in formation of memory T cells. Re-exposure to the antigen leads to recruitment of CD4 lymphocytes releasing cytokines that mediate the inflammatory reaction. Classic cases of contact dermatitis appear within 24 to 72 hours after antigen exposure.

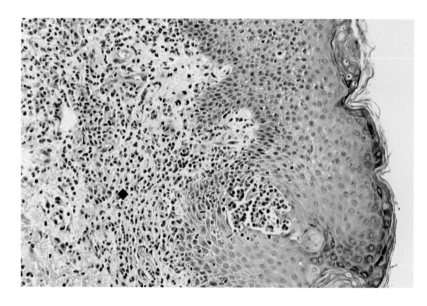

Figure 16-56 Acute eczematous dermatitis, microscopic

A pronounced eosinophilic infiltrate (◆) is present, along with lymphocytes extending from the epidermis to deep dermis in this acute allergic reaction, typically occurring with exposure to drugs and other ingested chemical agents. There is some residual epidermal spongiosis with early hyperkeratosis and acanthosis, as the lesion evolves from oozing to scaling over days.

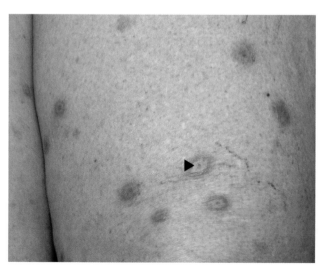

Figure 16-57 Erythema multiforme, gross

Various skin lesions (multiform) shown here range from macules to papules to vesicles to bullae. The classic target lesion has a central vesicle (▶) surrounded by a zone of erythema and usually appears on the hands after infection (e.g., cold sores in the mouth). This uncommon, but usually self-limited, disorder may arise from a hypersensitivity reaction to an infection, drugs, neoplasia, or collagen vascular disease. The skin is targeted by CD8 cytotoxic lymphocytes. The condition is classified as minor, with less than 10% total body surface area affected, often including symmetrical involvement of the extremities.

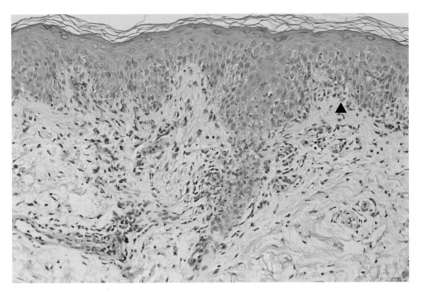

Figure 16-58 Erythema multiforme, microscopic

This cytotoxic CD8 cell-mediated inflammatory reaction is characterized by squamous epithelial cell dissolution (▲) at the dermal-epidermal junction (interface dermatitis). These lesions are "multiforme" because macules, papules, vesicles, and bullae may be seen grossly, with symmetrical involvement of the extremities. Stevens-Johnson syndrome is a febrile illness that is a more severe, generalized form of erythema multiforme, most often occurring in children, which can also involve mucous membranes and typically follows administration of a drug (e.g., a sulfa drug or an anticonvulsant).

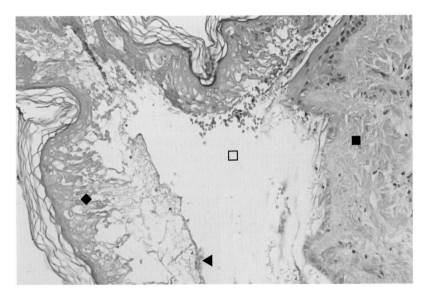

Figure 16-59 Toxic epidermal necrolysis, microscopic

There are few dermatologic emergencies. This is one of them, known as *toxic epidermal necrolysis*. This severe febrile disorder causes blistering and extensive sloughing of skin and mucosal surfaces as a consequence of full-thickness epidermal necrosis. Shown here is a necrotic epidermis (◆) lifting off (◄) the dermis (■) to form a subepidermal bulla (□). There are several variations on this theme; the condition may be the result of a reaction inducing keratinocyte apoptosis secondary to an infection or administration of a drug.

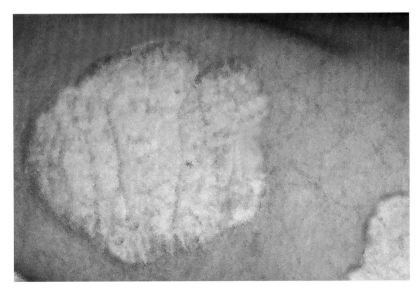

Figure 16-60 Psoriasis, gross

Of people of all ages, 1% to 2% may develop psoriasis. Some may also develop psoriatic arthritis (resembling rheumatoid arthritis), spondylitis, or myopathy. About two thirds of affected individuals have the HLA-Cw*0602 allele. Interaction of CD4 cells with epidermal dendritic cells and CD8 cells leads to cytokine release, including tumor necrosis factor, interleukin-12 (IL-12), IL-17, and interferon-γ, driving keratinocyte proliferation with inflammation. The thick, silvery, scaling lesions shown here are most often found over bony prominences, scalp, genitalia, and hands. The epidermal turnover is reduced from a month to only 4 days for a cell to traverse from the basal layer to the surface, accounting for the buildup of these scales.

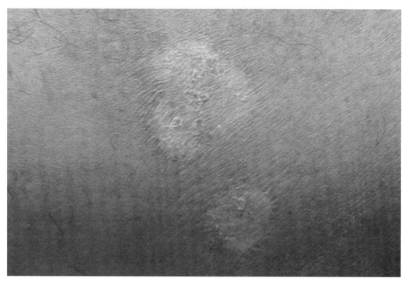

Figure 16-61 Psoriasis, gross
This is psoriasis after phototherapy with UVB. The scaling lesions are less florid on the background of this tanned skin. The long-term morbidity from the increased risk for skin cancer with UVB is probably not as great as the morbidity with psoriasis itself. Serious complications of psoriasis include extensive erythema and scaling, termed *erythroderma,* and extensive pustule formation with secondary infection accompanied by fever and leukocytosis, termed *pustular psoriasis.* A minor problem occurring in one third of patients is yellow-brown nail discoloration with pitting and separation from the nail bed (onycholysis).

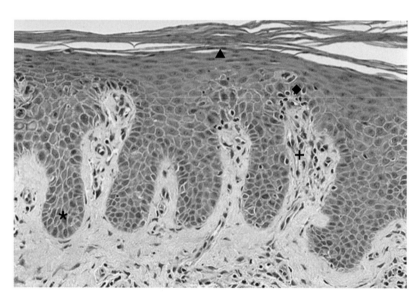

Figure 16-62 Psoriasis, microscopic
Microscopically, psoriasis shows downward elongation of the rete ridges (★) with thinning to absence of the overlying stratum granulosum, with prominent parakeratosis (▲) above this. Small aggregates of neutrophils (◆) with surrounding spongiform change appear in the superficial epidermis and parakeratotic region. Capillaries (✚) within dermal papillae are brought close to the surface, and lifting the scale from a plaque produces pinpoint areas of hemorrhage, known as *Auspitz sign.*

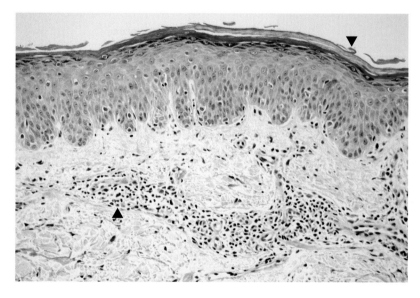

Figure 16-63 Seborrheic dermatitis, microscopic
Up to 5% of persons may have a chronic dermatitis that mainly involves skin with many sebaceous glands, including scalp, forehead, retroauricular area, nasolabial folds, presternal area, and skin folds in axillae and groin region. Scaling and crusting overlie oily macules and papules. Many cases are associated with presence of the fungus *Malassezia.* Early lesions have upper dermal lymphocytic infiltrates (▲) with epidermal spongiosis, parakeratosis, and hyperkeratosis (▼). Chronic lesions may resemble psoriasis.

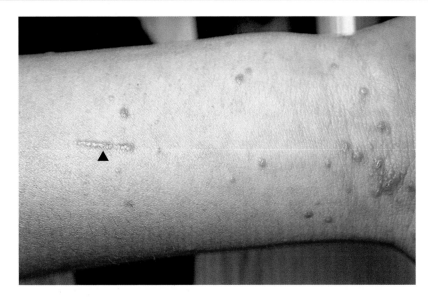

Figure 16-64 Lichen planus, gross
During the course of this disease, there are pruritic papules with a pink to violaceous appearance, as shown here. These lesions are symmetrically distributed, most often at the elbows and wrists, or the glans penis in men. The linear arrangement (▲) of the lichenoid lesion at the left is an example of the Koebner phenomenon (also occurring with psoriasis), in which lesions appear on the skin at the sites of trauma. White dots or lines known as *Wickham striae* appear at the right in papular lesions.

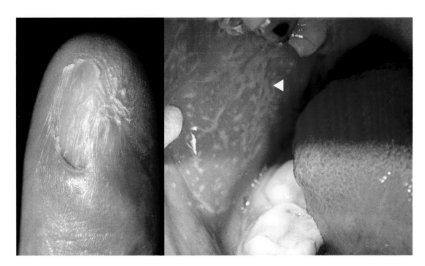

Figure 16-65 Lichen planus, gross
On the oral mucosa *(right panel)* the lesions appear as white, reticulated, netlike areas (◀), and these may persist for years. Skin lesions typically spontaneously resolve in 1 to 2 years, leaving hyperpigmented areas where the lesions were present. Nail findings *(left panel)* occurring in 10% of patients include longitudinal grooving and ridging, onycholysis (shown), and subungual hyperkeratosis.

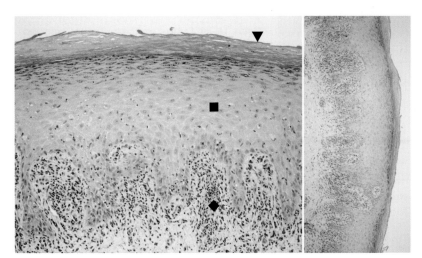

Figure 16-66 Lichen planus, microscopic
Shown here is irregular acanthosis (■), orthokeratotic hyperkeratosis (▼), and hypergranulosis of the epidermis along with a bandlike upper dermal infiltrate (◆) of CD8+ T lymphocytes. This bandlike lymphocytic infiltrate involves the dermal-epidermal junction (interface), and the basal layer of keratinocytes may undergo degeneration and necrosis, whereas the stratum granulosum often increases in thickness. The rete ridges take on a sawtooth appearance.

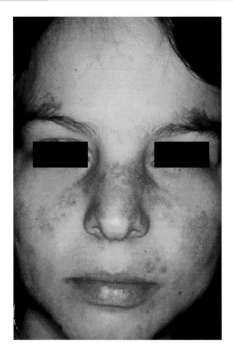

Figure 16-67 Lupus erythematosus, gross

This young woman has a red malar rash (the so-called *butterfly rash* because of the shape of the reddened skin across the cheeks) that suggests lupus erythematosus. More sharply demarcated discoid scaling plaques may also occur. The variant of lupus known as *discoid lupus erythematosus* (DLE) involves mainly just the skin and is benign compared with systemic lupus erythematosus (SLE), which typically is a systemic disease that affects internal organs such as the kidney but may initially manifest with skin rashes in a third of cases. In either DLE or SLE, sunlight exposure accentuates this rash. A few DLE patients (5% to 10%) go on to develop SLE (usually DLE patients with a positive antinuclear antibody test result).

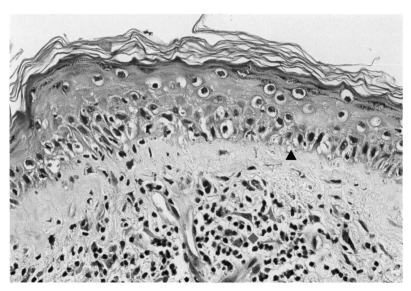

Figure 16-68 Lupus erythematosus, microscopic

A marked inflammatory skin infiltrate (♦) is present in the upper dermis of a patient with SLE in which the basal layer (▲) is undergoing vacuolization and dissolution, and there is purpura with red blood cells spilling out of blood vessels into the upper dermis (which is the cause for the rash). Autoimmune serologic markers include antinuclear antibody, anti–double stranded DNA, and anti-Smith.

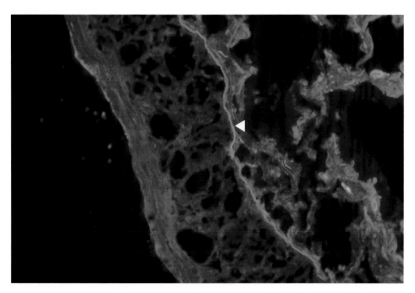

Figure 16-69 Lupus erythematosus, immunofluorescence

Shown here is a bright green band (◄) of fluorescence from staining with antibody to IgG. The localization at the dermal-epidermal junction is typical of immune complex deposition. These complexes are formed from antigens and antibodies (type III hypersensitivity) and tend to be trapped along the basement membranes. Complement activation enhances the inflammatory reaction further. Skin diseases with this immunofluorescence pattern include SLE, DLE, and bullous pemphigoid.

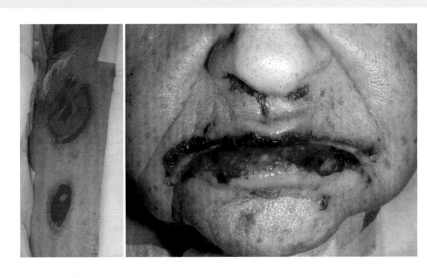

Figures 16-70 Pemphigus vulgaris, gross

In this blistering skin disease the stratum spinosum separates from the basal layer to form a flaccid bulla that often ruptures, as shown here. Oral mucosal ulcerative lesions may be present for months before the onset of skin involvement. Areas affected include the scalp, face, axilla, groin, trunk, and points of pressure. The vesicles and bullae rupture easily, leaving shallow erosions covered with dried serum and crust. Affected persons are usually 30 to 60 years of age.

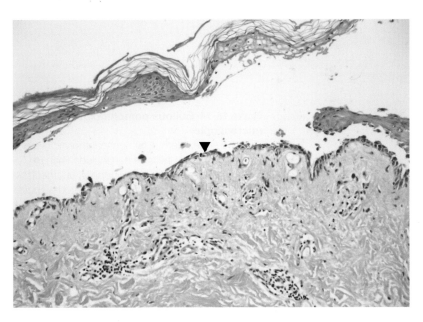

Figure 16-71 Pemphigus vulgaris, microscopic

The blister is forming above the basal layer (▼) within the epidermis, a suprabasal acantholytic blister. These lesions can become progressively larger, and more lesions can appear, leaving considerable skin surface denuded after rupture. Corticosteroid therapy halts progression of the disease, and immunosuppressive therapy may be required for maintenance therapy. Some cases of pemphigus represent a paraneoplastic syndrome, most often with a non-Hodgkin lymphoma.

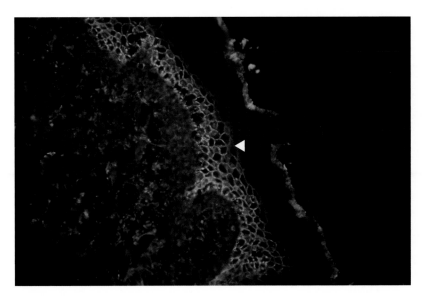

Figure 16-72 Pemphigus vulgaris, immunofluorescence

This autoimmune disease is produced by IgG antibodies directed against desmoglein proteins, a component of desmosomes that aid in keratinocyte binding. With immunofluorescence using antibodies directed against IgG, an intercellular staining pattern is observed here, producing a netlike pattern (◄). Circulating antibody can also be detected.

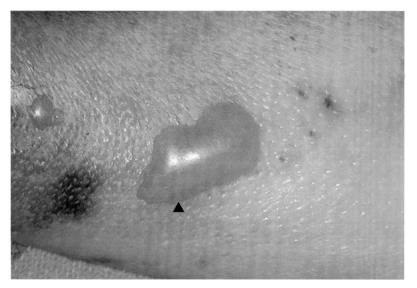

Figure 16-73 Bullous pemphigoid, gross
A large, tense bulla (▲) is visible in the center, and a smaller bulla appears at the left. These bullous skin lesions may occur in association with infections and drugs. The lesions shown here developed with *bullous pemphigoid,* which typically affects older individuals and involves cutaneous and mucosal surfaces. These lesions filled with clear fluid may reach several centimeters in size, but they do not rupture as easily as the lesions of pemphigus. Flexural regions of the axillae, groin, forearms, abdomen, and inner thighs are most often involved.

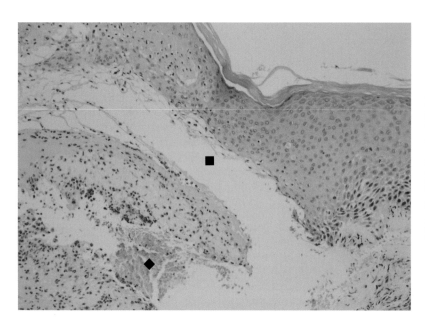

Figure 16-74 Bullous pemphigoid, microscopic
This is a subepidermal (■) nonacantholytic blister. The inflammatory infiltrate can include fibrin (◆) along with lymphocytes, eosinophils, and neutrophils. The superficial dermis is edematous. There may be pruritus. These lesions may heal without scarring. Oral lesions may occur in 10% to 15% of cases, and they follow the appearance of skin lesions.

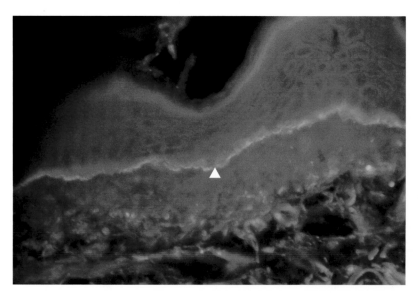

Figure 16-75 Bullous pemphigoid, immunofluorescence
Immunoglobulin and complement are usually distributed in a linear fashion (▲) along the basement membrane in this blistering disease. The antibody (IgG) is directed against bullous pemphigoid antigens (BPAGs) found in hemidesmosomes in the squamous epithelium. Autoantibodies to BPAG 2 in these hemidesmosomes result in complement fixation with recruitment and activation of inflammatory cells.

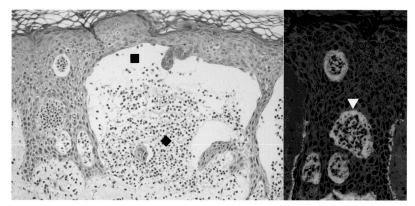

Figure 16-76 Dermatitis herpetiformis, microscopic

Grossly, areas of urticaria with grouped vesicle formation can occur, typically over extensor surfaces, elbows, knees, upper back, and buttocks. Middle-aged individuals are usually affected, mostly men. An association with intestinal celiac disease is shown with IgA and IgG antibodies formed against ingested gliadin protein found in gluten of grains such as wheat, barley, and rye, and also directed against reticulin with marked bright green (▼) immunofluorescence *(right panel)*. The reticulin is part of anchoring fibrils that connect epidermal basement membrane to the dermis. The characteristic microscopic finding shown here is collections of neutrophils (◆) within the dermal papillae, forming papillary microabscesses. Over time, these areas can coalesce, with subepidermal blister (■) formation *(left panel)*.

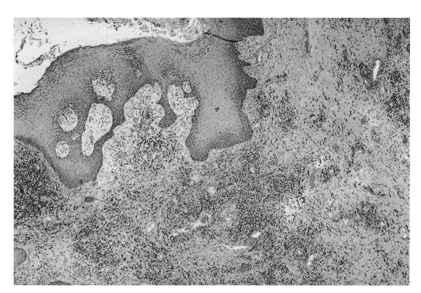

Figure 16-77 Acne vulgaris, gross

These mild acne lesions on the skin of the back consist of scattered inflammatory papules and occasional pustules. Acne occurs in nearly all teenagers and young adults after puberty to some degree. It results from increased sebaceous gland sebum production with an increase in androgenous steroid hormone production. Sebum and keratinaceous debris block hair follicles, leading to comedone formation. Bacteria such as *Propionibacterium acnes* in the comedones cause inflammation and enlargement, forming a pustule or nodule. This can rupture to produce a cystic area, generally a lesion larger than 0.5 cm, in which the purulent lesion extends with inflammation into the surrounding dermis.

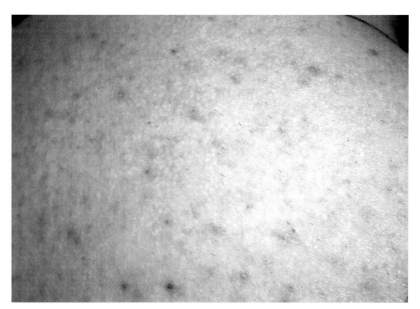

Figure 16-78 Acne vulgaris, microscopic

There is marked, acute and chronic inflammation extending all the way through the dermis. Acne is most often self-limited and generally abates in young adulthood, but about 10% to 20% of adults may continue to manifest acne. Boys are affected more than girls, although acne may persist longer in young women. A small subset of patients develop the severe lesion shown here. The result of severe acne can be scarring, which is more likely to occur in men. Breakdown of lipids by *P. acnes* bacteria to irritating fatty acids may drive the inflammatory process. Treatment with a synthetic vitamin A derivative (isotretinoin) is often successful.

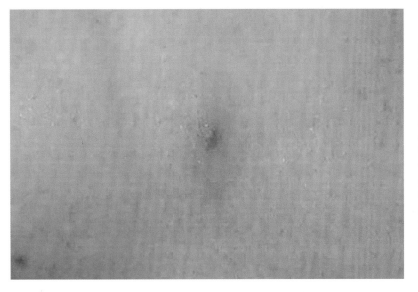

Figure 16-79 Erythema nodosum, gross
Here is a central tender nodule with a surrounding zone of erythema. Such lesions may reach several centimeters in size over weeks to months and then fade. Lesions are most common on the skin of the anterior leg and thigh. In time, they become purple, then flat and brown, then fade out. In some cases an underlying systemic inflammatory condition, such as a granulomatous disease (e.g., tuberculosis, fungal infection), is present, whereas other cases occur in association with drug therapy (sulfonamides), malignancies, and inflammatory bowel disease. In many cases this condition is idiopathic.

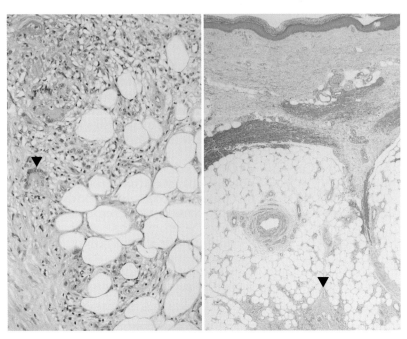

Figure 16-80 Erythema nodosum, microscopic
Erythema nodosum is a type of panniculitis. Note the extensive inflammation (▼) of subcutaneous adipose tissue with infiltration by lymphocytes, histiocytes, multinucleated giant cells (▼), and septal fibrosis *(left panel)*. The process extends deep into the subcutaneous fat *(right panel)*. Affected persons may have fever and malaise. On resolution there may be scarring.

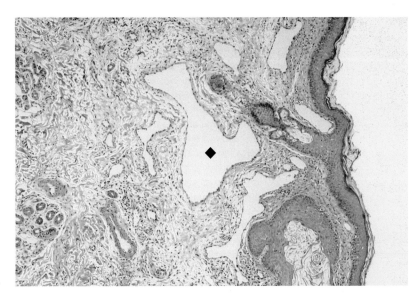

Figure 16-81 Telangiectasia, microscopic
There are dilated venules (◆) in the upper dermis, giving the lesion a reddish color. Telangiectasias may be solitary incidental findings. They may be part of systemic sclerosis. If part of a spectrum of persistent erythema and telangiectasia known as *rosacea,* telangiectasia progresses to pustules and papules, and finally rhinophyma with permanent thickening of the nasal skin. Rosacea occurs most often in adult women, mediated by abnormally high levels of cathelicidin contributing to cutaneous innate immunity. The rare autosomal dominant Osler-Weber-Rendu syndrome (hereditary hemorrhagic telangiectasia) affects blood vessels throughout the body and results in a bleeding tendency.

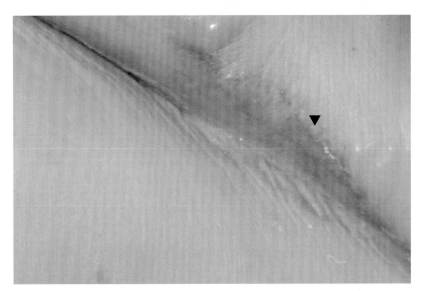

Figure 16-82 Intertrigo, gross
The erythematous region (▼) present in this lower abdominal skin fold is known as *intertrigo.* The rubbing of skin surfaces in the fold makes them more prone to chafing of the epidermis, and the warm, moist environment encourages fungal and bacterial growth. Secondary infection may occur. This is most often a complication of obesity.

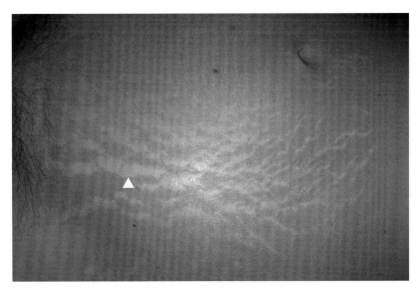

Figure 16-83 Abdominal striae, gross
The pale, linear, depressed, white scarlike marks (▲) appearing here on the lower abdomen are striae (more formally called *striae atrophicae* or *striae distensae*). They can be pink to purple when they first appear. These striae can arise on the abdomen, breasts, buttocks, and thighs in association with weakening of the dermal elastic tissue. Predisposing conditions include pregnancy, obesity, and Cushing syndrome.

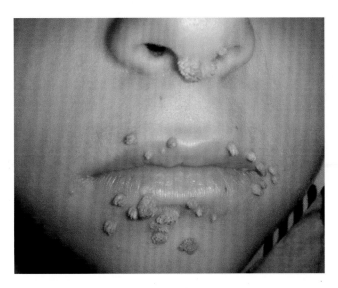

Figure 16-84 Verruca vulgaris, gross
Verruca vulgaris is a warty nodule very common on the skin, particularly in children and adolescents. They most often occur on the hands but can occur anywhere. They can be solitary or multiple, as shown. They have a rough surface and may be gray to tan to brown. These warts are caused by infection with HPV and occur from direct contact between individuals or by autoinoculation from one skin site to another. These lesions tend to grow slowly over several years before they begin to regress over 6 months to 2 years.

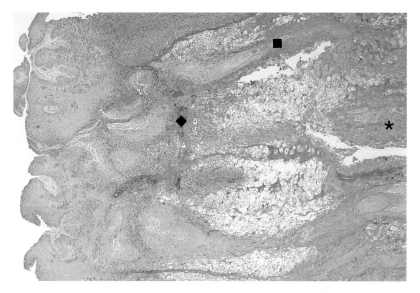

Figure 16-85 Verruca vulgaris, microscopic
A common wart, or verruca vulgaris, has prominent epithelial hyperplasia marked by hyperkeratosis (★) along with papillomatosis (■) to produce
the rough, warty gross appearance. The epidermal granular layer (◆) is prominent. These lesions
are usually a few millimeters to 1 cm in size and
are most often located on the dorsa of the hands.
Lesions can also appear on the face (verruca
plana), on the soles of the feet (verruca plantaris),
or on the palms of the hands (verruca palmaris).

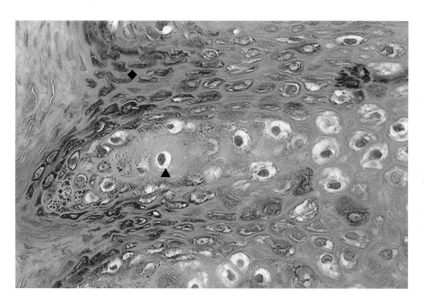

Figure 16-86 Verruca vulgaris, microscopic
At higher magnification, the vacuolization (▲) of
nuclei along with large basophilic keratohyaline
granules (◆) of the epidermal cells (koilocytotic
change) in this verruca vulgaris is prominent and
indicates the viral origin of this lesion. Viral particles are present within the epidermal cell nuclei.
These warts are usually caused by subtypes of
HPV that are not associated with malignant transformation. HPV subtype 16 has been associated
with development of SCC, however.

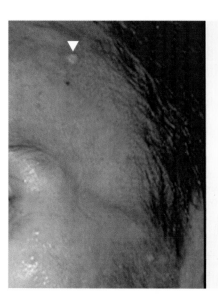
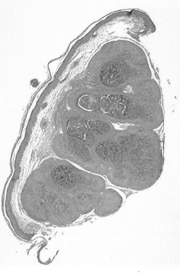

**Figure 16-87 Molluscum contagiosum, gross
and microscopic**
Multiple, 2- to 4-mm, dome-shaped, flesh-
colored firm papules (▼) caused by molluscum
contagiosum, a type of poxvirus, are visible
grossly in the *left panel.* These lesions can also
be umbilicated. They are most often found on
the skin of the trunk and anogenital region but
may appear elsewhere, as here on the face. The
biopsy specimen in the *right panel* shows pink
cuplike verrucous hyperplasia. This infection is
spread by direct contact between individuals.
This is a self-limited disease and the lesions
usually resolve within 18 months in immunocompetent persons.

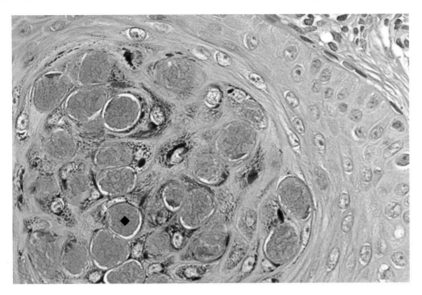

Figure 16-88 Molluscum contagiosum, microscopic

At high magnification there are large pink ovoid inclusions (♦) in epidermal cells. These are the cytoplasmic inclusions called *molluscum bodies* of molluscum contagiosum, which is caused by a large brick-shaped DNA-containing poxvirus. These lesions spontaneously involute over a period of months. These molluscum bodies may be identified with Giemsa staining of the cheesy material expressed from the center of a lesion.

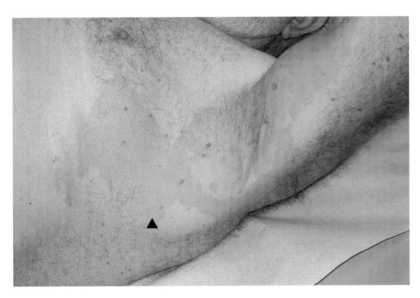

Figure 16-89 Superficial fungal infection, gross

Shown here is an irregularly shaped, lightly hyperpigmented confluent patch (▲) on the upper trunk characteristic of pityriasis versicolor *(tinea versicolor)* caused by *Malassezia furfur.* Various dermatophytes can produce irregular areas of eczema or irregular pigmentation, crusting, or scaling. Dermatophytes can include the genera *Trichophyton* and *Epidermophyton.* The lesions are called *tinea* and further described by the location, such as *tinea corporis* (body), *tinea capitis* (head), *tinea cruris* (groin, or jock itch), *tinea barbae* (male beard area), and *tinea pedis* (athlete's foot).

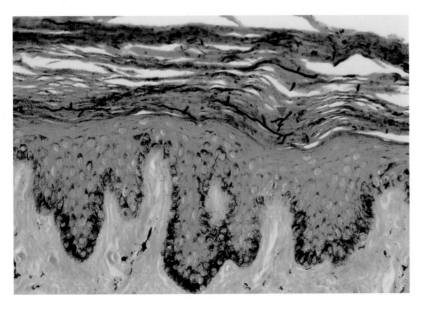

Figure 16-90 Superficial fungal infection, microscopic

Note the thin, black, elongated, branching hyphae (▼) of fungal organisms within the stratum corneum, appearing here with Gomori methenamine silver stain. Warm, moist environments aid in promoting fungal growth. Involvement of the nails is called *onychomycosis.* Viewing the areas with fluorescent light (Wood lamp) may reveal the autofluorescence of these fungi.

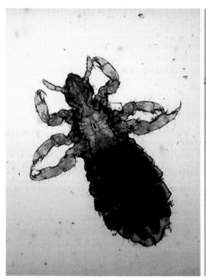
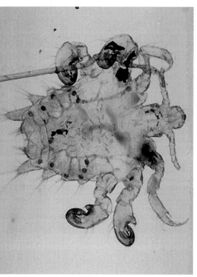

Figure 16-91 Pediculosis, microscopic
A crab louse is shown in the *right panel* hanging onto a pubic hair shaft. The more elongated body louse (or head louse, which is similar) is shown in the *left panel.* These wingless insects (note the six legs) live by biting and sucking on the blood of the human host. They are an annoyance and difficult to eradicate. The focal irritation they cause can lead to scratching and excoriation that may become secondarily infected. The body louse *(Pediculus humanus corporis)* is also the vector for *Rickettsia prowazekii* (epidemic typhus), *Borrelia recurrentis* (relapsing fever), and *Bartonella quintana* (trench fever, bacillary angiomatosis, endocarditis, lymphadenopathy).

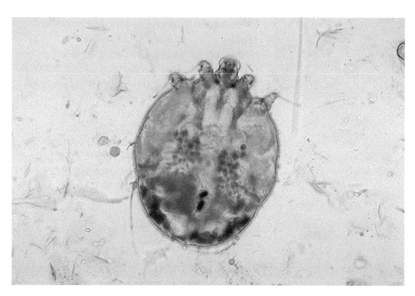

Figure 16-92 Scabies, microscopic
A skin scraping from between the fingers on the hand of a patient with linear reddish lesions 0.2 to 0.6 cm in length that had been excoriated (scratched) yielded this scabies mite *(Sarcoptes scabiei).* The female mite burrows under the stratum corneum, typically on the hands, but also in the genital region of males and periareolar region of females. The lesions itch intensely, and scratching leads to excoriation. The mode of transmission is direct human skin-to-skin contact, but these organisms can survive on clothing for 2 to 3 days. A variant called crusted scabies and resembling psoriasis occurs with numerous mites over extensive areas of skin; persons with immune compromise or poor health are at risk.

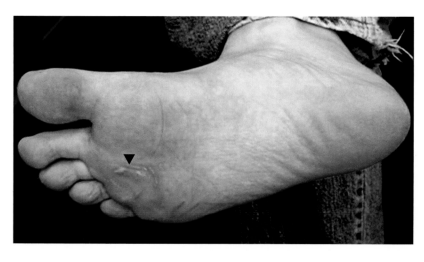

Figure 16-93 Cutaneous larva migrans, gross
Cutaneous larva migrans is the most common tropically acquired dermatosis. It manifests as pruritic, erythematous, serpiginous, slightly raised tracks (▼) averaging 2 to 3 mm wide × 3 to 4 cm long. The lesions are caused by accidental percutaneous penetration and subsequent migration of larvae of various nematode parasites found in soils, such as *Ancylostoma, Necator,* and *Strongyloides.* This condition is benign and self-limited. (Be careful where you step barefoot.)

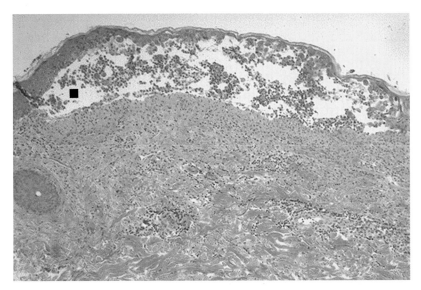

Figure 16-94 Herpes simplex, microscopic
Herpes simplex virus (HSV) types 1 and 2 primarily infect skin and mucous membranes (mucocutaneous infections) to produce inflammation, often vesicular (■) as shown, with grossly visible crops of clear vesicles, which can rupture, progressing to sharply demarcated ulcerations. HSV-1 mainly involves the oral cavity, whereas HSV-2 more often involves the genital region as a sexually transmitted disease. Either body region may be infected, however, by either subtype to produce clinically and histologically indistinguishable disease. Diagnosis can be aided by cytologic smears of lesions, by serologic titers, and by viral culture.

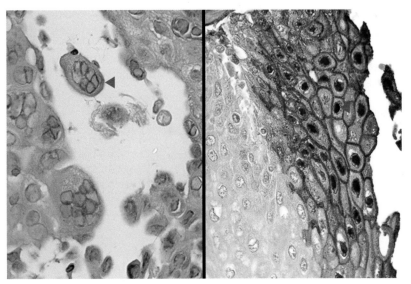

Figure 16-95 Herpes simplex, microscopic
Note ground-glass intranuclear inclusions and multinucleation (◀). In the *right panel,* keratinocyte intranuclear inclusions (◀) are highlighted in dark brown with immunohistochemical staining. HSV infection initially occurs through mucosa or abraded skin via contact with a person excreting virus through active, usually ulcerative, lesions. Viral replication begins within epithelium and underlying dermis or submucosa and spreads to nerve endings, where it is transported intra-axonally to neurons in ganglia. HSV spreads via peripheral sensory nerves back to other, usually adjacent, skin and mucosal sites. After an initial host response with cell-mediated and humoral mechanisms, the infection usually becomes latent, with HSV present but not actively replicating within ganglia.

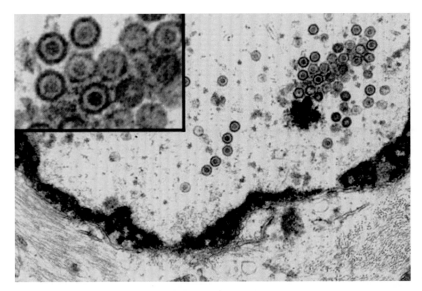

Figure 16-96 Herpes simplex, electron microscopy
On electron microscopy, the rounded, target-like viral particles (shown at higher magnification in the *inset*) of this DNA virus are visible inside the cell nuclear membrane. It is unclear how reactivation of HSV infection occurs, but lack of cell-mediated immunity in immunocompromised patients may be implicated. Antiviral agents, such as acyclovir and valacyclovir, help to suppress viral replication but cannot eliminate latent virus.

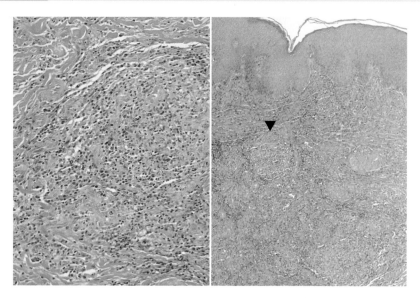

Figure 16-97 Bacillary angiomatosis, microscopic
This uncommon condition may involve internal organs such as liver and spleen, as well as skin, along with mucus membranes of the oral cavity and genital tract, most often in persons with HIV infection. Grossly, red-to-blue papules may increase to protruding or subcutaneous nodules, with some resemblance to Kaposi sarcoma. Shown here beneath the skin are mixed inflammatory infiltrates (▼) with extensive vascularity, similar to a pyogenic granuloma *(right panel)*. The prominent plump epithelioid-like endothelial cells of the many capillaries are shown in the *left panel*, along with lymphocytes, macrophages, and neutrophils.

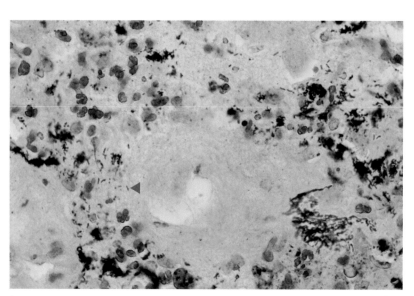

Figure 16-98 Bacillary angiomatosis, microscopic
The causative organism is *Bartonella henselae*. Shown here with Warthin-Starry silver stain are the small rodlike organisms (◀) that appear black, both singly and in aggregates, in the interstitium around a vascular space. Organisms tend to be most numerous where neutrophils are most prominent. Culture of this organism is difficult, and identification is aided by polymerase chain reaction (PCR) assay.

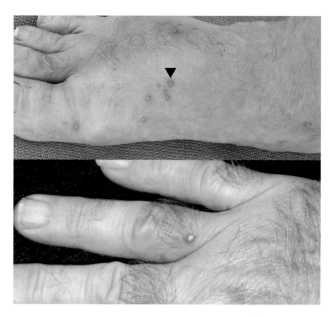

Figure 16-99 Insect bite, gross
The small sterile pustules (▼) shown here on the foot *(upper panel)* and the solitary lesion on the ring finger *(lower panel)* arose a day after fire ant envenomation. The venom contains piperidines that cause a burning sensation and incite an acute inflammatory response. The lesions regressed over the ensuing week, leaving no residual scarring. A sting by ants of the insect family Formicidae can produce a focal skin lesion, but some persons develop IgE specific to an insect venom, with risk for subsequent allergic reactions, including anaphylaxis, from type I hypersensitivity. Bee stings are particularly known to produce this phenomenon.

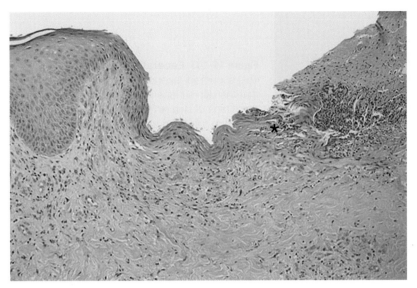

Figure 16-100 Brown recluse spider bite, microscopic
The bite of the brown recluse spider (*Loxosceles* spider) initially produces a mild stinging sensation, but within hours there is intense pain along with erythema and then bulla formation. This can be followed by formation of a deep ulcer with a necrotic base (★). Most of these ulcerative lesions heal spontaneously, although weeks to months may pass, and some cases require débridement or skin grafting.

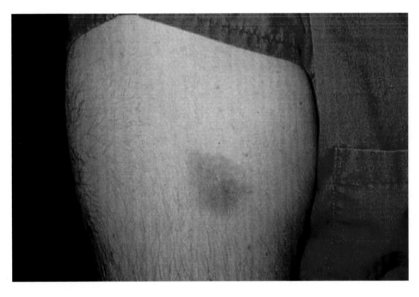

Figure 16-101 Contusion, gross
Blunt force injury that does not break the skin can rupture small blood vessels in the dermis and underlying soft tissue, resulting in the extravasation of red blood cells. Initially the contusion appears dull red to blue, but over time the red cells are broken down, releasing bilirubin and heme (which is processed by macrophages to hemosiderin) to give the yellow-brown hue shown here 1 week after the injury to the upper outer arm.

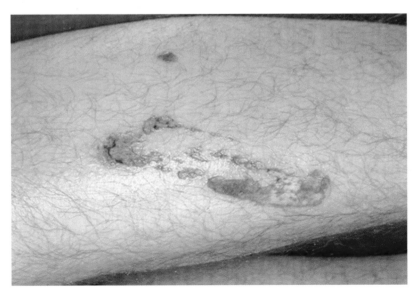

Figure 16-102 Abrasion, gross
Abrasions are made by a scraping injury to the skin surface, typically in an irregular fashion, as shown here over the skin of the leg. Note the superficial tearing of the epidermis, but no break in the skin surface. Sometimes the pattern of the abrasion can indicate what kind of surface the skin contacted when the force was applied. Sometimes foreign material can become embedded in the abraded surface.

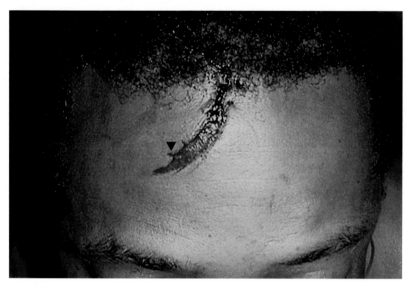

Figure 16-103　Laceration, gross
This superficial laceration of the forehead shows that the skin surface is broken. There are some small tags of skin (▼) where the surface was irregularly torn. The tearing may be linear to stellate, depending on the direction and amount of force applied. Lacerations typically occur by contact with an irregular object, either from blunt force or sharp force, with enough force applied to break the skin surface. Lacerations are deeper than abrasions and are more irregular than incised wounds.

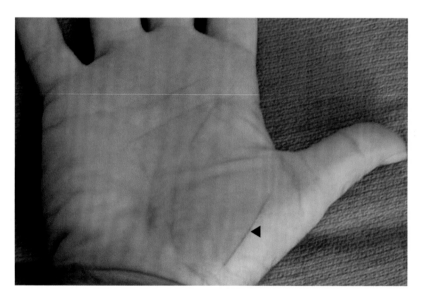

Figure 16-104　Incised wound, gross
An incision is defined as a very regular cut made by a sharp object, such as a knife. An incised wound (◄) of the skin of the hand is shown here. An incision has clean, straight edges made by the sharp object, in this case a rose thorn. It is easier to approximate the edges of an incision, such as a surgical incision, with sutures so that the wound heals by primary intention and leaves little or no scar.

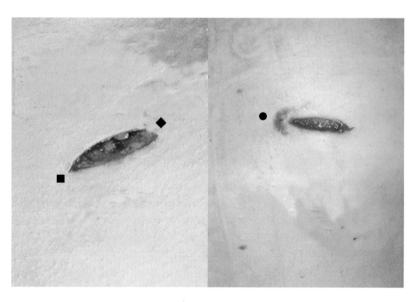

Figure 16-105　Stab wound, gross
This is a stab wound made with a single-edge knife blade. Note the sharp edge of the blade (■) and the notch of the opposite side of the knife (◆). The shape of stab wounds can vary considerably, depending on whether the incision is along the axis of, or perpendicular to, Langer lines. Incisions that are perpendicular tend to pull apart and gape open, whereas incisions parallel to the lines of stress tend to remain slitlike. Both wounds shown here are the result of a single-edge blade. The stab wound in the *right panel* has a "hilt" mark (●) opposite the sharp blade edge.

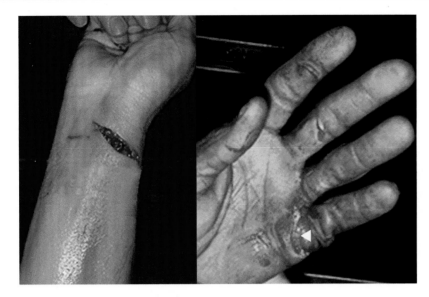

Figure 16-106 Defensive wounds, gross
Typical defensive wounds (◀) are shown on the forearm and hand of the victim of an assault with a sharp weapon, which produced the lacerations. The assailant was attacking with a knife. Such wounds result from an attempt by the victim to ward off the assailant. The victim holds up forearms and hands in front of the body as a shield.

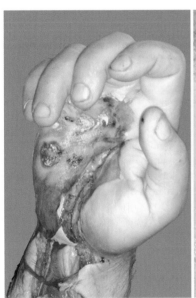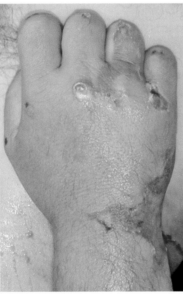

Figure 16-107 Electrocution injury, gross
This man accidentally grabbed a high-voltage electrical line, producing the entrance wound injury appearing on the palm of the hand, with subsequent soft-tissue damage and swelling extending to the forearm. The appearance is similar to a localized burn. The wounds produced as the current exited the hand can be seen on the dorsum of the hand.

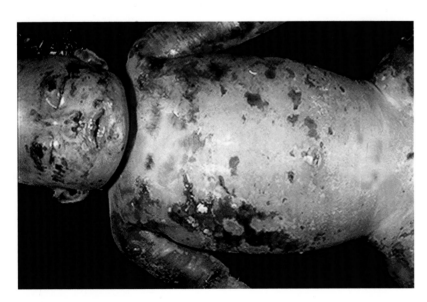

Figure 16-108 Thermal burn injury, gross
Thermal burn injuries occur with exposure to a hot local environment. The burned skin shown here over the torso and head of a child resulted from a fire. Flames are not required to produce the injury; heat can be conducted through air, liquids, and solids. Liquids, such as hot water or oil for cooking, are particularly injurious. The treatment and prognosis often depend largely on the extent of the burn injury—the total body surface area involved. Other factors include older age of the patient; underlying diseases; and the presence of an "inhalation injury" from breathing in hot gases, which typically occurs with fires in an enclosed space such as a building.

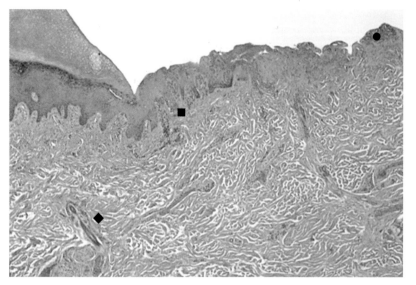

Figure 16-109 Thermal burn injury, microscopic

Thermal burn injuries can be classified as full thickness or partial thickness based on the ability of the skin to regenerate. The injury shown is partial thickness on the left because there are basal cells (■) and adnexal structures (◆) in the dermis that are viable and from which new epithelium could grow. The viable skin at the left merges with an area of full-thickness thermal burn injury without any viable epithelium either on the surface (●) or in dermal appendages on the right. The patient would require a skin graft to this full-thickness burn area for recovery.

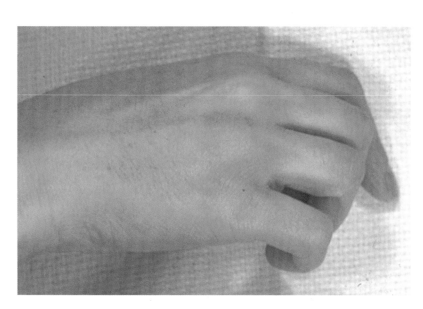

Figure 16-110 Carbon monoxide poisoning, gross

This bright cherry-red or pink lividity to the hand is characteristic of carbon monoxide poisoning, a form of asphyxia. Poorly ventilated houses with faulty heaters, house fires, and motor vehicle exhaust are the most common sources. Even small atmospheric concentrations of carbon monoxide are dangerous because carbon monoxide binds to hemoglobin 200 times more avidly than oxygen. Drowsiness and headache occur at carboxyhemoglobin concentrations of 10% to 20%. Levels of 20% to 30% can be fatal to individuals with preexisting cardiac or respiratory disease. Levels greater than 30% to 40% can be fatal to anyone. Similar lividity could be the result of cyanide poisoning or monofluoroacetate poisoning.

Bones, Joints, and Soft-Tissue Tumors

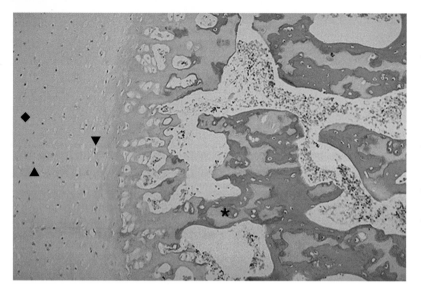

Figure 17-1 Normal fetal bone, microscopic
This normal fetal growth plate of long bones shows features of endochondral ossification. Hyaline cartilage (◆) on the left contains chondroblasts that secrete an extracellular matrix with glycosaminoglycans and proteoglycans along with type II collagen fibers and some elastic fibers. The chondroblasts (▲) become chondrocytes (▼) within lacunae defined by a pericellular capsule and surrounded by the cartilaginous matrix. The cartilage template transforms into bone spicules (★) of osteoid that become calcified. As this process continues, the bone lengthens. The hyaline cartilage remaining at the ends of long bones forms the articular cartilage of joints.

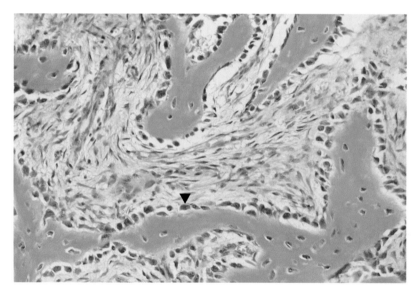

Figure 17-2 Normal bone osteoblasts, microscopic
The woven bone trabeculae at a healing fracture site have numerous osteoblasts (▼) lining surfaces and generating new osteoid, or uncalcified organic bone matrix, which is formed of type I collagen on which hydroxyapatite crystal (hydrated calcium phosphate) is deposited. Osteoblasts have parathyroid hormone (PTH) receptors and when stimulated by PTH release RANKL, which binds onto pre-osteoclast RANK (receptor activator for NF-κB) receptors to initiate osteoclastogenesis. Osteoblasts also secrete osteoprotegerin (OPG), a decoy receptor that favors bone formation.

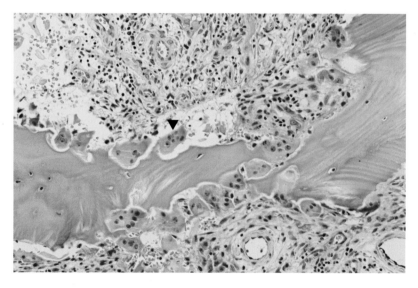

Figure 17-3 Normal bone osteoclasts, microscopic
Remodeling of bone is done through bone resorption with release of enzymes such as carbonic anhydrase, matrix metalloproteases, and alkaline phosphatase by osteoclasts (▼). Numerous multinucleated cells are visible here occupying Howship lacunae in bone spicules undergoing dissolution. The transmembrane receptor RANK is expressed on osteoclast precursors. PTH and glucocorticoids favor osteoclast activation, whereas sex steroids promote OPG production to reduce osteoclast activity.

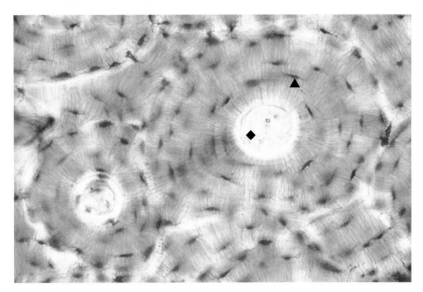

Figure 17-4 Normal adult bone, microscopic
This cross-section through unstained adult long compact bone cortex reveals round osteons formed of concentric layers of hydroxyapatite crystal around a central Haversian canal (◆) containing the neurovascular supply. Within the crystal are entrapped osteocytes (▲) inside their lacunae. Canaliculi radiate from these lacunae to allow communication between osteocytes. These osteocytes can respond to mechanical forces and can influence local calcium and phosphorus levels to maintain optimal bone structure. In adults, mineralization of osteoid takes about 2 weeks. Bone is a warehouse for body minerals, including 99% of calcium, 85% of phosphorus, and 65% of sodium found in the human body.

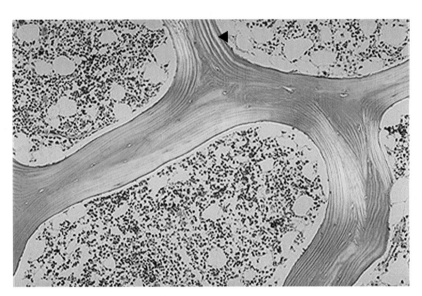

Figure 17-5 Normal adult bone, microscopic
Normal trabecular (cancellous) bone, visible here with polarized light, has a regular lamellar (◀) architecture. The lamellae of bone form by remodeling from primitive woven bone into a complex three-dimensional structure in response to stresses of gravity and movement to provide strength and support. Bone is constantly, albeit slowly, remodeling throughout the life span through the actions of osteoblasts and osteoclasts. Children have greater bone growth in size primarily from endochondral ossification with increasing length and girth of long bones until the epiphyses close. Between the bone trabeculae are marrow spaces, shown here with hematopoietic elements and adipocytes.

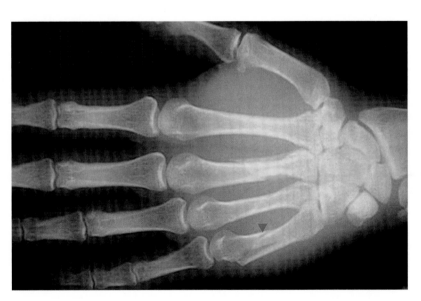

Figure 17-6 Bones of hand, fracture, radiograph
The normal radiographic appearance of bone is shown here (left hand). The outer rim of cortical bone is denser and appears brighter. Soft tissues have a light- to dark-gray appearance. Note the appearance of a recent unhealed and displaced fracture (▼) of the fifth metacarpal as a consequence of external trauma.

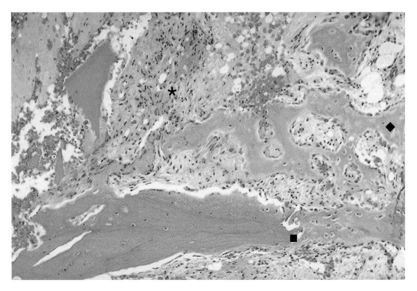

Figure 17-7 Fracture callus, microscopic
The region of fracture shows disrupted bony trabeculae (■) at the left and bottom. The paler pink new woven bone (◆) is forming in response to the injury at the right and top in areas of hemorrhage with early granulation tissue (★). In the region of fracture, the new woven bone is called *callus.* After 6 to 8 weeks, enough healing has occurred to support weight and movement. Eventually, over months to years, this new bone is remodeled into more regular lamellar bone that attains the original shape and strength. Fracture healing is more complete in children than adults. Orthopedic procedures to stabilize fractures and provide proper alignment with plates and screws are often performed.

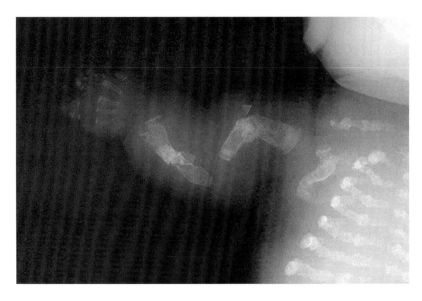

Figure 17-8 Osteogenesis imperfecta, radiograph
There are multiple fractures (▼) in these bones, which are markedly osteopenic, represented here as diminished brightness. The formation of type I collagen, a major constituent of the bone matrix, is impaired by either reduced synthesis or production of an abnormal triple helix of collagen. This leads to bone fragility and a propensity for fractures. Shown here is the perinatal lethal form (type II) of osteogenesis imperfecta (OI). Most cases are caused by a short pro-α1(1) collagen chain that leads to an unstable collagen triple helix ("dominant negative" mutation). The chest cavity is poorly formed, leading to pulmonary hypoplasia and respiratory distress at birth, if liveborn.

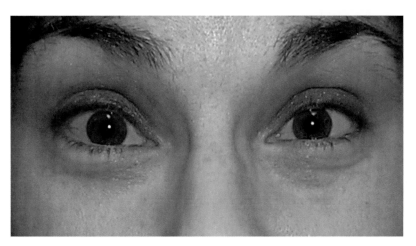

Figure 17-9 Osteogenesis imperfecta, gross
There is a bluish gray appearance to these sclerae, which reflects the deficient collagen structure with abnormal type I collagen synthesis. This condition is most often the result of an acquired mutation, but some cases are inherited in an autosomal dominant fashion and may be caused by either decreased or abnormal pro-α1(1) or pro-α2(1) collagen chains. OI type I is compatible with normal survival and stature, but affected patients have an increased risk for fractures and osteoarthritis and have dental and hearing problems.

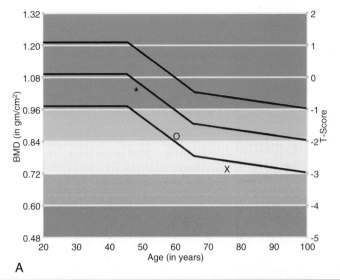

A

Figure 17-10 Osteoporosis, DEXA chart and gross

Bone mineral density (BMD) is best assessed with radiologic imaging, and dual-energy x-ray absorptiometry (DEXA) scans provide a standardized way of assessing risk for fracture from osteoporosis. **A,** A graphical display of a DEXA scan for the hip (femur) is shown, comparing BMD with age and T-score (in standard deviations above or below the comparable healthy young adult woman's mean BMD). The *asterisk* representing a woman at age 48 is within the expected range for age. The *circle* marks the BMD for a woman age 60 and is concerning for greater bone loss from osteopenia (–1 to –2.5) but not yet osteoporosis. The X marks the BMD for a woman age 76 and is in the range of osteoporosis (exceeding –2.5) with increased risk for fracture.

B, The bone in these vertebral bodies shows marked osteoporosis with fewer thin bony trabeculae. One vertebral body shows a greater degree of compression fracturing (▼) than the others. Osteoporosis is accelerated bone loss for age, greater than the usual 0.7% loss per year after the fourth decade. It is most common among postmenopausal women with reduced estrogen levels, putting them at risk for fractures, particularly involving hip, wrist, and vertebrae. Continued physical activity and a good diet help build bone mass in youth and maintain that mass with aging. Vitamin D deficiency in adults can lead to osteomalacia, which has gross and radiographic appearances similar to osteoporosis.

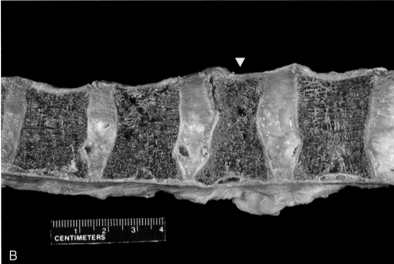

B

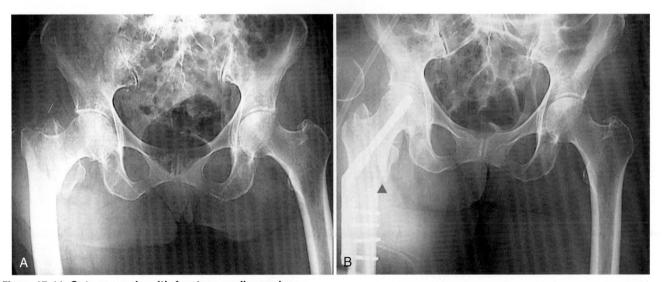

A   B

Figure 17-11 Osteoporosis with fracture, radiographs

There is severe osteoporosis involving the femurs of this elderly woman, and as a consequence a right intertrochanteric fracture (▼) has occurred and has been repaired (▲) surgically. This bone should be much denser and brighter, but instead displays greater lucency in these radiographic views because of the osteopenia. Up to a third of elderly persons with such a fracture may not survive a year.

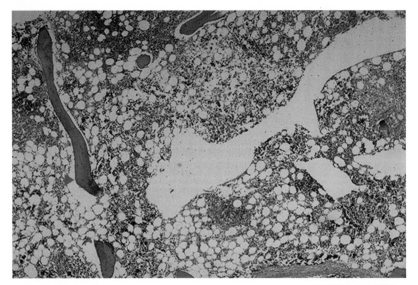

Figure 17-12 Osteoporosis, microscopic
The bone trabeculae (▶) in this vertebral body are thin and sparse from osteoporosis. The bone structure is normal, but there is less of it. The bone cortex becomes thinner, and trabeculae have less complex branching, providing less three-dimensional support. Laboratory values for serum calcium, phosphorus, alkaline phosphatase, and PTH all are normal. In contrast, in primary hyperparathyroidism, PTH levels are increased or high normal, calcium is increased, and phosphorus is decreased. Osteocalcin synthesized by osteoblasts is incorporated into extracellular bone matrix, and circulating levels correlate with osteoblast activity.

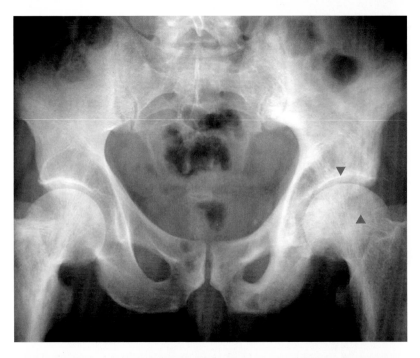

Figure 17-13 Paget disease of bone (osteitis deformans), radiograph
The left hip reveals a more irregular appearance to the bone than the right because of osteosclerosis (▼) with greater density and osteolysis with greater lucency (▲). This is the mixed osteoclastic and osteoblastic stage of Paget disease of bone, which most often occurs in elderly whites of European ancestry. A slow paramyxovirus infection may increase interleukin-6 (IL-6) secretion to drive osteoclast activity. In addition, osteoclasts may become more sensitive to RANKL and vitamin D. The serum alkaline phosphatase is increased, but the serum calcium and PTH levels are normal. This increased bone proliferation carries an increased risk for malignant neoplasia—a Paget sarcoma, typically an osteosarcoma—in 1% of all affected patients.

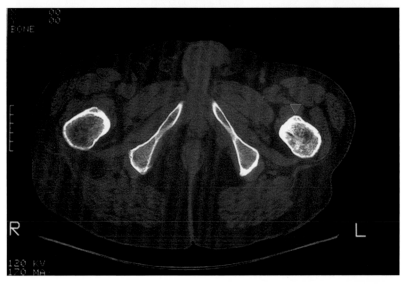

Figure 17-14 Paget disease of bone (osteitis deformans), MRI
There is more irregularity to this upper left femur, with increased brighter bony sclerosis (▼) along with areas of lucency. Paget disease mainly occurs in older individuals, and the course of the disease extends over many years. Initially there may be more osteolysis, but this is followed by the most diagnostic phase—mixed osteolytic and osteoblastic. Eventually the final phase results in prominent osteosclerosis. The clinical hallmark is pain with diminished joint range of motion and arthritis. The abnormally thickened bone is paradoxically weaker and prone to fracture. Skull involvement can lead to cranial nerve entrapment.

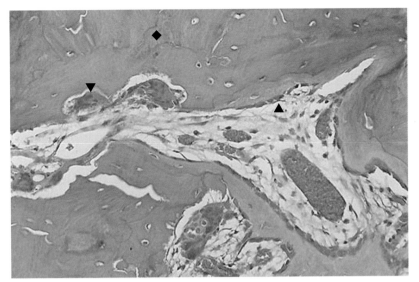

Figure 17-15 Paget disease of bone (osteitis deformans), microscopic

There is more bone turnover, with an uncoupling of osteoblast and osteoclast coordination in bone remodeling, leading to a haphazard microscopic appearance. Prominent osteoclast (▼) and osteoblast (▲) activity is shown here. The result is a thicker but weaker bone that has irregular cement lines (◆), producing a mosaic pattern instead of an organized lamellar pattern. This proliferating bone is highly vascularized, and the increased vascular flow can lead to high-output congestive heart failure. Localized disease may require no therapy other than occasional use of analgesics. More extensive polyostotic disease can be treated with osteoclast-inhibiting bisphosphonates.

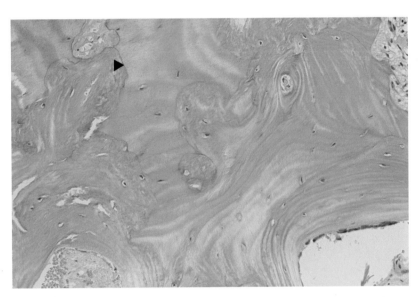

Figure 17-16 Paget disease of bone (osteitis deformans), microscopic

With polarized light microscopy the mosaic pattern is evident, with irregular lamellae and cement lines (▶) from increased bone turnover with dyssynchronous remodeling in the mixed lytic and blastic phase. Up to half of familial cases and 10% of sporadic cases may involve *SQSTM1* gene mutations that enhance NF-κB–dependent osteoclast formation. Most cases are polyostotic (multiple sites), and a sixth are monostotic. Serum markers include increased alkaline phosphatase and deoxypyridinoline.

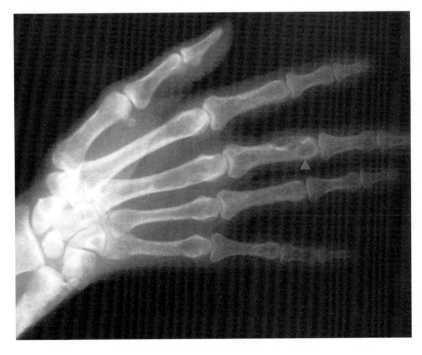

Figure 17-17 Hyperparathyroidism, radiograph

This patient has a parathyroid adenoma and increased serum calcium, decreased phosphorus, and elevated PTH. This is osteitis fibrosa cystica of bone, with expansile areas of lucency (▲), shown here as deformities involving the metatarsals and phalanges of this right hand. Such lesions can cause pain, but the focal decrease in bone mass also predisposes to fracture. In contrast, secondary hyperparathyroidism is caused by chronic renal failure with retention of phosphate that depresses serum calcium to stimulate PTH release; secondary hyperparathyroidism produces osteitis fibrosa cystica. Hyperparathyroidism also promotes osteomalacia, osteoporosis, osteosclerosis, and growth retardation. All of these features are collectively known as *renal osteodystrophy.*

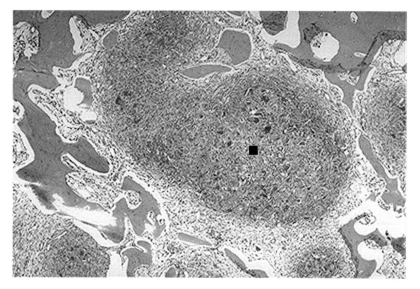

Figure 17-18 Hyperparathyroidism, brown tumor, microscopic

Note the nodular lesion (■) within bone. This area of reactive fibrous tissue proliferation with admixed multinucleated giant cells is called a *brown tumor* because of the grossly apparent brown color imparted by the vascularity, hemorrhage, macrophage infiltration, and hemosiderin deposition that often accompany this proliferation. These lesions can undergo cystic degeneration and produce focal pain and predispose to fracture. The radiograph of this lesion can show a focal radiolucency in the category of osteitis fibrosa cystica.

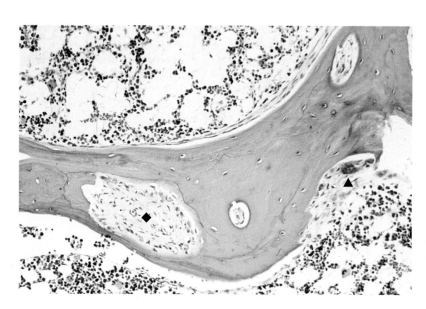

Figure 17-19 Hyperparathyroidism, dissecting osteitis, microscopic

A bone spicule with pronounced osteoclastic and osteoblastic activity (◆) is shown. This is accelerated bone remodeling with osteoclasts (▲) that tunnel into the bone trabeculae and form pockets of fibrovascular tissue. The fibrovascular tissue also is increased in the peritrabecular spaces. In secondary hyperparathyroidism from chronic renal failure, the metabolic renal tubular acidosis also stimulates bone resorption and drives osteomalacia. Increased circulating β_2-microglobulin with long-term hemodialysis can lead to amyloid deposition in bone.

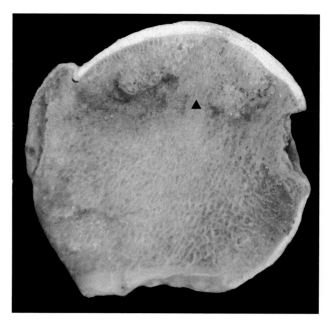

Figure 17-20 Avascular necrosis, gross

Beneath the articular cartilage of this femoral head is a pale yellow, wedge-shaped area of osteonecrosis (▲) in a patient with pain in the hip that developed after long-term use of corticosteroids. Additional risk factors include traumatic vascular disruption, thrombosis, barotrauma, vasculitis, sickle cell disease, and radiation therapy. The usual initial symptom is pain with movement, but this progresses to constant pain. Replacement of necrotic bone with new bone (creeping substitution) does not proceed fast enough to prevent focal collapse with disruption of articular cartilage and fracture. Infarction within the medullary cavity is more likely to be clinically silent.

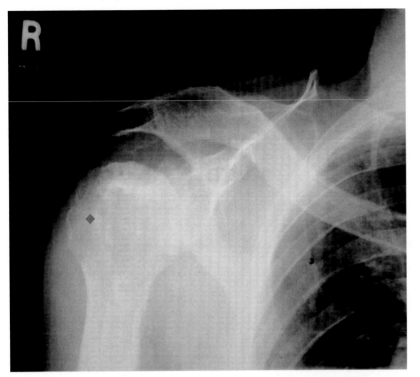

Figure 17-21 Avascular necrosis, radiograph
Note the irregular remodeling (◆) of the head of this proximal humerus as a result of osteonecrosis. The bones of the humeral head and the femoral head have a tenuous blood supply that can be traumatically disrupted. The devitalized bone undergoes remodeling and bone distortion, and the adjacent joint becomes painful with increased use and decreased function. The remodeling process is inefficient and slow, and there is eventual collapse with distortion of the overlying articular cartilage, leading to secondary osteoarthritis of the joint.

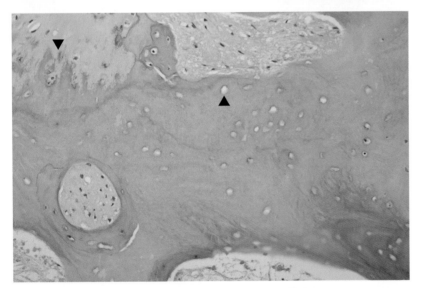

Figure 17-22 Avascular necrosis, microscopic
Osteocyte nuclei are absent from their lacunae (▲) in the bony trabeculae, and lamellae are not well defined. Adjacent cartilage may break down and fragment (▼). Marrow adipocytes are replaced by debris and reactive proliferating cartilage and fibrous connective tissue. This proliferative response leads to scarring without revascularization of the bone, so that remodeling is abnormal and the joint surface altered to produce abnormal joint motion. Treatment may consist of joint replacement.

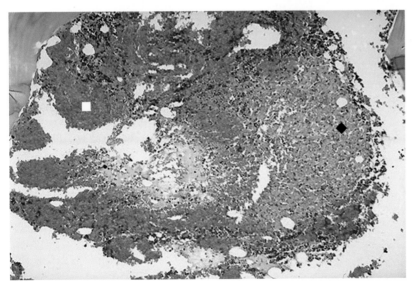

Figure 17-23 Bone marrow infarct, microscopic
Hemorrhage (■) with necrosis (◆) involving the marrow of a vertebral body is shown. This lesion occurred in a patient experiencing a sickle cell crisis and severe back pain. Microvascular occlusions by the "sticky" sickled red blood cells lead to release of hemoglobin that binds nitric oxide. Reduced nitric oxide favors vasoconstriction and platelet aggregation. These vaso-occlusive crises can affect multiple organs, including acute chest syndrome with pulmonary vascular bed occlusion. The pain of bone infarcts mimics acute osteomyelitis.

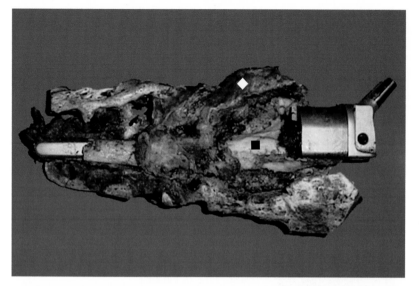

Figure 17-24 Osteomyelitis, gross

Extensive bone destruction with irregular re-modeling results in the appearance of a lighter colored (■) necrotic sequestrum, appearing here immediately adjacent to the prosthetic device, surrounded by the darker involucrum (◆) that is the reactive new bone in this chronic process. Osteomyelitis may result from penetrating injury with introduction of organisms, typically bacteria, into bone. More commonly, osteomyelitis is ac-quired by hematogenous dissemination. In grow-ing bones of children, most bone infections begin predominantly in the metaphyseal region, with the greatest blood flow. Osteomyelitis in adults most often begins in epiphyseal and subchondral locations.

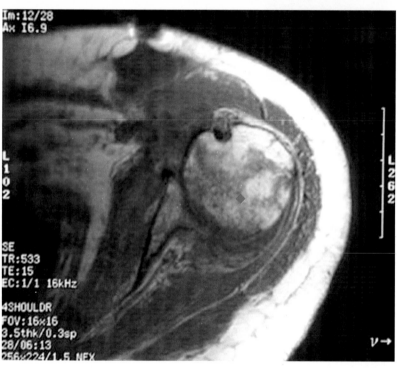

Figure 17-25 Osteomyelitis, MRI

This proximal humeral head shows irregular lysis and sclerosis (◆) from infection. Patients with acute osteomyelitis have pain, fever, and leuko-cytosis, but radiographic findings are subtle. A blood culture may be positive. About 5% to 25% of acute cases fail to resolve and go on to chronic osteomyelitis. There may be acute exacerba-tions. The weakened bone is prone to fracture. A fracture complicated by osteomyelitis may fail to heal, with development of a pseudarthrosis. An uncommon complication is development of a draining sinus tract, and rarer still is development of a squamous cell carcinoma within such a sinus tract.

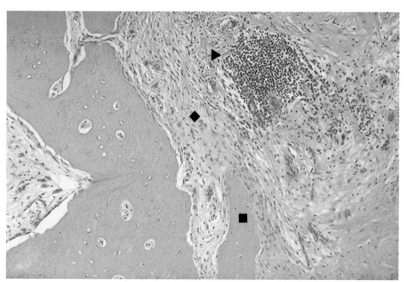

Figure 17-26 Osteomyelitis, microscopic

Shown here in the marrow is fibrosis (◆) accom-panied by chronic inflammatory cell infiltrates (▶). The bony trabeculae have become disorganized, and the bone is devitalized (■). Osteomyelitis is difficult to treat and may require surgical drain-age and antibiotic therapy. The most common causative organism is *Staphylococcus aureus*. Neonates may have *Haemophilus influenzae* and group B streptococcal bone infections. Patients with sickle cell anemia are at risk for *Salmonella* osteomyelitis. Patients with urinary tract infections and injection drug users are at risk for osteomy-elitis with *Escherichia coli* and *Pseudomonas* and *Klebsiella* species.

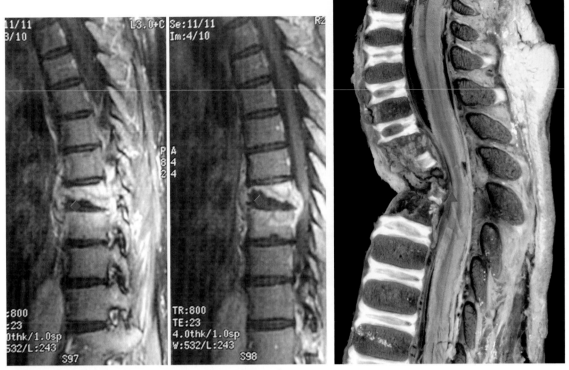

Figures 17-27 and 17-28 Tuberculous osteomyelitis, MRI and gross
Extensive bone destruction (◆) is shown involving the T8 and T9 mid-thoracic vertebrae in a patient with disseminated *Mycobacterium tuberculosis* infection. Hematogenous spread is most likely, although there may be direct extension from the lung. This is Pott disease of the spine. The vertebral body destruction here has resulted in impingement (▲) on the spinal cord. The infection may spread into adjacent paraspinal or psoas muscles to form a cold abscess.

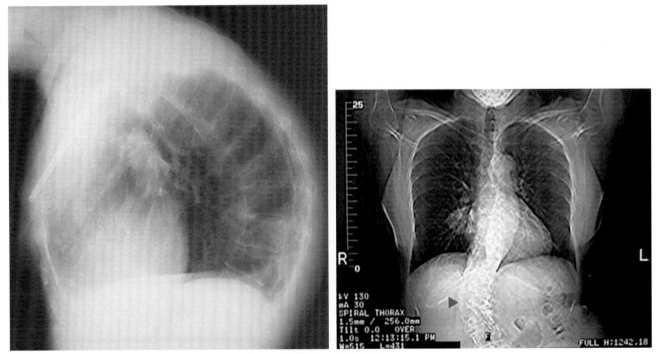

Figures 17-29 and 17-30 Kyphosis, radiograph, and scoliosis, CT image
The lateral chest radiograph in the *left panel* shows marked kyphosis of the vertebral column, so that the head and neck are bent forward and the total chest volume is markedly reduced. This patient had severe osteoporosis, and a fall with trauma resulted in a fracture of the humerus that required open reduction and internal fixation, evidenced by the bright metal rod shown here. The chest CT scout image in coronal view in the *right panel* shows marked scoliosis of the lower thoracic vertebral column, with a major curve (▶) to the right. The superior-inferior axis and the anterior-posterior axis of the vertebral column show rotation. (Note that this patient also has a mass lesion within the right lung—bronchogenic carcinoma).

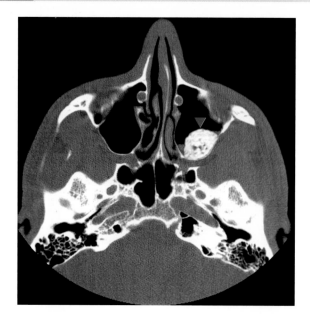

Figure 17-31 Osteoma, CT image
A rounded bony cortical irregularity known as an *osteoma* (▼) is extending into the left maxillary sinus. Such a lesion may occur in a patient with Plenk-Gardner syndrome caused by an *APC* gene mutation. The osteomas are typically an incidental finding in this syndrome. Solitary osteomas occur in middle-aged adults as sessile periosteal or endosteal masses. Osteomas are composed of a dense mixture of woven and lamellar bone.

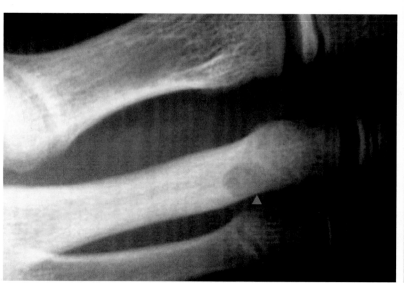

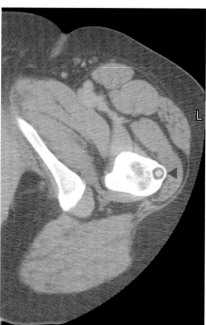

Figure 17-32 and 17-33 Osteoid osteoma, radiograph and CT image
The discrete round lucency surrounded by a thin rim of sclerosis in this proximal phalanx (▲, *left panel*) and proximal femur (◄, *right panel*) is an osteoid osteoma. Despite their size (usually <2 cm), they can produce considerable pain from prostaglandin production, which can be blocked by analgesics such as aspirin. Osteoid osteomas most commonly arise in the second or third decade. They are most often found in the bone cortex of the femur or tibia.

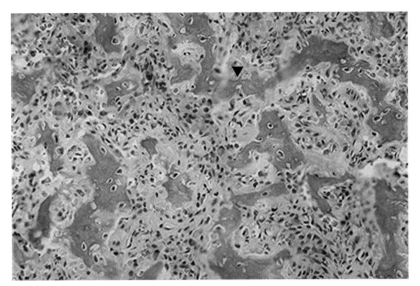

Figure 17-34 Osteoid osteoma, microscopic
This is the central nidus, or radiolucent portion, of an osteoid osteoma, composed of irregular reactive new woven bone (▼). Osteoid osteomas usually occur in the bone cortex. An osteoblastoma is a well-circumscribed mass that has an identical microscopic appearance but is larger (defined as >2 cm) and more likely to be present in a posterior vertebral body. These lesions are benign and cured by local resection, but they may recur if not completely resected. They may also be treated with radiofrequency ablation.

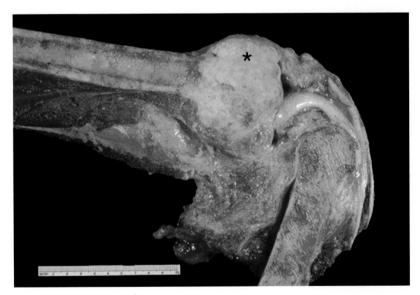

Figure 17-35 Osteosarcoma, gross
This irregular mass lesion (★) is arising within the metaphysis at the upper tibia in this cross-section of the lower extremity. It breaks through the bone cortex and extends into adjacent soft tissue. The tumor tissue is firm and tan-white. Glistening white articular cartilage of the uninvolved femoral condyle can be seen just to the right of the tumor. Osteosarcoma is the most common primary malignant bone tumor. Most arise during the first two decades of life. Males are affected more than females. More than half the tumors occur around the knee. Other sites of origin include the pelvis, proximal humerus, and jaw. Familial osteosarcomas often have *RB* gene mutations. Most are sporadic and also have *RB, TP53, CDK4, INK4a,* and *MDM2* mutations.

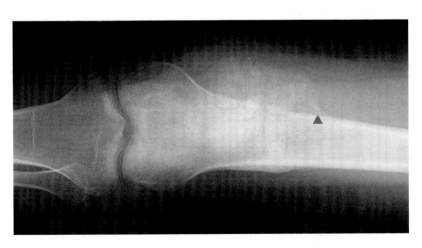

Figure 17-36 Osteosarcoma, radiograph
This malignancy (▼) involves the metaphyseal region of the distal femur. Long bones are more often affected in young individuals, probably because bone growth with mitotic activity increases risk for genetic mutations. This tumor erodes and destroys the bone cortex, extending into soft tissue where irregular reactive bone formation with calcification is visible as brighter areas in the normally dull-gray soft tissues. The periosteum here is lifted off (▲) to form a Codman triangle.

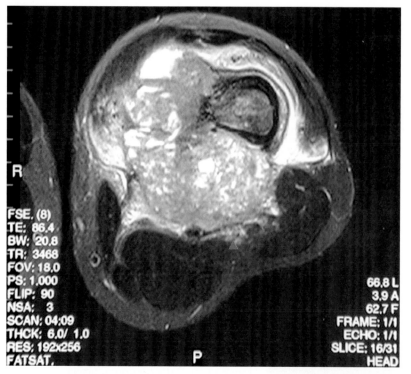

Figure 17-37 Osteosarcoma, MRI
A mass with increased signal intensity in the distal femur is visible with axial T2-weighted fast spin echo MRI with fat saturation. There is extensive cortical bone disruption with extension (▲) of the tumor into the adjacent soft tissue. Areas of hemorrhage and cystic degeneration impart the variegation appearing here as different areas of brightness. The first clinical manifestation is often pain as the tumor breaks through the bone cortex and lifts off the periosteum. Osteosarcomas, similar to sarcomas in general, are most likely to metastasize hematogenously, most often to lungs.

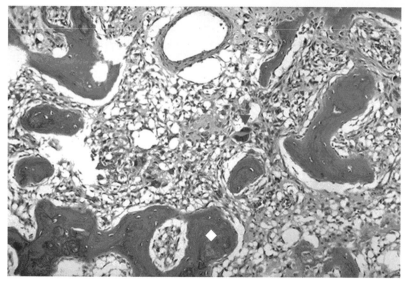

Figure 17-38 Osteosarcoma, microscopic
This tumor is composed of very pleomorphic cells, many with a spindle shape. One large, bizarre multinucleated cell (▼) with very large nuclei is present. Nuclear hyperchromatism and cellular pleomorphism are features of malignant neoplasms. There are islands (◆) of reactive new woven bone forming in response to the infiltration and destruction of normal bone by the tumor.

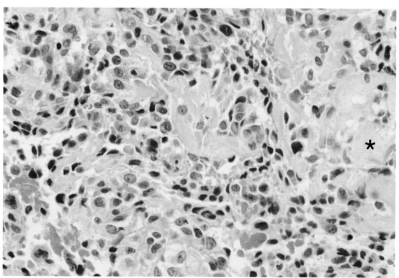

Figure 17-39 Osteosarcoma, microscopic
The neoplastic pleomorphic cells of osteosarcoma are shown to be making pink osteoid (★). Osteoid production by a sarcoma is diagnostic of an osteosarcoma. This osteoid matrix vaguely resembles primitive woven bone. Additional microscopic elements of an osteosarcoma include vascular proliferation, cartilaginous matrix, and fibrous connective tissue. There may be considerable microscopic variation within a single tumor, and metastases may not exactly resemble the primary site microscopic appearance.

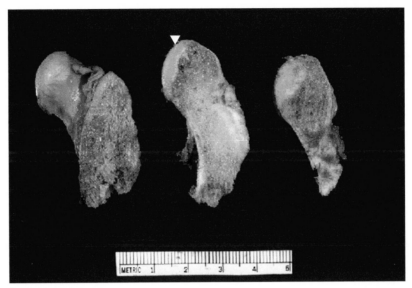

Figure 17-40　Osteochondroma, gross

Longitudinal cross-sections through this excised exostosis reveal a bluish-white cartilaginous cap (▼) overlying a bony cortex. These lesions are probably not true neoplasms but are likely an aberration of endochondral bone formation with lateral displacement of the growth plate. They form a slowly growing mass lesion that extends outward from the metaphyseal region of a long bone—an exostosis. They are typically solitary, arising most often in the metaphyseal region of a long bone before growth plate closure. The knee is the most common site, but the pelvis, scapula, and ribs may be involved. Less commonly, more than one lesion can appear at multiple sites, with an onset in childhood.

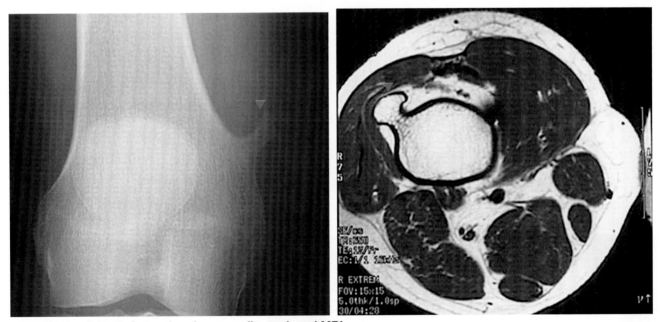

Figures 17-41 and 17-42　Osteochondroma, radiograph and MRI

An osteochondroma (▼) of the metaphyseal region projects laterally from the distal femur in the radiographic coronal view in the *left panel* and in the axial T1-weighted MRI image in the *right panel,* and has a composition very similar to the normal bone. About 15% of these lesions can be multiple, with loss-of-function mutations in either the *EXT1* or the *EXT2* gene, and part of an inherited condition such as the autosomal dominant multiple hereditary exostosis syndrome, with increased risk for development of osteosarcoma.

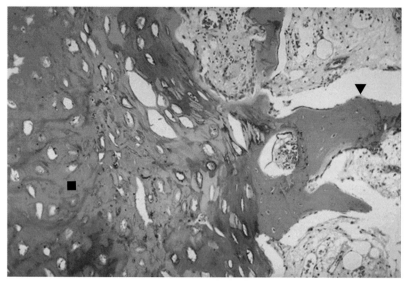

Figure 17-43 Osteochondroma, microscopic
Shown here is a benign cartilaginous cap (■) on the left with underlying bony cortex (▼) on the right. This abnormal growth enlarges very slowly and usually stops growing when the epiphyseal plate closes. Although benign, osteochondromas can sometimes lead to pain and irritation if the exostosis causes nerve compression, is traumatized, or is fractured. Lesions that are symptomatic may be surgically removed. Malignant transformation to a sarcoma, such as a chondrosarcoma, is uncommon in solitary lesions.

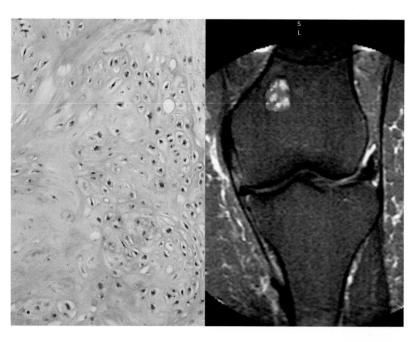

Figure 17-44 Enchondroma, MRI and microscopic
The mass (◄) in the medullary cavity (right panel) is a circumscribed benign cartilaginous tumor. Such enchondromas are true neoplasms, with mutations in the *IDH1* and *IDH2* genes. Solitary lesions are usually less than 3 cm in size and typically arise in metaphyseal regions of tubular bones, such as the distal femur here, but more likely in the hands and feet. Cellularity is greater than that of normal cartilage, but the cells are not highly atypical *(left panel)*. Multiple enchondromas may be seen with hereditary Ollier disease, with risk for development of a sarcoma.

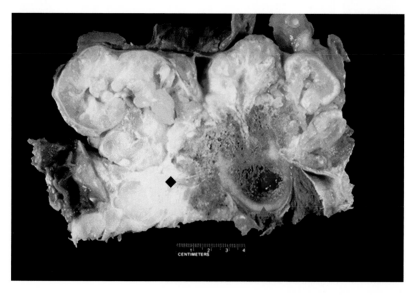

Figure 17-45 Chondrosarcoma, gross
This large, irregular mass (♦) is arising within pelvic bone (▲) and extending into soft tissues. Most chondrosarcomas arise in the central (axial) skeleton. A cartilaginous tumor arising more peripherally is more likely to be benign. Note the extensive nodules of white to bluish-white cartilaginous tumor tissue eroding bone and extending outward from the residual bone. Chondrosarcomas can occur over a wide age range, and there is a slight male predominance. Many of them are low grade and slow growing, with symptoms present for a decade or more. Larger tumors are more aggressive than smaller ones. This is the second most common primary bone tumor.

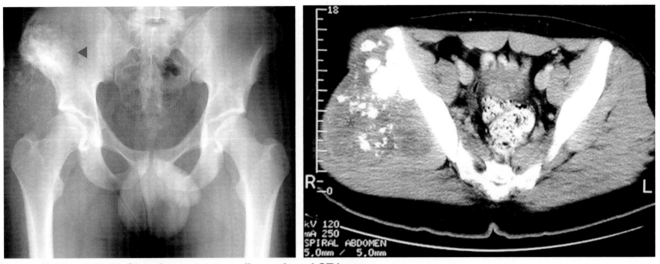

Figures 17-46 and 17-47 Chondrosarcoma, radiograph and CT image
In the *left panel,* a chondrosarcoma (◀) arising in the right iliac wing and extending to soft tissues exhibits irregular brightness. In the *right panel,* the CT scan shows extensive soft-tissue involvement (✱) with brightly calcified areas. These appearances reflect the heterogeneous tissue composition of these tumors. They cause local pain. Metastases from high-grade tumors typically occur in the lungs.

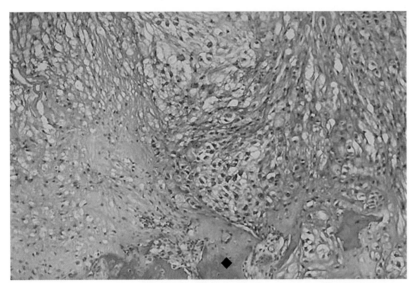

Figure 17-48 Chondrosarcoma, microscopic
At low magnification, the tissue is still recognizable as cartilage, and there are chondrocytes within clear lacunae, surrounded by a bluish matrix, but there is no orderly pattern, and there is increased cellularity and atypia. At the bottom the chondrosarcoma is invading and destroying bone (◆). Most chondrosarcomas are low grade and indolent, but a focus of high-grade (dedifferentiated) sarcoma may be present in some of them. Some arise within an intraosseous cartilaginous tumor known as an *enchondroma,* typically when multiple enchondromas (enchondromatosis) are present.

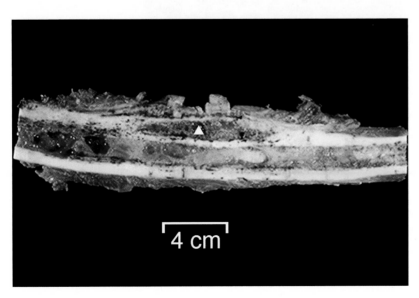

Figure 17-49 Ewing sarcoma, gross
This primary bone tumor mainly arises within the medullary cavity in the diaphysis of long bones and pelvis in the first two decades of life, with a slight male predominance. The fibular tumor mass shown here is breaking through (▲) the cortex. The tan tumor tissue has prominent areas of reddish hemorrhage and brownish necrosis. More normal long bone fatty marrow appears at the far right. Such an enlarging mass may manifest with local tenderness, warmth, and swelling at the affected site. Some patients have fever and leukocytosis, suggesting an infection.

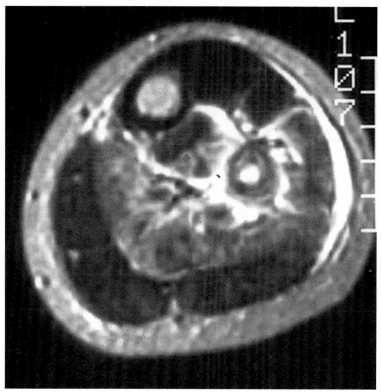

Figure 17-50 Ewing sarcoma, MRI

This T2-weighted MRI image shows irregular bright tumor (◆) extending from the fibula into surrounding soft tissue. The normal bone cortex of the tibia is dark, whereas the marrow cavity filled with fatty marrow is bright. With a standard radiograph, this lesion often appears lytic, with cortical destruction. The Ewing sarcoma family of tumors (ESFTs) also includes primitive neuroectodermal tumors (PNETs) that occur in soft tissues, usually in children.

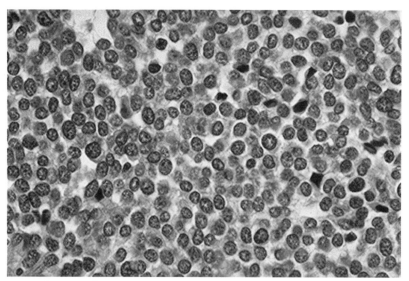

Figure 17-51 Ewing sarcoma, microscopic

This is a small round blue cell tumor of childhood. Note the marked cellularity and the high nuclear-to-cytoplasm ratio of these tumor cells, which are slightly larger than lymphocytes. There is little intervening stroma. Mitoses are present. PAS stain may reveal abundant glycogen within tumor cell cytoplasm. These malignancies often arise when there is a t(11;22) chromosomal translocation that produces the *EWS-FLI1* fusion gene acting as a transcription factor to drive cellular proliferation. Ewing sarcoma and PNET have a similar molecular origin, but a PNET has more neural differentiation.

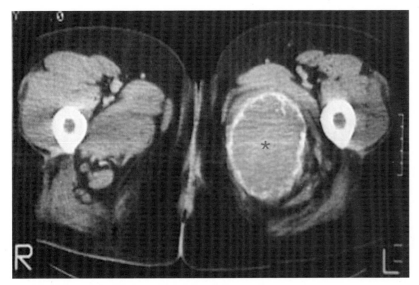

Figure 17-52 Giant cell tumor, CT image
The mass appearing here involves the left ischial ramus of the pelvis and appears as an eccentric, expansile, lytic tumor (✱) with extension into adjacent soft tissue. As the tumor expands, it produces a bright rim of overlying reactive new bone. This locally aggressive lesion is most likely to arise in the epiphyseal region and extend to the metaphyseal region of bone, most often around the knee, in the third to fifth decades. These tumors often appear benign histologically but may recur after local resection. A few act in a malignant fashion, with sarcomatous transformation, and can have distant metastases.

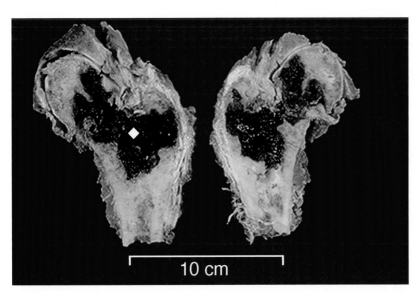

Figure 17-53 Giant cell tumor, gross
This proximal femur has been amputated and sectioned longitudinally to reveal an irregular, dark red-black hemorrhagic mass (◆) arising within the epiphyseal region and extending into the metaphysis. The expansion of this tumor near a joint can produce arthritic pain. The weakened bone may fracture (pathologic fracture) or become deformed.

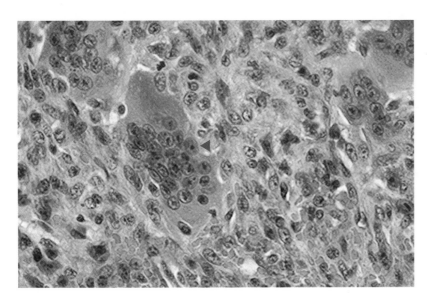

Figure 17-54 Giant cell tumor, microscopic
Giant cell tumors of bone are composed of osteoclast-like multinucleated giant cells (◀) in a sea of round-to-oval mononuclear stromal cells. There may also be lipid-laden macrophages along with hemorrhage and hemosiderin deposition within the stroma. The tumor cells are primitive osteoblast precursors that, though few in number, are producing large amounts of RANKL, which promotes proliferation of osteoclast precursors that differentiate into mature osteoclasts.

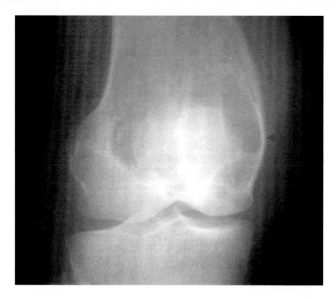

Figure 17-55 Aneurysmal bone cyst, radiograph

The aneurysmal bone cyst (ABC) shown here radiographically in distal femur is an eccentric, expansile, lytic lesion with a well-defined margin composed of a thin shell (◀) of reactive bone. There are internal septations. Grossly, there are multiloculated blood-filled cystic spaces. Rearrangements in chromosome 17p13 result in fusion of the coding region of *TRE17* to the promoter regions of genes involved in osteoblastic function that induce abnormal expression of *TRE17* in the stromal cells of ABC. *TRE17* encodes a ubiquitin-specific protease that, through NF-κB, activates matrix metalloproteases, potentially accounting for the cystic resorption of bone.

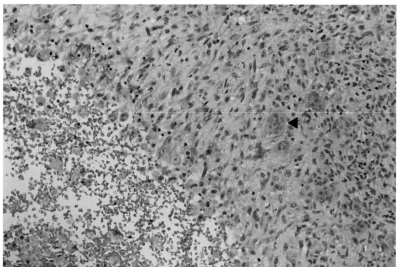

Figure 17-56 Aneurysmal bone cyst, microscopic

ABCs most often arise in the first two decades, most often in long bone metaphyses. Microscopically there are red blood cells in lakes along with pale brown hemosiderin, giving the red-to-brown gross appearance. These lakes are bounded by septal proliferations of fibroblasts, mitotically active spindle cells with *TRE17* expression, osteoid in woven bone, and osteoclast-like multinucleated giant cells (◀). Recurrence after resection is uncommon, and malignant behavior is rare.

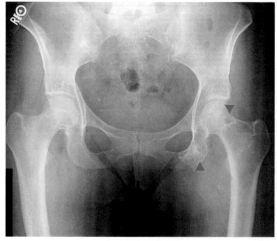

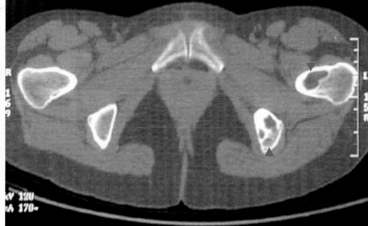

Figures 17-57 and 17-58 Fibrous dysplasia, radiograph and CT image

A single irregular area of bone lucency is visible in the region of the left femoral neck (▼) and in the left ischium (▲). In the pelvic CT scan in the *right panel,* lucency in the femoral neck on the left and another lucency in the left ischium can be seen. Polyostotic (multiple bone site) lesions associated with endocrinopathies and café-au-lait spots on the skin constitute McCune-Albright syndrome, representing about 3% of all cases. Most cases of fibrous dysplasia are monostotic (involve just one bone site) and appear in adolescence. This is a condition in which there is progressive replacement of bone by a disorganized proliferation of fibrous tissue and woven bone. Skeletal deformity and fracture can occur.

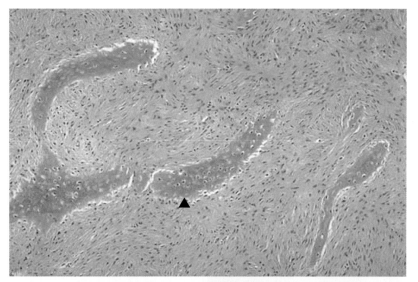

Figure 17-59 Fibrous dysplasia, microscopic
Shown here is a proliferative process with haphazard spicules (▲) of woven bone in a cellular stroma. There is little osteoblastic activity. As the localized area of irregular woven bone proliferates, it does not develop into solid lamellar bone, but leaves a weakened area that can produce deformity or fracture. Transformation of this process into a sarcoma is rare. This lesion arises from a somatic gain-of-function mutation in the GNAS1 gene producing a G protein–coupled receptor activating adenylyl cyclase, leading to excess cyclic adenosine monophosphate, which drives cellular proliferation.

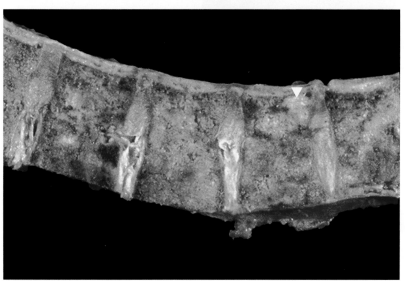

Figure 17-60 Metastases, gross
This sagittal section of vertebral bone at autopsy shows multiple foci (▼) of pale and irregular metastatic tumor. Overall, the most common neoplasm involving bone is a metastasis. Virtually all bone metastases occur from carcinomas, and the most common primary sites are remembered with the "lead kettle" mnemonic (PBKTL): prostate, breast, kidney, thyroid, lung. Metastases from renal cell carcinomas and most other carcinomas tend to be osteolytic (they destroy the bone) and are radiolucent, whereas metastases from prostatic carcinomas tend to be osteoblastic (they initiate prominent new bone formation) and are radiodense.

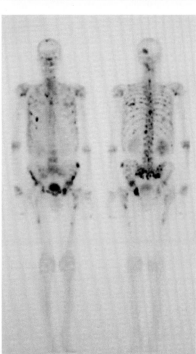
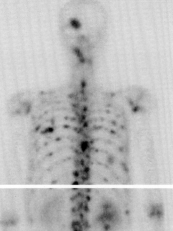
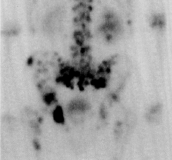

Figure 17-61 Metastases, bone scan
This radionuclide bone scan reveals numerous areas of increased uptake—the dark foci, or hot spots—from metastases, which are usually multifocal. Note the darker right kidney, which is hydronephrotic from obstruction by the primary tumor—a urothelial carcinoma of the bladder involving the right ureteral orifice. The increased cellularity and vascularity of the metastatic foci compared with normal bone produce this differential uptake of the radioactive compound. Osteolytic lesions can occur when metastases produce prostaglandins, cytokines, and parathormone-related peptide (PTHrP) that upregulate RANKL on osteoblasts to stimulate osteoclast activity. Most metastases have a mixture of osteoclastic and osteoblastic activity because bone lysis often elicits reactive new bone formation, but osteolysis predominates.

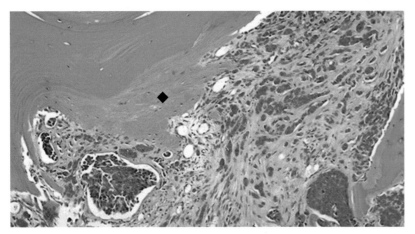

Figure 17-62 Metastases, microscopic
Metastatic infiltrating ductal carcinoma of breast appears within vertebral bone, and it is filling the marrow cavity. There is reactive new bone (◆) at the margin of the carcinoma, with pale pink osteoid being laid down next to a bony spicule at the upper left. Metastases may produce pain. They may weaken the bone to an extent that a pathologic fracture occurs. The serum alkaline phosphatase is often elevated with metastatic bone disease.

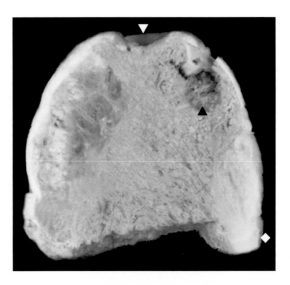

Figure 17-63 Osteoarthritis, gross
This sagittal cross-section of the femoral head shows surface erosion (▼), a subchondral cyst (▲), and an osteophyte (◆). The changes of osteoarthritis are most often reported by the patient as pain or difficulty with movement at the involved joint. The abnormal movement exacerbates joint damage at the involved joint and in distal joints. "Primary" osteoarthritis, as with wear and tear of aging, usually involves just a few joints (oligoarticular). "Secondary" osteoarthritis follows an underlying disease or poorly healed fracture with misalignment that often affects adjacent bone.

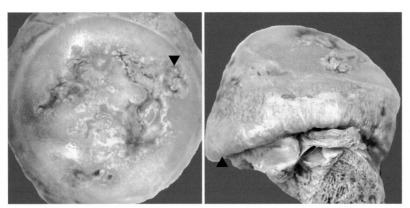

Figure 17-64 Osteoarthritis, gross
There is often minimal outward deformity, and osteoarthritis causes little inflammation. In these panels the femoral head on the *left* shows a rough, eburnated, irregular appearance of eroded articular cartilage (▼) typical of osteoarthritis. In the *right panel* there is prominent osteophyte formation (▲) with widening of the femoral head margin. Early in the pathogenesis, chondrocyte injury leads to chondrocyte proliferation with release of inflammatory mediators and proteases that remodel matrix and subchondral bone, but when symptomatic the process has evolved to chondrocyte and matrix loss with bone damage and the appearance shown here.

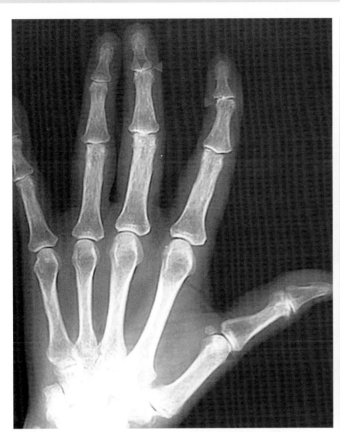
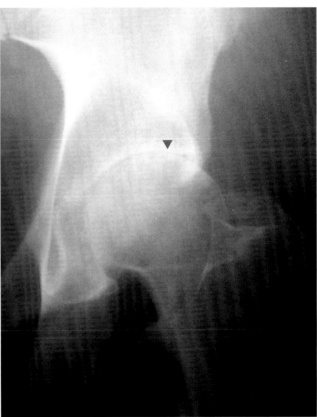

Figures 17-65 and 17-66 Osteoarthritis, radiographs

The hand in the *left panel* shows degenerative osteoarthritis with joint space narrowing (▼) and greater lateral widening (◀) at the distal interphalangeal (DIP) joints than the proximal interphalangeal (PIP) joints. There is subluxation (▶) at the DIP joints as well, most marked in the second digit. The base of the thumb (▲) has marked osteoarthritis. The pelvis in the *right panel* shows joint space narrowing (▼) of the left hip with osteoarthritis. Hip joints and knees are commonly involved because they are heavy weight-bearing joints. These degenerative changes are progressive with aging, but joint ankylosis is unlikely.

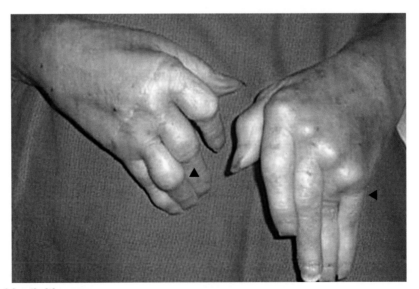

Figure 17-67 Rheumatoid arthritis, gross

Prominent ulnar deviation (◀) of the hands and flexion-hyperextension (swan neck) deformities (▲) of the fingers are present. This autoimmune disease leads to inflammation with synovial proliferation (pannus formation) that causes joint destruction, typically in a symmetrical pattern that first involves small joints of the hands and feet, followed by wrists, ankles, elbows, and knees. Many patients have certain *HLA-DRB1* alleles, suggesting a genetic susceptibility. Exposure to an infectious agent may initiate an inflammatory response that continues as an autoimmune reaction to various tissues, principally synovium, but also vasculature and soft tissues. CD4 lymphocyte activation leads to cytokine production, principally tumor necrosis factor α (TNF-α) and IL-1.

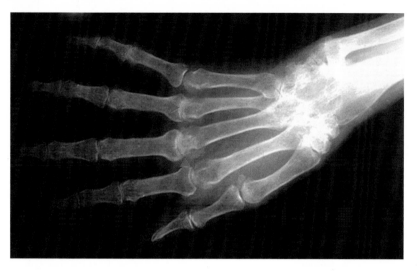

Figure 17-68 Rheumatoid arthritis, radiograph

This hand shows joint space narrowing (▶) with marginal erosions (▲) and osteopenia, mainly involving the proximal PIP joints and metacarpophalangeal joints. The carpal bones are nearly indistinguishable from ankylosis. Bone loss is primarily juxta-articular. Activated CD4 lymphocytes help B cells produce antibodies, mainly IgM, directed at the Fc portion of IgG, known as *rheumatoid factor*. Anti–cyclic citrullinated peptide antibodies are often present. Rheumatoid arthritis (RA) may begin insidiously with malaise, fever, and generalized aches and pains before joint swelling, warmth, and tenderness appear. RA tends to follow a course of remissions and exacerbations. Significant morning stiffness is often present.

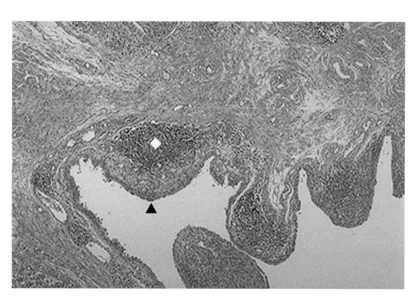

Figure 17-69 Rheumatoid arthritis, microscopic

This synovium shows marked chronic inflammation with aggregates of lymphocytes and plasma cells that produce the blue areas (◆) appearing within the nodular proliferations beneath synovium (▲). This process forms a proliferative "pannus" that is destructive through release of collagenases and produces erosion of the adjacent articular cartilage, eventually destroying the joint and leading to deformity and ankylosis. Inflammation increases RANKL, which activates osteoclasts to promote bone destruction. An aspirate of joint fluid typically shows increased turbidity, decreased viscosity, increased protein, and leukocytosis with predominance of neutrophils.

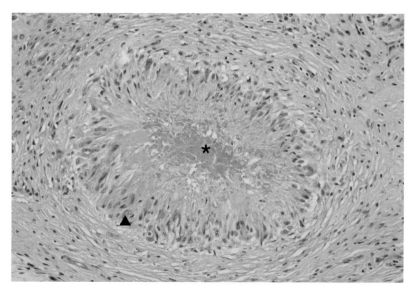

Figure 17-70 Rheumatoid nodule, microscopic

This nodule has a central area of fibrinoid necrosis (★) surrounded by palisading epithelioid macrophages (▲) and other mononuclear cells. Such firm, nontender nodules occur in about one fourth of patients with RA, typically those with more severe involvement. They appear in soft tissues beneath the skin over bony prominences such as the elbow. They occasionally appear in visceral organs, including lungs and heart. RA affects about 1% of the population. Women are affected more often than men. The onset is often in the second to fourth decades, but RA occurs over a wide age range. About half the risk for RA comes from a genetic susceptibility.

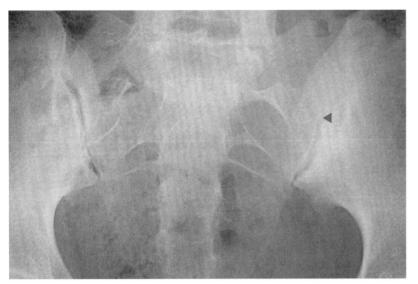

Figure 17-71 Ankylosing spondylitis, radiograph
This pelvis has sacroiliitis on the left, with narrowing and sclerosis (◀) of the sacroiliac joint. The sacroiliac joint on the right appears relatively normal by comparison. One third of patients have involvement of other joints, including hips, knees, and shoulders. This is a chronic progressive inflammatory arthritis producing spinal immobility with low back pain. The chronic synovitis leads to loss of articular cartilage with progressive bony ankylosis that limits range of motion. Low back pain is a frequent feature. About 90% of affected patients have the *HLA-B27* allele.

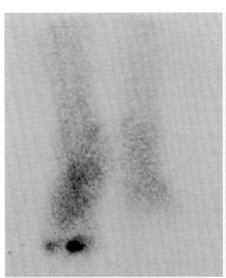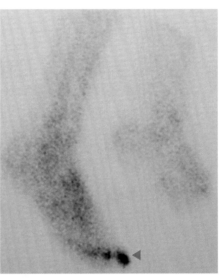

Figure 17-72 Suppurative arthritis, bone scan
Note the increased uptake (◀) in the region of the great toe in a patient having intense pain with swelling and reduced range of motion, as well as fever and leukocytosis. This is typically caused by bacterial infection. *S. aureus* is the most common agent past childhood, whereas *H. influenzae* is commonly seen in children younger than 2 years. Sexually active individuals are at risk for *Neisseria gonorrhoeae* infection. Patients with sickle cell disease are prone to develop *Salmonella* infections.

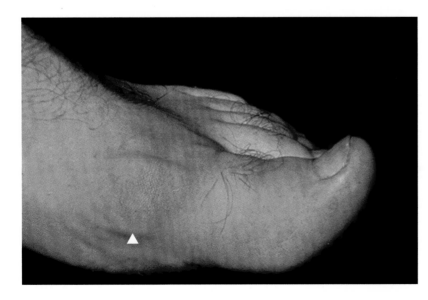

Figure 17-73 Gouty arthritis, gross
The first metatarsophalangeal joint (big toe), as shown here, is most often affected by acute attacks characterized by severe pain, swelling (▲), and erythema of the involved joint, but multiple joints may be involved. Gout results from deposition of sodium urate crystals in joints, and sometimes other soft tissues. In most cases there is hyperuricemia. Uric acid is the end point of purine metabolism, and a decrease in hypoxanthine-guanine phosphoribosyltransferase (HGPRT) in the purine salvage pathway increases de novo urate pathway production. Increased cell turnover and/or decreased renal uric acid excretion also can increase the serum uric acid.

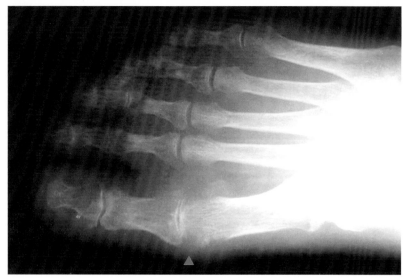

Figure 17-74 Gouty arthritis, radiograph
Chronic gout occurs about 12 years after the initial acute attack. It is marked by deposition of urates into a chalky mass known as a *tophus*. Tophi can appear around a joint and the adjacent bone, as visible here (▲) radiographically. The tophus can erode and destroy adjacent bone. A joint aspirate during an acute gouty attack shows increased turbidity, decreased viscosity, and leukocytosis with many neutrophils. On microscopy, needle-shaped birefringent monosodium urate (MSU) crystals appear in the fluid. The crystals activate complement and attract neutrophils that phagocytize the crystals and then release leukotrienes, prostaglandins, free radicals, and lysosomal enzymes to produce inflammation.

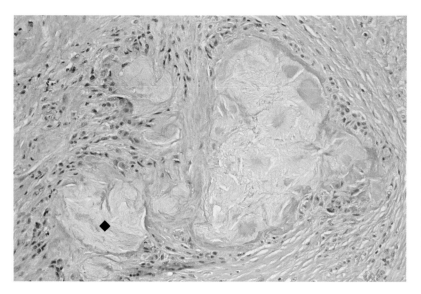

Figure 17-75 Gouty arthritis, microscopic
Tophaceous gout results from continued precipitation of MSU crystals during attacks of acute gout. The MSU crystals incite a surrounding destructive inflammatory response. The pale areas (♦) visible here are aggregates of urate crystals surrounded by chronic inflammatory infiltrates of lymphocytes, macrophages, and foreign-body giant cells. Tophi most often form around joints, in soft tissues, including tendons and ligaments, and less commonly in visceral organs. Urate deposition also can occur in the kidneys, and about 20% of patients with gout may eventually develop renal failure.

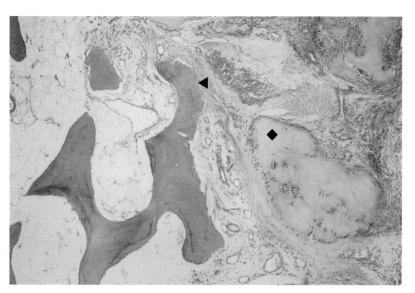

Figure 17-76 Gouty arthritis, microscopic
Destruction of bone spicules (◀) by gouty tophi (♦) is shown here. Gout may result from overproduction or reduced excretion of MSU. Most primary cases of gout involve overproduction, with increased serum uric acid. The rare absence of HGPRT in Lesch-Nyhan syndrome has severe neurologic sequelae and is known as *secondary gout*. Chemotherapy with marked turnover of purines from malignant cell death (lysis syndrome) is another form of secondary gout.

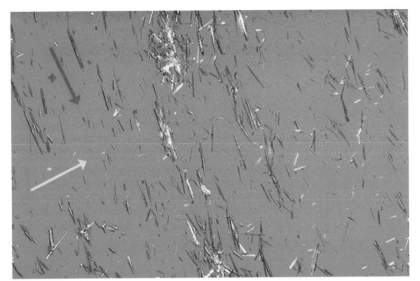

Figure 17-77 Gouty arthritis, microscopic
Synovial fluid aspirated from a joint in a patient with gout can be examined for the presence of needle-shaped MSU crystals. If these crystals are observed under polarized light with a red compensator, they appear negatively birefringent (yellow) similar to the (→) in the main ("slow") axis of the compensator and blue in the opposite perpendicular direction. Risks for gout include increased alcohol consumption, obesity, drugs such as thiazides, and lead poisoning.

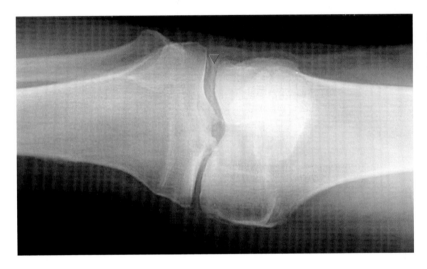

Figure 17-78 Calcium pyrophosphate crystal deposition, radiograph
Calcium pyrophosphate crystal deposition (CPPD) disease, also called *pseudogout,* is more common in individuals older than 50 years and can lead to acute, subacute, or chronic arthritis of knees, wrists, elbows, shoulders, and ankles. The articular damage is progressive, although in most cases not severe. This knee reveals extensive chondrocalcinosis involving the menisci (▼) and articular cartilage. The relationship to osteoarthritis is unclear, but CPPD can contribute to osteoarthritic changes, and both diseases can be present simultaneously.

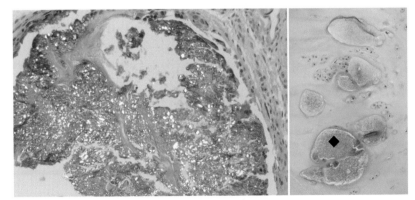

Figure 17-79 Calcium pyrophosphate crystal deposition, microscopic
Focal calcium and crystalline deposits (◆) appear in articular cartilage in the *right panel.* With polarized light the weakly negatively birefringent (pale blue) rhomboid crystals of CPPD disease are shown in the *left panel.* A joint aspirate may show crystals along with neutrophils. Microscopic findings in the articular cartilage include calcium deposition. Most cases are idiopathic, but increased adenosine triphosphate breakdown or increased nucleoside triphosphate pyrophosphohydrolase activity may play a role. Some cases may occur in persons with thyroid disease, hyperparathyroidism, diabetes mellitus, or hemochromatosis.

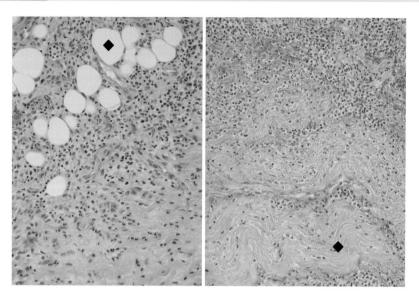

Figure 17-80 Necrotizing fasciitis, microscopic

Infection with inflammation involving soft tissue may begin within fascial planes and spread to adjacent soft tissues. Extensive neutrophilic infiltrates are present in the *right panel,* with destruction of residual dense connective tissue (◆) at the bottom. In the *left panel* the acute inflammatory infiltrates involve connective tissue and extending into adipose tissue (◆). A polymicrobial infection is often present, including gas-forming anaerobes, producing subcutaneous crepitus. This surgical emergency requires débridement along with antibiotics.

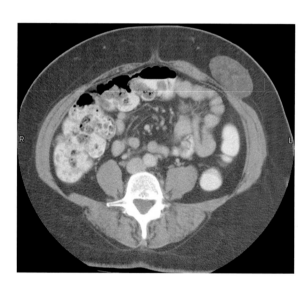

Figure 17-81 Fibromatosis, CT image

These aggressive fibroblastic proliferations can occur within the shoulder, chest wall, neck, and thigh, producing pain as well as a mass lesion (◀). Such a deep fibromatosis is called a *desmoid tumor.* They arise most often in the second to fourth decades. *APC* or β-catenin gene mutations can be present. In women during or just after pregnancy, they may appear as a mass lesion in the abdominal wall as shown here.

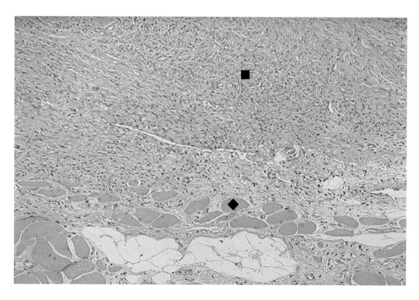

Figure 17-82 Fibromatosis, deep, microscopic

Desmoid tumors are poorly demarcated and often invade surrounding soft tissues, so they must be excised with a wide margin. Microscopically, they are composed of a cellular proliferation of spindle-shaped fibroblastic cells (■) in a collagenous stroma, visible here at the top, which extend into adjacent skeletal muscle (◆) and adipose tissue at the bottom, making resection difficult. Their infiltrative nature predisposes to recurrence after resection, but they do not metastasize.

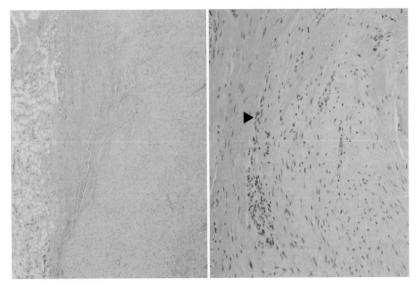

Figure 17-83 Fibromatosis, superficial, microscopic
In contrast to desmoids, superficial fibromatoses are less cellular and less aggressive. Such lesions include palmar (Dupuytren contracture), plantar, and penile (Peyronie disease) fibromatoses. Note the irregular border *(left panel)* and the poorly defined broad fascicles of fibroblasts (▶) along with abundant dense collagen *(right panel)*. As they enlarge, they may produce contracture with deformity. Some may remain stable, whereas some regress. They may recur after resection.

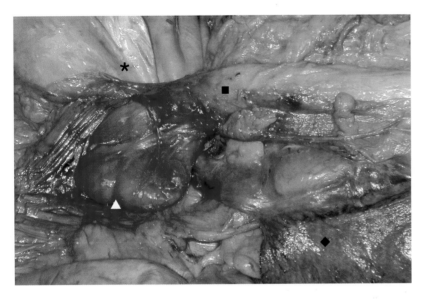

Figure 17-84 Lipoma, gross
Here is a yellow mass (▲) on the external surface of the esophagus (■) above the diaphragm (★) near the right lung (◆), as seen at autopsy. It has the characteristics of a benign neoplasm: It is well circumscribed and resembles the tissue of origin (fat). Lipomas consist of mature adipocytes forming a slowly growing, soft, mobile, localized mass, which is often an incidental finding. Any symptoms may relate to a mass effect with compression on an adjacent structure. Most lipomas are small subcutaneous masses. They can occur anywhere adipose tissue is present. They can easily be excised.

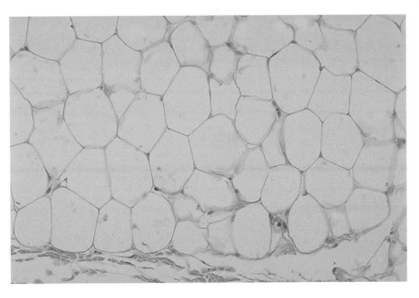

Figure 17-85 Lipoma, microscopic
This lipoma is composed of cells that are so well differentiated that they are indistinguishable from normal adipocytes. Lipomas can be found in many places, often in superficial locations, but rarely reach more than a few centimeters in size. Lipomas are the most common soft-tissue tumor.

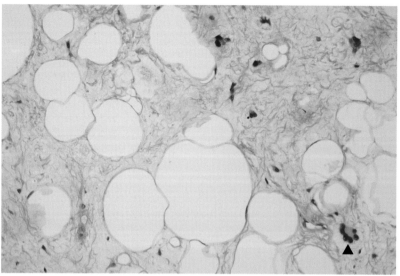

Figure 17-86 Atypical lipoma, microscopic

Compared to lipoma, an atypical lipoma has more irregularity of adipocyte size and shape, cell numbers, and nuclear size and shape. Floret cells with a ring (▲) or semicircle of nuclei, as at the lower right, may be present. There is more fibrous connective tissue. The borders of the mass may be more irregular. They tend to arise in deep soft tissues and are larger than 4 cm. They may recur locally but are not aggressive and do not metastasize.

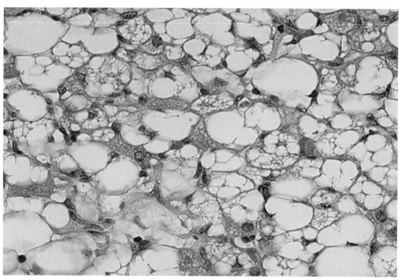

Figure 17-87 Liposarcoma, microscopic

Soft-tissue sarcomas are uncommon. They usually occur in older adults in sites such as the retroperitoneum, thigh, and lower extremities. This liposarcoma has enough differentiation to determine the cell of origin, large bizarre lipoblasts, but there is still significant pleomorphism. Sarcomas are best treated surgically because most respond poorly to chemotherapy or radiation. Sarcomas tend to be much larger masses than their benign counterparts. They often invade locally, but there can be distant hematogenous metastases.

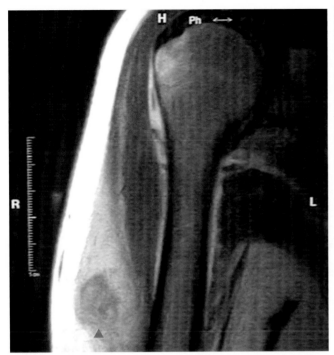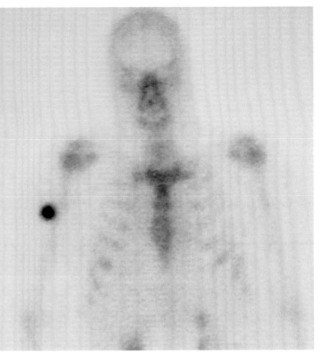

Figures 17-88 and 17-89 Myositis ossificans, MRI and bone scan
The rounded lesion (▲) of the upper arm adjacent to the humerus in the T1-weighted MR image in the *left panel* is a tumorlike mass within skeletal muscle called *myositis ossificans.* It is a benign form of connective tissue metaplasia that results from a florid healing response to injury. In the *right panel,* the lesion appears as a discrete "hot spot" in soft tissue in a bone scan.

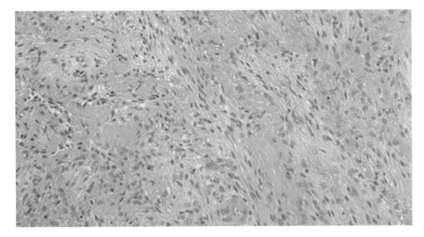

Figure 17-90 Myositis ossificans, microscopic
Myositis ossificans is an uncommon condition and occurs not within bone, but in adjacent muscle; lesions can reach several centimeters in size. Shown here is the central core of exuberant, cellular granulation tissue that can mimic a sarcoma. The correct diagnosis is suggested by radiographs. In contrast to a true neoplasm, this lesion decreases in size over time. It can cause pain and local irritation.

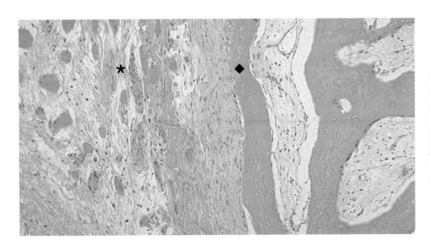

Figure 17-91 Myositis ossificans, microscopic
Peripheral to the cellular core (★) of the lesion is a zone of reactive new bone formation with a rim (◆) of dense trabecular bone appearing here on the right. This outer shell of bone blends with adjacent muscle fibers visible here on the left. The whole process eventually calcifies and shrinks over weeks to months.

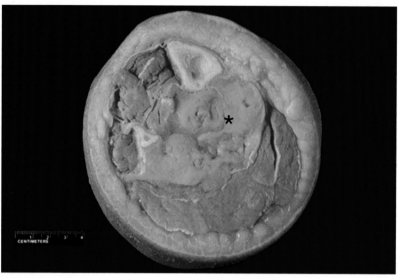

Figure 17-92 Soft-tissue sarcoma, gross

This high-grade undifferentiated pleomorphic sarcoma is a gray-white fleshy mass (★) arising within soft tissues of the lower leg behind the knee, with the tibia and fibula shown here in transverse section. Sarcomas tend to be bulky masses that invade locally, as can be seen here by the ill-defined margins of this mass. Hematogenous metastases can occur, but lymphatic metastases from sarcomas are uncommon.

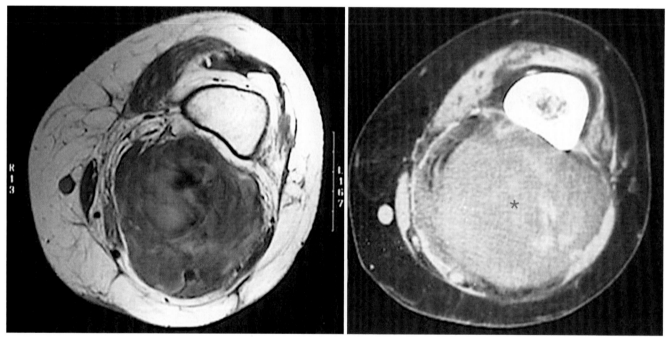

Figure 17-93 Sarcoma, MRI and CT image

This sarcoma (★) posterior to the knee at the lower femur is shown in the *left panel* with MRI and in the *right panel* with CT. This mass is arising and growing separate from the bone.

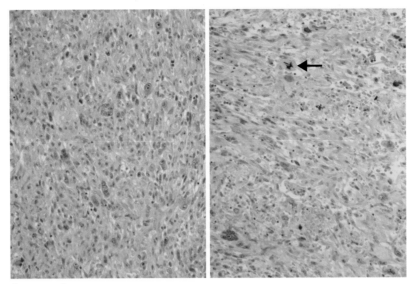

Figure 17-94 Sarcoma, microscopic

This high-grade undifferentiated pleomorphic sarcoma has a spindle cell pattern. Some of the cells are very pleomorphic, hence the name. A very large abnormal mitotic figure (←) is seen on the right. The cell of origin of sarcomas is often difficult to determine because of their tendency to be poorly differentiated or even anaplastic. Immunohistochemical staining can help determine their origin. Most sarcomas are vimentin positive, whereas carcinomas are cytokeratin positive.

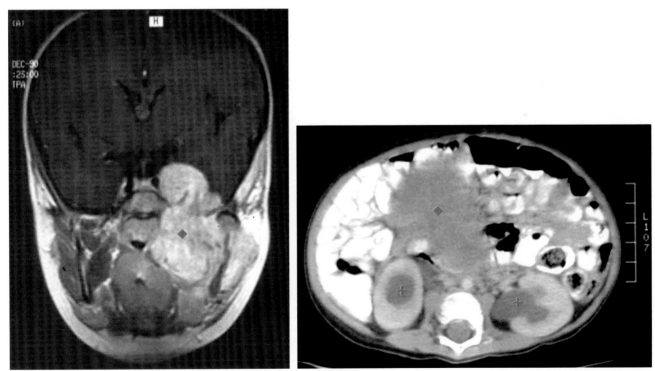

Figures 17-95 and 17-96 Rhabdomyosarcoma, MRI and CT image

This coronal MRI image of a child reveals a soft-tissue mass (◆) beneath the cranial cavity and expanding upward. Although still rare, rhabdomyosarcomas are one of the more frequent soft-tissue malignancies in children. The head and neck area is a common site for a pediatric rhabdomyosarcoma. The pelvis or abdomen may be involved, as shown in the CT scan by a large mass (◆) leading to hydronephrosis (+). These masses are often locally infiltrative and difficult to remove completely.

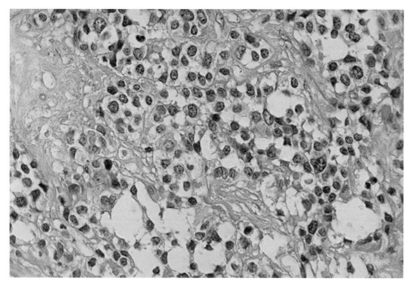

Figure 17-97 Rhabdomyosarcoma, microscopic

This alveolar rhabdomyosarcoma is composed of primitive round blue cells (rhabdomyoblasts) arranged in nests with spaces and surrounded by a fibrous stroma. A variant of this neoplasm that occurs in the genital tract is the sarcoma botryoides. A common genetic alteration is a chromosomal translocation producing a chimeric PAX3-FKHR protein that is involved in muscle differentiation.

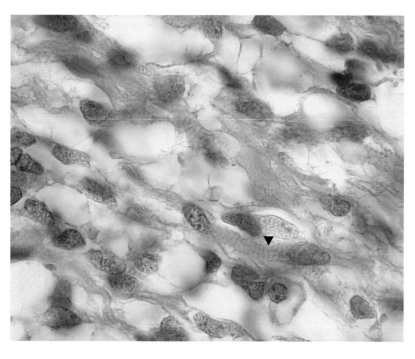

Figure 17-98 Rhabdomyosarcoma, microscopic

In adults, rhabdomyosarcomas can arise in large muscles, such as those of the thigh. At high magnification, this rhabdomyosarcoma reveals pleomorphism and hyperchromatism of the nuclei, along with variable amounts of pink cytoplasm. Note the appearance of a characteristic "strap cell," which has recognizable cross-striations (▼) mimicking a skeletal muscle fiber.

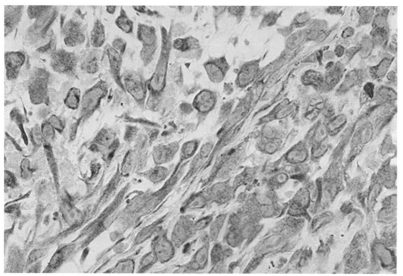

Figure 17-99 Sarcoma, microscopic

Immunohistochemical staining with antibody to vimentin reveals positive red-brown reaction product within the cytoplasm of these neoplastic cells. Positive vimentin staining is a characteristic of many types of sarcomas. Note the spindle shape of many of these cells, another feature of neoplasms of mesenchymal derivation.

CHAPTER

18

Peripheral Nerve and Skeletal Muscle

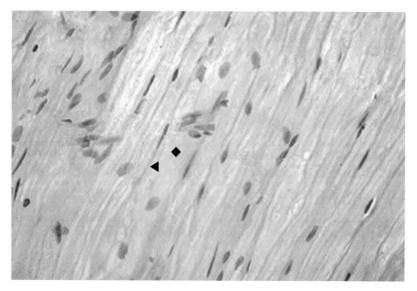

Figure 18-1 Normal peripheral nerve, microscopic

This normal peripheral nerve in longitudinal section shows slightly wavy, elongated cell bodies (axons [♦]) of the nerve fibers. A thin connective tissue layer, the endoneurium (◀), surrounds individual nerve fibers. A perineurium encloses a fascicle of nerve fibers and forms a blood-nerve barrier. The epineurium surrounds a whole nerve. Motor fibers are myelinated. Most sensory fibers are unmyelinated, although fibers for fine discriminatory senses, such as touch and vibration, are myelinated. The major component of an axonal myelin sheath is myelin protein zero, and myelin basic protein is the second most common structural protein.

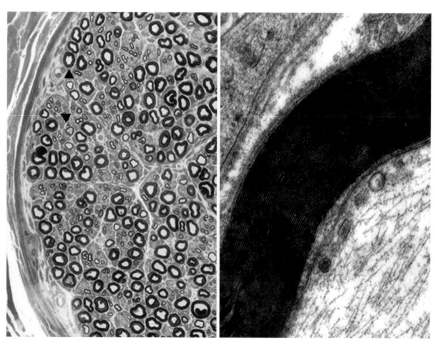

Figure 18-2 Normal peripheral nerve, microscopic

This normal peripheral nerve in transverse section with toluidine blue stain in the *left panel* has blue-black myelin around a normal number and distribution of thickly (▲) and thinly (▼) myelinated fibers. Pale background areas have the unmyelinated fibers. Overall, unmyelinated axons 0.4 to 2 μm in diameter are more numerous than myelinated axons 1 to 20 μm in diameter. Myelinated fibers transmit impulses with higher conduction velocity (6 to 120 m/sec) than nonmyelinated fibers (0.5 to 2 m/sec). The larger the fiber, the faster the conduction velocity. Note the even spacing between the dark myelin lamellae around an axon in the electron micrograph in the *right panel.*

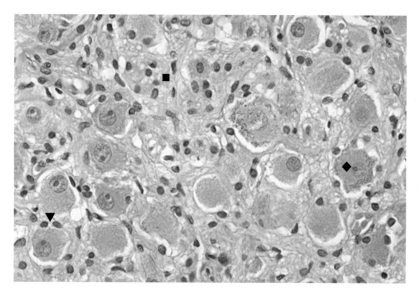

Figure 18-3 Normal peripheral ganglion, microscopic

This peripheral ganglion has nerve cell bodies (♦) and surrounding satellite cells (▼) and interstitial fibroblasts (■). The nerve cell bodies have fine pink Nissl granules, and some nerve cells display light-brown lipochrome pigment within their cytoplasm. There is no blood-nerve barrier around a ganglion. The sensory and the postganglionic autonomic nerve fibers have neuronal cell bodies located in ganglia associated with cranial nerves, dorsal spinal roots, and autonomic nerves. Ganglia and Schwann cells are embryologically derived from the neural crest.

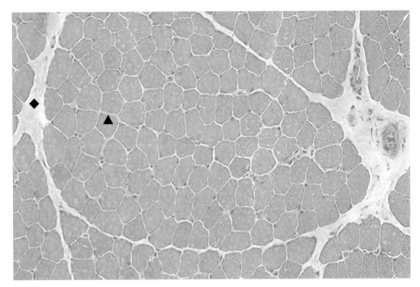

Figure 18-4 Normal skeletal muscle, microscopic
Skeletal muscle fibers are shown here in cross-section at low magnification. There are several fascicles. A connective tissue band, the *perimysium* (◆), surrounds each individual fascicle. An individual muscle fiber within the fascicle is invested by the endomysium (▲). The entire muscle is surrounded by a connective tissue band called the *epimysium*. The muscle cell nuclei are located at the periphery of the fibers. Each fiber is bounded by a sarcolemma, which projects into the cytoplasm as T tubules containing a high concentration of calcium ions. A nerve impulse causes depolarization with release of the calcium ions to initiate muscle contraction.

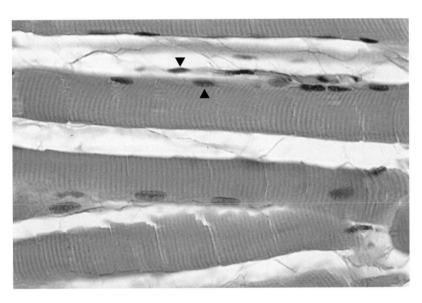

Figure 18-5 Normal skeletal muscle, microscopic
In longitudinal section, a skeletal muscle fiber has prominent cross-striations formed by the Z discs. The thin actin filaments are attached to Z discs and interdigitate with the thick myosin filaments to allow muscle contraction. The functional contractile unit is a sarcomere between two Z discs. The additional proteins tropomyosin and troponin complex regulate actin, myosin, and calcium binding. The skeletal muscle fiber is a multinucleated cell with numerous sarcolemmal nuclei (▲) at the periphery of each muscle fiber. Occasional satellite cells (▼) provide for maintenance, repair, and regeneration of injured fibers.

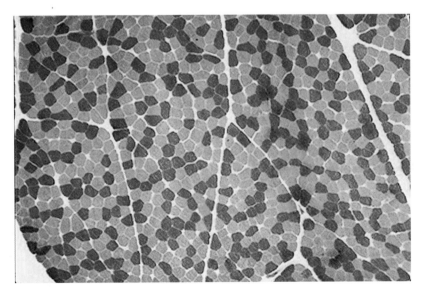

Figure 18-6 Normal skeletal muscle, microscopic
In cross-section with adenosine triphosphatase (ATPase) stain at pH 9.4, the normal pattern of type 1 and type 2 skeletal muscle fibers within fascicles is shown. These fibers are intermixed to form a checkerboard pattern. The type 1 fibers (slow twitch, oxidative) are light tan, and the type II fibers (mainly glycolytic) stain dark brown at this pH. Type I fibers have more mitochondria and more myoglobin for sustained contraction. A lower motor neuron innervates a group of myofibers, known as *motor units*. The motor units are small in number (<50 myofibers) when fine motor control is required (extraocular muscles) and large (hundreds of myofibers) in postural muscles, such as the quadriceps femoris.

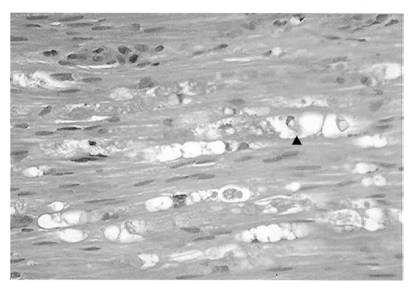

Figure 18-7 Wallerian degeneration, microscopic

Wallerian degeneration occurs distal to the site of an injury with axonal disruption by a crush injury or traumatic transection of a peripheral nerve. In this distal nerve segment in longitudinal section, small axonal and myelin fragments lie within myelin ovoids as vacuolar digestion chambers (▲). Regeneration may be possible because the proximal nerve stump undergoes axonal sprouting, and Schwann cells proliferate to remyelinate the nerve fiber. Regeneration proceeds along the course of the degenerated axon at a rate of about 2 mm/day.

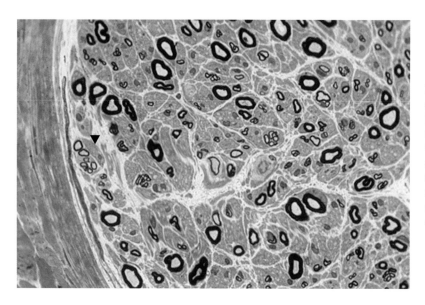

Figure 18-8 Peripheral nerve with axonal sprouting, microscopic

Here is axonal regrowth in a plastic-embedded cross-section of a peripheral nerve after transection, with clusters of regrowing axons (▼) surrounded by the basement membrane of a Schwann cell. Such small clusters of thinly myelinated fibers represent regrowth (axonal sprouting). With ongoing neuropathies, axonal degeneration and regeneration may coexist.

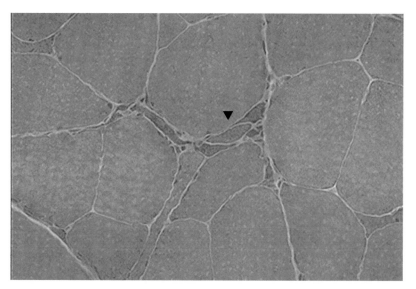

Figure 18-9 Denervation atrophy, microscopic

This modified Gomori trichrome stain shows the neurogenic form of skeletal muscle atrophy, with the characteristic pattern of "grouped atrophy" (▼) of muscle fibers that have lost their innervation from a lower motor neuron. These affected muscle fibers do not die, but downsize with loss of actin and myosin, becoming small and angular. Denervation could result from traumatic nerve injury, peripheral neuropathy, or a motor neuron disease, such as amyotrophic lateral sclerosis (ALS). Remaining axons may reinnervate myofibers as a single fiber type (type grouping).

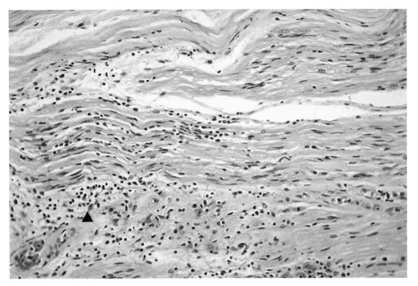

Figure 18-10 Guillain-Barré neuropathy, microscopic

Neuritis secondary to an acute inflammatory demyelinating polyneuropathy (Guillain-Barré syndrome) is shown in a longitudinal section of peripheral nerve with lymphocytic infiltrates (▲) that damage the nerve, followed by macrophages that strip off the myelin lamellae, leading to demyelination with relative preservation of axons in most cases. There is an acute ascending paralysis that occurs over days, advancing distally to proximally. Respiratory paralysis is life-threatening. A bacterial *(Campylobacter jejuni)* or viral (cytomegalovirus) illness may precede the onset of this disease. Recovery occurs in most patients receiving ventilatory support.

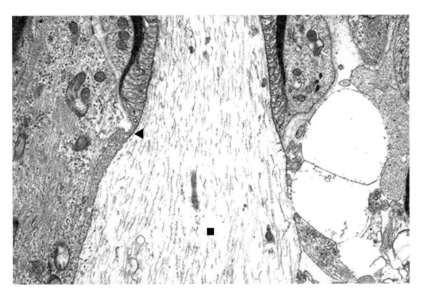

Figure 18-11 Demyelination, electron microscopy

This peripheral nerve shows a demyelinated axon next to an internode (◄). The axoplasm in the lower demyelinated portion (■) is swollen. The Schwann cell is attracted to the demyelinated axon and remyelinates it. In Guillain-Barré syndrome, there is segmental demyelination between internodes. During recovery from this form of inflammatory neuropathy, these areas become remyelinated. Examination of the cerebrospinal fluid shows few inflammatory cells, little or no pleocytosis, but an elevated protein.

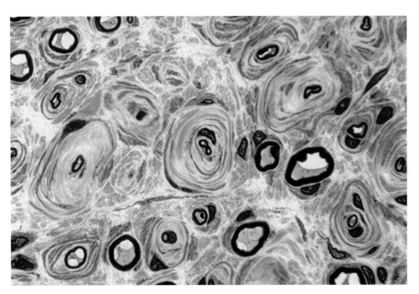

Figure 18-12 Chronic inflammatory demyelinating polyneuropathy, microscopic

In this sural nerve biopsy specimen on cross-section note the "onion bulb" formation from excessive proliferation of Schwann cells after recurrent demyelination and remyelination from macrophage response to immunoglobulin deposition. This is the most common chronic acquired inflammatory peripheral neuropathy, lasting from months to years, usually with relapses and remissions. There is a symmetrical, mixed sensorimotor polyneuropathy. An underlying autoimmune disorder may be present.

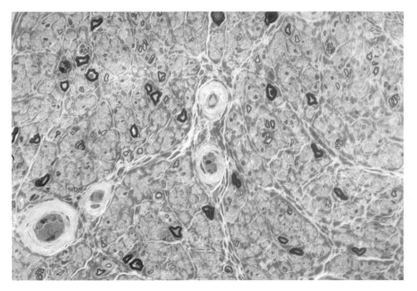

Figure 18-13 Diabetic neuropathy, microscopic

This plastic embedded cross-section of nerve shows diffuse loss of darkly staining thickly and thinly myelinated fibers typical of the progressive neuropathy that accompanies diabetes mellitus. Note the microvascular disease with thickened walls of small vessels. End glycosylation of proteins and sorbitol accumulation in cells not requiring insulin for glucose uptake can underlie the pathogenesis of this neuropathy, driven by hyperglycemia.

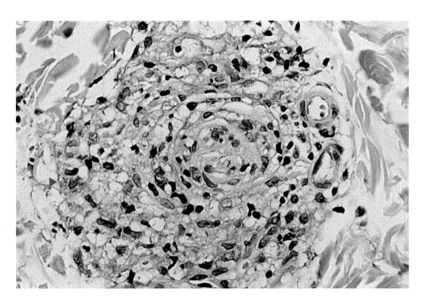

Figure 18-14 Hansen disease, microscopic

A poorly formed granuloma appears around a peripheral nerve within the dermis. The leprosy bacilli *(Mycobacterium leprae)* grow best just below body temperature, preferring the cooler skin and peripheral nerves. Hypopigmented patches or macular lesions with decreased sensation develop on the face, extremities, and trunk. Nodular disfiguring lesions can appear, with the lepromatous form having many macrophages filled with numerous acid-fast bacilli (globi) (▶). In the tuberculoid form, acid-fast organisms are sparse. Shown here is the borderline form, with some organisms and some epithelioid cells. It is possible to control leprosy with drug therapy (rifampin and dapsone).

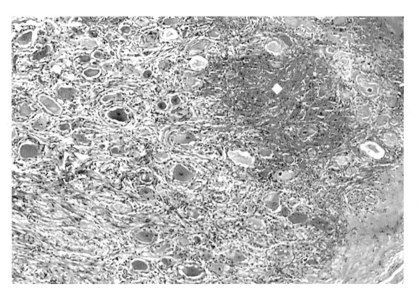

Figure 18-15 Varicella-zoster virus infection, microscopic

Chickenpox, a common childhood infection, is caused by the varicella-zoster virus. It is typically self-limited, but the virus persists and becomes latent in dorsal root ganglia. A postherpetic neuralgia syndrome persists in about 10% of infected individuals. In some patients, activation of the virus later in life, particularly with immune compromise, can produce the painful condition known as *shingles,* a vesicular eruption in a dermatome innervated by an infected ganglion. Reactivated varicella-zoster virus produces hemorrhagic lesions (◆) of these ganglia, as shown here. In some immunocompromised patients, acute encephalitis can occur.

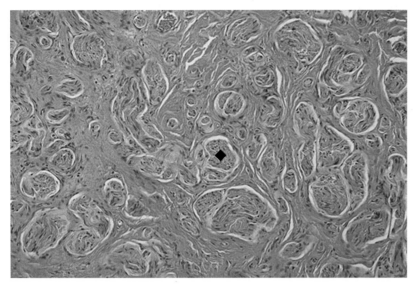

Figure 18-16 Traumatic neuroma, microscopic

This disorganized jumble of sprouting neurites or axons in bundles (◆) that have become embedded within a dense reactive connective tissue stroma is a *traumatic neuroma*. This non-neoplastic lesion occurs when a peripheral nerve is severed or damaged, and the proximal axons try to regrow but are unable to connect with the distal axonal sheaths, forming the haphazard mass of nerve and fibrous connective tissues. The resulting neuroma can become a painful nodule. A common location for this lesion is between the bases of the second and third digits of the foot because a characteristic human folly is fashion over function, with choice of footwear such as pointed-toe shoes and high heels that produce compression injury.

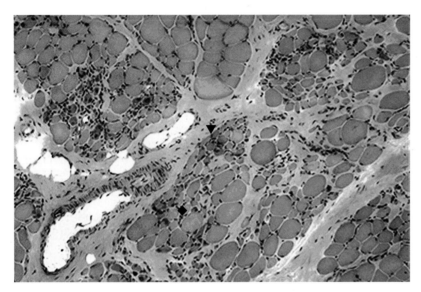

Figure 18-17 Duchenne muscular dystrophy, microscopic

Degeneration (◆) of muscle fibers is shown along with some small purple regenerating fibers (▼), scattered chronic inflammatory cells, fibrosis, adipocytes, and hypertrophy of remaining muscle fibers. Duchenne muscular dystrophy (DMD) is caused by a defective dystrophin gene on the X chromosome that leads to an inability to produce the striated muscle sarcolemmal membrane structural protein dystrophin. This is an X-linked recessive disorder. About one third of cases of DMD arise from spontaneous new mutations rather than maternal inheritance. This very large gene may have mutations involving different exons, giving rise to phenotypic variable expressivity.

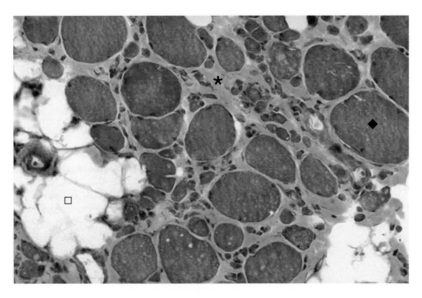

Figure 18-18 Duchenne muscular dystrophy, microscopic

Adipose tissue (□) and increased endomysial pale blue-green connective tissue (★) are revealed by this modified Gomori trichrome stain. Large oval hypertrophic fibers (◆) are interspersed with smaller atrophic degenerating or regenerating fibers, typical of a myopathic disease process. Early in the course, such large fibers can lead to pseudohypertrophy of calf muscles. Patients with DMD initially develop more proximal muscle weakness early in childhood by age 5 years, but they are typically wheelchair-bound by age 10 and die of respiratory failure by the third decade.

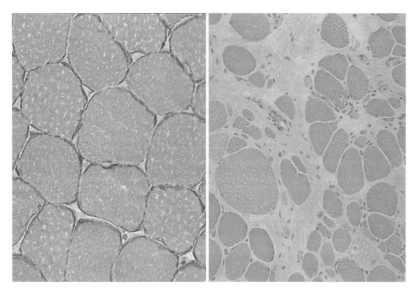

Figure 18-19 Duchenne muscular dystrophy, microscopic
This immunohistochemical stain with antibody to the sarcolemmal protein dystrophin appears here to be localized at the periphery of the normal muscle fibers *(left panel)* but absent in the atrophic fibers of a patient with DMD *(right panel).* Dystrophin, encoded by a gene in the chromosome Xp21 region, stabilizes the membrane. Female carriers may have elevated serum creatine kinase (CK) but little or no muscular weakness. Affected males have elevated CK in childhood, but with eventual extensive muscular atrophy, the CK returns to normal. Affected males also often develop cardiomyopathy and cognitive impairment.

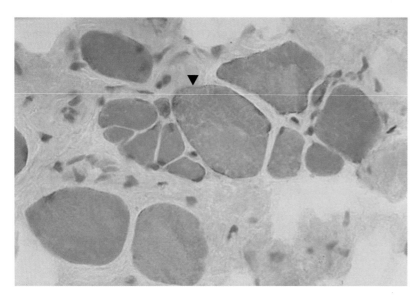

Figure 18-20 Becker muscular dystrophy, microscopic
This immunohistochemical stain reveals only small amounts of dystrophin (▼), typical of Becker muscular dystrophy (BMD), which is less common but less severe than DMD. The same dystrophin gene is involved in BMD but with a different mutation than in DMD. Some dystrophin is made in BMD but not normal amounts. The atrophic fibers and fibrosis here are from a middle-aged man. Patients with BMD have an onset of muscular weakness in adolescence to young adulthood and have a less severe course than patients with DMD.

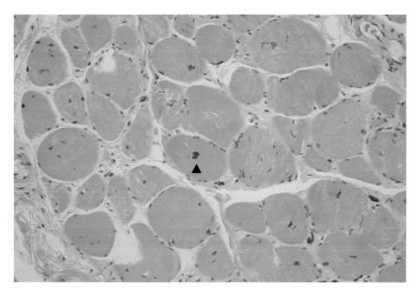

Figure 18-21 Myotonic dystrophy, microscopic
Note the central nuclei (▲) in these myofibers in cross-section, along with variation in fiber size and fibrosis, typical of myotonic dystrophy, the most common form of adult-onset muscular dystrophy, affecting 1 in 10,000 people. Forms of the disease include (1) congenital, symptomatic at birth or in the first year of life; (2) classic, with onset between 10 and 60 years; and (3) minimal, with onset after 50 years and causing only myotonia and a mild degree of muscle weakness. In the classic form there may also be cataracts, intellectual changes, hypersomnia, gonadal atrophy, insulin resistance, decreased esophageal and colonic motility, and cardiomyopathy. Frontal balding is a common phenotypic feature.

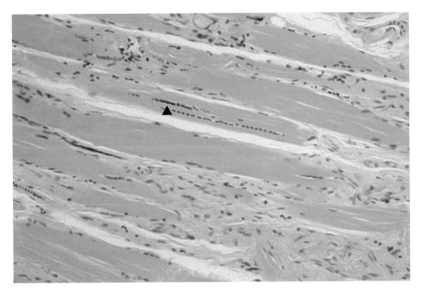

Figure 18-22 Myotonic dystrophy, microscopic

These myofibers in longitudinal section have long strings (▲) of nuclei. This autosomal dominant disorder stems from expanded CTG trinucleotide repeat sequence (tandem repeats) within the noncoding portion of the dystrophia myotonica protein kinase *(DMPK)* gene. Repeats may accumulate in successive generations (anticipation). Skeletal muscle, liver, and brain can be affected. Muscular weakness is apparent early in the neck muscles (e.g., sternocleidomastoids) and distal limb muscles. The palate, tongue, and pharyngeal muscles also become involved, producing dysarthric speech and swallowing problems.

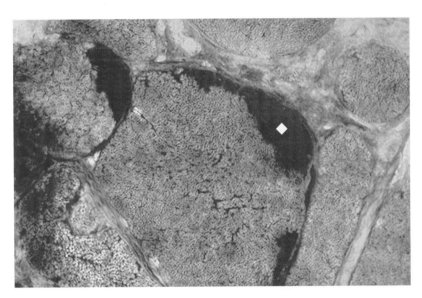

Figure 18-23 McArdle disease, microscopic

This is type V glycogen storage disease. The onset can be in childhood or adulthood. The myophosphorylase enzyme (part of glycolytic metabolism) is deficient, and excess glycogen becomes deposited within muscle, appearing here as the red subsarcolemmal deposits (◆) highlighted in red with PAS stain. This myopathic disease results in muscular weakness, muscle cramps after exercise, myoglobinuria, and lack of an exercise-induced increase in blood lactate. Although the serum CK can be elevated, there is little or no muscle fiber degeneration or inflammation.

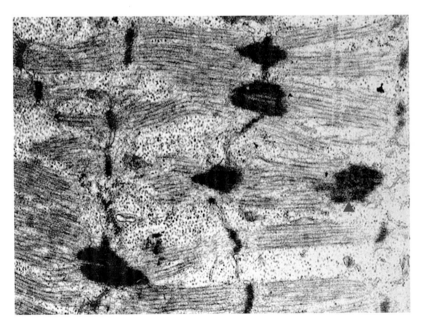

Figure 18-24 Nemaline myopathy, electron microscopy

Some "floppy infants" have a congenital myopathy. Clinical findings include hypotonia, muscle weakness, joint contractures (arthrogryposis), and a nonprogressive to slowly progressive course. Some of these myopathies have been described by their characteristic histologic features. The dark rod-shaped subsarcolemmal inclusions (▲) appearing in this electron micrograph are known as *nemaline rods*. The rods appear to arise from Z bands and are composed of a protein (α-actinin) found in the Z bands.

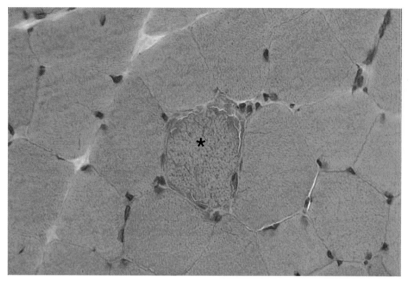

Figure 18-25 Mitochondrial myopathy, microscopic

Mitochondrial myopathies are rare diseases marked by "ragged red fibers" containing aggregates of abnormal mitochondria that appear subsarcolemmally and scattered through some muscle fibers. They appear as granular red areas (★) on H&E staining. Mitochondrial proteins are necessary for oxidative metabolism to maintain normal skeletal muscular, cardiac, and nervous system function. Synthesis of these proteins is directed either by nuclear DNA or mitochondrial DNA. With the latter, the inheritance pattern is maternal; one example is the disorder known as *mitochondrial encephalomyopathy with lactic acidosis and strokelike episodes* (MELAS).

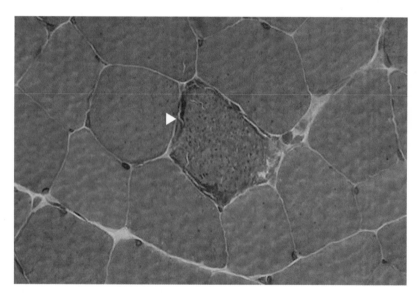

Figure 18-26 Mitochondrial myopathy, microscopic

With the modified Gomori trichrome stain, the abnormal mitochondrial deposits here appear as reddish granular deposits (▶), the so-called *ragged red fibers*. Mitochondrial myopathy may manifest clinically in several ways: proximal muscular weakness, ophthalmoplegia, encephalopathy, and cardiomyopathy. The onset of these diseases often occurs in childhood or young adulthood but can also occur in infancy. The increased numbers of mitochondria have an abnormal shape and size. By electron microscopy, some mitochondria can have "parking lot" inclusions.

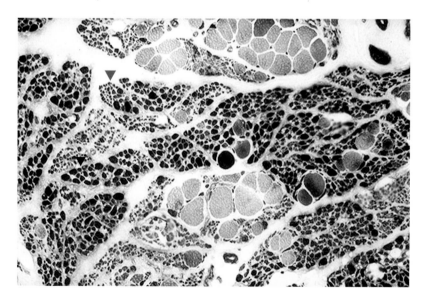

Figure 18-27 Spinal muscular atrophy, microscopic

This is grouped atrophy (▼) of rounded infantile muscle fibers, shown with ATPase stain at pH 9.4. This neurogenic atrophy has resulted from Werdnig-Hoffmann disease, the most common form of spinal muscular atrophy, although still a rare condition. It is one of several autosomal recessive disorders resulting from homozygous mutations in the survival motor neuron 1 (*SMN1*) gene. There is severe loss of lower motor neurons during infancy. These "floppy infants" generally die of respiratory failure during infancy or within the first 3 years of life. Other forms of spinal muscular atrophy are milder, and affected patients die in childhood.

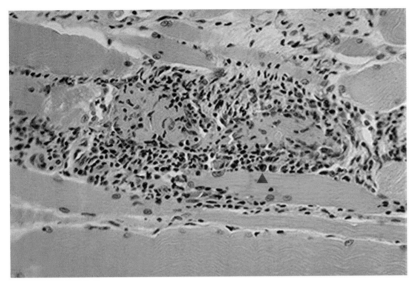

Figure 18-28 Polymyositis, microscopic
Shown are marked chronic inflammatory cell infiltrates (▲) with degeneration of muscle fibers as part of this autoimmune disease. Serum CK is markedly increased. Polymyositis results from the cytotoxic effects of CD8+ lymphocytes recognizing HLA class I major histocompatibility complex molecules on myofiber sarcolemmal membranes. Of the autoantibodies, anti–Jo-1 is the most common with this disorder. In contrast, dermatomyositis is mainly mediated through a CD4 cell-mediated vasculitis affecting small capillaries; it is accompanied by a skin rash (typically the violaceous heliotrope rash of eyelids) and an increased risk for visceral cancers.

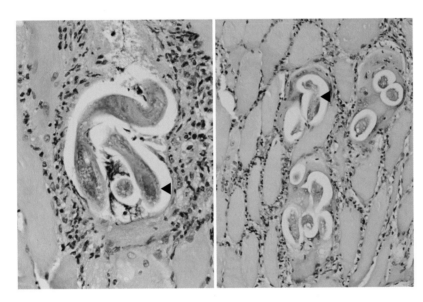

Figure 18-29 Trichinosis, microscopic
Encysted *Trichinella spiralis* larvae (◄) are shown here within skeletal muscle. Humans act as an intermediate host when larvae are ingested while eating poorly cooked or uncooked meat from an infected animal, such as a pig. These larvae mature into adults in the gastrointestinal tract, releasing larvae that penetrate tissues and spread hematogenously to striated muscle where they can elicit an inflammatory reaction with myositis *(left panel)*. The early phase of infection is marked by fever, muscle pain, and peripheral blood eosinophilia with a T_H2 immune response. A heavy infestation of larvae *(right panel)* can lead to death. Most cases go unnoticed, however, and the encysted larvae undergo dystrophic calcification over months to years.

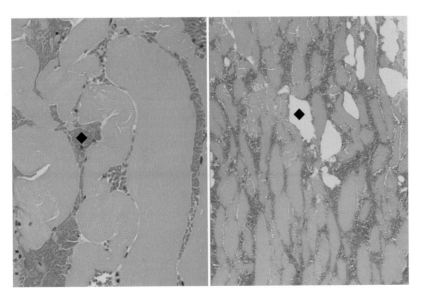

Figure 18-30 Myonecrosis, microscopic
The clear spaces (◆) in the *right panel* are areas of gas formation from growth of *Clostridium perfringens* organisms in the muscle after trauma that introduced this infectious agent, an anaerobe. The gas formation may produce crepitus on examination. There are some residual cross-striations, but degenerative changes with loss of myofiber integrity and interstitial hemorrhage (◆) as in the *left panel*. The process continues to extensive necrosis known as *gas gangrene*.

The Central Nervous System

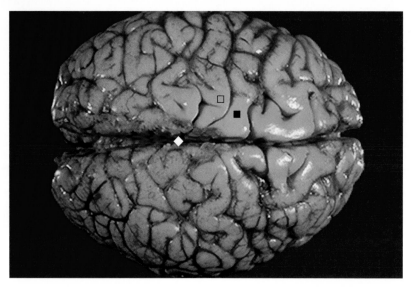

Figure 19-1 Normal brain, gross
The superior aspect at the vertex of an adult brain is shown here with the central sulcus (◆) between the right and left hemispheres. Note the pattern of gyri and sulci beneath the thin, filmy meninges (pia and arachnoid layers; the overlying dura has been removed). The rolandic fissure with the precentral gyrus (■) (motor cortex) and the postcentral gyrus (□) (somesthetic cortex) are shown here. The normal adult brain weighs 1100 to 1700 g.

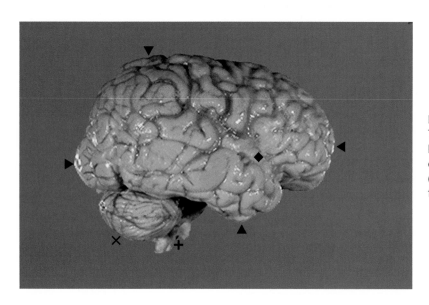

Figure 19-2 Normal brain, gross
The lateral view of the brain reveals the frontal lobe (◀), parietal lobe (▼),temporal lobe (▲), occipital lobe (▶), cerebellum (✗), and brain stem (✚). Note the sylvian fissure (◆) separating the frontal lobe from the temporal lobe.

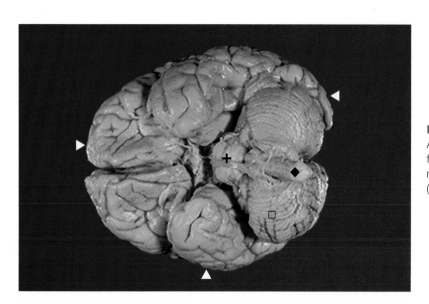

Figure 19-3 Normal brain, gross
At the base of the brain can be seen the inferior frontal lobes (▶), temporal lobes (▲), pons (✚), medulla oblongata (◆), cerebellar hemispheres (□), and occipital lobes (◀).

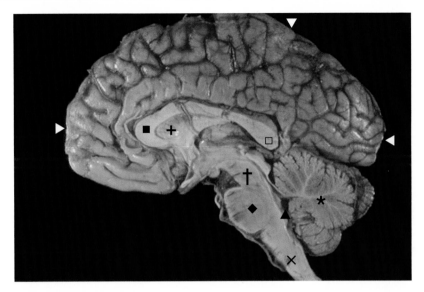

Figure 19-4 Normal brain, gross
A sagittal section through the midline of the brain reveals the frontal lobe (▶), parietal lobe (▼), and occipital lobe (◀). The genu (■) and the splenium (□) of the corpus callosum appear above the third ventricle, divided by the thin membrane, the septum pellucidum (✚). The midbrain (†), pons (◆), and medulla oblongata (✕) form the brain stem. The aqueduct of Sylvius connects the third ventricle to the fourth ventricle (▲). The fourth ventricle lies below the cerebellum (★) and above the medulla.

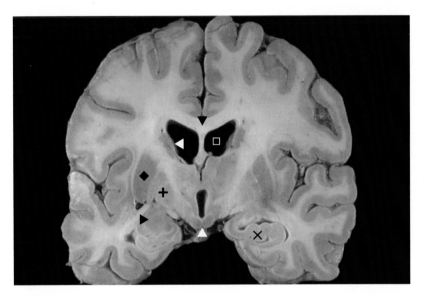

Figure 19-5 Normal brain, gross
This coronal section through the center of the brain reveals the mammillary bodies (▲), globus pallidus (✚), putamen (◆), caudate nucleus (◀), lateral ventricles (□), corpus callosum (▼), and hippocampus (✕). This section is not completely symmetrical (as is the case with many CT scans and MRI images), so the amygdala (▶) appears on just one side.

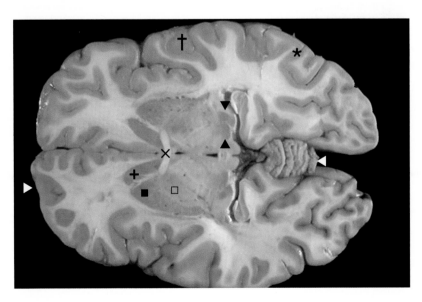

Figure 19-6 Normal brain, gross
This axial (transverse) section through the brain reveals the frontal lobe (▶), caudate nucleus (✚), anterior commissure (✕), putamen (■), globus pallidus (□), medial (▲) and lateral (▼) geniculate nuclei, temporal lobe (†), parietal lobe (★), and anterior vermis (◀) of the cerebellum.

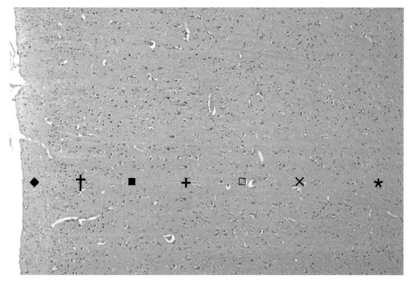

Figure 19-7 Normal neocortex, microscopic
The neocortex (gray matter) of the cerebral hemispheres has six layers that are microscopically indistinct with H&E staining. Beneath the pia-arachnoid on the far left is an outer plexiform (◆) layer with nerve cells arranged horizontally. Next is the outer granular layer (†) containing small pyramidal neurons. Next is the outer pyramidal cell layer (■) with medium-sized pyramidal neurons. Below this is the inner granular layer (✦) of larger pyramidal neurons. Beneath this is the inner pyramidal layer (□) of larger pyramidal neurons. The innermost cortical layer is the polymorphous layer (✕), which lacks pyramidal cells. Beneath the cortex is the white matter (★).

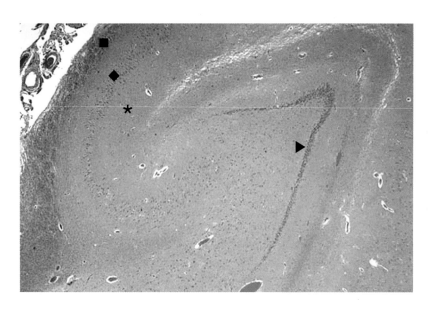

Figure 19-8 Normal hippocampus, microscopic
The normal appearance of the hippocampus is shown here at low magnification. Hippocampus consists of "paleocortex" with three layers: polymorphic (■), pyramidal neuronal (◆), and molecular (★) layers. The granule cell layer (▶) of the dentate gyrus is present.

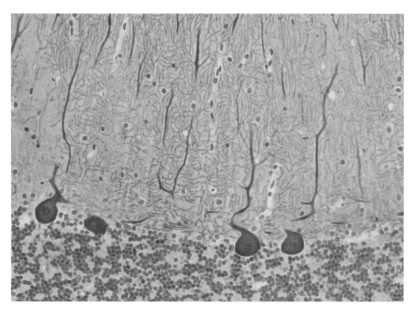

Figure 19-9 Normal cerebellum, microscopic
The normal appearance of the cerebellum is shown here at low magnification with immunostaining for calcineurin, highlighting the large brown Purkinje cells with their extensive arborizing dendritic network into the molecular layer above, like that drawn by Prof. Ramón y Cajal. The granule layer is below.

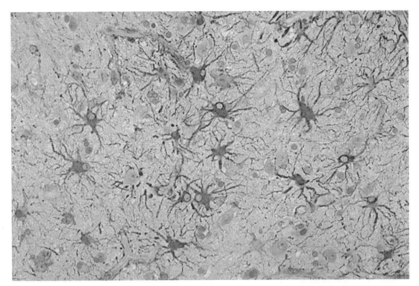

Figure 19-10 Normal brain, microscopic
This immunohistochemical stain for intermediate filaments known as *glial fibrillary acidic protein* (GFAP) highlights astrocytes with their prominent processes that extend between neurons. At least one process either extends to the overlying pia or surrounds a capillary to form the blood-brain barrier along with endothelial cells and pericytes, a diffusion barrier that prevents the influx of most compounds from blood to brain. Pericytes encircle endothelial cells, providing structural support and aiding in controlling blood flow. Tight junctions between endothelial cells form the selective diffusion barrier. Astrocytic foot processes closely adherent to small vessels aid in the induction and maintenance of the tight junction barrier.

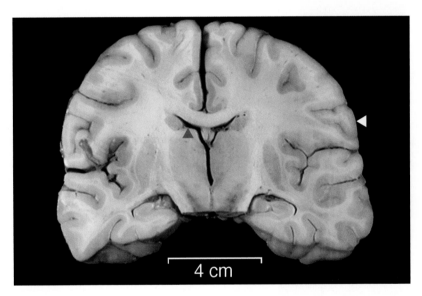

4 cm

Figure 19-11 Cerebral edema, gross
This coronal section of cerebrum shows marked compression with effacement of lateral ventricles (▲) and flattening of gyri (◀) from extensive bilateral cerebral edema. This patient was climbing a 5000-m mountain peak and ignored the warning sign of a persistent, worsening headache. The hypoxia leads to endothelial damage with an increase in intracellular edema (cytotoxic edema). In contrast, vasogenic edema results from disruption of the blood-brain barrier by inflammation or neoplasia, or generalized ischemia, so the two forms often overlap. In either case, edema increases intracranial pressure (ICP), with risk for herniation.

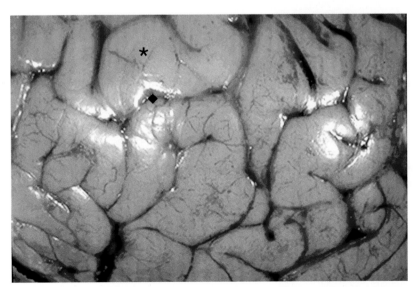

Figure 19-12 Cerebral edema, gross
The cortical surface beneath the meninges of this brain with cerebral edema shows widened, flattened gyri (★) with narrowed sulci (◆). Disruption of the blood-brain barrier by inflammation or neoplasms can lead to vasogenic edema with fluid leakage into intercellular spaces. Ischemia results in cytotoxic edema from direct cell injury and an increase in intracellular fluid. Both of these conditions can be localized. When there is extensive edema, in general both injury patterns are present. There are no intracranial lymphatics to scavenge the excess fluid, but glial cells may assist in fluid movement.

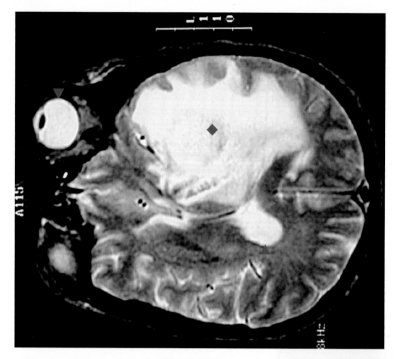

Figure 19-13 Cerebral edema, MRI
An abscess (◆) with inflammation that compromises the blood-brain barrier to produce surrounding edema appears bright in this T2-weighted axial MRI image of the brain at the level of the orbits. Fluid appears bright, as in the globe of the eye (▼) and in the lateral ventricles (▲) compressed by the mass effect of the edema, with shift of the midline to the right. The brain tissue with edema appears brighter as well. This edema is most pronounced in the white matter.

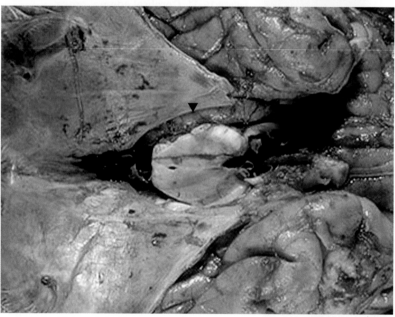

Figure 19-14 Herniation, gross
This brain shows medial temporal lobe (uncinate) herniation on the left. Note the resulting compression of the left side of the midbrain. The medial temporal lobe tissue is pushed beneath the tentorium (▼), called *transtentorial herniation.* This can occur either by a mass effect or from edema on the ipsilateral side of the brain. Impingement on cranial nerves (CNs) can occur, particularly oculomotor (CN III) nerve palsy.

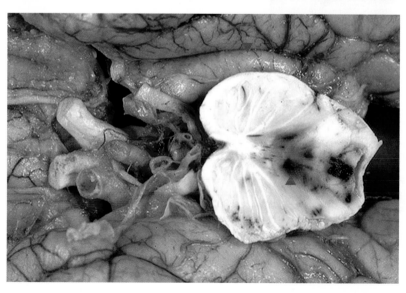

Figure 19-15 Herniation with Duret hemorrhages, gross
Medial temporal lobe (uncal) herniation (▼) has caused bleeding (▲) into the pons, known as *Duret hemorrhage.* When the herniated tissue pushes the brain stem further down into the posterior fossa and stretches and tears the perforating vessels into the pons and midbrain, this type of secondary brain stem bleeding occurs. Note the deep groove on the right medial temporal lobe (uncus) caused by pressure against the tentorium. When the degree of herniation is pronounced, hemiparesis ipsilateral to the side of the herniation may be caused by compression of the contralateral cerebral peduncle.

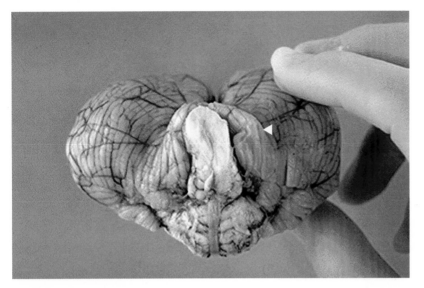

Figure 19-16 Cerebellar tonsillar herniation, gross
Acute brain swelling above the tentorium or within the posterior fossa can force posterior fossa contents downward toward the foramen magnum, and this can often produce herniation of the cerebellar tonsils into the foramen magnum. Note the cone shape of the cerebellar tonsils (◄) around the medulla. Compression of the medulla compromises brain stem centers controlling respiration and cardiac activity, leading to death from herniation.

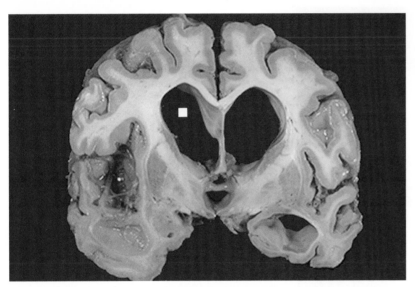

Figure 19-17 Hydrocephalus, gross
Note the marked dilation (■) of these cerebral ventricles; the adjacent white matter may have interstitial edema. Hydrocephalus can be caused by a lack of absorption of cerebrospinal fluid (CSF), called *communicating hydrocephalus,* or by an obstruction to flow of CSF, called *noncommunicating hydrocephalus.* Hydrocephalus can be a long-term complication of infection, such as a basilar meningitis, which leads to scarring that obstructs CSF outflow through the foramina of Luschka and Magendie. Inflammation with scarring of arachnoid granulations at the vertex may diminish CSF absorption.

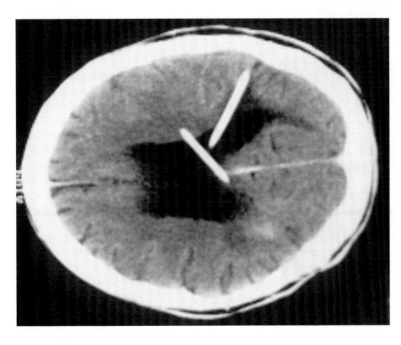

Figure 19-18 Hydrocephalus, CT image
This axial view shows enlarged lateral ventricles. This condition has been treated by placing two shunts (the linear bright objects). Temporary ventricular shunts can be placed acutely to relieve hydrocephalus, or a permanent shunt can be placed with routing of the fluid to the peritoneum, where it is resorbed and recycled. The choroid plexuses normally produce about 0.5 to 1.5 L of CSF per day. This CSF is an ultrafiltrate of plasma that provides a "shock absorber" and cleansing function for the brain. The CSF circulates through the ventricles and spinal canal. At any time, about 150 mL of CSF fills the ventricular system. CSF is normally reabsorbed at the arachnoid granulations at the vertex of the brain.

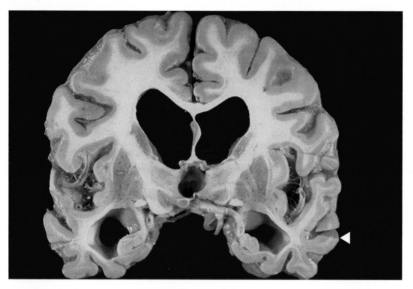

Figure 19-19 Hydrocephalus ex vacuo, gross
This coronal section shows a moderate degree of cerebral atrophy, which is more severe in the temporal lobe (◄) regions. The sylvian fissures appear enlarged. Note the moderate dilation of the cerebral ventricles, including the temporal horns, secondary to parenchymal loss. The condition called *hydrocephalus ex vacuo* results from enough loss of brain parenchyma (with atrophy) to cause compensatory ventricular enlargement. There is no intrinsic abnormality of CSF production, flow, or absorption. This patient had Alzheimer disease (AD), which led to the cerebral cortical atrophy.

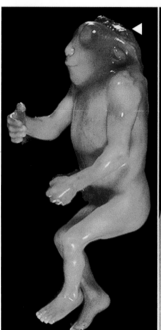
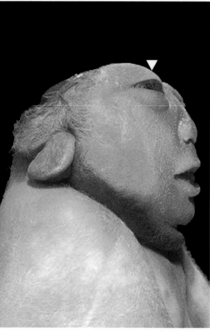

Figure 19-20 Anencephaly, gross
The most dramatic form of neural tube defect (NTD) is anencephaly. This malformation of the caudal portion of the neural tube leads to failure of formation of the fetal cranial vault. The unprotected brain cannot form when exposed to amniotic fluid. The eyes (▼) appear proptotic *(right panel)* because of the lack of a forehead for perspective. The reddish tissue (◄) at the base of the brain *(left panel)* represents the area cerebrovasculosa, a residual disorganized mass of glial, meningeal, and vascular tissue. A small amount of brain stem tissue may be spared, providing for short survival after birth. The open defect predisposes to infection. Supplementing the maternal diet with folate before and during early pregnancy can help to reduce the risk for NTDs, which otherwise occur at a rate of about 1 to 5 of 1000 live births.

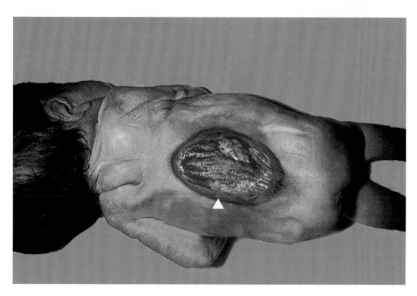

Figure 19-21 Meningomyelocele, gross
NTDs result from improper embryonic neural tube closure. The most minimal defect is called *spina bifida,* in which the posterior arch of a vertebral body fails to fuse completely, but the defect is not open to the skin. Open NTDs extending to and through the thin layer of skin covering the defect and can include meningocele with just meninges protruding through the defect. The meningomyelocele (▲) shown here is large enough to allow meninges and a portion of spinal cord to protrude through the defect, with loss of spinal cord function from that level down. Open defects predispose to CNS infection. Such defects can be suspected prenatally by finding elevated maternal serum or amniotic fluid α-fetoprotein and acetylcholinesterase levels.

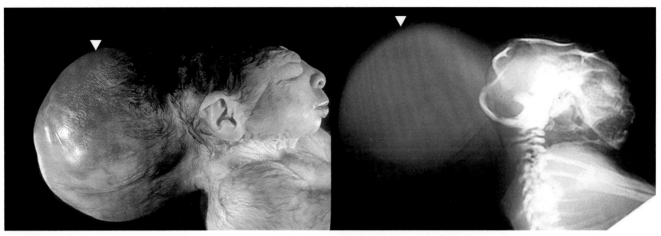

Figure 19-22 Encephalocele, gross
This is an occipital encephalocele with brain tissue extending through a posterior skull defect and forming a saclike structure (▼) that is covered by skin. The cranial vault is present but appears flattened because there is less brain tissue developing within the cranial cavity. The herniated brain tissue is not functional.

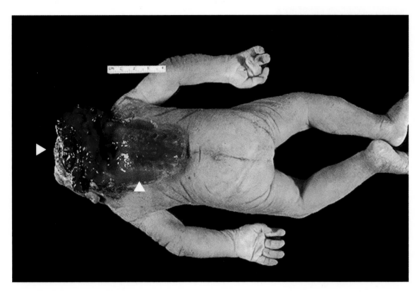

Figure 19-23 Rachischisis, gross
The most common form of NTD is failure of closure of the posterior (caudal) neural tube, leading to spinal dysraphism, or spina bifida. This condition may not be severe, with only a portion of the vertebral arches missing (spina bifida occulta), but with an overlying skin covering, evidenced by a small skin dimple that may contain a tuft of hair over the site of the defect. A more severe form, known as *rachischisis*, is shown here with a large open defect (▲) involving the upper thoracic and cervical vertebrae, along with absence of the occipital bone. Because the cranial vault (▶) also appears to be absent, the condition shown here is best termed *craniorachischisis*.

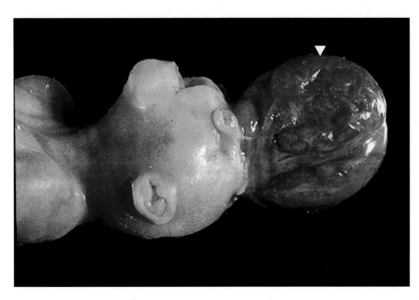

Figure 19-24 Exencephaly, gross
This is the rarest form of NTD, known as *exencephaly*. Note here the absence of the cranial vault, but the presence of brain tissue (▼) covered only by thin meninges. In this condition, all or part of the fetal cranial vault may be missing, but there is still enough tissue covering the brain to allow its development in utero. Exencephaly is most likely to occur in conjunction with an early amnion disruption sequence, or limb–body wall complex, often with amnionic bands involving the head.

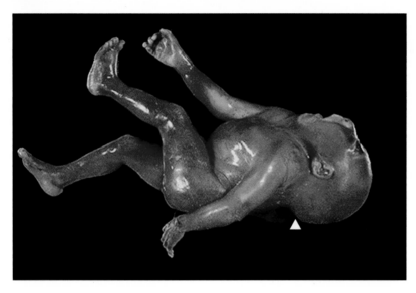

Figure 19-25 Iniencephaly, gross
This variation of NTD results from lack of proper formation of occipital bones, along with a short neck and defect of the upper spinal cord. The head is tilted back (▲), giving the appellation "stargazer" to infants with this rare condition. An encephalocele or rachischisis typically accompanies iniencephaly. In any form of NTD, the amount of CNS tissue that fails to form or is disrupted or secondarily affected by infection or trauma determines the extent of neurologic deficits, including motor and sensory loss. Bowel and bladder function can be lost. High NTDs involving the spinal cord can lead to quadriplegia, whereas NTDs in the thoracic or lumbar regions may lead to paraplegia.

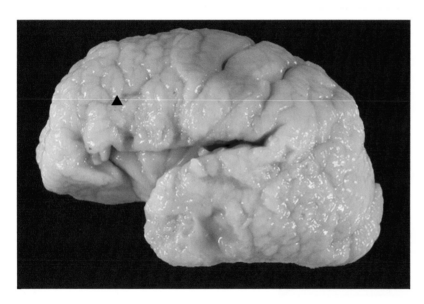

Figure 19-26 Polymicrogyria, gross
The developmental abnormality in this newborn brain appearing from the left lateral aspect, with loss of normal contours of the cerebral hemispheric convolutions, is called *polymicrogyria*. Note the numerous small gyral bumps (▲) over the lateral surface of this left hemisphere. These are not separated by sulci microscopically. In this anomaly the gyri are abnormally fused together, with entrapment of meningeal tissue, and there are no more than four layers instead of the normal six-layered neocortex. This entire brain is too small (microcephaly). Genetic, teratogenic, and material factors may play a role in such an appearance.

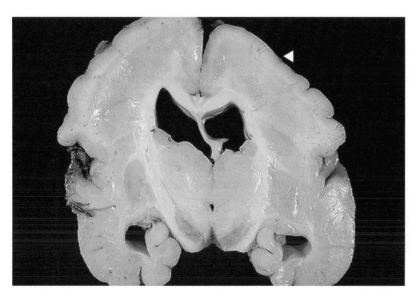

Figure 19-27 Lissencephaly, gross
This coronal section of a child's brain shows markedly diminished gyral development (◄), along with marked thickening of the underlying cerebral cortex. The hippocampi and the deep gray matter structures appear normal. Lissencephaly (agyria) here led to severe developmental delay. A 17p13.3 deletion with loss of the *LIS1* gene occurs in the rare Miller-Dieker syndrome with agyria, seizures, and mental retardation. In normal fetal brain development, gyri first become visible at about 20 weeks' gestation, so lissencephaly before 20 weeks is expected. After 20 weeks, gyral development continues to term in an orderly manner.

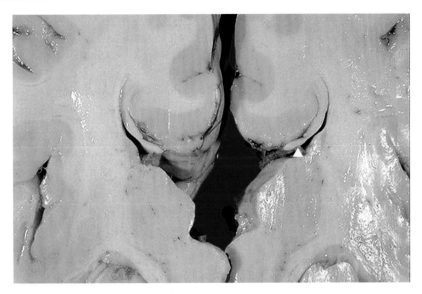

Figure 19-28 Agenesis of the corpus callosum, gross

In this coronal section of brain, no corpus callosum can be seen. Only the small bundles of callosal fibers visible laterally, the Probst bundles (▲), remain. The cingulate gyri appear displaced downward bilaterally. Agenesis of the corpus callosum, which is one of the most common anomalies that occurs in the CNS, about 1 in 1000 persons, may occur as an isolated event or in association with other anomalies. It may be complete or partial. It may be completely asymptomatic and detectable only with specialized testing. The much smaller but adaptable anterior commissure can assume the duties of the missing corpus callosum, part of the plasticity of neural development.

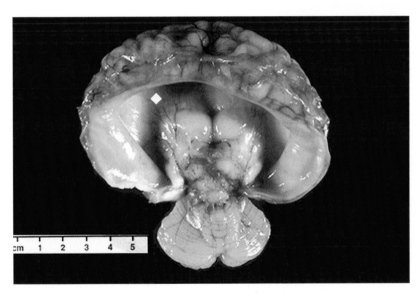

Figure 19-29 Alobar holoprosencephaly, gross

The alobar form of holoprosencephaly shown here has only a single large ventricle (◆) and no attempt at formation of separate cerebral hemispheres. Holoprosencephaly is often accompanied by the failure of fetal facial midline structures to form properly, with midline facial defects, such as cleft lip, cleft palate, and cyclopia, typically with a chromosomal abnormality, such as trisomy 13. It can also occur with maternal diabetes mellitus or sporadically. Some cases are associated with mutation of the human Sonic Hedgehog gene.

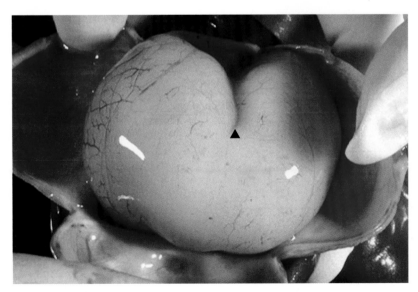

Figure 19-30 Semilobar holoprosencephaly, gross

The fetal skull is opened here at autopsy to reveal the semilobar form of holoprosencephaly, so named because there is a small cleft (▲) representing partial development of the hemispheres. There is no apparent gyral pattern here because this stillborn fetus was less than 20 weeks' gestation, and the lissencephaly is appropriate for this gestational age. Holoprosencephaly is a grave condition with little or no brain function.

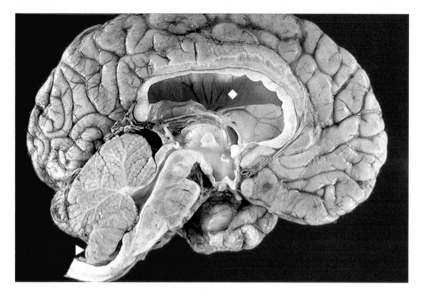

Figure 19-31 Arnold-Chiari I malformation, gross

This sagittal section shows the cerebellar tonsils (▶) herniated downward over the cervical spinal cord. There is hydrocephalus (◆), thought to be secondary to poor flow of CSF out the foramina of Luschka and Magendie, caused by the compression of brain tissue within the posterior fossa. Neurosurgical repair can be done.

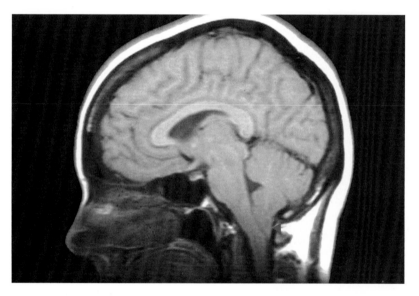

Figure 19-32 Arnold-Chiari I malformation, MRI

This MRI image of the brain in a sagittal view shows a small posterior fossa, and the cerebellar tonsils (◀) herniate through the foramen magnum. The third ventricle is enlarged, and the lateral ventricles may be enlarged. This is the milder form of the malformation, and many patients do not have any symptoms.

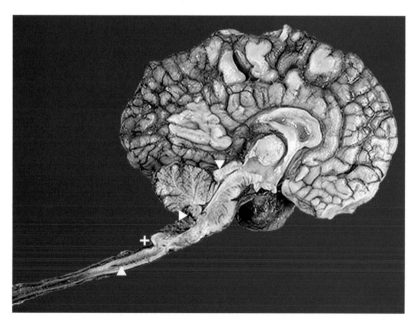

Figure 19-33 Arnold-Chiari II malformation, gross

In Arnold-Chiari type II malformation, there is also a small posterior fossa with tonsillar herniation (▶). This more severe form of the Chiari malformation shows kinking (✚) of the medulla over the cervical cord, and there is a syrinx (▲) in the cervical cord as well. The collicular plate (▼) is pulled up (called *tenting*), and there is invariably an associated hydrocephalus. Most children affected by this anomaly also have a lumbar meningomyelocele.

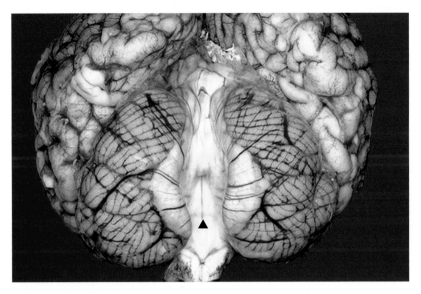

Figure 19-34 Dandy-Walker malformation, gross

Note the enlargement of the posterior fossa beneath the tentorium, accompanied by agenesis of the vermis of the cerebellum. There is replacement of the vermis by a midline cyst lined by ependyma and contiguous with leptomeninges, forming a roofless fourth ventricle. Shown here is the cerebellum with the floor (▲) of the enlarged fourth ventricle. There may be dysplasias of brain stem nuclei as well.

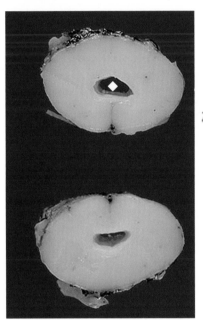

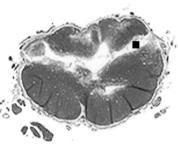

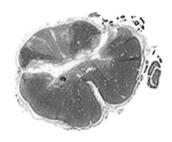

Figure 19-35 Hydromyelia, gross, compared with syringomyelia, microscopic

The cross-sections of spinal cord *(left panel)* show a prominent dilation (◆) of the central canal known as *hydromyelia*. This cavity most often forms in the cervical cord and is lined by ependyma. With syringomyelia *(right panel)* there is a slitlike cavity (■) extending across the spinal cord, which often cuts across the anterolateral system tracts, leading to loss of upper extremity pain and temperature sensation. Extension of the lesion superiorly into the medulla is termed *syringobulbia*. This lesion is most often associated with Chiari I malformation. Other associations include cord trauma or intraspinal tumors. If the cavity continues to enlarge, a drain can be placed to relieve the symptoms.

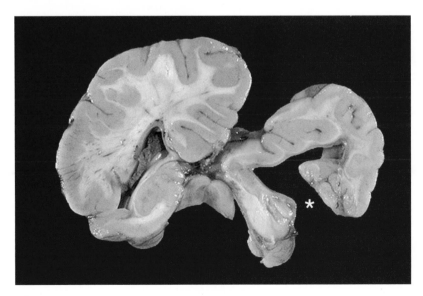

Figure 19-36 Porencephaly, gross

Shown here is a large defect (★) involving the left cerebral hemisphere of a child. Porencephaly is defined by an abnormal opening through the cerebral hemisphere between the ventricular system and the subarachnoid space. This condition can be developmental or secondary to an insult, thought to be vascular, early in utero that destroys the tissue and produces the defect. In contrast, schizencephaly is a developmental disorder of neuronal migration producing a CSF-filled cleft lined by gray matter that extends across the entire cerebral hemisphere, from the ventricular surface to the pial surface of the brain.

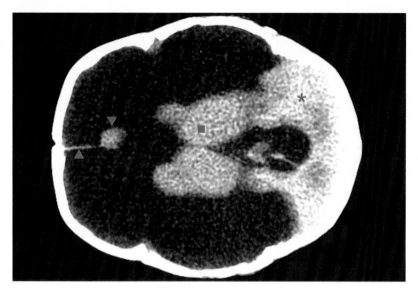

Figure 19-37 Hydranencephaly, CT image
All that remains of this fetal brain in the supratentorial compartment are the basal ganglia (■), the inferior occipital lobes (✱), and a small remnant of frontal lobe (▼) adjacent to the falx cerebri (▲). This is a more dramatic example of the result of a developmental or secondary insult in utero in which a large portion of the developed brain is destroyed. Affected infants are missing most of their cerebral hemispheres. The consequence is a fluid-filled space covered by meninges, mimicking hydrocephalus, but the size of the head may not be increased, because CSF pressure is not increased.

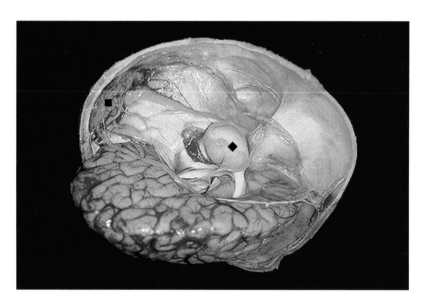

Figure 19-38 Hydranencephaly, gross
This is an example of unilateral hydranencephaly, observed at autopsy of a child, with the cranial cavity opened superiorly. The cranial cavity is almost empty on the left. There is a small remnant of the left occipital lobe (■), and there is a bump representing the basal ganglia (◆). The right cerebral hemisphere is formed properly. An ischemic event in utero may have led to this finding.

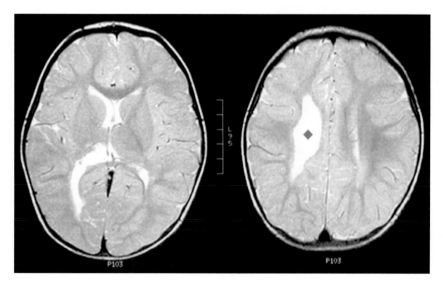

Figure 19-39 Cerebral palsy, MRI
This developmental disorder of motor function is present from infancy or early childhood, probably the result of a vascular accident with localized infarction occurring prenatally or intrapartum. The actual event may go unrecognized until a motor problem, such as spasticity, dystonia, or paresis, is noted early in development. In this case the child had impaired motion, particularly of extensor muscles, on the left. Visible here is asymmetrical mild loss of white matter, basal ganglia, and thalamus on the right with ventricular ex vacuo dilation (◆). Cerebral palsy is nonprogressive, and the childhood brain has an amazing plasticity with ability to rewire itself, minimizing the deficit over time.

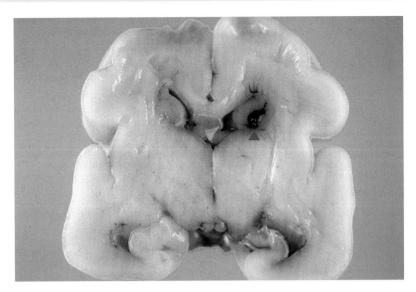

Figure 19-40 Germinal matrix hemorrhage, gross

This coronal section of brain from a 25-week–gestational age premature infant shows a germinal matrix hemorrhage (▲) that occurred shortly after birth. The germinal matrix is a highly vascularized area bordering the caudate nucleus and thalamus that is very sensitive to injury from variations in blood pressure and hypoxia. The risk for hemorrhage is greatest for premature infants born at 23 to 32 weeks' gestation, with a peak at 28 weeks' gestation.

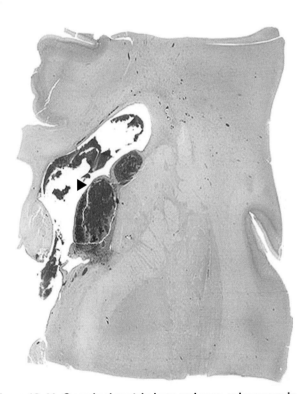

Figure 19-41 Germinal matrix hemorrhage, microscopic

This transverse section of fetal brain shows a subependymal hemorrhage (▶) arising within the darker blue, very cellular and metabolically active subependymal germinal matrix. Hemorrhage extends into the ventricular space. This subependymal region has a high proliferation of neuroblasts that migrate into the cerebral parenchyma by 20 weeks' gestation; then glioblasts proliferate, differentiate, and migrate until 32 weeks. This hemorrhage can rupture into the adjacent lateral ventricle to produce intraventricular hemorrhage, which is a feared complication of prematurity.

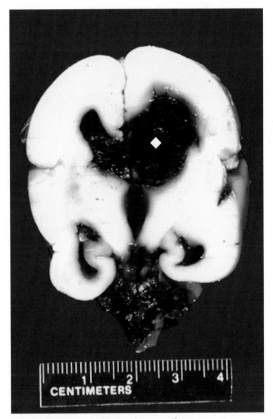

Figure 19-42 Intraventricular hemorrhage, gross

This coronal section of a newborn brain shows a very large subependymal hemorrhage extending into and dilating the ventricular system. Intraventricular hemorrhage (◆) can be severe, as shown here with blood filling and distending all the lateral ventricles, extending into brain parenchyma, and extending down the third ventricle and out into the subarachnoid space. The prognosis with this extent of hemorrhage is grim. If the infant survives, resolution of the hemorrhage with scarring can lead to obstructive hydrocephalus.

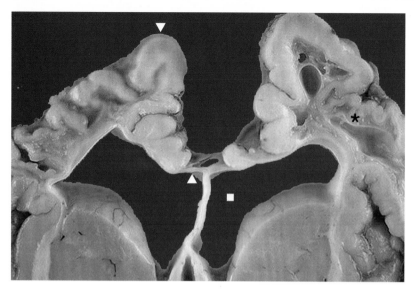

Figure 19-43 Leukomalacia, gross
Shown here in the brain of a child is severe leukomalacia in which the white matter has become cystic and markedly shrunken (✶). The corpus callosum (▲) has become only a thin band of tissue, and there is marked ex vacuo ventricular dilation (■) from loss of the hemispheric parenchyma. The overlying gray matter (▼) appears better preserved, although there is loss in the cortex as well. Affected patients usually experience an anoxic insult around the time of birth, or congenital infection, and are severely impaired neurologically. Periventricular leukomalacia may be marked by radiographic appearance of bright dystrophic calcifications in addition to the necrosis.

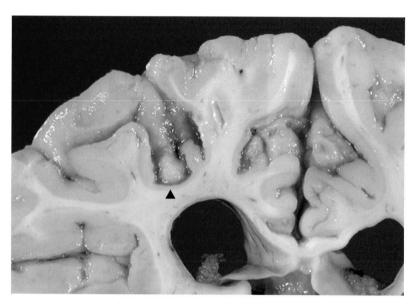

Figure 19-44 Ulegyria, gross
In this brain of a child, there is extensive loss of the cortical gray matter (▲) at the depths of these sulci. The remaining thin gyri become gliotic. Ulegyria is usually the result of an anoxic-ischemic event at or around the time of birth. The injury is most pronounced at the depths of the sulci.

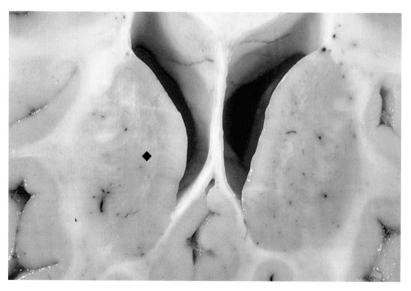

Figure 19-45 Status marmoratus, gross
This coronal section of brain through the basal ganglia with caudate and putamen shows an increased irregular white color (◆) of the basal ganglia. This is status marmoratus, or "marbled state," owing to anoxia, which causes malfunction of the myelinating cells, the oligodendroglia, leading to abnormal myelination and the abnormal white areas visible here within the basal ganglia. There is also neuronal loss and gliosis, which adds to the increased white color. These patients can have severe extrapyramidal movement problems, such as choreoathetosis.

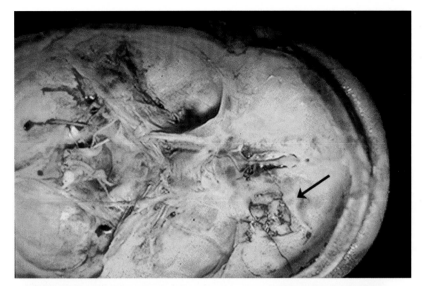

Figure 19-46 Skull fracture, gross
Blunt force trauma to the head can lead to skull fracture. The right orbital plate at the base of this skull shows multiple fractures (◄) in an older patient who fell backward. The force of the blow was transmitted forward, resulting in a contre-coup injury pattern. Such basilar skull fractures may also occur with a blow to the side of the stationary head (coup injury pattern). A basal skull fracture may be suspected in a patient with a periorbital hematoma or CSF rhinorrhea or otorrhea.

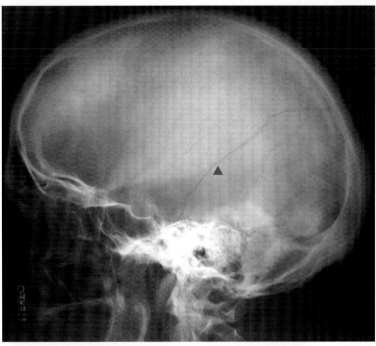

Figure 19-47 Skull fracture, radiograph
After a fall, this patient incurred a linear skull fracture, the long dark line (▲) in this lateral skull radiograph. The fainter branching gray lines represent the normal cranial vascular pattern along the inner skull surface.

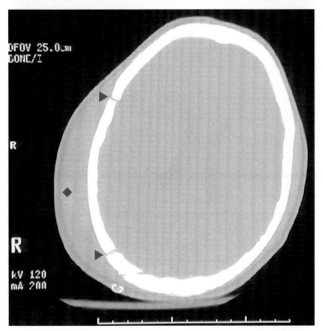

Figure 19-48 Skull fracture, CT image
Head CT scan in "bone window" shows a skull fracture (▶) on the right with diastasis of the sutures. This is not a depressed skull fracture, however, and it is not displaced; a displaced fracture results in skull bone extending into the cranial cavity for a distance greater than the skull thickness. A fracture in this location could result from a coup injury as a consequence of a direct blow to that portion of skull. Note the marked overlying soft-tissue swelling (◆) in the scalp, and that a small overlying skin laceration has been closed with a staple.

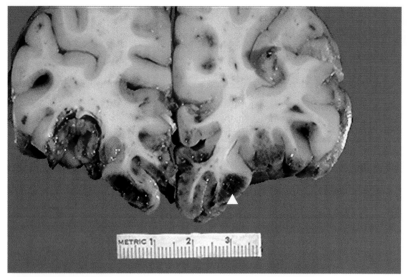

Figure 19-49 Cerebral contusions, gross
A coronal section through the frontal lobes reveals extensive recent contusions (bruises) with multiple superficial gyral hemorrhages (▲), most pronounced at the crests of the gyri, with relative sparing of cortex in the sulci. More severe lesions have extension of hemorrhage to underlying white matter. This contrecoup injury resulted from a fall backward in which the victim struck the occiput, so that the force was transmitted anteriorly to produce the contusions shown here. In contrast, a coup type of brain injury occurs with a direct blow to the head and force delivered to the region of the brain adjacent to the site of impact. There can be subarachnoid hemorrhage and edema in cortex in the region of contusion, producing a local mass effect.

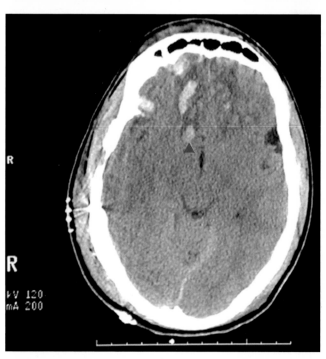

Figure 19-50 Cerebral contusions, CT image
The brighter areas (▲) of attenuation shown here in the cerebral parenchyma represent subfrontal contusions resulting from a contrecoup injury sustained in a fall backward. This patient also had a subdural hemorrhage that was drained through a burr hole marked by the starburst artifact, with overlying sutures appearing on the right. More hemorrhage and edema are present on the right, with a midline shift to the left and narrowing of ventricles.

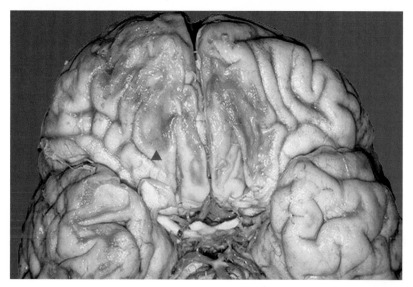

Figure 19-51 Cerebral contusions, gross
The inferior surfaces of these frontal lobes and the right inferior temporal lobe tip display old hemosiderin-stained contusions (▲). They are slightly depressed from removal of necrotic cortex by macrophages and subsequent gliosis. These old lesions have been called *plaques jaunes* because of the yellow-to-brown discoloration from accumulation of hemosiderin derived from breakdown of blood in the superficial cortical hemorrhages. Patients with such contusions may develop a focal or partial seizure disorder years after the accident. There may be loss of smell (anosmia) if the olfactory bulbs and/or tracts are involved.

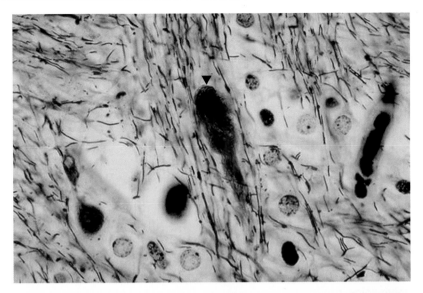

Figure 19-52 Diffuse axonal injury, microscopic
This silver stain of the centrum semiovale shows dark axonal retraction balls (▼) within white matter. These retraction balls can be formed after shearing force injuries. Such injuries can occur with rotational forces (angular acceleration or deceleration) or with violent shaking, as in "shaken infant" syndrome, or in individuals ejected from motor vehicles at high speed. The axons are stretched and broken at nodes of Ranvier, then undergo retraction, causing the axoplasm to compress into an enlarged ball. Such involved axonal fibers eventually degenerate. Focal hemorrhages may accompany these lesions. Half of patients in coma after trauma have these lesions.

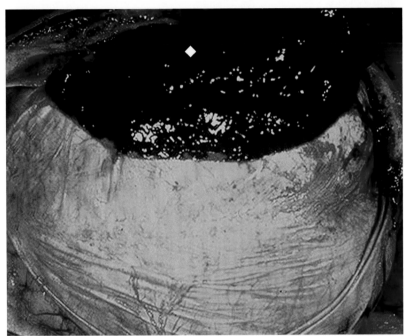

Figure 19-53 Epidural hematoma, gross
Blunt force head trauma causing a tear in a meningeal artery, most often the middle meningeal artery, leads to a collection of blood (◆) in the epidural space. This acute arterial bleeding occurs between the dura and the skull and quickly leads to hematoma formation, visible here on the right after opening the cranial vault at autopsy. There is often a skull fracture accompanying this lesion. Because the bleeding from the artery is brisk, these patients may have a short lucid interval after the injury, but quickly lapse into coma because of the brain compression by the expanding hematoma. If not emergently evacuated, the expanding mass of blood leads to herniation and death.

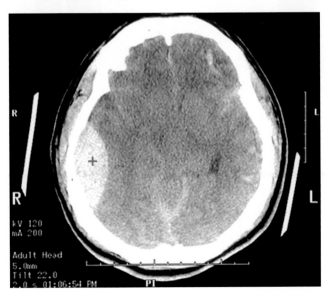

Figure 19-54 Epidural hematoma, CT image
Note the large right epidural hematoma with a lens-shaped outline (✚), as the smooth dura becomes indented against the underlying cortex on the right lateral aspect of the cerebrum. The epidural hematoma is confined within an area bounded by cranial sutures where the dura is firmly adherent to the skull. This acute blood collection appears bright on CT scan. Note the mass effect with effacement of the lateral ventricles and the shift of midline to the left. In this case the patient fell from a height and struck the right side of his head, severing the middle meningeal artery. This epidural hematoma collected within hours.

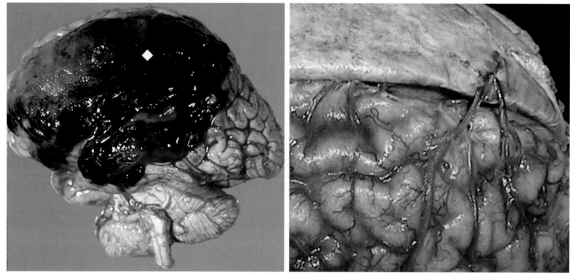

Figure 19-55 Subdural hematoma, gross, and bridging veins, gross

A large subdural hematoma (◆) is shown in the *left panel* overlying the left frontoparietal region. A subdural hematoma forms after head trauma that severs the bridging veins from dura to brain, shown in the *right panel* where the dura has been reflected to reveal the normal appearance of the bridging veins (◀) that extend across to the superior aspect of the cerebral hemispheres. Elderly patients and very young patients are at greater risk because their cerebral veins are more vulnerable to injury. Because the bleeding is venous, blood collects over hours to weeks, with variable onset of symptoms. Because the blood is present beneath the dura, a subdural hematoma can be seen to cross the region of cranial sutures and interdigitate with underlying cortex.

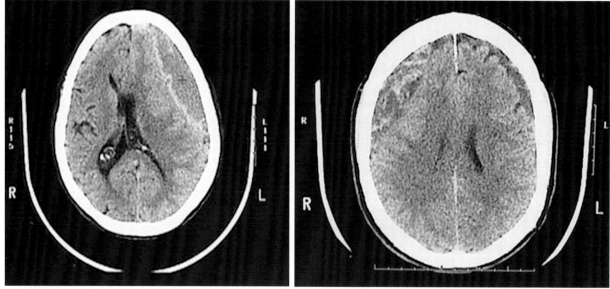

Figure 19-56 Subdural hematomas, CT images

In the *left panel*, there is a large left subdural hematoma (✚) with left-to-right shift (◀) and ventricular narrowing. This subdural hematoma interdigitates with the adjacent gyri and sulci but compresses the brain. In the *right panel,* bilateral subdural hematomas can be seen, the right one (✚) greater in size than the left (✖). There are irregular bright areas within these subdural hematomas, indicating that the hemorrhage was relatively recent but is not completely bright, so some organization of the hematoma has begun. Clot lysis generally occurs 1 week after hematoma formation, with granulation tissue, including fibroblastic proliferation from the dura, occurring over the next week, and formation of a neomembrane of connective tissue within 1 to 3 months after the original injury. Symptoms of subdural hematoma have a variable onset of hours to weeks, depending on the amount of bleeding. Rebleeding from delicate vessels within the granulation tissue is common, leading to chronic subdural hematoma.

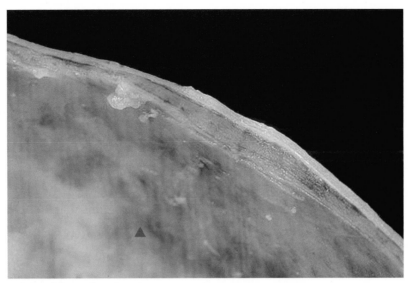

Figure 19-57 Organizing subdural hematoma, gross
A subdural hematoma gradually organizes with granulation tissue formation and forms a vascularized membrane of reactive connective tissue. There may be rebleeding or fluid collection within this membrane, producing a mass effect that impinges on the brain. Note the brownish discoloration (▲) of the chronic subdural membrane appearing here from hemosiderin staining derived from the blood. These old membranes are only loosely attached to the dura and can be easily peeled away.

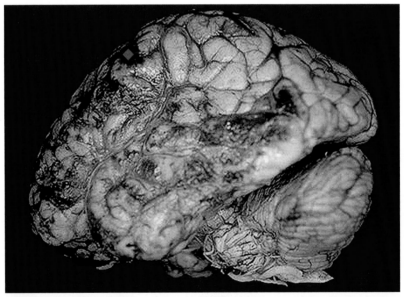

Figure 19-58 Subarachnoid hemorrhage, gross
Acute subarachnoid hemorrhage (SAH) may follow trauma. Many of the areas of subarachnoid hemorrhage (◆) shown here are associated with underlying contusions. Simple subarachnoid hemorrhage without contusions also can occur from superficial damage to vessels or vascular disease over the surface of the brain. Atraumatic cases of SAH over the cerebral convexities may result from cerebral vasoconstriction syndrome in younger patients and cerebral amyloid angiopathy in older patients.

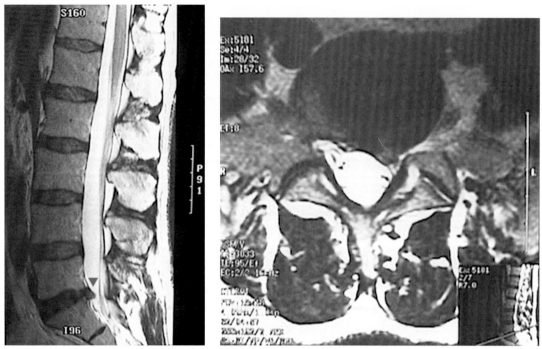

Figures 19-59 and 19-60 Herniated intervertebral disc, MRI

The *left panel* shows in sagittal view herniation of the nucleus pulposus of the intervertebral disc between L5 and S1, with compression (▼) of the lumbar spinal cord. A herniated disc can compress spinal nerve roots to produce pain and motor weakness. In the *right panel,* an axial view at L4 shows herniation and compression (▼) of the nerve roots on the left.

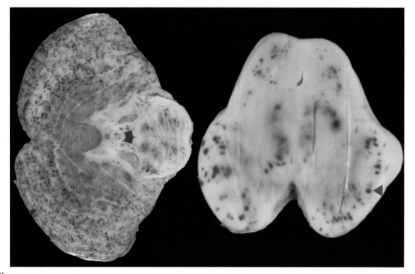

Figure 19-61 Fat embolism, gross

Note the numerous red petechial hemorrhages (◄), mainly in white matter, of brain stem and cerebellum. Fat embolism syndrome (FES) is the presence of fat or marrow elements (or both) within the microvasculature, usually involving lung and brain, but other organs, such as kidneys, may be affected to cause oliguria and renal failure. Neurologic symptoms range from confusion and stupor to deep coma. FES, even with severe cerebral symptoms, often resolves with supportive therapy, leaving no permanent sequelae. There can be fragments of bone marrow, with fat and hematopoietic elements in small vessels. The fat globules are usually of different sizes and may aggregate; there is little, if any, associated inflammation. FES occurs in many clinical settings, including burn injuries, pancreatitis, frostbite, fatty liver, seizures, decompression illness, sickle cell crisis, and hepatic necrosis, and as a complication of surgical procedures, including intramedullary rod placement and liposuction procedures.

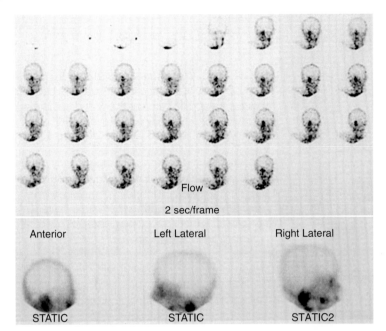

Flow

2 sec/frame

Anterior   Left Lateral   Right Lateral

STATIC   STATIC   STATIC2

Figure 19-62 Brain death, perfusion scan
This cerebral scan shows no apparent perfusion to the cerebral hemispheres, indicative of brain death. The patient remains in a persistent vegetative state with no higher cerebral function. This can occur after many types of injuries—traumatic, toxic, metabolic, ischemic. Although there may be some residual brain stem function, and the patient can be kept alive with mechanical ventilation and through tube feedings, there will be no recovery. Advance directives for health care communicated by the patient before this situation are paramount to resolving the dilemma of what decision to make regarding continuation, or not, of this state. You never know what may happen. Make the most of each day, and appreciate those individuals you meet in the course of daily activities.

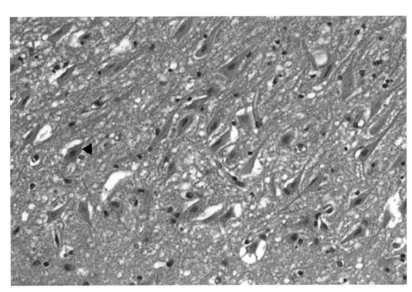

Figure 19-63 Hypoxic encephalopathy, microscopic
Neurons are highly differentiated cells that depend on glucose and oxygen for continued function, and they are very sensitive to hypoxic injury. Shown here are red neurons (◀) in cortex, which are dying 12 to 24 hours after onset of hypoxia. One of the most sensitive areas in the brain to hypoxic injury is the hippocampus. Cerebellar Purkinje cells and neocortical pyramidal neurons are also very sensitive to ischemic events. A global hypoxic encephalopathy occurs with reduction of all cerebral perfusion with reduced cardiac output and with hypotension. Intracranial vascular diseases may reduce blood flow focally to the brain, and the extent of injury depends on collateral circulation

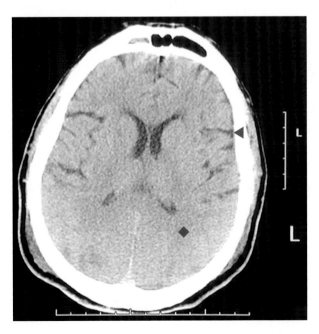

Figure 19-64 Acute cerebral ischemia, CT image
Shown here are recent bilateral occipital lobe acute infarctions that developed as a result of focal ischemic injury, characterized by loss of gyral distinction, along with decreased attenuation (a darker appearance) of the white matter (◆). Compare with the uninfarcted parietal and frontal lobes, with gyri and sulci (◀) still visible.

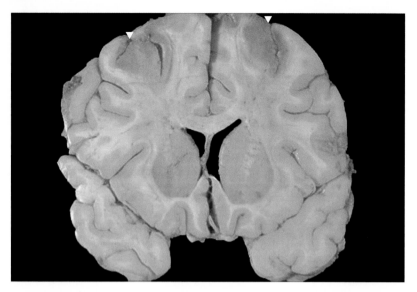

Figure 19-65 Watershed infarction, gross
The bilaterally symmetrical darker red (▼) discolored areas shown here superiorly and just lateral to the midline in this coronal section of the brain at autopsy represent areas of recent infarction in the watershed (border) zone between distal regions of the anterior and middle cerebral arterial circulations. Such watershed infarctions can occur with relative or absolute hypoperfusion of the brain. Hypoperfusion can occur with a decrease in cardiac output from cardiac diseases.

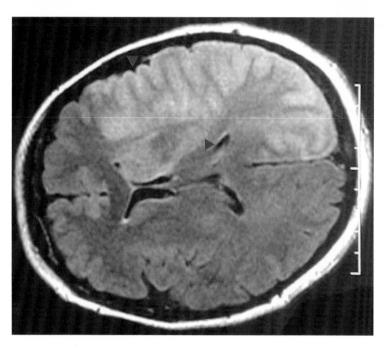

Figure 19-66 Cerebral acute infarction, MRI
This FLAIR-mode MRI image reveals an area of massive infarction in the left cerebral hemisphere, mostly involving the left middle cerebral (▼) arterial distribution, but also in the left posterior cerebral (◄) distribution. This infarct is of recent formation, with brain swelling and a slight midline shift to the right causing compression (▶) of the ventricular system. Cerebral infarction is most often caused by embolic occlusion of a cerebral arterial branch, but thrombotic occlusion can also occur, typically in an area of marked cerebral arterial atherosclerosis. Embolic infarcts are more likely to appear hemorrhagic from reperfusion of the damaged vessels and tissue, either from collateral circulation or after dissolution with breakup of the embolus.

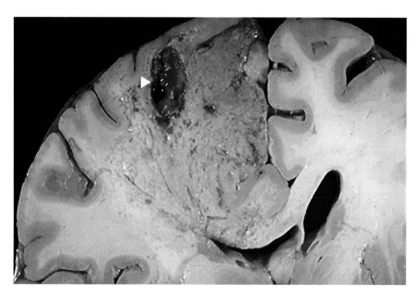

Figure 19-67 Cerebral subacute infarction, gross
In this coronal section, a subacute infarct of the frontal lobe shows liquefactive necrosis with beginning formation of cystic spaces (▶) as resolution occurs 10 days to 2 weeks after the initial ischemic event. The initial subacute changes begin 24 hours after the initial ischemic injury with influx of macrophages to remove the necrotic tissue, followed by progressively increasing vascular proliferation and reactive gliosis.

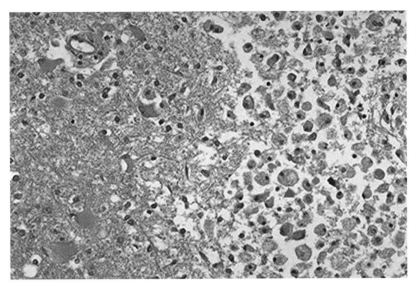

Figure 19-68 Subacute infarction, microscopic

On the right are many macrophages (▲) that are present in this subacute infarct to phagocytize lipid debris from the ongoing liquefactive necrosis. Gliosis is beginning to appear on the left. Ischemic injury leads to infarction. Focal ischemic infarction (stroke) can result from either arterial thrombosis or embolism. The location and extent of the infarction depend on the part of the cerebral circulation affected and determine the clinical findings and resulting neurologic dysfunction.

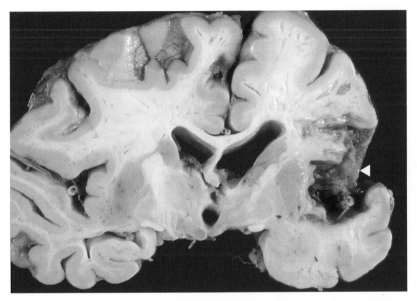

Figure 19-69 Cerebral remote infarction, gross

This coronal section shows that a portion of one cerebral hemisphere has been destroyed, with a large residual defect (◄) in the region of the insular cortex. This remote infarction has occurred in the distribution of the middle cerebral artery. Resolution of liquefactive necrosis leads to formation of a cystic space surrounded by remaining gliotic brain tissue. This repair reaction begins 2 weeks after the ischemic injury and proceeds for months.

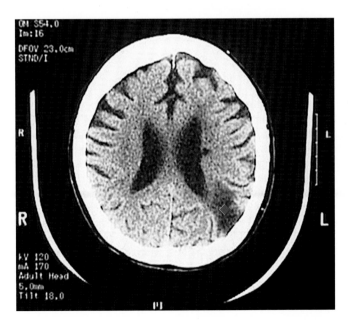

Figure 19-70 Cerebral remote infarction, CT image

The decreased area of attenuation (♦) shown here in the region of the left occipital lobe is a cystic area from healing of a remote cerebral infarction as a consequence of a thromboembolus to the left posterior cerebral artery. Resolution of the liquefactive necrosis leaves a cystic space. The neurologic deficits after infarction depend on the location and size of the infarct. Patients may be left with motor and sensory deficits. Over time there may be partial recovery of some lost functions, but this is inconstant and unpredictable. Plasticity to recover function becomes more limited with aging. In this case the patient was left with visual field defects.

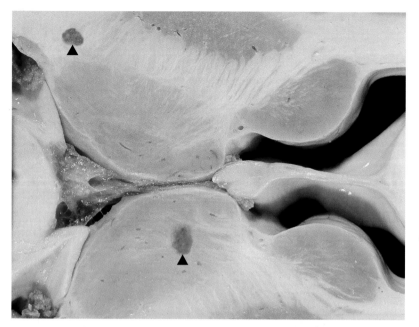

Figure 19-71 Lacunar infarction, gross
The arteriolar sclerosis that results from chronic hypertension leads to small lacunar infarcts (▲), or lacunes, two of which are shown here within the internal capsule at the top and the thalamus at the bottom. Such lesions are most common in lenticular nuclei, thalamus, internal capsule, deep white matter, caudate nucleus, and pons. Although these infarcts are typically smaller than 15 mm, and many result in no clinical findings, they can sometimes be strategically located where they damage important tracts, especially the descending corticospinal tracts, leading to hemiparesis, or the thalamus, leading to sensory problems.

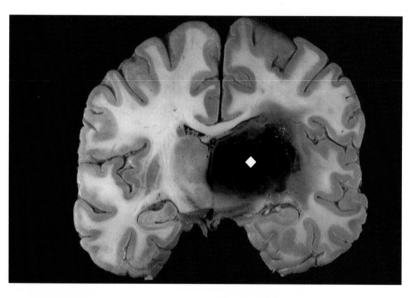

Figure 19-72 Cerebral hypertensive hemorrhage, gross
Hypertension is the most common cause of intraparenchymal brain hemorrhage, accounting for more than half of all such bleeds.
An intracerebral hemorrhage is one form of stroke. Hemorrhages involving the basal ganglia area (◆) as shown here (the putamen in particular) tend to be nontraumatic and caused by chronic hypertension, which damages and weakens the small penetrating arteries. A mass effect from the blood with midline shift, often with secondary edema, may lead to herniation. Hypertensive cerebral hemorrhages originate in the putamen in 50% to 60% of cases, but the thalamus, pons, and cerebellar hemispheres can also be sites of involvement.

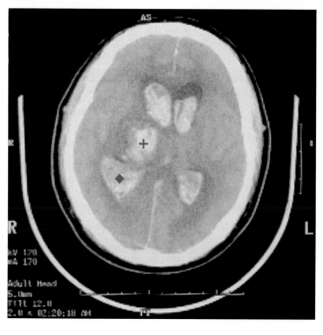

Figure 19-73 Cerebral hypertensive hemorrhage, CT image
A hypertensive hemorrhage is present here in the right thalamic region (✚). In a few such cases, the hemorrhage may extend into the ventricular system (◆), as shown here. Hemorrhages involving the basal ganglia, thalamus, and brain stem are not generally amenable to surgical intervention with removal of the blood. The arteriosclerosis that accompanies chronic hypertension predisposes small arterial vessels to rupture and produce the hemorrhage. In addition, chronic hypertension is associated with the development of minute aneurysms (<300 μm in diameter), termed *Charcot-Bouchard microaneurysms,* which can also rupture.

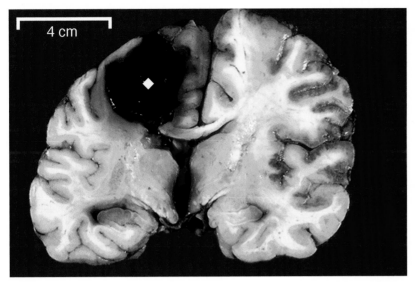

Figure 19-74 Lobar hemorrhage, gross
Note the large parietal lobe recent hemorrhage
(◆). Cerebral intraparenchymal hemorrhages
involving the lobes of the cerebral hemispheres
may have many different causes, including a
neoplasm, a coagulopathy, infections, vasculitis,
amyloid angiopathy, and drug abuse
(e.g., cocaine ingestion). A large bleed can
produce a mass effect with risk for herniation.
Resolution of a large hemorrhage may leave a
cystic region similar to an infarct.

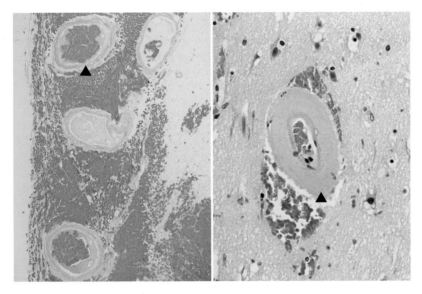

**Figure 19-75 Amyloid angiopathy
hemorrhage, microscopic**
There is marked thickening with a pink hyaline
appearance (▲) of the small peripheral cerebral
artery *(right panel)* with leakage of red blood cells
(RBCs). The amorphous pink amyloid (▲) within
medium-sized arteries *(left panel)* has weakened
the vascular walls to allow either "microbleeds" or
more extensive lobar hemorrhage. About 10% of
persons with AD have a terminal stroke with lobar
or subarachnoid hemorrhage over the hemispheres, particularly when *APP* mutations or the
ApoE ε4 allele is present.

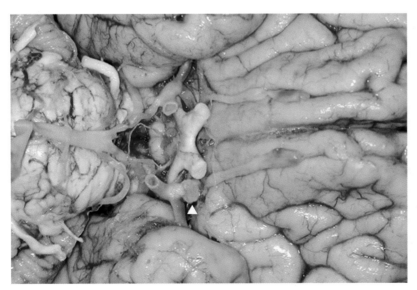

Figure 19-76 Berry aneurysm, gross
A nonruptured saccular (berry) aneurysm
(▲) is visible at the bifurcation of the left middle
cerebral and anterior communicating arteries
of the circle of Willis at the base of the brain.
These aneurysms form at one or more points of a
developmental weakness in the arterial wall, most
commonly at the bifurcation of the anterior communicating, middle cerebral, or internal carotid
arteries. These aneurysms occur sporadically and
may be present in 1% to 2% of people. Saccular
aneurysms are more frequent with some genetic
conditions, such as autosomal-dominant polycystic kidney disease, vascular-type Ehlers-Danlos
syndrome (type IV), neurofibromatosis type 1,
and Marfan syndrome. Half of people with a berry
aneurysm have risks that include hypertension
and smoking.

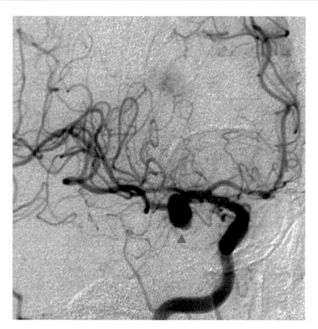

Figure 19-77 Berry aneurysm, angiogram
This lateral view with contrast material filling a portion of the cerebral arterial circulation shows a berry aneurysm (▲) involving the middle cerebral artery of the circle of Willis at the base of the brain. As the weak wall of an artery lacking an internal elastic lamina and a media expands to form the aneurysm, there may initially be leakage of blood that produces headaches, but there is risk for sudden rupture to produce a severe headache. A sudden increase in ICP may predispose to rupture. The blood irritates the arteries to produce vasospasm and promote cerebral ischemia. A later consequence of this bleeding is organization with fibrosis at the base of the brain to block outflow of CSF through the foramina of Luschka and Magendie, leading to an obstructive hydrocephalus.

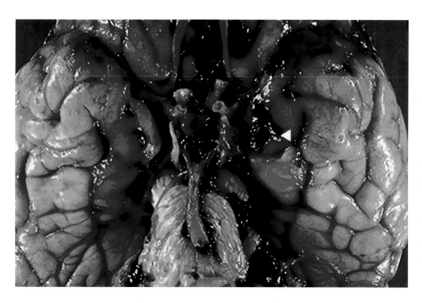

Figure 19-78 Subarachnoid hemorrhage, gross
Berry aneurysms take years to increase in size, and larger aneurysms are more prone to rupture, particularly aneurysms reaching 1 cm in diameter, so that rupture is most likely to occur in young to middle-aged adults. Neurosurgery can be performed with embolization or clipping of the aneurysm at its base to prevent bleeding or rebleeding. The subarachnoid hemorrhage (◄) from a ruptured aneurysm is more of an irritant producing vasospasm than a mass lesion. In some cases, this arterial blood under pressure may dissect upward into the brain parenchyma. The result is often a sudden, severe headache followed by loss of consciousness.

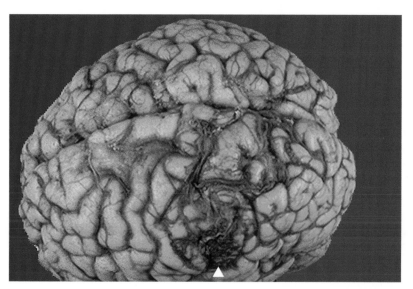

Figure 19-79 Vascular malformation, gross
A mass of irregular, tortuous vessels (▲) over the left posterior parietal region of the brain is shown here. Arteriovenous malformations and cavernous hemangiomas are prone to bleed and may cause significant intracranial hemorrhage, particularly in individuals 10 to 30 years old, more often in men. Most occur in a cerebral hemisphere in the distribution of the middle cerebral artery. Two other malformations, *capillary telangiectasia,* or *venous angioma,* are less likely to bleed. Localized lesions can be resected.

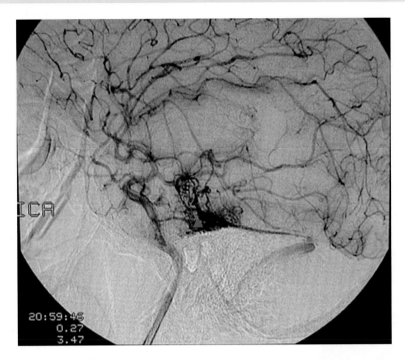

Figure 19-80 Vascular malformation, angiogram
Contrast material is filling a tortuous collection of irregular small vessels (▲) in the temporal region of the brain. A vascular malformation may bleed, resulting in symptoms that range from new-onset seizures or headache to sudden loss of consciousness. The bleeding is most often intraparenchymal but may extend to the overlying subarachnoid space.

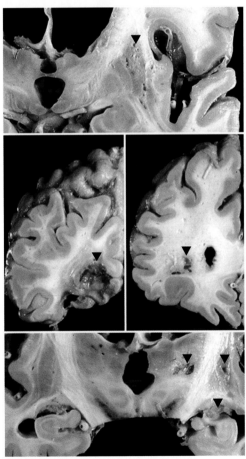

Figure 19-81 Vascular (multi-infarct) dementia, gross
Multiple vascular events, including embolic arterial occlusion, atherosclerosis with vascular narrowing and thrombosis, and hypertensive arteriolar sclerosis, may lead to focal but additive loss of cerebral tissue. The cumulative effect of multiple small areas of infarction (▼) may result in clinical findings equivalent to AD along with focal neurologic deficits or gait disturbances. Vascular dementia is marked by the loss of higher mental function in a stepwise, not continuous, fashion. Shown is a collage of cerebral coronal sections in which variably sized remote infarcts are present. Another variation of this process is Binswanger disease, characterized by extensive subcortical white matter loss.

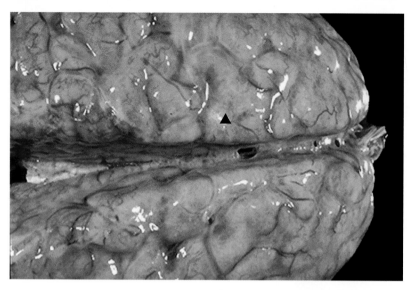

Figure 19-82 Acute meningitis, gross
The yellow-tan clouding of the meninges over gyri (▲) shown here, which obscures the sulci, is caused by an inflammatory exudate from acute meningitis. This is most often the result of a bacterial (pyogenic) infection. Routes for intracranial infection include hematogenous dissemination (the most common cause), extension from an adjacent paranasal sinus or mastoid air cells, retrograde flow through facial veins into the cavernous sinus, and trauma with direct implantation by a penetrating injury through the skull. Lumbar puncture reveals increased ICP and CSF showing a marked leukocytosis with a preponderance of neutrophils. Patients often have headache, nuchal rigidity, and changes in mental status.

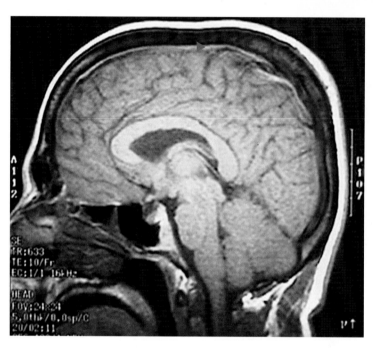

Figure 19-83 Acute meningitis, MRI
Shown in sagittal view is bright meningeal enhancement (▶) as a consequence of formation of an exudate covering the meninges in a case of acute bacterial meningitis with *Streptococcus pneumoniae*. The inflammation leads to dilation of meningeal vessels, causing the bright enhancement shown here. The most likely causative organisms are age related, with *Escherichia coli* and group B streptococci occurring in neonates, *Haemophilus influenzae* in children, *Neisseria meningitidis* in adolescents and young adults, and *S. pneumoniae* in older adults. Immunization has markedly reduced the incidence of *H. influenzae* and *S. pneumoniae* meningitis. *Listeria monocytogenes* remains a significant congenital and food-borne infection.

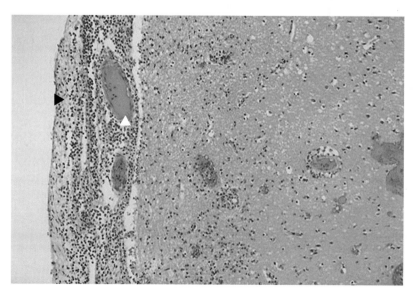

Figure 19-84 Acute meningitis, microscopic
A neutrophilic exudate (▶) involves the meninges on the left, with prominent dilated vessels (▲). Edema and focal inflammation (extending into superficial brain parenchyma through the Virchow-Robin space) are present in the neocortex to the right. This acute meningitis is typical of a bacterial infection. This edema can lead to brain swelling with herniation and death. Resolution of infection may be followed by adhesive arachnoiditis with obliteration of the subarachnoid space leading to obstructive hydrocephalus. Diagnosis is aided by performing lumbar puncture to obtain CSF that typically shows increased leukocytes, mainly neutrophils, decreased glucose, and increased protein. Gram stain, serologies, and culture help identify specific microorganisms.

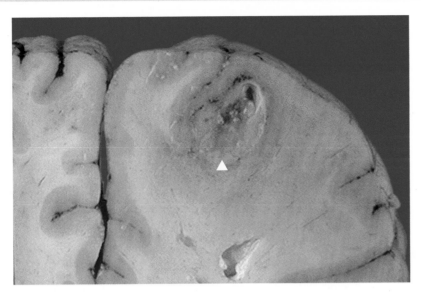

Figure 19-85 Cerebral abscess, gross
This coronal section through the superior parietal lobe shows a focal lesion (▲) with a liquefactive center containing yellow pus and surrounding thin wall. Cerebral abscesses usually result from hematogenous spread of a bacterial infection, typically from infective endocarditis or from pneumonia, but may also occur from direct penetrating trauma or extension from adjacent infection in paranasal sinuses or mastoid. Patients may have a fever along with focal but progressive neurologic deficits. The mass effect with surrounding edema can increase the ICP, with risk for herniation.

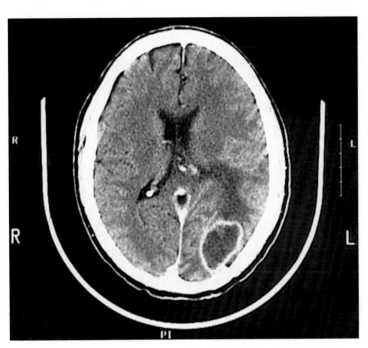

Figure 19-86 Cerebral abscess, CT image
This abscess of the left occipital lobe displays prominent "ring enhancement" with a bright border (▼) caused by the surrounding highly vascular granulation tissue that contains many small vessels at the periphery of the abscess. Most of these cases result from staphylococcal or streptococcal infections. In addition to being destructive of brain tissue, an abscess is a mass lesion, often with surrounding edema that can increase ICP and cause herniation. The elevated ICP may manifest with papilledema observed on funduscopy. If it is safe to perform a lumbar puncture, an increased ICP is usually observed, and examination of the CSF may show leukocytosis with neutrophilia, along with elevated protein, but often without a decrease in glucose. The abscess may be complicated by rupture and spread to cause ventriculitis, meningitis, or cerebral venous sinus thrombosis.

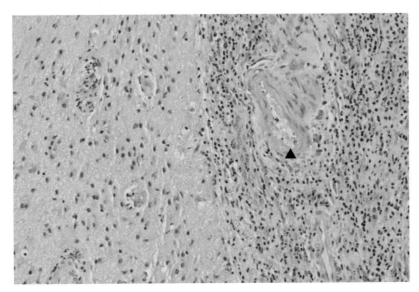

Figure 19-87 Cerebral abscess, microscopic
The acute inflammatory cells in the abscess are at the right, with adjacent cerebral cortex at the left. Note the prominent small artery (▲) with thickened wall and dilated lumen, which imparts the ring enhancement visible with radiologic scans.

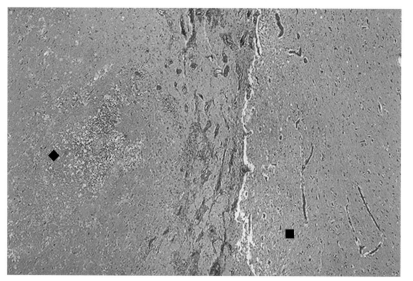

Figure 19-88 Cerebral abscess, microscopic
A key microscopic feature of a brain abscess, shown here with trichrome stain, is the organizing wall that contains collagenous fibrosis (the blue-staining tissue) in addition to adjacent gliosis (■) in brain. The necrotic center (◆) of the abscess is on the left, and the adjacent surrounding brain is on the right, with the granulation tissue in between. Patients with such an abscess may develop progressive neurologic deficits, headache, and seizures days to weeks after the initial infection. Antibiotic therapy and surgical drainage can be effective treatment options.

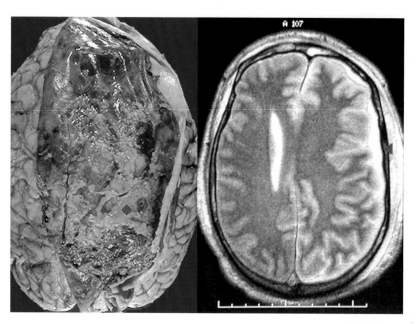

Figure 19-89 Subdural empyema, gross and MRI
Spread of infection to the subdural space in children is usually a complication of bacterial meningitis; in adults, it often represents spread of infection from sinusitis or otitis media. There is bright signal intensity (◀) of the left subdural space *(right panel)* indenting the gyri and producing a mass effect effacing the left lateral ventricle. Note the overlying scalp swelling. The increased ICP, if unilateral, can cause left papilledema. The reflected dura *(left panel)* shows extensive yellow exudate (◆). Clinical findings include fever, headache, and nuchal rigidity. Vascular structures, including bridging cerebral veins, may be involved with thrombophlebitis, leading to venous cerebral infarction.

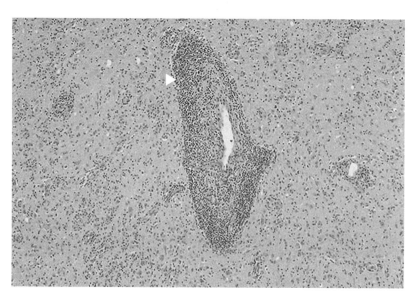

Figure 19-90 Viral encephalitis, microscopic
Note prominent perivascular (▶) and parenchymal lymphocytic infiltrates. Viral infections of the brain typically involve the cortex (encephalitis), sometimes with meningeal involvement as well (meningoencephalitis). Some viruses, such as rabies virus, involve very specific areas, whereas others, such as echovirus, coxsackievirus, or West Nile virus, have more general involvement. Shown here are characteristic parenchymal and perivascular lymphocytic infiltrates. Patients may have fever and altered mental status that can persist for days to weeks. Examination of CSF may show a lymphocytic pleocytosis, moderately increased protein, and normal glucose; the Gram stain is negative.

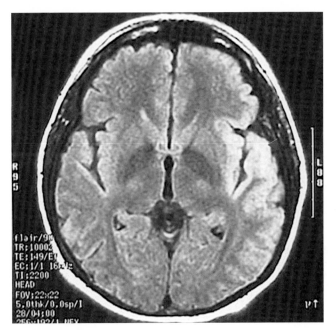

Figure 19-91 Viral meningoencephalitis, MRI

In this axial view, there is markedly abnormal signal hyperintensity, mainly in the left temporal lobe (◀) and adjacent insular cortex, extending to the meninges. This is consistent with a diffuse viral meningoencephalitis. This may be termed *aseptic meningitis* because bacterial organisms are not shown by routine Gram stain and culture, but there can be an acute onset, similar to a pyogenic bacterial meningitis, although it is often caused by viral organisms. Some drugs, such as nonsteroidal anti-inflammatory drugs and antibiotics, may produce similar findings, termed *drug-induced aseptic meningitis.* The CSF shows a leukocytic pleocytosis with a predominance of lymphocytes, moderately elevated protein of <0.5 g/dL, and normal glucose.

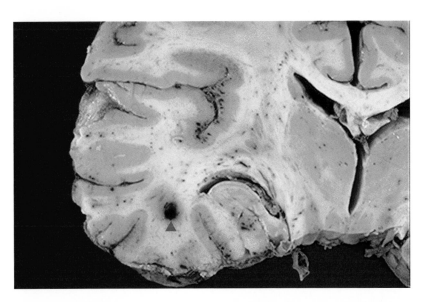

Figure 19-92 Herpes simplex virus encephalitis, gross

Herpes simplex virus (HSV) infection of the brain often produces hemorrhages (▲) within the temporal lobe, as shown here. HSV encephalitis is uncommon but distinctive. Most cases are sporadic, but some cases can occur in immunocompetent individuals. A prior history of HSV infection is elicited in only 10% of patients. Similar to other viral infections, there are mononuclear cell infiltrates, sometimes with necrosis. Either HSV-1 or HSV-2 can produce these findings in adults, and in newborns as a congenital infection. Most cases of adult HSV encephalitis are caused by HSV-1, and the course may extend over 4 to 6 weeks. HSV-2 causes most perinatal cases.

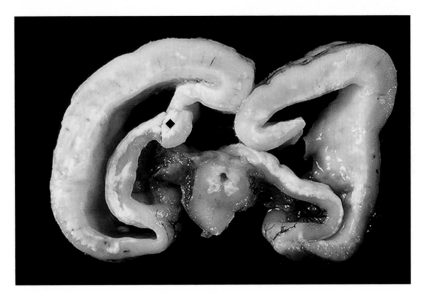

Figure 19-93 Congenital cytomegalovirus infection, gross

Cytomegalovirus (CMV) infection acquired in utero may cause marked destruction of the brain by hemorrhagic necrotizing ventriculoencephalitis. Appearing here at autopsy are many chalky white (◆) periventricular calcifications. There was no fetal movement in utero, and CMV was disseminated in multiple organs. In adults who are immunocompromised, such as individuals with HIV infection, CMV may produce widespread encephalitis, primarily in a subependymal or periventricular distribution. Prominent involvement of white matter is described as periventricular leukomalacia.

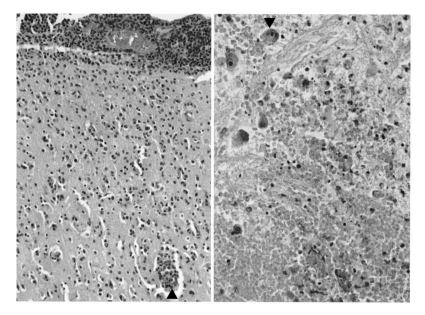

Figure 19-94 Cytomegalovirus meningoen-cephalitis, microscopic

There is an intense lymphocytic infiltrate in the meninges and underlying cerebral cortex, including perivascular (▲) location *(left panel)*. More extensive inflammation can lead to necrosis and hemorrhage, along with large (cytomegalic) glial cells containing intranuclear inclusions (▼) of CMV *(right panel)*.

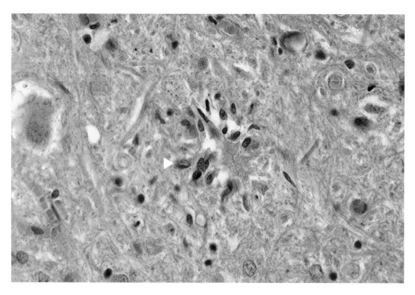

Figure 19-95 Poliomyelitis, microscopic

Poliovirus infection destroys motor neurons in the gray matter of the spinal cord. Neurono-phagia occurs during acute poliomyelitis, visible here with a small group of inflammatory cells (▶) surrounding the remnants of an anterior horn cell. Poliomyelitis is an enterovirus that can lead to anterior horn cell loss or bulbar lower motor neuron loss during the acute stage of the disease. Flaccid paralysis with muscle wasting occurs in the distribution of affected neurons. The severity of the infection determines the degree of impairment. A postpolio syndrome with progressive weakness may occur decades after initial infection.

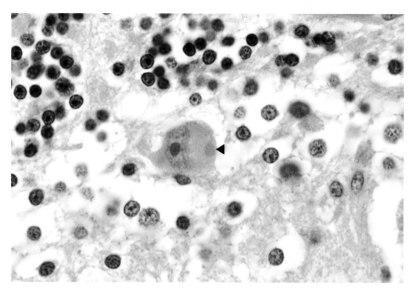

Figure 19-96 Rabies, microscopic

Rabies is still prevalent in parts of the world with animal reservoirs. Shown here is a Negri body (◀) within Purkinje cell cytoplasm, the most common site, but Negri bodies can also be identified within the pyramidal cells of the hippocampus. This virus travels intra-axonally from the site of the animal bite, taking 1 to 3 months to travel from peripheral sites to the CNS. Virus spreads within the CNS to cause initial symptoms of malaise, headache, and fever; paresthesias may persist at the site of the bite. Hyperexcitability with convulsions, pharyngeal spasm, and meningismus follow. Eventually a flaccid paralysis occurs, followed by coma and death.

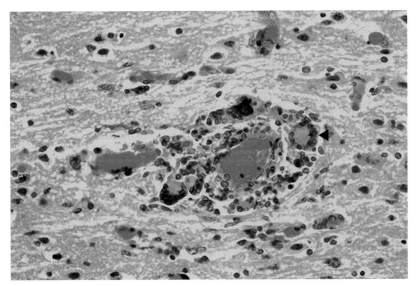

Figure 19-97 HIV encephalitis, microscopic
HIV infection often involves the brain through macrophages that are carried there from reservoirs of infection within lymphoid tissues. Shown here is an encephalitis with a focal lesion (microglial nodule) showing perivascular multinucleated cells (◄), which can be infected by HIV. There are few lymphocytes because of the markedly reduced number of CD4 lymphocytes with progression of HIV infection. Brain injury is potentiated by microglial activation and cytokine release. The encephalitis can lead to progressive loss of cognitive and motor function, termed *HIV-associated dementia*. Aseptic meningitis may also occur with acute HIV infection.

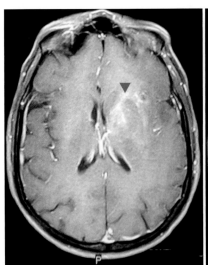
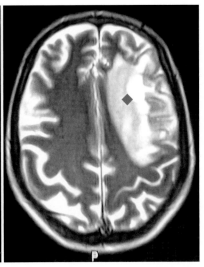

Figure 19-98 Progressive multifocal leukoencephalopathy, MRI
Progressive multifocal leukoencephalopathy (PML) occurs in immunocompromised patients, such as those with AIDS, from reactivation of JC polyomavirus infection. Shown here are areas of markedly increased signal intensity (♦) in the left hemispheric centrum semiovale *(right panel)* with T2 weighting, fat saturation. The extensive white matter involvement (▼) is subtle with T1 weighting, postgadolinium *(left panel)*. The multifocal lesions may also involve the cerebellum. PML appears grossly as irregular, multifocal areas of granularity in white matter, similar to the demyelinating plaques of multiple sclerosis (MS).

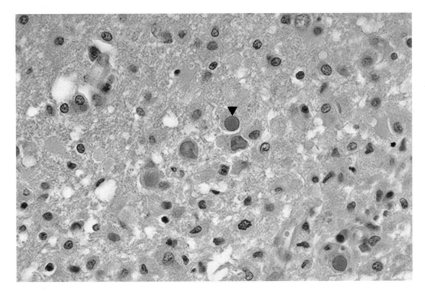

Figure 19-99 Progressive multifocal leukoencephalopathy, microscopic
PML lesions have perivascular monocyte infiltrates, astrocytosis with bizarre or enlarged astrocytes (with occasional mitotic figures), and central lipid-laden macrophages. The virus preferentially infects oligodendrocytes in white matter, leading to demyelination. Shown here at the periphery of the lesions are large "ballooned" oligodendrocytes infected with JC polyoma virus that have enlarged dark pink, ground-glass nuclei (▼) containing viral antigen.

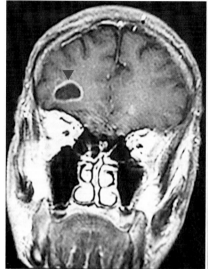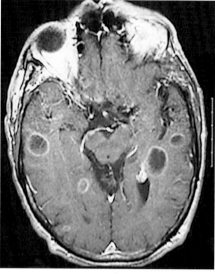

Figure 19-100 Cysticercosis, MRI
In the coronal view in the *left panel,* there is a solitary cysticercus cyst (▼) of the brain, and in the transverse view in the *right panel,* there are multiple cysticercus cysts. In both views the cysts display diminished signal intensity (dark centers) and distinct bright borders with gadolinium enhancement. These patients both had new-onset seizures on presentation. A cyst enlarging beneath the ependyma or within meninges (racemose variety) might produce obstructive hydrocephalus. More than 90% of infected patients have CNS involvement (neurocysticercosis)

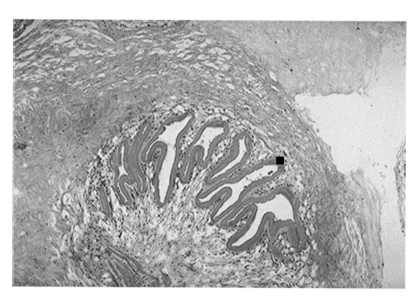

Figure 19-101 Cysticercosis, microscopic
Cysticercosis is caused by ingestion of poorly cooked pork containing the cysticerci of the tapeworm *Taenia solium.* Humans are the definitive host in which the cysticerci develop into adult tapeworms releasing eggs. Normally the eggs pass with feces, but they may hatch in the stomach (autoinfection) or they may be ingested with fecal contamination of food. The eggs hatch and become oncospheres that penetrate the gut wall and can migrate to various tissues, including the brain, and encyst. Note the undulating border (■) of the cyst shown, with surrounding gliotic reaction. The organism dies in a few years and undergoes dystrophic calcification.

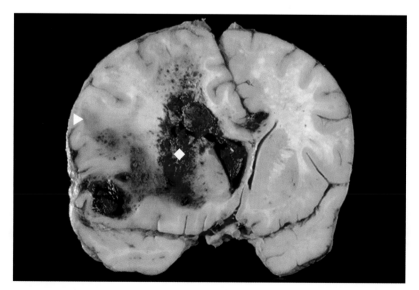

Figure 19-102 Aspergillosis, gross
In this coronal section of brain are focal areas of hemorrhage (◆) with prominent brain swelling and a midline shift. This resulted from a disseminated *Aspergillus* infection in an immunocompromised patient who was markedly neutropenic. The postmortem green discoloration (▶) has resulted from bile pigments (oxidized to biliverdin by formalin fixation) leaking past a blood-brain barrier destroyed by the invasive fungal hyphae. The branching, septate hyphae of *Aspergillus* are prone to cause vascular invasion with thrombosis and subsequent infarction.

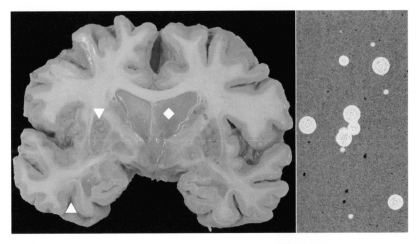

Figure 19-103 Cryptococcal meningitis, gross and microscopic
The coronal section shows a thick mucoid exudate within the subarachnoid space (▲), ventricles (◆), and brain parenchyma (▼) in an immunocompromised patient with *Cryptococcus neoformans* meningitis. Perivascular collections of the organisms can cause small cystic spaces within the brain. An India ink stain of CSF *(right panel)* reveals the thick, clear capsule of these organisms surrounding these yeasts. The CSF may have a mild to moderate leukocytosis, elevated protein, and decreased glucose.

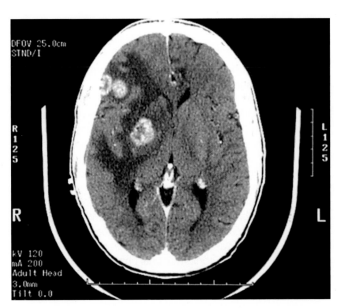

Figure 19-104 *Toxoplasma* encephalitis, CT image
Toxoplasma gondii infection can be congenital in neonates or an opportunistic infection of immunocompromised adults. This CT scan shows several ring-enhancing lesions (▲) with darker areas of surrounding edema that are typical of toxoplasmosis producing multiple abscesses in adults. The vascularity in the organizing wall of an abscess leads to the observed bright ring enhancement with CT and MRI. Congenital *Toxoplasma* infections can produce a cerebritis with multifocal cerebral necrotizing lesions that may calcify. Microscopic examination may reveal *Toxoplasma* pseudocysts containing bradyzoites, but immunohistochemical staining may be needed to identify the small free tachyzoites within the tissues.

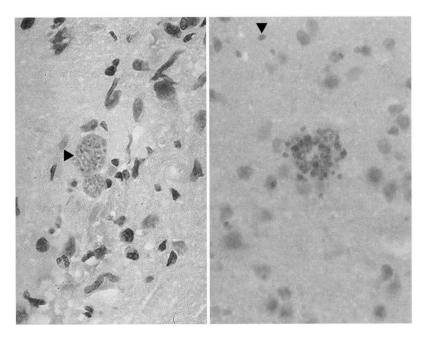

Figure 19-105 Toxoplasmosis, microscopic
T. gondii infection can result in the formation of pseudocysts, which occur within an infected cell, with the cell membrane forming the cyst wall. Pseudocysts (▶) are visible in the *left panel* within the cerebrum in a microglial nodule of a patient with AIDS. In the *right panel* the immunohistochemical staining with antibody to *T. gondii* highlights the brown bradyzoites within the pseudocyst and adjacent free tachyzoites (▼). The organisms become progressively harder to detect as the abscessing lesions become more chronic and organized.

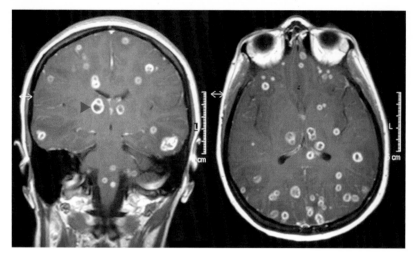

Figure 19-106 Nocardiosis, microscopic
Nocardia asteroides infection typically starts in the lung and may disseminate to the brain, appearing as the multiple small ring-enhancing lesions (▶) shown. Lesions have central suppuration with surrounded granulation tissue with fibrosis: organizing abscesses. Most cases occur in persons with defective cell-mediated immunity, including those with HIV infection and those undergoing chemotherapy or corticosteroid therapy. The long filamentous branching organisms are gram-positive and faintly acid fast.

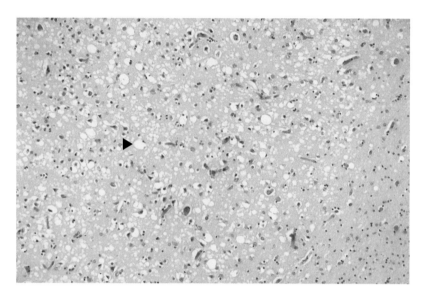

Figure 19-107 Creutzfeldt-Jakob disease, microscopic
The numerous clear vacuoles (▶) in the cerebral cortical gray matter shown here are the spongiform encephalopathy with Creutzfeldt-Jakob disease (CJD), a form of rapidly progressive dementia. As CJD progresses and neurons drop out, there is marked gliosis and atrophy from neuronal loss. It has potential for infectious spread, but cases appear sporadically. The agent of CJD is a prion protein (PrP), a neuronal cell surface sialoglycoprotein encoded by the *PRNP* gene. The normal prion protein, PrPc, can undergo conformational change to an abnormal PrPSc, which is protease resistant (PrPres) and can accumulate and lead to loss of neuronal cell function, vacuolization, and death.

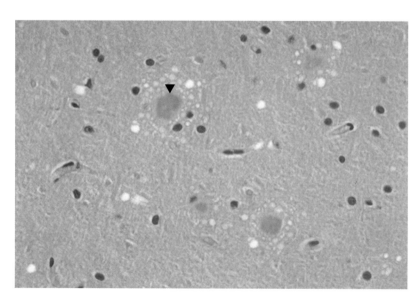

Figure 19-108 Variant Creutzfeldt-Jakob disease, microscopic
The relationship of bovine spongiform encephalopathy (BSE), also called *mad cow disease,* to human spongiform encephalopathy is unclear. An outbreak of BSE among cattle in England in the 1980s was followed by the appearance in the 1990s of rare cases of a CJD-like illness characterized by younger age of onset, lack of characteristic EEG findings, longer course of disease, and a halo of extensive spongiform change with plaques (▼) (shown here) compared with typical cases of CJD. These cases, known as *variant Creutzfeldt-Jakob disease* (vCJD), suggest the possibility of a relationship, and cases of vCJD continue to appear in regions where BSE was prevalent.

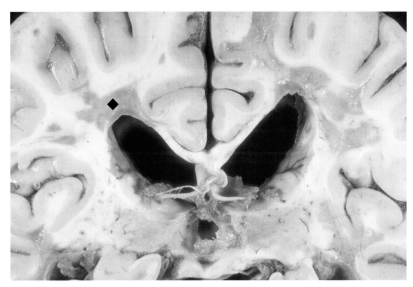

Figure 19-109 Multiple sclerosis, gross

Shown here in periventricular white matter are multiple large "plaques" (◆) of demyelination that have a sharp border with adjacent normal white matter. Such gray-to-tan plaques are typically associated with the clinical course of remitting and eventual progressive loss of neurologic function in MS. Because MS is often multifocal and the lesions appear in various white matter locations in the CNS over time, the clinical course and findings can be quite varied. The finding of chronic inflammation around MS plaques suggests an immune mechanism, and CD4+ T_H1 and T_H17 lymphocytes reacting against myelin antigens, with secretion of cytokines such as interferon-γ that activate macrophages, can be shown.

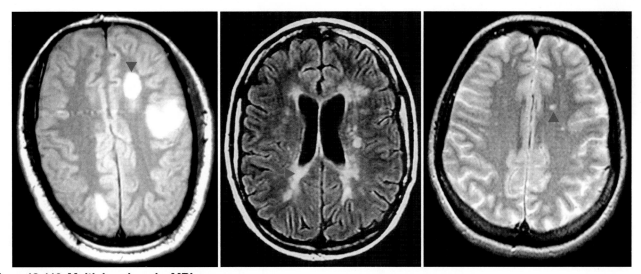

Figure 19-110 Multiple sclerosis, MRI

These MRI images in axial view show multiple bilateral small bright foci (▲) in the *right panel* that represent areas of demyelinating plaque formation in a patient with an exacerbation of MS. In the *center panel* is shown extensive demyelination (▶) of periventricular white matter. Larger lesions (▼) appear in the *left panel*. White matter anywhere within brain and spinal cord can be involved. The CSF often has increased protein, mainly from IgG that shows oligoclonal bands on electrophoresis. Myelin basic protein may also be present in the CSF with active demyelination. A moderate CSF pleocytosis is found in one third of cases. A common clinical finding is visual disturbance from optic neuritis. The prevalence of MS is about 1 per 1000 population in the United States and Europe. Most cases occur after adolescence and before age 50, with a female-male ratio of 2:1. Most patients have a relapsing and remitting course, with eventual neurologic deterioration and sensory and motor impairments.

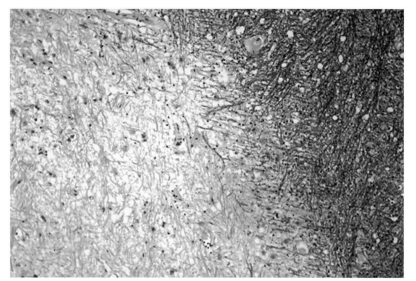

Figure 19-111 Multiple sclerosis, microscopic
This Luxol fast blue (LFB) stain for myelin shows lack of staining with demyelination on the left in a sharply demarcated MS plaque, with residual blue-staining myelinated white matter at the right. Note the individual myelinated axons still remaining at the edge of the plaque. Axons remain relatively preserved. As the plaque becomes quiescent (inactive) and inflammation decreases, astrocytes are found in the lesion responding to the loss of myelin, and oligodendrocytes are decreased. The pale thin strands within the lesion shown here represent the remaining axons.

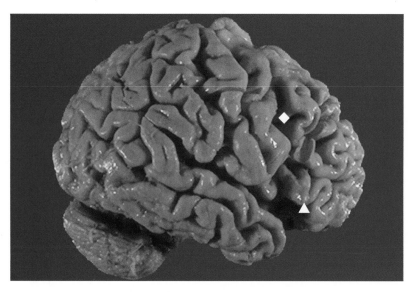

Figure 19-112 Alzheimer disease, gross
After removal of the meninges at autopsy, the cerebral atrophy appearing here mainly involves the frontal and parietal regions, but also temporal, with sparing of the occipital region. This atrophy is characterized by narrowed gyri (▲) and widened sulci (◆). This atrophy is due to AD, the most common form of dementia in elderly individuals. There is a progressive decline in cognition with memory loss and eventual aphasia and immobility. The prevalence of AD increases with age; more than 40% of individuals older than 85 years are affected. AD is rarely symptomatic before age 50 except in individuals with Down syndrome. Five percent to 10% of cases are familial. The typical course from onset to death is 5 to 10 years.

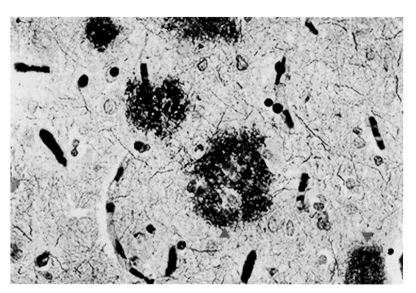

Figure 19-113 Alzheimer disease, microscopic
The neocortical neuritic plaques (▲) of AD appear here with a silver stain. There are extracellular deposits of amyloid β-protein (Aβ), a peptide derived from amyloid precursor protein (APP). In the more numerous, smaller diffuse plaques (▼), Aβ alone is present as filamentous masses. The diagnostic neuritic plaques also have dystrophic dilated and tortuous neurites, microglia, and surrounding reactive astrocytes. Such plaques are most numerous in the cerebral neocortex and in the hippocampus, but the diagnosis of AD is made on finding increased numbers of neocortical plaques for age. This form of dementia is marked mainly by progressive memory loss with increasing inability to perform activities of daily living.

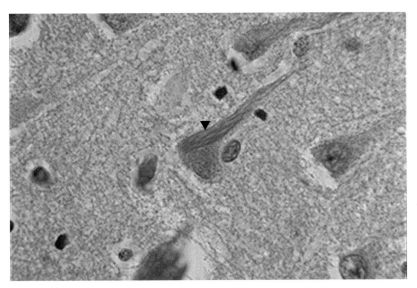

Figure 19-114 Alzheimer disease, microscopic

This is a neurofibrillary "tangle" of AD. The tangle (▼) appears as long pink filaments within the neuronal cytoplasm. Neurofibrillary tangles are composed of cytoskeletal intermediate filaments in the form of hyperphosphorylated microtubule-associated protein known as *tau.* Ubiquitin is also present. The major biochemical defect in AD is a loss of acetylcholine as a neurotransmitter in the cerebral cortex. Genetic defects associated with AD include mutations involving the *APP* gene on chromosome 21, the presenilin 1 and 2 genes on chromosomes 14 and 1, and the ε4 allele of the apolipoprotein E gene on chromosome 19.

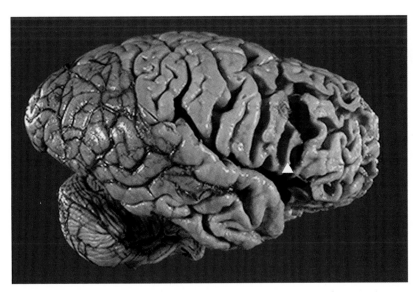

Figure 19-115 Pick disease, gross

The marked frontal and temporal lobe (lobar) atrophy with knifelike thinning of the gyri (▲) shown here in sagittal view of the brain is a result of a less common form of dementia known as *Pick disease,* a form of frontotemporal lobar degeneration (FTLD). Cerebral atrophy may be asymmetrical. Clinical features are similar to those of AD, but with more pronounced behavioral changes and language disturbances. Microscopically, there is marked loss of cortical neurons with gliosis. Pick bodies, cytoplasmic inclusions that are highlighted by silver stain, are present in the neocortex. Mutations can be found in the *tau* gene, which codes for a microtubular protein associated with the Pick bodies.

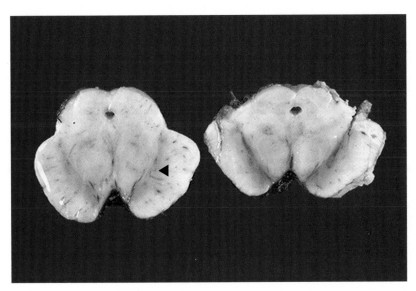

Figure 19-116 Parkinson disease, gross

Note the loss of dark pigmentation in substantia nigra (◄) of the midbrain on the left compared with normal at the right. Parkinson disease (PD) includes several conditions of different causes that affect primarily pigmented neuronal groups, including dopaminergic neurons within the substantia nigra. Patients usually have movement problems, such as a festinating gait, cogwheel rigidity of the limbs, poverty of voluntary movement, masklike facies, and a pill-rolling tremor at rest. Mental deterioration does not often occur, but some patients may become demented as the disease progresses. Idiopathic PD commonly begins in late middle age, and the course is slowly progressive.

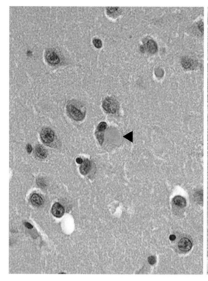
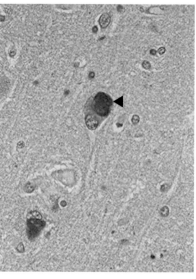

Figure 19-117 Dementia with Lewy bodies, microscopic

Shown are homogeneous pink bodies (◀) on H&E stain, with a surrounding halo *(left panel)*. Immunohistochemical staining with antibody to ubiquitin *(right panel)* or to α-synuclein is positive in these Lewy bodies. About 10% to 15% of patients with parkinsonian symptoms also develop dementia, and in these patients, Lewy bodies appear in the cerebral cortex and within the cytoplasm of pigmented neurons of the substantia nigra. When dementia is the primary feature, the disease can be termed *dementia with Lewy bodies,* with clinical findings similar to those of AD. For diagnosis, the Lewy bodies must be widespread in the neocortex.

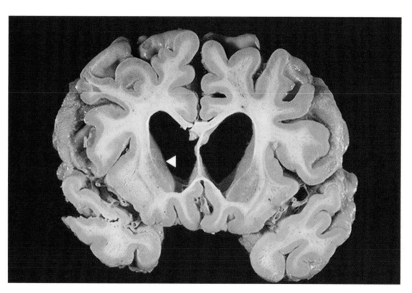

Figure 19-118 Huntington disease, gross

The head of the caudate (◀) shown here has become shrunken, with ex vacuo dilation of lateral ventricles. A dominant mutation in the *HD* gene on chromosome 4 encoding for a protein called *huntingtin* leads to HD. Between the ages of 20 and 50 years, patients begin to demonstrate choreiform movements, character change, or psychosis. The abnormal gene contains increased trinucleotide CAG repeat sequences. There is anticipation, with a greater number of repeats predicting earlier the onset of the disease in successive generations of a family. Spontaneous new mutations are uncommon. There is severe loss of spiny neurons in caudate and putamen with reactive astrocytosis. There is a loss of γ-aminobutyric acid, enkephalin, and substance P.

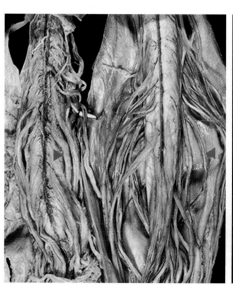
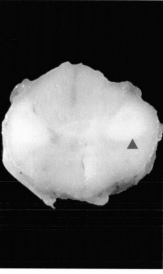

Figure 19-119 Amyotrophic lateral sclerosis, gross

Amyotrophic lateral sclerosis (ALS) usually begins in middle age and leads to death in several years. There is loss of spinal cord anterior horn cells and bulbar motor neurons in CN nuclei (lower motor neurons) as well as neocortical upper motor neurons (Betz cells) projecting to corticospinal tracts, leading to progressive muscular weakness and spasticity proceeding to paralysis from neurogenic muscular atrophy. Anterior (ventral) spinal nerve roots show atrophy (◀), shown here in comparison with normal spinal cord nerve roots (▶). Lateral corticospinal tracts, shown here in thoracic spinal cord, have a pale white appearance (▲)

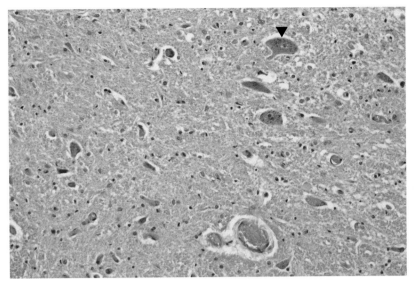

Figure 19-120 Amyotrophic lateral sclerosis, microscopic

There is loss of the anterior horn cells in this section of spinal cord, with a few residual lower motor neuron nuclei (▼). As a consequence there also is lateral column degeneration with gliosis—the "sclerosis" of ALS. Patients exhibit progressive symmetrical muscular weakness. Superoxide dismutase 1 (*SOD1*) gene mutations may be present, including some in the 20% of familial ALS cases. FTLD occurs in association with other cases, with neuronal inclusions that contain TDP-43, an RNA-binding protein.

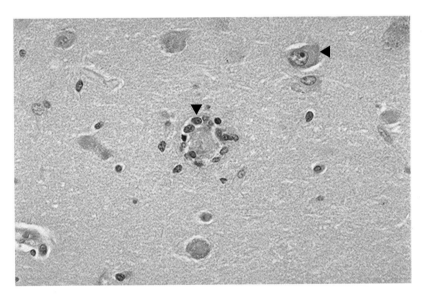

Figure 19-121 Neuronophagia, microscopic

Neuronophagia is a process in which the neuron dies and in the process is surrounded by microglial cells (▼). Compare with an intact neuron (◄). Such single-cell neuronal necrosis can be a feature of viral infections. It may also occur in association with paraneoplastic encephalomyelitis (with polyclonal IgG anti-Hu antibodies or type 1 antineuronal nuclear antibodies appearing in about half of cases). In either case, it is probably mediated by cytotoxic T lymphocytes.

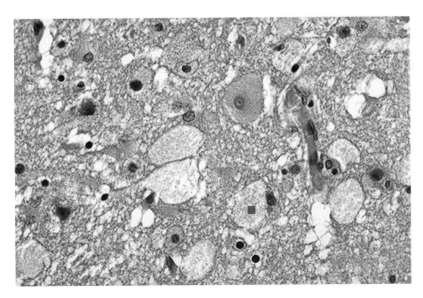

Figure 19-122 Tay-Sachs disease, microscopic

Enlarged, pale neurons (■) appear in the neocortex. This autosomal recessive condition is caused by deficiency of hexosaminidase A enzyme. A mutation within exon 11 is found in 80% of the carriers of Tay-Sachs disease from the Ashkenazi Jewish population, an ethnic group with a 10-fold higher gene frequency for a severe form of this disorder than the general population. By 6 months of age an affected infant is not meeting developmental milestones, and over the first 2 years of life there is relentless neurologic deterioration with motor incoordination and flaccidity, resulting in death. Other storage diseases involving the CNS, such as Niemann-Pick disease (decreased sphingomyelinase), have similar findings.

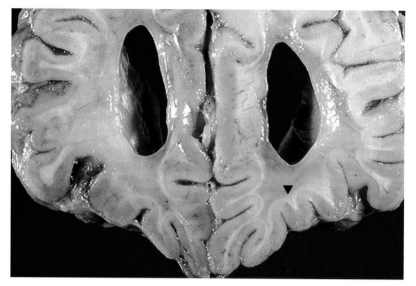

Figure 19-123 Metachromatic leukodystrophy, gross
This coronal section of the frontal lobes shows marked thinning and gray discoloration (▼) of the white matter, with sparing of the white-appearing U fibers at the depths of sulci. This rare autosomal recessive storage disorder is caused by the deficiency of arylsulfatase A, resulting in macrophage lysosomal storage of the sphingolipid cerebroside sulfate as sulfatides that impart the metachromasia with toluidine blue stain. This lipid is abundant in myelin, and increased storage mainly affects white matter. Patients have progressive demyelination causing various neurologic symptoms. The condition is fatal, and no treatment is available.

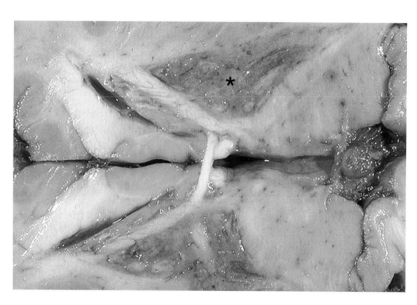

Figure 19-124 Leigh disease, gross
This axial section shows necrotic-appearing lesions (✱) in the putamen bilaterally that correspond to areas of increased signal intensity on T2-weighted MRI. This form of subacute necrotizing encephalopathy has clinical findings in children including lactic acidosis, psychomotor retardation, feeding difficulties, hypotonia or weakness, and ataxia. Dystonias, tremor, chorea, and myoclonus are also frequently found. This disorder results from abnormalities in mitochondrial oxidative phosphorylation. Autosomal recessive and mitochondrial pattern inheritance forms of the disease occur.

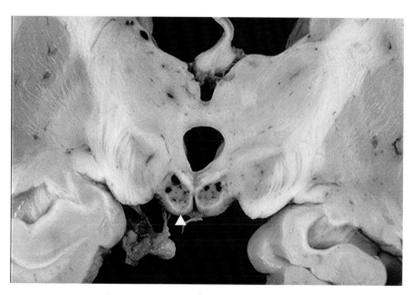

Figure 19-125 Wernicke disease, gross
In this coronal section the small dark petechial hemorrhages appearing in the mammillary bodies (▲) (and also found throughout the nuclear groups of the brain stem) are characteristic of Wernicke disease, a complication of thiamine deficiency, most often occurring in patients with a history of chronic alcohol abuse. The ophthalmoplegia observed in these patients can be reversed with thiamine replacement. In the chronic form of the disease, called *Korsakoff psychosis,* the mammillary bodies are atrophic. The entire spectrum of this disease is usually referred to as *Wernicke-Korsakoff syndrome.*

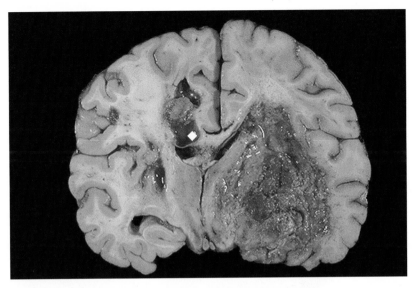

Figure 19-126 Glioblastoma, gross
Gliomas account for more than 80% of all primary brain tumors in adults. Most are located above the tentorium and within the cerebral hemispheres. They are poorly circumscribed. Shown here is the worst form of glioma—a glioblastoma. In this coronal section the large mass has extensive necrosis and infiltrates across the cerebral midline (◆) to the opposite hemisphere. Patients may initially have a new-onset seizure disorder, headaches, or focal neurologic deficits. Although this neoplasm is highly aggressive within the brain, metastases outside the CNS are rare.

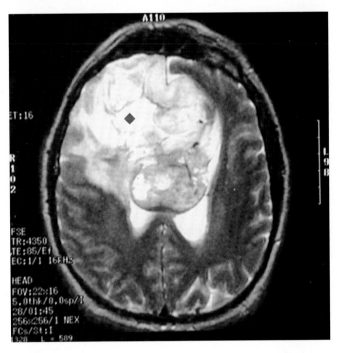

Figure 19-127 Glioblastoma, MRI
This T2-weighted MRI image in axial view shows a large mass (◆) involving much of the right anterior cerebral hemisphere. The brightly enhancing tumor is variegated and has central necrosis, edema, and an irregular border. It crosses the midline by the corpus callosum and extends into the opposite cerebral hemisphere. Such a tumor is not resectable, although radiation and chemotherapy may add months to patient survival. Gliomas may begin as low-grade neoplasms that often have *TP53* mutations, and as they progress to higher-grade lesions, there is *PDGFRA* amplification, a pattern termed *secondary glioblastoma,* which is most likely to occur in younger patients. In contrast, the primary glioblastoma pattern in older individuals does not arise in a lower-grade glioma and is characterized by genetic defects including *EGFR* gene amplification, *p16INK4A* deletion, or *PTEN* mutation.

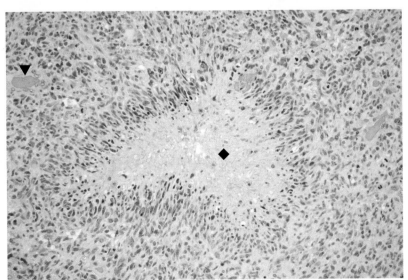

Figure 19-128 Glioblastoma, microscopic
This malignant glioma is highly cellular with marked hyperchromatism and pleomorphism. Note the prominent vascularity (▼) and the area of pale necrosis (◆) in the center, with neoplastic cells concentrated around it. This pseudopalisading necrosis is characteristic of glioblastoma. The cells can infiltrate widely, particularly along white matter tracts, and even through the CSF. Such highly anaplastic cells may be difficult to differentiate from metastases, but gliomas should be GFAP positive with immunohistochemistry.

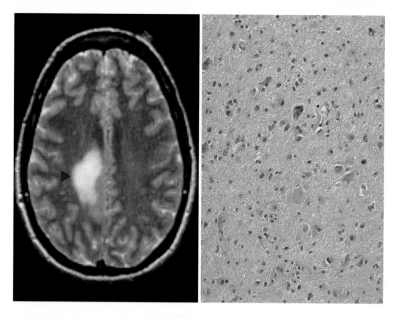

Figure 19-129 Astrocytoma, MRI and microscopic
A diffuse fibrillary astrocytoma (▶) is a form of glioma that is lower grade and not as extensively invasive as a glioblastoma, but it is still not a highly discrete mass, as visible in the T2-weighted axial MRI image *(left panel)*. These gliomas tend to enhance brightly because of their abnormal vascularity. In the *right panel* this astrocytoma shows increased cellularity and pleomorphism compared with normal brain, but far less than a high-grade glioma. Note the one very pleomorphic cell at the top center. The clinical course may be slowly progressive for years, but astrocytomas have a tendency to become more anaplastic with time as genetic alterations accumulate within the neoplastic cells, and then more rapid deterioration ensues.

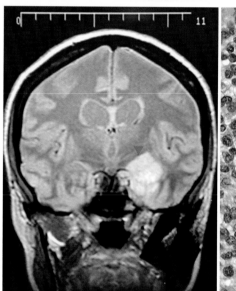
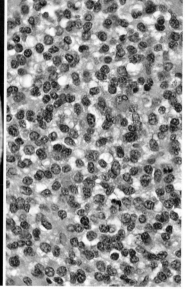

Figure 19-130 Oligodendroglioma, MRI and microscopic
The enhanced MRI image in coronal view *(left panel)* shows a mass (▼) within the left temporal lobe. This type of glioma tends to be well circumscribed, with cystic areas and focal calcification. It enhances as a result of the rich vascular network of anastomosing capillaries within the tumor. Oligodendrogliomas constitute about 5% to 15% of all gliomas; they typically occur within the cerebral hemispheres, usually in white matter, of adults in their 30s and 40s. Typical oligodendrogliomas have round blue nuclei with clear cytoplasm *(right panel)*. Most have cytogenetic abnormalities involving chromosomes 1p and 19q. They tend to be slowly progressive over years and can have a better prognosis than other adult gliomas.

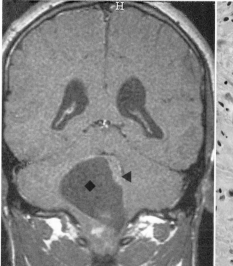
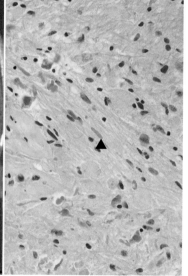

Figure 19-131 Pilocytic astrocytoma, MRI and microscopic
The coronal MRI image *(left panel)* shows a large cerebellar cyst (◆) with a small mural nodule (◀), the typical appearance of a pilocytic astrocytoma, which most often occurs in children below the tentorium in sites such as the cerebellum. It may also occur in optic nerves, floor of the third ventricle, or cerebral hemispheres. These are often slow-growing, low-grade astrocytic tumors that are minimally infiltrative and have a very good prognosis after surgical removal. Shown in the *right panel* are microcystic change, pilocytic cells with long thin processes that are GFAP positive, similar to cells of other gliomas, and red Rosenthal fibers (▲).

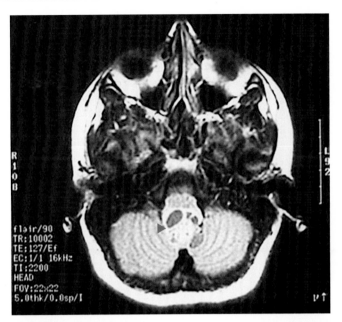

Figure 19-132 Ependymoma, CT image
A discrete, bright mass (▶) with cystic areas fills the fourth ventricle. This is the most common site of an ependymoma in children. This neoplasm arises from the ependymal lining cells. Enlargement of the tumor with blockage of the CSF flow in the fourth ventricle may produce obstructive (noncommunicating) hydrocephalus. Although ependymomas tend not to be invasive, they can be close to vital brain stem structures, and they can spread into the CSF and can be difficult to eradicate. In adults, most ependymomas are found within the spinal cord, and some are associated with neurofibromatosis type 2.

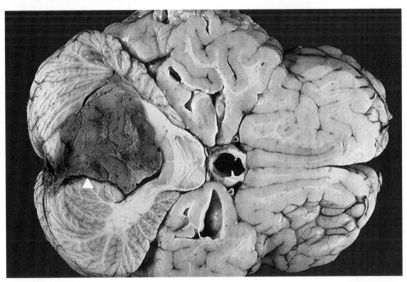

Figure 19-133 Ependymoma, gross
This horizontal (axial) section of the brain reveals a large reddish ependymoma (▲) with discrete borders that is filling and expanding the fourth ventricle. Ependymomas are usually slow-growing neoplasms, but their location within the fourth ventricle makes complete removal difficult, so the overall prognosis at this location is poor.

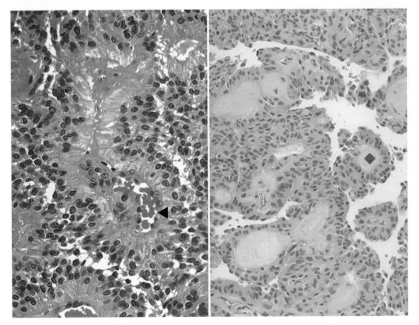

Figure 19-134 Ependymoma, microscopic
The microscopic appearance in the *left panel* of an ependymoma from the fourth ventricle reveals a rosette pattern with the tumor cells arranged around a central vascular space (◀) (perivascular pseudorosette). The ependymal processes stain positively for GFAP. In the *right panel* is a myxopapillary ependymoma that typically arises in the filum terminale of the spinal cord of an adult. The cuboidal tumor cells are arranged around papillations that have a myxoid (◆) connective tissue core.

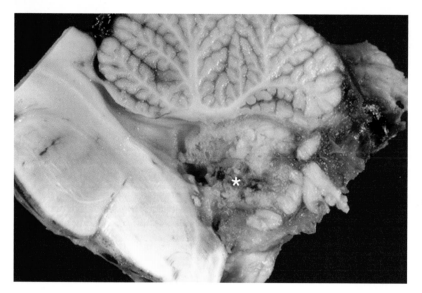

Figure 19-135 Medulloblastoma, gross
This sagittal section shows an irregular posterior fossa mass (★) arising near the midline of the cerebellum and extending into the fourth ventricle above the brain stem. A medulloblastoma is one of the small round blue cell tumors that most often occur in children. These highly malignant, poorly differentiated tumors commonly spread into the subarachnoid space and seed by the CSF into the spinal canal. Those associated with mutations in the WNT signaling pathway have the best prognosis.

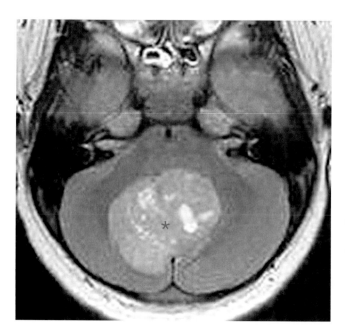

Figure 19-136 Medulloblastoma, MRI
This axial MRI image through the posterior fossa shows an irregular, variegated mass (✳) with some enhancement arising within the cerebellum. Medulloblastomas are of neuroectodermal origin and occur in the cerebellar vermis in children, where they can occlude the fourth ventricle to cause hydrocephalus. In older patients, these tumors more commonly arise within the cerebellar hemispheres. These primitive tumors are very radiosensitive. About a third of medulloblastomas occur in patients 15 to 35 years old. Two thirds are found in patients younger than 15 years.

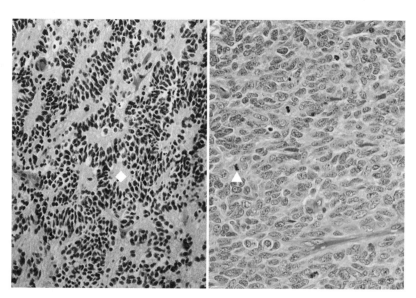

Figure 19-137 Medulloblastoma, microscopic
Poorly differentiated round blue cells with scant cytoplasm and hyperchromatic nuclei are shown. On occasion the cells form pseudorosettes (◆) (called *Homer Wright rosettes*) with cells surrounding eosinophilic circular zones. The nodular desmoplastic variant *(left panel)* has areas of stromal response with "pale islands" that have more neuropil and show greater expression of neuronal markers. The large cell variant *(right panel)* has large irregular vesicular nuclei, prominent nucleoli, and frequent mitoses (▲).

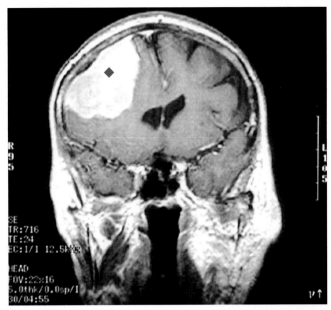

Figure 19-138 Meningioma, MRI
This MRI image in coronal view shows bright enhancement of a meningioma (◆) arising in the parasagittal region over the right frontal lobe. Meningiomas often act in a benign manner, growing very slowly, and are rarely associated with herniation. The most common locations for a meningioma are the parasagittal convexity, lateral convexity, sphenoid wing, olfactory groove beneath the frontal lobe, sella turcica, and foramen magnum. Less commonly they arise within the ventricular system.

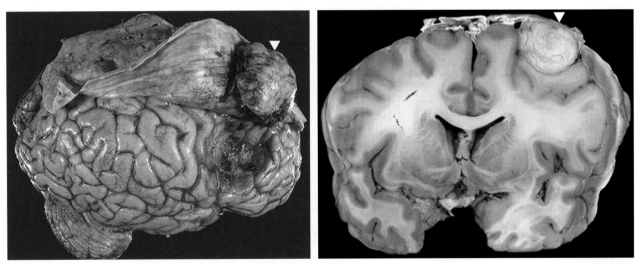

Figures 19-139 and 19-140 Meningioma, gross
Note how each of these meningiomas (▼) beneath the dura has compressed the underlying cerebral hemisphere. These neoplasms, which arise from meningothelial arachnoid cap cells, are typically well-circumscribed masses that are amenable to resection. Sometimes they produce a flattened mass, and sometimes the overlying bone shows hyperostosis. Rarely, meningiomas can be more atypical and recur, or aggressive (anaplastic) and invade the underlying brain.

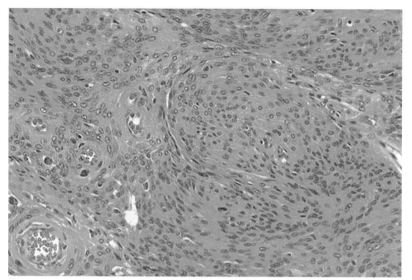

Figure 19-141 Meningioma, microscopic
Meningiomas exhibit many different microscopic patterns. Here the cells are arranged in a tight, whorled pattern, with oval nuclei containing dispersed chromatin, giving them an open and vesicular appearance. They may also contain psammoma bodies or fibroblastic elements. Some meningiomas, particularly when multiple, occur with neurofibromatosis 2, and sporadic meningiomas often have a mutation involving the *NF2* gene on the 22q chromosome. Atypical meningiomas have a higher mitotic index, increased cellularity, and increased nuclear-to-cytoplasmic ratio; they are associated with local invasion and increased risk for recurrence after resection. Meningiomas are uncommon in children. The female-male ratio is 3:2.

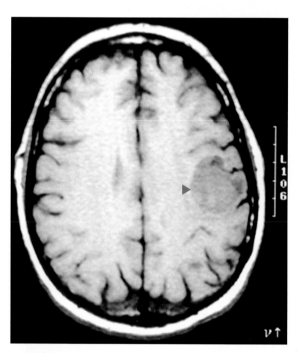

Figure 19-142 Metastasis, MRI
This axial T1-weighted MRI image shows a solitary peripheral brain mass (▶) with minimal adjacent edema located in the cortex near the gray-white junction. This lesion in a middle-aged man proved to be a metastasis from a pulmonary bronchogenic carcinoma, the most common primary site of brain metastases. Lung, breast, skin melanoma, kidney, and gastrointestinal tract primaries account for 80% of all metastases to the brain. In some cases, more specific patterns are observed, such as meningeal carcinomatosis. In some cases the metastases become clinically apparent before the primary site is discovered.

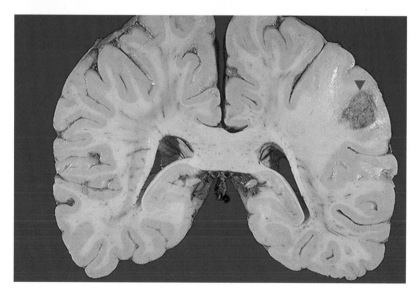

Figure 19-143 Metastasis, gross
In this coronal section of brain, there is a red-brown mass (▼) located at the gray-white junction. This proved to be a metastasis from a renal cell carcinoma of the kidney. A solitary brain mass in an adult could be either primary or metastatic. The borders of a metastasis tend to be more discrete than the borders of a primary glioma. A biopsy may be required to discern the difference.

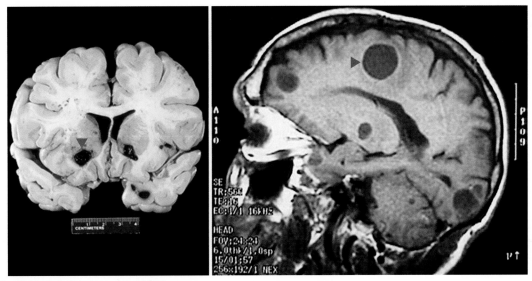

Figure 19-144   Metastases, gross and MRI

Multiple tumor masses, as shown here, suggest metastases rather than a primary neoplasm. In the *left panel* are darkly pigmented metastases (▼) from a malignant melanoma, with the corresponding sagittal MRI image showing multiple cerebral masses (▶) in the *right panel*. Sometimes there is a zone of vasogenic edema around the metastatic lesion, accentuating the mass effect.

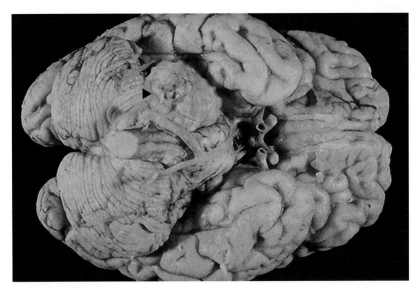

Figure 19-145   Schwannoma, gross

At the base of the brain there is a mass lesion (▶) arising in the vestibular branch of CN VIII at the cerebellopontine angle on the right. This is best termed a *schwannoma* (a so-called acoustic neuroma). Patients often present with hearing loss or tinnitus. Other intracranial sites of involvement include branches of the trigeminal nerve and dorsal roots. These benign neoplasms can be removed. Extradural schwannomas tend to arise in large peripheral nerve trunks. Some cases, particularly with bilateral masses, are associated with neurofibromatosis 2.

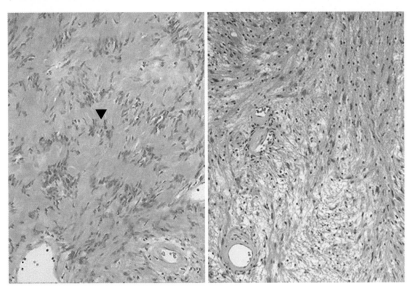

Figure 19-146   Schwannoma, microscopic

Note the more cellular "Antoni A" pattern in the *left panel* with palisading nuclei (▼) surrounding pink areas (Verocay bodies). Shown in the *right panel* is the "Antoni B" pattern with a looser stroma, fewer cells, and myxoid change. *NF2* gene mutations with loss of merlin protein are typically present in both the sporadic and rarer familial occurrences of this neoplasm. Immunohistochemical staining for S100 protein is usually positive in these cells.

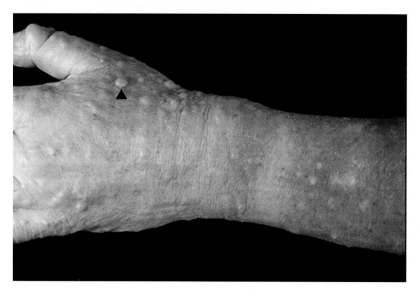

Figure 19-147 Neurofibromatosis, gross
Shown here are multiple nodules (▲) on the skin surface of the forearm and hand of a patient with neurofibromatosis 1. There is loss of function of the *NF1* tumor suppressor gene and its protein product neurofibromin that stimulates activity of a GTPase inhibiting RAS activity. The yellow-orange staining of the skin is an iodine solution applied in surgery (this is an amputation specimen) because a neurofibrosarcoma was present in the deep soft tissue of the wrist. The presence of pale brown macules on the skin, known as *café au lait spots,* particularly when there are six or more of these spots that are 1.5 cm or larger, is highly indicative of neurofibromatosis type 1.

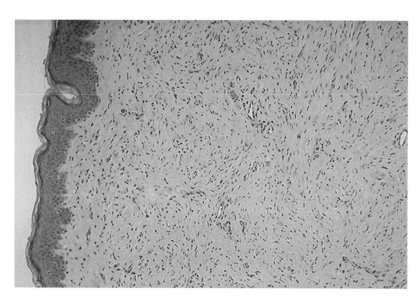

Figure 19-148 Neurofibroma, microscopic
The skin overlying a cutaneous neurofibroma may show some hyperpigmentation, but the actual lesion is in the dermis. This most common type of neurofibroma consists of bundles of wavy, elongated spindle cells with small, dark, oblong nuclei and a lot of intervening pink collagen. This lesion is benign and may occur sporadically or in association with neurofibromatosis type 1. Patients with neurofibromatosis type 1 may develop the plexiform type of neurofibroma in large nerve trunks. With neurofibromatosis type 1, there is an increased risk for development of malignant neoplasms, including malignant degeneration of neurofibromas, malignant peripheral nerve sheath tumors, and gliomas.

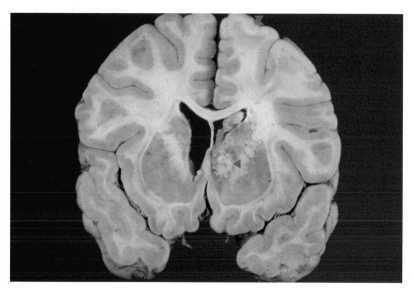

Figure 19-149 Tuberous sclerosis, gross
Tuberous sclerosis, or Bourneville disease, is an autosomal dominant condition with an estimated frequency of 1 in 6000. Neoplasms include hamartomatous growths and low-grade neoplasms in various organs, including facial angiofibromas, cerebral cortical tubers, subependymal nodules, giant cell astrocytomas, retinal glial hamartomas and astrocytomas, cardiac rhabdomyomas, renal angiomyolipomas, and subungual fibromas. *TSC1* or *TSC2* gene mutations are found. This coronal section shows a superior cortical tuber (▼). Note the grayish discoloration in the area of the tuber. There are calcified subependymal glial nodules (◄) by the lateral ventricle. Patients may have intellectual disability and seizures.

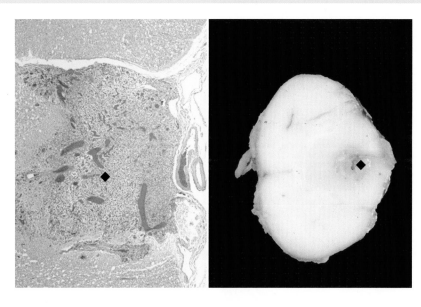

Figure 19-150 Hemangioblastoma, microscopic and gross
The axial section of cervical spinal cord in the *right panel* shows a small dorsal mass (◆) that in the *left panel* consists of abundant capillaries with intervening stromal cells. Hemangioblastomas occur sporadically (usually in the cerebellum), but a fourth arise in von Hippel–Lindau (VHL) disease, an autosomal dominant condition with a frequency of 1 in 40,000. The *VHL* gene acts as a tumor suppressor. The typical neoplasms with von Hippel–Lindau disease are hemangioblastomas, pheochromocytomas, retinal angiomas (often similar histologically to hemangioblastomas), cystadenomas, and renal cell carcinomas.

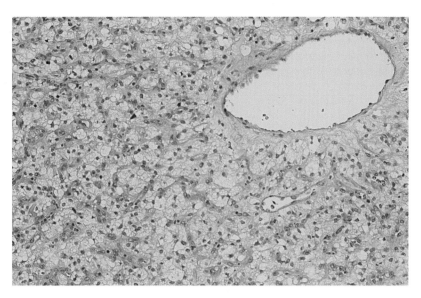

Figure 19-151 Hemangioblastoma, microscopic
The stromal cells are polygonal with clear to pale eosinophilic cytoplasm and small round nuclei. There is an extensive capillary network around small nests of the neoplastic stromal cells. Intracytoplasmic lipid and glycogen impart the clear appearance. Stromal cells exhibit immunohistochemical staining for neuron-specific enolase and neuroendocrine markers. About 10% of hemangioblastomas are associated with polycythemia. Clinical features of cerebellar lesions include ataxia or increased ICP from hydrocephalus.

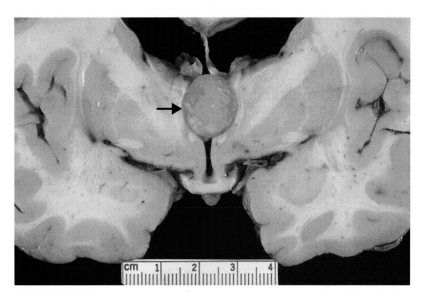

Figure 19-152 Colloid cyst, gross
The discrete round mass lesion (→) occluding the third ventricle is a non-neoplastic lesion known as a *colloid cyst.* Such cysts are better termed *neuroepithelial* cysts because they are lined by cells resembling choroid plexus or ependyma. They contain thick, gelatinous, viscous fluid that is PAS positive microscopically. Most of them are discovered in the third to fifth decades.

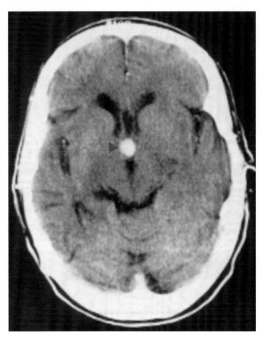

Figure 19-153 Colloid cyst, CT image
Note the hyperdense mass lesion (▶) in the region of the third ventricle. They vary in size from 0.3 to 4 cm, and they are most often incidental findings. However, even small ones may be symptomatic. Headache is the most common presentation and often associated with a change in body position. Rarely they may cause sudden death from acute obstructive hydrocephalus.

The Eye

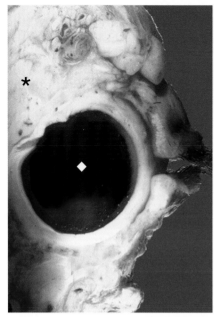
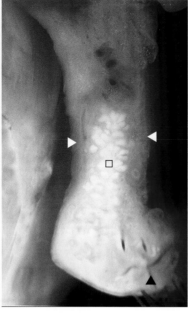

Figure 20-1 Normal eye, gross
A sagittal section through the orbit (◆) is shown in the *left panel,* with the relationship of the eyeball to the eyelid apparatus. The orbit in which the eyeball is located contains adipose tissue (★). In the *right panel* is a closer sagittal view of the upper eyelid. The outer squamous epithelial covering of skin (◀) is on the right. Beneath this are connective tissue and the palpebral part of the orbicularis oculi muscle. There is a dense plate of connective tissue called the *tarsus* (□), beneath which to the left are the meibomian glands (▶), which secrete fluids forming the tear film. Eyelashes (▲) are visible at the lower right margin of the eyelid.

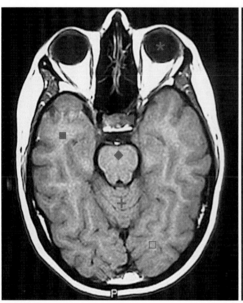
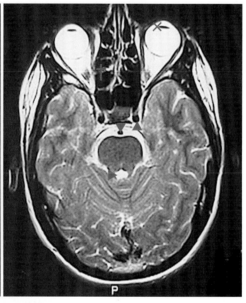

Figure 20-2 Normal eyes and orbits, MRI
Normal axial MRI images (T1 in the *left panel,* with fat having the brightest attenuation, and T2 in the *right panel,* with fluid the brightest) show the temporal lobe (■) and occipital lobe (□), basilar artery (▼), internal carotid artery (▲), basis pontis (◆), aqueduct of Sylvius (▶), cerebellar vermis (✚), ethmoid sinus (†), pituitary (◀), globe of eye (★), and lens of eye (✖).

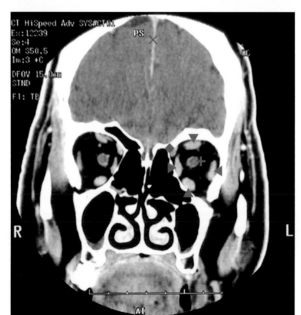

Figure 20-3 Normal eye, CT image
Normal sinus CT scan shows structures in the orbit, including the optic nerve (✚), superior rectus muscle (▼), superior oblique muscle (◆), medial rectus muscle (▶), inferior rectus and inferior oblique muscles (▲), and lateral rectus muscle (◀) in the anterior skull. Within the cranial cavity above are the right and left frontal lobes divided by the falx cerebri (✖).

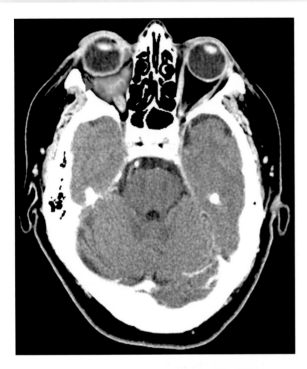

Figure 20-4 Idiopathic orbital inflammation, CT image
The orbital mass (▶) with bright attenuation posterior to the globe is an inflammatory pseudotumor. This idiopathic condition may be unilateral or bilateral. Tissues involved include the lacrimal gland, extraocular muscles, or the fascial layer around the eye. There is a mixed inflammatory infiltrate with fibrosis. Some cases arise in conjunction with IgG4-related disease.

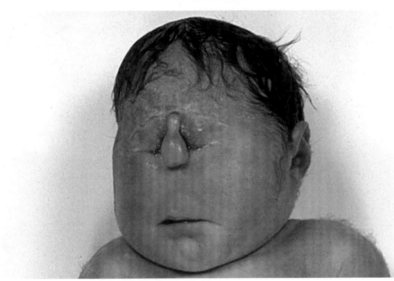

Figure 20-5 Cyclopia, gross
This infant with trisomy 13 (Patau syndrome) has cyclopia (single midline eye) with a proboscis (the projecting tissue just above the eye). The "eye" often consists of nothing more than a slitlike space without a globe. Other ocular anomalies with trisomy 13 when a globe is present include colobomas, cataracts, persistent hyperplastic primary vitreous, and retinal dysplasia.

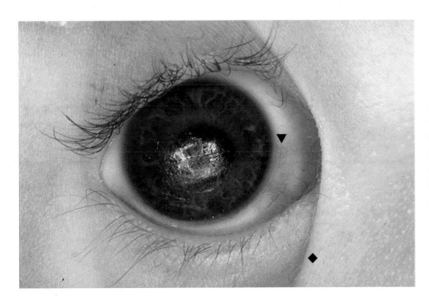

Figure 20-6 Trisomy 21, gross
This is a prominent epicanthal fold (◆) covering the medial aspect of the eye. Also present is a Brushfield spot (▼). Other ocular findings that can be present with trisomy 21 (Down syndrome) include hypertelorism, keratoconus, and oblique palpebral fissures.

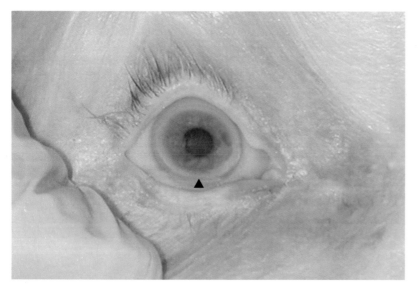

Figure 20-7 Arcus senilis, gross
The thin white ring (▲) around the periphery of the cornea shown here is a condition known as *arcus senilis,* or *arcus lipoides.* This is a finding seen with aging in some individuals and has no pathologic significance. It is caused by increased lipid deposition in the periphery of the cornea and may appear with hyperlipidemia.

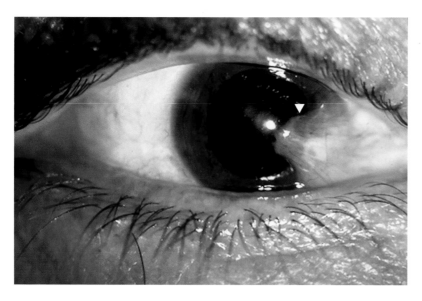

Figure 20-8 Pterygium, gross
This submucosal proliferation is composed of fibrovascular connective tissue encroaching (▼) onto the cornea, which can interfere with vision but does not cause blindness because the process does not cross the midline. In contrast, a pinguecula would be found only on the conjunctiva. The appearance of this raised, whitish yellow lesion is associated with advancing age and is thought to be the result of environmental or solar exposure with solar elastosis over a lifetime. Inflammation induced within a pinguecula by a foreign body in the eye can produce an actinic granuloma.

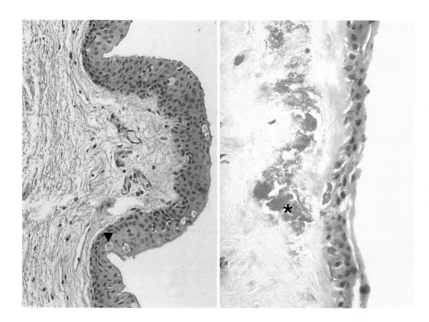

Figure 20-9 Normal conjunctiva and pterygium, microscopic
The appearance of normal conjunctival epithelium is shown in the *left panel.* The conjunctiva forms the mucous membrane of the eyelid, extending posteriorly to the tarsal plate and around the fornix to form the bulbar conjunctiva that extends to the cornea. Note the scattered goblet cells (▼) in this stratified epithelium. At the *right* is a pterygium. Beneath the thinned conjunctival epithelium is an area of elastosis (★) with basophilic degeneration of the substantia propria collagen.

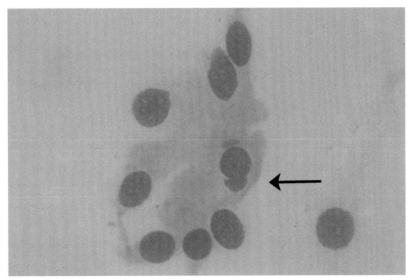

Figure 20-10 Trachoma, microscopic
This conjunctival scraping from the eye, with Giemsa stain, reveals an intracytoplasmic elementary body of *Chlamydia trachomatis* (←). This is a chronic, progressive infection of the upper tarsal plate that produces scarring of the conjunctiva and cornea through inversion of the upper eyelid to direct the eyelashes inward (trichiasis). This is a process that eventually may lead to partial or complete blindness. In contrast, chlamydial infection acquired by passage through the birth canal can produce a purulent conjunctivitis known as *inclusion blennorrhea*. In children and adults, inclusion conjunctivitis results from limited conjunctival inflammation with *C. trachomatis*.

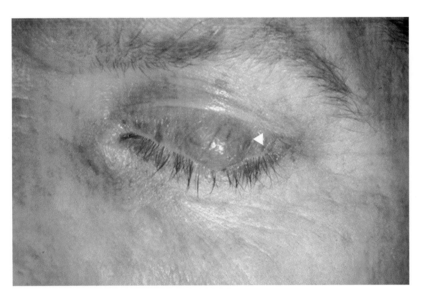

Figure 20-11 Chalazion, gross
This localized swelling (◄) involves the upper eyelid. A chalazion forms when plugging of a duct from meibomian glands leads to chronic lipogranulomatous inflammation. This is an irritating, but benign, process. A recurrent chalazion should undergo biopsy to rule out the possibility of a sebaceous carcinoma.

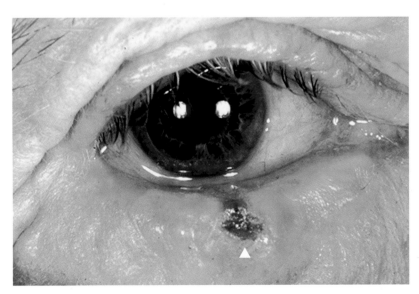

Figure 20-12 Basal cell carcinoma, gross
There is a small nodule (▲) with central ulceration at the edge of the lower eyelid. This is the most common malignant neoplasm of the eyelid, and it arises in the setting of sun damage from chronic ultraviolet light exposure. The nodule has a central rounded ulceration and raised pink margins. A basal cell carcinoma is slow growing, but in this location it presents a problem in removal because adequate margins are needed to prevent recurrence, whereas enough eyelid must be preserved to be functional.

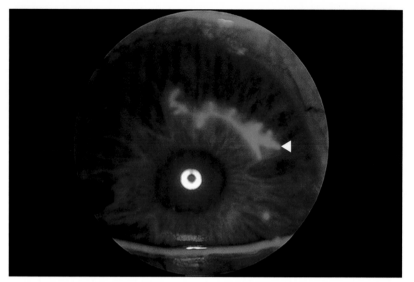

Figure 20-13 Herpetic keratitis, gross
Fluorescein dye has been placed onto the surface of the eye, and this is the appearance of the cornea on slit-lamp examination under fluorescent light. The dye is collecting at the top and bottom conjunctival margins. The lesion shown is a dendritic ulceration (◀) of the corneal epithelium, which is a coalescence of smaller punctate ulcerations. Such a dendritic ulcer is characteristic of infection with herpes simplex virus. Herpetic keratitis is a serious infection because it can be recurrent and can penetrate through the cornea to involve the stroma.

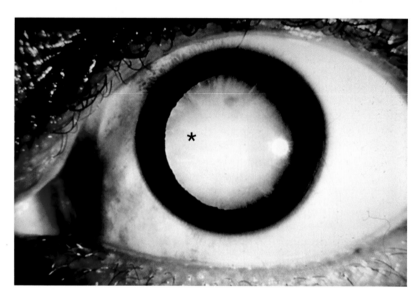

Figure 20-14 Cataract, gross
An opacification (★) of the crystalline lens results from a series of events starting in the lens cortex with rarefaction, then liquefaction, of cortical cells. This leads to fragmentation of lens fibers and extracellular globule formation. In the lens nucleus, there is a progressive increase in the amount of insoluble proteins, which leads to hardening (sclerosis) and brownish discoloration (brunescence). Cataracts are more common in elderly individuals and patients with diabetes mellitus. Cataracts can be removed and replaced by a lens implant.

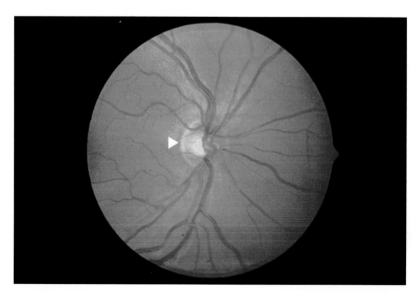

Figure 20-15 Normal retina, funduscopy
The normal funduscopic appearance of the retina is shown. Note the arteries (brighter red) emanating from the central optic disc (▶). The larger-caliber and darker retinal veins extend back to the optic disc. These vessels are evenly distributed. The margins of the optic disc are sharp and clear. The normal posterior chamber vitreous is avascular. With aging, liquefaction and collapse of the vitreous can lead to floaters in the field of vision.

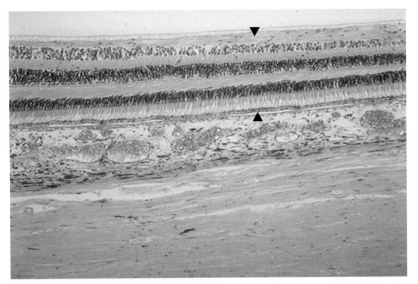

Figure 20-16 Normal retina, microscopic
The normal histologic appearance of the retina shows many layers. The lowest layer just above the retinal pigment (▲) epithelium and supporting connective tissue is the layer of rods and cones (photoreceptors). Above this are layers of external and internal plexiform and nuclear lamina. The nerve fibers (▼) are at the top and collect together to enter the optic nerve at the optic disc. The retinal pigment epithelium aids in maintenance of the photoreceptors, and disturbances of this interface may occur with inherited forms of retinitis pigmentosa.

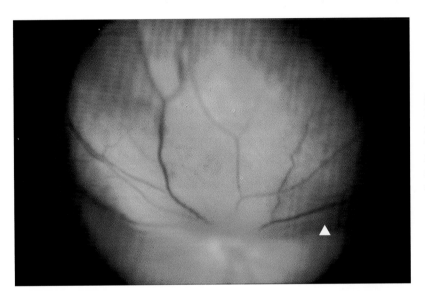

Figure 20-17 Ocular melanoma, funduscopy
Bearing a passing resemblance to Jupiter's moon Io is this view of an irregular mass lesion that is producing discoloration and bulging (▲) underneath the retina on funduscopy. An ocular melanoma usually arises within the pigmented choroidal layer. Melanoma is the most common intraocular neoplasm of adulthood.

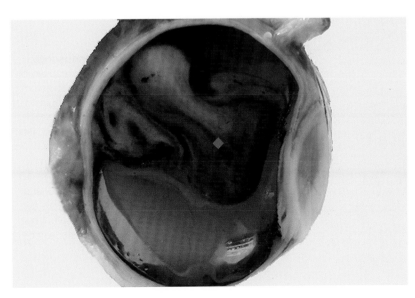

Figure 20-18 Ocular melanoma, gross
This cross-section of an enucleated eye shows a darkly pigmented mass (◆) extending into the vitreous. This is a choroidal melanoma. Most noncutaneous melanomas arise in the eye. The melanoma may sometimes breach the sclera and invade into orbital soft tissues. The expansion of the melanoma may lead to retinal detachment with sudden visual loss.

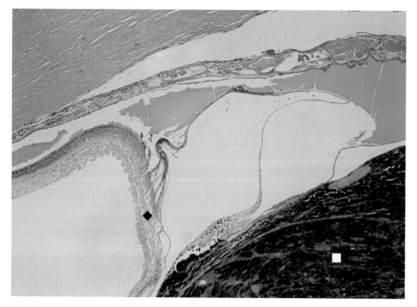

Figure 20-19 Ocular melanoma, microscopic
A darkly pigmented mass (■), a choroidal melanoma, is shown at the lower right, beneath the detached retina (◆). In the eye, in contrast to the skin, it is the lateral extent of growth, not the depth, that is the greatest factor determining prognosis. Tumors containing epithelioid cells have a worse prognosis than those composed exclusively of spindle cells. Because there are no intraocular lymphatic channels, the spread of this neoplasm from the eye typically occurs initially through the scleral vascular channels, and hematogenous metastases can then occur. The liver is the most common site of distant metastases.

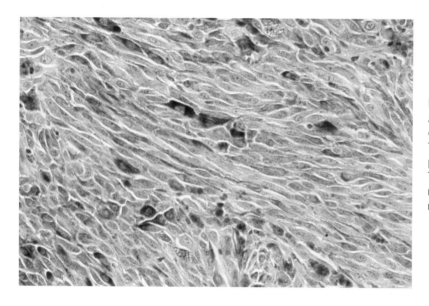

Figure 20-20 Ocular melanoma, microscopic
At higher magnification these spindle-shaped cells contain abundant brown melanin pigment. This ocular melanoma would likely have a better prognosis than a melanoma with epithelioid cells. Tumors confined to the iris have a better prognosis. Complications from increasing size of the mass include retinal detachment and glaucoma.

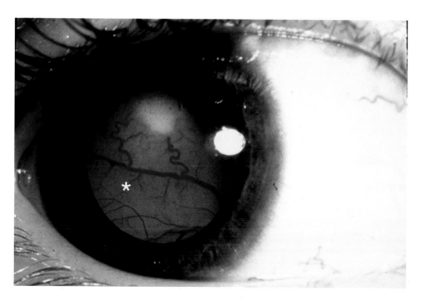

Figure 20-21 Retinoblastoma, funduscopy
This is leukocoria, or "white pupil" (★), caused by the presence of a mass lesion—a retinoblastoma. This is the most common intraocular neoplasm of childhood. Retinoblastomas arise as a consequence of mutations in the *RB* gene. If the patient inherits one mutated allele (the *RB* gene on chromosome 13), either by a point mutation or by deletion of the locus q14 on chromosome 13, the other allele is typically lost in childhood, and a retinoblastoma develops. Such individuals are at risk for retinoblastoma arising in the other eye and additional neoplasms, such as osteosarcoma or pineoblastoma.

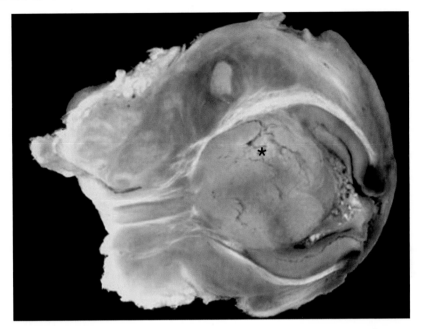

Figure 20-22 Retinoblastoma, gross
This sagittal section of an enucleated eye shows a large white mass (★) pushing into the vitreous and filling most of the globe. This produces the appearance known as "white pupil" (leukocoria) on funduscopic examination. Patients with sporadic, nonfamilial retinoblastomas are not at increased risk for bilateral retinoblastoma or other neoplasms. In familial cases, there is inheritance of an abnormal *RB* tumor suppressor gene and a classic example of a neoplasm arising from a "two-hit" genetic defect.

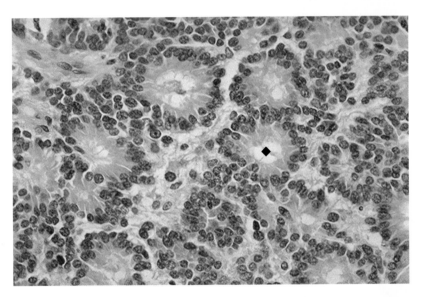

Figure 20-23 Retinoblastoma, microscopic
Retinoblastoma is one of the "small blue cell tumors" of childhood. The characteristic microscopic pattern is the circular arrangement of the small blue cells into Flexner-Wintersteiner "rosettes" (◆) shown here. Focal dystrophic calcifications can occur. The spread of this neoplasm from the eye typically occurs through the optic nerve, but hematogenous metastases, often to bone marrow, may occur.

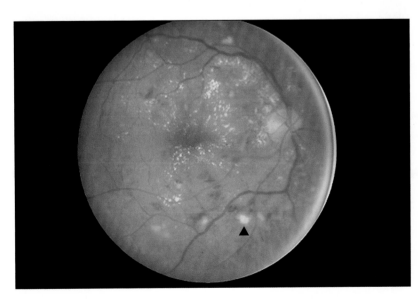

Figure 20-24 Diabetic retinopathy, funduscopy
Note the extensive hard exudates (▲), typical of the "background retinopathy" of diabetes mellitus. The microangiopathy that occurs with diabetes mellitus is associated with edema and retinal exudates that are "soft" microinfarcts or "hard" yellowish waxy exudates, which are deposits of plasma proteins and lipids. These hard exudates are more a feature of older individuals with type 2 diabetes mellitus. Additional findings with background retinopathy include capillary microaneurysms, dot and blot hemorrhages, flame-shaped hemorrhages, and cotton-wool spots (soft exudates).

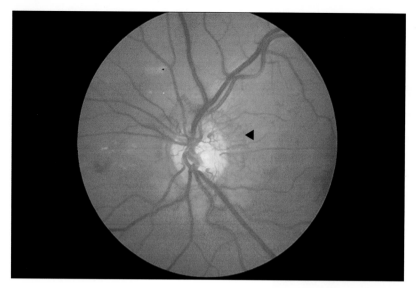

Figure 20-25 **Diabetic retinopathy, funduscopy**
Neovascularization with diabetic proliferative retinopathy is shown here. Note the proliferation (◀) of small vessels near the optic disc. These delicate new vessels grow toward the vitreous humor. They are prone to bleed, producing vitreal hemorrhages that obscure vision. A proliferation of fibrovascular and glial tissue ensues, and when this abnormal tissue contracts, there is a risk for retinal detachment. Involvement of the macula by this process markedly diminishes vision. Diabetic proliferative retinopathy may appear after more than 10 years of poorly controlled or uncontrolled hyperglycemia.

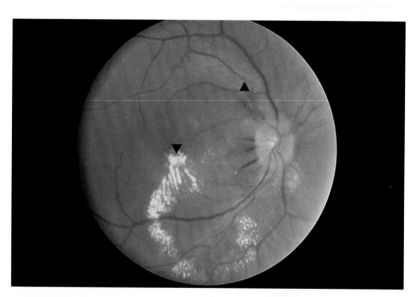

Figure 20-26 **Hypertensive retinopathy, funduscopy**
Shown here is retinal arteriolar narrowing (▲). There are also cotton-wool spots (▼), which represent microinfarcts of the nerve fiber layer with accumulation of mitochondria at the swollen ends of damaged axons forming collections of cytoid bodies. Damage to the choroidal vasculature predisposes to retinal attachment. Additional findings with hypertension include flame-shaped hemorrhages into the retinal nerve fiber layer and papilledema. Other findings include hard (waxy) exudates.

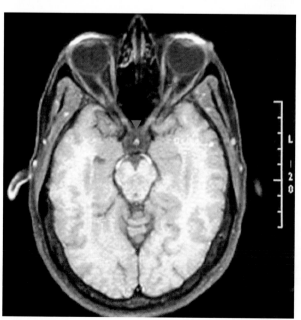

Figure 20-27 **Optic nerves, MRI**
The location of the optic nerves (✛) extending to the optic chiasm (▼) is shown in this axial fluid-attenuated inversion recovery (FLAIR) MRI image. Because the optic nerve is surrounded by meninges, it is affected by changes in cerebrospinal fluid pressure.

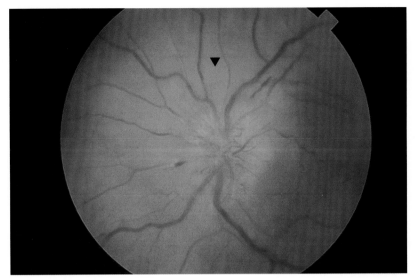

Figure 20-28 Papilledema, funduscopy
The margins (▼) of the optic disc are indistinct with blurring because there is swelling with elevation of the optic nerve head. Any condition that increases intracranial pressure (e.g., edema, hemorrhage, mass lesions) may produce papilledema because the optic nerve is actually a white matter tract extension of the CNS diencephalon. The presence of papilledema suggests that cerebrospinal fluid pressure has exceeded 200 mm H_2O and that a lumbar puncture should not be performed or removal of cerebrospinal fluid may be followed by herniation.

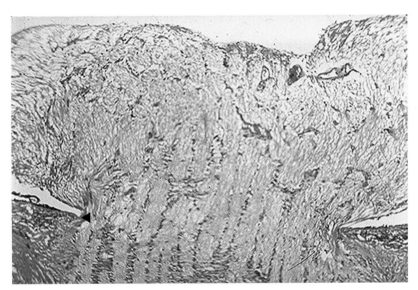

Figure 20-29 Papilledema, microscopic
This microscopic section through the head of the optic nerve displays papilledema. Note the bulging of the nerve head above the level (◄) of the surrounding retina, with forward bowing of the lamina cribrosa. The increase in pressure encircling the nerve contributes to venous stasis both at the nerve head and in axoplasmic transport, leading to nerve head swelling. The intracranial pressure causing this effect must be relieved, or the patient may experience herniation (at locations such as the cerebellar tonsils, uncus of hippocampus, or cingulate gyrus).

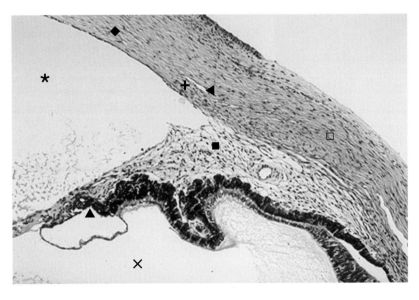

Figure 20-30 Normal eye, microscopic
The structures of a fetal eye (small enough to put key structures in close proximity) are shown here at low magnification, including the cornea (◆), the anterior chamber (✱), the posterior chamber (×), the trabecular meshwork (✚), the canal of Schlemm (◄), the iris (▲), the ciliary body (■), and the sclera (□). In primary angle-closure glaucoma, most likely to occur in small, hyperopic eyes, the angle between the iris and the trabecular meshwork is narrowed, impeding absorption of aqueous humor. Most cases of glaucoma are of the primary open-angle type, in which there is no obvious point of obstruction, but the mechanism for aqueous absorption malfunctions.

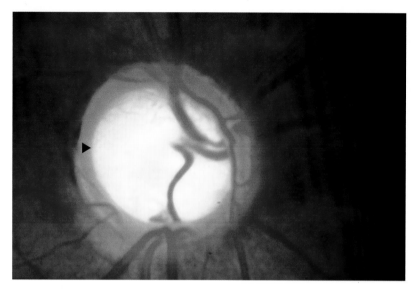

Figure 20-31 Glaucoma, funduscopy
This is marked cupping of the optic disc, indicative of glaucoma. Glaucoma most often results from increased intraocular pressure with damage to the ganglion cells and their axons with thinning of the retinal nerve layer. This increased ocular pressure over time in most patients leads to deepening (▶) of the optic cup with excavation. The vessels shown here appear to "fall into" the deepened optic cup. "Primary" glaucoma occurs without another eye or medical condition, and "secondary" glaucoma consequent to another disease such as diabetes mellitus.

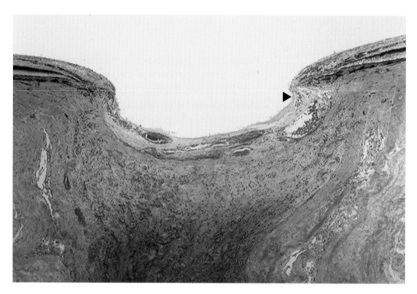

Figure 20-32 Glaucoma, microscopic
There is deepening of the optic cup with excavation (▶). The atrophy of the optic nerve leads to progressive loss of vision, regardless of the cause of the increased intraocular pressure. Glaucoma is described as open-angle when nothing physically blocks outflow of aqueous humor and as closed-angle when the position of the lens and iris blocks aqueous outflow (hyperopia). Open-angle glaucoma tends to progress slowly and silently, whereas some cases of closed-angle glaucoma may manifest acutely with a painful red eye and markedly elevated intraocular pressure. Some cases of primary open-angle glaucoma are associated with mutations in the *MYOC* gene encoding for the myocilin protein found in the ciliary body and trabecular meshwork.

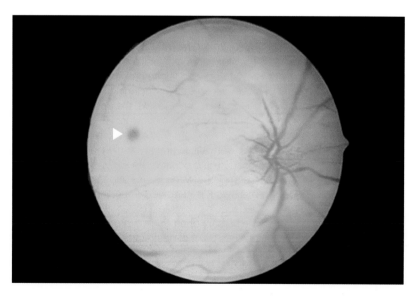

Figure 20-33 Tay-Sachs disease, funduscopy
Note the paleness of the retina, with extensive opacification more characteristic of Tay-Sachs disease, although retinal artery occlusion has a similar appearance. Tay-Sachs disease results from a deficiency in hexosaminidase A enzyme with accumulation of G_{M2} gangliosides in retinal ganglion cells, producing the pale appearance that obscures the vascularity. The greatest density of ganglion cells in the macular area leads to greater opacification except in the foveal pit, which is devoid of ganglion cells, so that a solitary "cherry red" spot (▶) is visible here at the left of the image. The lipids accumulating in retinal ganglion cells lead to ganglion cell hypertrophy, followed by cell death and eventual gliosis and blindness.

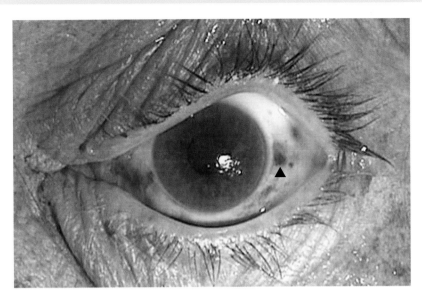

Figure 20-34 Petechiae, gross
Mechanical asphyxia, including strangulation, can be marked by the appearance of petechial hemorrhages (▲) within the conjunctiva, as shown on the sclera here. Such a finding is not specific for this injury, however, and can occur with other conditions. Finding ligature marks on the neck, hyoid bone fracture, or soft-tissue hemorrhages in the neck and larynx may help to determine the mechanism of injury.

Figure Credits

Chapter 1

Figure 1-17 Courtesy Dr. M. Elizabeth H. Hammond, University of Utah. **Figure 1-20** Courtesy Department of Pathology, University of Hong Kong. **Figure 1-33** Courtesy Dr. Walter H. Henricks, Cleveland Clinic Foundation. **Figure 1-49** Courtesy Department of Pathology, University of Hong Kong. **eFigure 1-6** Courtesy Dr. Richard Conran, Uniformed Services University.

Chapter 2

Figure 2-11 Courtesy Dr. Mary Ann Sens, University of North Dakota. **Figures 2-47, 2-48,** and **2-50** Courtesy Department of Pathology, University of Hong Kong.

Chapter 3

Figures 3-15 Courtesy Dr. Sherrie L. Perkins, University of Utah. **Figures 3-33, 3-35,** and **3-36** Courtesy Dr. Carl R. Kjeldsberg, University of Utah. **Figures 3-40, 3-41,** and **3-54** Courtesy Dr. Sherrie L. Perkins, University of Utah. **Figure 3-57** Courtesy Dr. Carl R. Kjeldsberg, University of Utah. **Figure 3-80** Courtesy Department of Pathology, University of Hong Kong. **eFigure 3-2** Courtesy Dr. Sherrie L. Perkins, University of Utah.

Chapter 5

Figure 5-91 Courtesy Dr. Mary Ann Sens, University of North Dakota.

Chapter 6

Figure 6-9 Courtesy Department of Pathology, University of Hong Kong.

Chapter 7

Figure 7-12 Courtesy Department of Pathology, University of Hong Kong. **Figures 7-64** and **7-65** Courtesy Dr. Richard Conran, Uniformed Services University. **Figure 7-142** Courtesy

Dr. John Blackmon, Florida State University. **eFigures 7-3, 7-9, 7-10, 7-11,** and **7-13** Courtesy Dr. Tomas Slavik, University of Pretoria, South Africa. **eFigure 7-12** Courtesy Department of Pathology, University of Hong Kong.

Chapter 8

Figures 8-9 and **8-21** Courtesy Dr. Jeannette J. Townsend, University of Utah. **eFigure 8-10** Courtesy Dr. Tomas Slavik, University of Pretoria, South Africa.

Chapter 10

Figures 10-76, 10-95, and **10-99** Courtesy Department of Pathology, University of Hong Kong. **Figure 10-102** Courtesy Dr. Richard Conran, Uniformed Services University. **eFigure 10-4** Courtesy Arthur J. Belanger, Yale University.

Chapter 11

Figure 11-15 Courtesy Dr. Mary Ann Sens, University of North Dakota. **Figure 11-17** Courtesy Dr. Richard Conran, Uniformed Services University. **Figures 11-21** and **11-22** Courtesy Dr. David Cohen, Tel Aviv University. **eFigure 11-1** Courtesy Dr. Richard Conran, Uniformed Services University. **eFigure 11-2** Courtesy Dr. Ilan Hammel, Tel Aviv University.

Chapter 12

Figure 12-48 Courtesy Dr. John Blackmon, Florida State University.

Chapter 13

Figure 13-9, 13-27, 13-28, and **13-43** Courtesy Dr. David Cohen, Tel Aviv University. **Figures 13-27, 13-28,** and **13-43** and. **Figures 13-61** and **13-62** Courtesy Dr. Hiroyuki Takahashi, Jikei University School of Medicine. **Figure 13-69** Courtesy Dr. David Cohen, Tel Aviv University. **Figure 13-86** Courtesy Dr. Hiroyuki Takahashi, Jikei University School of Medicine. **Figure 13-88** Courtesy Dr. David Cohen, Tel Aviv University. **Figure 13-91** Courtesy Department of Pathology, University of Hong Kong. **Figures 13-92, 13-98,** and **13-99** Courtesy Dr. Hiroyuki Takahashi, Jikei University School of Medicine. **eFigure 13-3** Courtesy Dr. Richard Conran, Uniformed Services University. **eFigure 13-3** Courtesy Dr. Richard Conran, Uniformed Services University. **eFigure 13-4** Courtesy Dr. David Cohen, Tel Aviv University.

Chapter 14

Figure 14-19 Courtesy Dr. David Cohen, Tel Aviv University.

Chapter 15

Figure 15-28 Courtesy Department of Pathology, University of Hong Kong. **eFigure 15-8** Courtesy Dr. Jeannette J. Townsend, University of Utah.

Chapter 16

Figure 16-25 Courtesy Dr. Sate Hamza, University of Manitoba. **Figure 16-27** Courtesy Dr. David Cohen, Tel Aviv University. **Figures 16-29** and **16-31** Courtesy Dr. Sate Hamza, University of Manitoba. **Figure 16-32** Courtesy Dr. Ilan Hammel, Tel Aviv University. **Figure 16-37** Courtesy Dr. Lauren Hughey, University of Alabama at Birmingham. **Figure 16-38** Courtesy Dr. Sate Hamza, University of Manitoba. **Figure 16-43** Courtesy Dr. Ilan Hammel, Tel Aviv University. **Figure 16-44** Courtesy Dr. Amy Theos, University of Alabama at Birmingham. **Figures 16-47, 16-48, 16-49, 16-53, 16-57,** and **16-66** Courtesy Dr. Sate Hamza, University of Manitoba. **Figures 16-64** and **16-65** Courtesy Dr. Shane Silver, Winnepeg, Manitoba. **Figure 16-67** Courtesy Dr. M. Elizabeth H. Hammond, University of Utah. **Figures 16-70, 16-71, 16-72, 16-73, 16-74, 16-75,** and **16-77** Courtesy Dr. Sate Hamza, University of Manitoba. **Figures 16-84** Courtesy Dr. Omid Zargari, Rasht, Iran. **Figures 16-89** and **16-90, eFigure 16-3, eFigure 16-6,** Courtesy Dr. Sate Hamza, University of Manitoba. **eFigure 16-10** Courtesy

Dr. Omid Zargari, Rasht, Iran. **eFigure 16-14** Courtesy Arthur J. Belanger, Yale University, **eFigure 16-15** and **16-16** Courtesy Dr. Sate Hamza, University of Manitoba.

Chapter 17

Figures 17-28 and **17-63** Courtesy Department of Pathology, University of Hong Kong. **Figure 17-98** Courtesy Dr. David Cohen, Tel Aviv University, **eFigure 17-9** Courtesy Department of Pathology, University of Hong Kong.

Chapter 18

Figures 18-1, 18-2, 18-8, 18-12, 18-13, 18-15, 18-23, 18-24, and **18-28** and **eFigure 18-2** Courtesy Dr. Jeannette J. Townsend, University of Utah.

Chapter 19

Figures 19-16, 19-31, 19-33, 19-34, 19-35, and **19-36** Courtesy Dr. Jeannette J. Townsend, University of Utah. **Figure 19-38** Courtesy Dr. Todd C. Grey, University of Utah. **Figures 19-41, 19-43, 19-44,** and **19-45** Courtesy Dr. Jeannette J. Townsend, University of Utah. **Figure 19-46** Courtesy Dr. Todd C. Grey, University of Utah. **Figures 19-57, 19-58, 19-78, 19-79, 19-85, 19-92, 19-93, 19-95, 19-96, 19-97, 19-123, 19-124, 19-125, 19-133,** and **19-140, eFigure 19-2, eFigure 19-3,** and **eFigure 19-9** Courtesy Dr. Jeannette J. Townsend, University of Utah.

Chapter 20

Figures 20-1, 20-8, 20-9, 20-11 through **20-18, 20-21, 20-22, 20-24, 20-25, 20-26, 20-28, 20-29, 20-31,** and **20-32** Courtesy Dr. Nick Mamalis, University of Utah. **Figure 20-4** Courtesy Department of Pathology, University of Hong Kong.

Page numbers including an *e* are electronic content.